T0201007

CLINICAL MANUAL OF
Youth Addictive Disorders

CLINICAL MANUAL OF
Youth Addictive Disorders

Edited by

Yifrah Kaminer, M.D., M.B.A.

Ken C. Winters, Ph.D.

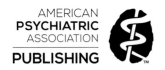

AMERICAN
PSYCHIATRIC
ASSOCIATION
PUBLISHING

If you wish to purchase 50 or more copies of the same title, please go to www.appi.org/specialdiscounts for more information.

Copyright © 2020 American Psychiatric Association Publishing

ALL RIGHTS RESERVED

Manufactured in the United States of America on acid-free paper

23 22 21 20 19   5 4 3 2 1

American Psychiatric Association Publishing
800 Maine Avenue SW
Suite 900
Washington, DC 20024-2812
www.appi.org

Library of Congress Cataloging-in-Publication Data
Names: Kaminer, Yifrah, editor. | Winters, Ken C., editor. | American Psychiatric Association Publishing, issuing body.
Title: Clinical manual of youth addictive disorders / edited by Yifrah Kaminer, Ken C. Winters.
Other titles: Clinical manual of adolescent substance abuse treatment.
Description: Washington, DC : American Psychiatric Association Publishing, [2020] | Includes bibliographical references and index.
Identifiers: LCCN 2019033775 (print) | LCCN 2019033776 (ebook) | ISBN 9781615372362 (paperback) | ISBN 9781615372812 (ebook)
Subjects: MESH: Substance-Related Disorders—diagnosis | Substance-Related Disorders—therapy | Behavior, Addictive | Comorbidity | Adolescent
Classification: LCC RJ506.D78 (print) | LCC RJ506.D78 (ebook) | NLM WM 270 | DDC 362.290835—dc23
LC record available at https://lccn.loc.gov/2019033775
LC ebook record available at https://lccn.loc.gov/2019033776

British Library Cataloguing in Publication Data
A CIP record is available from the British Library.

Contents

Contributors .... **xvii**

Introduction............................. **xxv**
Yifrah Kaminer, M.D., M.B.A.
Ken C. Winters, Ph.D.

PART I

Course, Prevention, and Pretreatment Considerations

1 Diagnosis, Epidemiology, and Course of Youth Substance Use and Use Disorders **3**
Gerald Montano, D.O.
Tammy Chung, Ph.D.

Adolescence as a Critical Developmental Period for
  Initiation of Substance Involvement.............. 4

Prevalence of Substance Use in Adolescents 5

Children of Substance Using Parents 8

Trajectories of Substance Use During Adolescence ... 9

Diagnosis of Substance Use Disorders 10

DSM-IV Prevalence of Substance Use Disorders in
  Adolescent Samples 11

Developmentally Informed Substance Use Disorder
  Assessment 13

Course of Adolescent-Onset
  Substance Use Disorders 14

Conclusion 19

Key Points 19

References................................. 20

2 **Prevention of Substance Use and Substance Use Disorders** **25**

Lawrence M. Scheier, Ph.D.
Richard Catalano, Ph.D.
Ken C. Winters, Ph.D.

Nature and Extent of the Problem 26
Background of Prevention Efforts. 26
Role of Risk and Protective Factors. 27
Evidence-Based Programs. 34
Implementation of Prevention Programs 38
Future of Prevention Efforts 41
Key Points 43
References................................. 44

3 **Screening and Assessing Youth With Substance Use Disorder** **51**

Ken C. Winters, Ph.D.
Randy Stinchfield, Ph.D.
Andria M. Botzet, M.A.

Principles of Assessment...................... 52
Self-Report Method 53
Alternatives to Self-Report 54
Core Clinical Content of a Comprehensive Assessment. . 55
Assessment Instruments 57
Treatment Outcome Assessment. 67
The Clinical Interview......................... 69
Key Points 69
References................................. 70

4 **Primary Care and Pediatric Settings: SCREENING, BRIEF INTERVENTION, AND REFERRAL TO TREATMENT (SBIRT)** **75**

Areej Hassan, M.D., M.P.H.
Sion K. Harris, Ph.D.
John Rogers Knight, M.D.

Screening and Screening Tools.................. 78
Brief Interventions 86

Case Vignettes. 88

Referral to Treatment. 91

Key Points 92

References. 93

**5 Bioassays and Detection of
Substances of Abuse in Youth 97**

Albert J. Arias, M.D.
Wendy Welch, M.D., C.P.E.
Yifrah Kaminer, M.D., M.B.A.

Social Context of Youth Drug Testing 98

School Drug Testing. 98

Home Drug Testing 99

Concordance Among Reports 100

Available Biomarkers 100

Overview of Testing by Sample Source 101

Testing for Specific Drugs of Abuse. 103

Conclusion 116

Key Points 116

Relevant Websites 117

References. 117

**6 Placement Criteria and Integrated Treatment
Services for Youth With Substance Use
Disorders 123**

Marc Fishman, M.D.

General Principles of Treatment Planning and
Placement 124

Dimensional Assessment and Treatment Planning
Using the ASAM Criteria 127

Treatment Matching and Placement 135

Key Points 136

References. 137

PART II

Description, Diagnosis, and Interventions for Specific Substances of Abuse

7 Youth Alcohol Use **141**
   Robert Miranda Jr., Ph.D.
   Ryan W. Carpenter, Ph.D.

   Pharmacological Treatment of
      Adolescent Alcohol Misuse 142
   Conclusion 152
   Key Points 152
   References 153

8 Youth Tobacco Use **157**
   Grace Kong, Ph.D.
   Suchitra Krishnan-Sarin, Ph.D.

   Noncigarette Tobacco/Nicotine Products 158
   Diagnosis 162
   Prevention 163
   Cessation Interventions 164
   Treatment Modality and Setting 168
   Conclusion 169
   Key Points 170
   References 170

9 Youth Cannabis Use **175**
   Christian Thurstone, M.D.
   Yifrah Kaminer, M.D., M.B.A.

   The Endocannabinoid System 176
   Definitions and Description of
      Cannabis Products 176
   Cannabis Drug and Medication Interactions 178
   Prevalence and Epidemiology of Cannabis Use 179
   Negative Consequences of Cannabis on Youth 180
   Specific Health Concerns 183

Prevention and Treatment 189

Impact of Liberalization of
   Cannabis Policies on Youth 192

Recommendations for Public Health Policies 194

Key Points 196

References 196

10 Youth Opioid Use 203
   Christopher J. Hammond, M.D., Ph.D.
   Brian Hendrickson, M.D.
   Marc Fishman, M.D.

Opioid Pharmacology and Neurobiology 204

Epidemiology 205

Negative Sequelae of Opioid Misuse and
   Opioid Use Disorder in Youth 206

Risk Factors for Development of Opioid Misuse
   and Opioid Use Disorder in Youth 206

Prevention Targeting Known Risk Factors 210

Clinical Management and Evidence-Based
   Interventions for Youth Opioid Use Disorder 211

Role for Medication-Assisted Treatment in
   Youth Opioid Use Disorder 213

Medications for Maintenance Treatment in
   Youth with Opioid Use Disorder 214

Medications for Opioid Withdrawal in Youth 217

Opioid Overdose Prevention 218

Alternative Medicines for Opioid Use Disorder and
   the Case of Kratom 219

Opioids and Pediatric Pain Management 220

Complex Relationship Between
   Youth Cannabis Use and Opioid Use Disorder . . . 220

Conclusion 222

Key Points 222

References 223

11 **Youth Club, Prescription, and Over-the-Counter Drug Use** **229**

    Charles Albert Whitmore, M.D., M.P.H.
    Christian Hopfer, M.D.

    Club Drugs 230

    Prescription and Over-the-Counter Medications 241

    Conclusion 247

    Key Points 248

    References 248

PART III

Specific Interventions for Youth With Substance Use Disorders

12 **Continuity of Care for Abstinence and Harm Reduction** **255**

    Yifrah Kaminer, M.D., M.B.A.
    Mark D. Godley, Ph.D.
    Ken C. Winters, Ph.D.
    Kara S. Bagot, M.D.

    Progress in Youth Treatment Research 256

    The Therapeutic Process, Mechanisms of
       Behavioral Change, and Outcomes 257

    Harm Reduction (Versus Abstinence)
       in Youth With Substance Use Disorders 266

    Conclusion and Future Directions 269

    Key Points 271

    References 271

13 **Brief Motivational Interventions, Cognitive-Behavioral Therapy, and Contingency Management** **277**

    Anthony Spirito, Ph.D., A.B.P.P.
    Yifrah Kaminer, M.D., M.B.A.
    Kimberly H. McManama O'Brien, Ph.D., L.I.C.S.W.

    Brief Motivational Interventions 278

Cognitive-Behavioral Therapy 288
Contingency Management Reinforcement Approach . . 290
Key Points 294
References. 295

14 Family and Community-Based Therapies 301
Molly Bobek, L.C.S.W.
Susan H. Godley, Rh.D.
Aaron Hogue, Ph.D.
Family Therapy. 302
Multicomponent Treatment. 308
Lessons Regarding Training Clinicians 312
Lessons Regarding Training Supervisors 312
Implementation and Outcomes With Subpopulations . . 312
Key Points 314
References. 315

15 Twelve-Step and Mutual-Help Programs 319
John F. Kelly, Ph.D.
Alexandra W. Abry, B.A.
Nilofar Fallah-Sohy, B.S.
Life Contexts and Youth-Specific 12-Step Groups. . . 321
Youth Mutual-Help Organization Participation 325
Evidence for Mutual-Help Organizations and
    12-Step Facilitation for Youth. 327
Moderators and Mediators of
    12-Step Participation Benefits 332
Cost-Effectiveness 336
Clinical Strategies to Increase
    12-Step Participation Among Youth. 340
Conclusion 343
Key Points 344
References. 344

16 **Electronic Tools and Resources for Assessing and Treating Youth Substance Use Disorders** ...**349**
Rachel Gonzales-Castaneda, Ph.D., M.P.H.
Kyle C. McCarthy, M.S.
Briana Thrasher, B.A.

Technology to Aid Screening and Prevention 350

Technological Considerations for Adolescents Along
the Treatment-Recovery Continuum 351

Trials and Empirical Contributions 354

Technology Applications for
Adolescents in Recovery 357

Future Directions 359

Conclusion 360

Key Points 361

References................................. 362

PART IV

Co-occurring Disorders in Youth

Introduction............................ **367**

The Etiology and Nature of the Association 368

Diagnostic Considerations 370

Clinical and Service Implications 371

References................................. 372

17 **Assessment and Treatment of Co-occurring Internalizing Disorders:** DEPRESSION, ANXIETY DISORDERS, AND PTSD ... **375**
Yifrah Kaminer, M.D., M.B.A.
Kristyn Zajac, Ph.D.
Ken C. Winters, Ph.D.

Depression................................. 376

Anxiety Disorders 385

Adolescent Posttraumatic Stress Disorder......... 392

Key Points 402

References................................. 403

18 **Assessment and Treatment of Co-occurring Suicidal Behavior** **413**

David B. Goldston, Ph.D.
Angela M. Tunno, Ph.D.
John F. Curry, Ph.D.
Karen C. Wells, Ph.D.
Michelle Roley-Roberts, Ph.D.

Definitions of Suicidal Behaviors 414

Characteristics and Epidemiology of
Suicidal Ideation and Behaviors............... 414

Suicidal Ideation and Behaviors and
Substance Use Disorders 416

Relationship Between Alcohol and Substance Use
Disorders and Suicidal Behaviors 416

Clinical Characteristics of Youth With Both
Substance Use Problems and Suicidal Behaviors .. 417

Assessment of Suicidal Behaviors Among Youth
With Substance Use Problems 418

Treatment of Substance Use Disorder and
Suicidal Ideation and Suicide Attempts 422

Conclusion 430

Key Points 430

References................................ 431

19 **Assessment and Treatment of Comorbid Psychotic Disorders:**
BIPOLAR DISORDER, SCHIZOPHRENIA, AND DRUG-INDUCED PSYCHOTIC DISORDERS **437**

Kara S. Bagot, M.D.
Robert Milin, M.D., F.R.C.P.C.
Desiree Shapiro, M.D.
Daphna Finn, M.D.
Shavon Moore, M.D.

Psychosis and Substance Use Disorders 437

Bipolar Disorder and Substance Use Disorders..... 451

Key Points 465

References. 466

20 **Assessment and Treatment of
Co-occurring Externalizing Disorders:
ATTENTION-DEFICIT/HYPERACTIVITY DISORDER
AND DISRUPTIVE BEHAVIOR DISORDERS 477**

Martha J. Ignaszewski, M.D.
K.A.H. Mirza, M.B., F.R.C.P.C.
Oscar G. Bukstein, M.D., M.P.H.

Epidemiology 478

Relationship Between ADHD and
Substance Use Disorders 478

Relationship Between Oppositional Defiant Disorder/
Conduct Disorder and Substance Use Disorders . . . 480

Assessment 482

Treatment. 484

Other Considerations 490

Conclusion 493

Key Points 494

References. 495

21 **Behavioral Addictions: GAMBLING DISORDER
AND INTERNET GAMING DISORDER 501**

Luis C. Farhat, M.D.
Jeffrey Derevensky, Ph.D.
Marc N. Potenza, M.D., Ph.D.

Gambling Disorder 504

Internet Gaming Disorder. 508

Treatment of Gambling and Gaming Addictions 512

Conclusion 513

Key Points 514

References. 515

PART V
Special Populations

**22 Management of Youth With Substance Use
Disorders in the Juvenile Justice System** **521**

Kristyn Zajac, Ph.D.
Tess K. Drazdowski, Ph.D.
Ashli J. Sheidow, Ph.D.

Overlapping Risk Factors for Substance Use and
Juvenile Justice System Involvement 522

Outcomes for Youth With Substance Use and
Juvenile Justice System Involvement 523

Screening and Assessment Within
the Juvenile Justice System. 524

Interventions for Youth With Substance Use and
Juvenile Justice System Involvement 527

Unique Challenges When Intervening With
Substance Use in the Juvenile Justice System . . . 529

Falling Through the Cracks: Transition-Age Youth . . 532

Key Points 536

References. 537

23 Maternal Substance Use in Pregnancy. **543**

Amy M. Johnson, M.D., F.A.C.O.G.
Courtney Townsel, M.D., M.Sc., F.A.C.O.G.

Screening. 544

Review of Substances and Pregnancy Risks. 545

Management During Pregnancy. 556

Key Points 561

References. 562

**Appendix A:
Resource Materials on Screening and
Assessment Instruments** **567**

Appendix B:
Parent Resources on
Adolescent Substance Use 569

Appendix C:
Websites for Self-Help and
Mutual-Help Organizations 571

Index. 573

Contributors

Alexandra W. Abry, B.A.
Senior Clinical Research Coordinator, Recovery Research Institute, Center for Addiction Medicine, Massachusetts General Hospital, Boston, Massachusetts

Albert J. Arias, M.D.
Associate Professor, Department of Psychiatry, Division of Addiction Psychiatry, Virginia Commonwealth University School of Medicine, Richmond, Virginia

Kara S. Bagot, M.D.
Assistant Professor, Department of Psychiatry, University of California, San Diego

Molly Bobek, L.C.S.W.
Director, Clinical Implementation, Center on Addiction, New York, New York

Andria M. Botzet, M.A.
Family Therapist, Department of Psychiatry, University of Minnesota Medical Center–Fairview, Minneapolis, Minnesota

Oscar G. Bukstein, M.D., M.P.H.
Professor of Psychiatry, Boston Children's Hospital, Harvard Medical School, Boston, Massachusetts

Ryan W. Carpenter, Ph.D.
Postdoctoral Fellow, Center for Alcohol and Addiction Studies, Brown University, Providence, Rhode Island

Richard Catalano, Ph.D.
Bartley Dobb Professor for the Study and Prevention of Violence, School of Social Work, University of Washington, Seattle

Tammy Chung, Ph.D.
Professor of Psychiatry, Western Psychiatric Institute and Clinic, University of Pittsburgh School of Medicine, Pittsburgh, Pennsylvania

John F. Curry, Ph.D.
Professor, Department of Psychiatry, Duke University School of Medicine, Durham, North Carolina

Jeffrey Derevensky, Ph.D.
Professor, Department of Educational and Counselling Psychology; Director, International Centre for Youth Gambling Problems and High Risk Behaviors, McGill University, Montreal, Quebec, Canada

Tess K. Drazdowski, Ph.D.
Early Career Scientist, Oregon Social Learning Center, Eugene, Oregon

Nilofar Fallah-Sohy, B.S.
Senior Clinical Research Coordinator, Recovery Research Institute, Center for Addiction Medicine, Massachusetts General Hospital, Boston, Massachusetts

Luis C. Farhat, M.D.
Department of Psychiatry, University of São Paulo Medical School (FMUSP), São Paulo, Brazil

Daphna Finn, M.D.
Resident Physician, Department of Psychiatry, University of California, San Diego

Marc Fishman, M.D.
Medical Director, Maryland Treatment Centers; Assistant Professor of Psychiatry, Department of Psychiatry and Behavioral Sciences, Johns Hopkins University School of Medicine, Baltimore, Maryland

Mark D. Godley, Ph.D.
Senior Scientist, Chestnut Health Systems, Normal, Illinois

Susan H. Godley, Rh.D.
Senior Research Scientist Emeritus, Chestnut Health Systems, Normal, Illinois

David B. Goldston, Ph.D.
Associate Professor, Department of Psychiatry, Duke University School of Medicine, Durham, North Carolina

Rachel Gonzales-Castaneda, Ph.D., M.P.H.
Professor, Azusa Pacific University, Psychology Department, Azusa, California; Associate Research Psychologist, University of California at Los Angeles, Integrated Substance Abuse Programs, Los Angeles, California

Christopher J. Hammond, M.D., Ph.D.
Assistant Professor of Psychiatry and Child Psychiatry, Division of Child and Adolescent Psychiatry, Behavioral Pharmacology Research Unit, and Department of Psychiatry and Behavioral Sciences, Johns Hopkins University School of Medicine, Baltimore, Maryland

Sion K. Harris, Ph.D.
Associate Professor of Pediatrics, Harvard Medical School, Division of Adolescent/Young Adult Medicine, Boston Children's Hospital, Boston, Massachusetts

Areej Hassan, M.D., M.P.H.
Assistant Professor of Pediatrics, Harvard Medical School, Division of Adolescent/Young Adult Medicine, Boston Children's Hospital, Boston, Massachusetts

Brian Hendrickson, M.D.
Child and Adolescent Psychiatry Fellow, Division of Child and Adolescent Psychiatry, Johns Hopkins University School of Medicine, Baltimore, Maryland

Aaron Hogue, Ph.D.
Director, Adolescent and Family Research, Center on Addiction, New York, New York

Christian Hopfer, M.D.
Professor, Division of Substance Dependence, Department of Psychiatry, University of Colorado, Denver

Martha J. Ignaszewski, M.D.
Clinical Fellow in Psychiatry, Boston Children's Hospital, Boston, Massachusetts

Amy M. Johnson, M.D., F.A.C.O.G.
Associate Professor of Obstetrics and Gynecology, Residency Program Director, University of Connecticut School of Medicine, Farmington, Connecticut

Yifrah Kaminer, M.D., M.B.A.
Professor of Psychiatry and Pediatrics, Alcohol Research Center, University of Connecticut Health Center, Farmington, Connecticut

John F. Kelly, Ph.D.
Elizabeth R. Spallin Professor of Psychiatry, Harvard Medical School; Director, MGH Recovery Research Institute, Center for Addiction Medicine, Massachusetts General Hospital, Boston, Massachusetts

John Rogers Knight, M.D.
Associate Professor of Pediatrics (Ret.), Harvard Medical School, Departments of Medicine and Psychiatry, Boston Children's Hospital, Milton, Massachusetts

Grace Kong, Ph.D.
Assistant Professor, Yale School of Medicine, New Haven, Connecticut

Suchitra Krishnan-Sarin, Ph.D.
Professor, Yale School of Medicine, New Haven, Connecticut

Kyle C. McCarthy, M.S.
Graduate Research Assistant, Azusa Pacific University, Psychology Department, Azusa, California

Kimberly H. McManama O'Brien, Ph.D., L.I.C.S.W.
Research Scientist, Boston Children's Hospital, Department of Psychiatry, Boston, Massachusetts

Robert Milin, M.D., F.R.C.P.C.
Associate Professor of Psychiatry, University of Ottawa, ON, Canada

Robert Miranda Jr., Ph.D.
Professor of Psychiatry and Human Behavior, Brown University; Director, Adolescent Co-occurring Disorders Program, Bradley Hospital; Center for Alcohol and Addiction Studies, Center for Alcohol and Addiction Studies, Providence, Rhode Island

K.A.H. Mirza, M.B., F.R.C.P.C.
Hon. Senior Lecturer and Consultant Psychiatrist, University Department of Child and Adolescent Psychiatry and South London and Maudsley NHS Trust, London, England

Gerald Montano, D.O.
Assistant Professor of Pediatrics, University of Pittsburgh School of Medicine, Pittsburgh, Pennsylvania

Shavon Moore, M.D.
Resident Physician, Department of Psychiatry, University of California, San Diego

Marc N. Potenza, M.D., Ph.D.
Professor, Department of Psychiatry, Child Study Center, Department of Neuroscience, Yale School of Medicine, New Haven, Connecticut; Director, Connecticut Council on Problem Gambling, Wethersfield, Connecticut

Michelle Roley-Roberts, Ph.D.
Postdoctoral Fellow, Department of Psychiatry, Ohio State University Medical Center, Columbus, Ohio

Lawrence M. Scheier, Ph.D.
President, LARS Research Institute, Scottsdale, Arizona; Senior Research Scientist, Prevention Strategies, LLC, Greensboro, North Carolina; Visiting Scholar, Department of Public Health Education, University of North Carolina, Greensboro

Desiree Shapiro, M.D.
Assistant Clinical Professor, Department of Psychiatry, University of California, San Diego

Ashli J. Sheidow, Ph.D.
Senior Research Scientist, Oregon Social Learning Center, Eugene, Oregon

Anthony Spirito, Ph.D., A.B.P.P.
Professor, Department of Psychiatry and Human Behavior, Alpert Medical School of Brown University, Providence, Rhode Island

Randy Stinchfield, Ph.D.
Clinical Psychologist, St. Paul, Minnesota

Briana Thrasher, B.A.
Research Associate, Azusa Pacific University, Psychology Department, Azusa, California

Christian Thurstone, M.D.
Professor, Department of Psychiatry, University of Colorado, Denver, Colorado

Courtney Townsel, M.D., M.Sc., F.A.C.O.G.
Assistant Professor, Department of Obstetrics and Gynecology, Division of Maternal Fetal Medicine, University of Michigan, Ann Arbor, Michigan

Angela M. Tunno, Ph.D.
Medical Instructor, Department of Psychiatry, Duke University School of Medicine, Durham, North Carolina

Wendy Welch, M.D., C.P.E.
Chief Medical Officer, Cardinal Innovations Healthcare, Charlotte, North Carolina

Karen C. Wells, Ph.D.
Associate Professor, Department of Psychiatry, Duke University School of Medicine, Durham, North Carolina

Charles Albert Whitmore, M.D., M.P.H.
Child and Adolescent Psychiatry Fellow, Vanderbilt University Medical Center, Nashville, Tennessee

Ken C. Winters, Ph.D.
Senior Scientist, Oregon Research Institute (Minnesota Location), Falcon Heights, Minnesota

Kristyn Zajac, Ph.D.
Assistant Professor of Medicine, Calhoun Cardiology Center—Behavioral Cardiovascular, Prevention Division, University of Connecticut School of Medicine, Farmington, Connecticut

Disclosure of Competing Interests

The following contributors to this book have indicated a financial interest in or other affiliation with a commercial supporter, a manufacturer of a commercial product, a provider of a commercial service, a nongovernmental organization, and/or a government agency, as listed below:

Oscar G. Bukstein, M.D., M.P.H.—*Royalties* (as author): Guilford Press, Routledge Press; *Contributor to Up-to-Date:* Wolters Kluwer Health

Richard Catalano, Ph.D.—The author was a board member of the Channing Bete Company, which distributes Guiding Good Choices, one of the parenting programs mentioned in the chapter.

Marc Fishman, M.D.—The author has received consultant fees and research funding from Alkermes and consultant fees from US WorldMeds; he has an ownership interest in Maryland Treatment Centers.

David B. Goldston, Ph.D.—American Foundation for Suicide Prevention; National Institutes of Health (NIAAA and NIMH); Substance Abuse and Mental Health Services Administration

Christopher J. Hammond, M.D., Ph.D.—*Research funding:* National Institute on Drug Abuse/American Academy of Child and Adolescent Psychiatry Physician Scientist Program in Substance Abuse (2K12DA000357).

Robert Milin, M.D., F.R.C.P.C.—*Consultant:* US WorldMeds (on protocol for pediatric lofexidine trial related to opioid withdrawal management)

Marc N. Potenza, M.D., Ph.D.—The author has consulted for and advised RiverMend Health, Lakelight Therapeutics/Opiant, and Jazz Pharmaceuticals; has received research support from the Mohegan Sun Casino and the National Center for Responsible Gaming; has participated in surveys, mailings, or telephone consultations related to drug addiction, impulse-control disorders, or other health topics; and has consulted for law offices and gambling entities on issues related to impulse-control disorders and addictive disorders.

Desiree Shapiro, M.D.—The author is a reviewer for Stahl's Essential Psychopharmacology: Prescriber's Guide—Children and Adolescents.

Ashli J. Sheidow, Ph.D.—The author is co-owner of Science to Practice Group, LLC, which provides the training and quality assurance for Multisystemic Therapy for Emerging Adults.

Karen C. Wells, Ph.D.—*Royalties:* Multi-Health Systems.

Ken C. Winters, Ph.D.—The author has commercial and financial interests in a brief intervention program cited in Chapter 2 and in assessment tools cited in Chapter 3.

The following contributors have indicated that they have no financial interests or other affiliations that represent or could appear to represent a competing interest with the contributions to this book:

Alexandra W. Abry, B.A.
Albert J. Arias, M.D.
Kara S. Bagot, M.D.
Molly Bobek, L.C.S.W.
Andria M. Botzet, M.A.
Ryan W. Carpenter, Ph.D.
Tammy Chung, Ph.D.
John F. Curry, Ph.D.
Jeffrey Derevensky, Ph.D.
Tess K. Drazdowski, Ph.D.
Nilofar Fallah-Sohy, B.S.
Luis C. Farhat, M.D.
Daphna Finn, M.D.
Mark D. Godley, Ph.D.
Susan H. Godley, Rh.D.
Rachel Gonzales-Castaneda, Ph.D., M.P.H.
Sion K. Harris, Ph.D.
Areej Hassan, M.D., M.P.H.
Brian Hendrickson, M.D.
Martha J. Ignaszewski, M.D.
Amy M. Johnson, M.D., F.A.C.O.G.
Yifrah Kaminer, M.D., M.B.A.

John F. Kelly, Ph.D.
John Rogers Knight, M.D.
Grace Kong, Ph.D.
Suchitra Krishnan-Sarin, Ph.D.
Kyle C. McCarthy, M.S.
Kimberly H. McManama O'Brien, Ph.D., L.I.C.S.W.
Robert Miranda Jr., Ph.D.
K.A.H. Mirza, M.B., F.R.C.P.C.
Gerald Montano, D.O.
Shavon Moore, M.D.
Michelle Roley-Roberts, Ph.D.
Lawrence M. Scheier, Ph.D.
Anthony Spirito, Ph.D., A.B.P.P.
Randy Stinchfield, Ph.D.
Christian Thurstone, M.D.
Courtney Townsel, M.D., M.Sc., F.A.C.O.G.
Angela M. Tunno, Ph.D.
Wendy Welch, M.D., C.P.E.
Charles Albert Whitmore, M.D., M.P.H.
Kristyn Zajac, Ph.D.

Introduction

Welcome to the *Clinical Manual of Youth Addictive Disorders*. It has been a decade since the publication of the clinical manual on which this new book is based.

This extended and updated manual has been devoted to youth. This subpopulation includes adolescents 12–17 years of age and "emerging adults," a term that refers to individuals ages 18–25 years. The common denominator of the youth subpopulation is its neurocognitive and socioecological developmental stage. Since youth are not "miniature adults," a developmentally informed approach is important in understanding the onset of substance use and the pathways (trajectory) to substance use disorders (SUDs) and behavioral addictive disorders. This plethora of high-risk behaviors and clinical disorders commonly leads to negative consequences. Drug and non-substance addictive behaviors have been characterized by elevated sensation seeking and often impulsive, nonproblematic behavior that is devoid of effective use of executive functions and inhibitions. These components have been attributed to developmental dysregulation, particularly in the prefrontal cortex, that occurs throughout adolescence and into the mid-20s of young adulthood. These findings underscore the importance of clinicians' knowledge of risk factors that predict progression from substance use to SUD as well as the challenges of developing age-appropriate prevention and treatment strategies to postpone, reduce, and/or eliminate substance use and SUDs.

Developmentally, not all adolescents who use substances escalate their use to levels described in DSM-IV as "abuse" or "dependence" and now defined in DSM-5 as substance use disorder with severity specified. For those adolescents who show escalating use, several full cycles spanning many years may be the norm rather than the exception. Nonetheless, emerging research on developmental psychopathology and adolescent development has implications for how we view current prevention, intervention, and treatment paradigms. The field can benefit from a greater understanding of how varying levels of substance use severity are viewed within etiological paradigms and optimally treated with different levels and intensities of prevention, intervention, treatment, and aftercare/continued-care strategies.

This manual not only captures the progress made in the domains of youth substance use and SUDs included in the 16 chapters of its 2010 predecessor, but also includes additional important topics that have emerged or expanded since then. The 23 chapters of this manual include 7 new chapters devoted to primary care and pediatric assessment and intervention; electronic tools and resources for treating youth with SUDs; and maternal-fetal addiction. Specific chapters on alcohol, tobacco, cannabis, and opioids have been added to include emerging new products and delivery systems and innovative patterns of use. This rapid expansion of knowledge is of great importance to clinicians (e.g., pediatricians/adolescent medicine experts, family physicians, mental health professionals, substance use specialists), applied researchers, and public health policy makers. Thus, the scope of this manual is to provide an updated, comprehensive, and clinically oriented text that includes research and policy implications.

This manual has been organized into five parts:

Part I: Course, prevention, and pretreatment considerations
Part II: Description, diagnosis, and interventions for specific substances of abuse
Part III: Specific interventions for youth with SUDs
Part IV: Co-occurring disorders in youth
Part V: Special populations

The manual also includes three appendixes: resources for screening and assessment instruments (Appendix A); a select list of websites for parents who are seeking advice and resources about drug prevention and intervention (Appendix B); and a listing of websites with general information about self-help, including how to find AA or NA meetings in someone's neighborhood (Appendix C).

Finally, we have assembled some of the most experienced authors in the field. Several new contributors have joined our authorship from the 2010 clinical manual and bring fresh perspectives on the domains of their expertise. Authors were invited because they excel in bridging the knowledge gap between research and its application in clinical practice. These contributors review the state of the art from an international data–based literature in order to advance clinical work and research in youth addictive disorders.

Happy reading!

Yifrah Kaminer, M.D., M.B.A.
Ken C. Winters, Ph.D.

PART I

Course, Prevention, and Pretreatment Considerations

1

Diagnosis, Epidemiology, and Course of Youth Substance Use and Use Disorders

Gerald Montano, D.O.

Tammy Chung, Ph.D.

Adolescence is a critical developmental period that involves pubertal maturation, continuing brain development, changes in social roles (e.g., initiating dating, obtaining a driver's license) and contexts (e.g., transition to high school, college, and employment), and an increase in risky behavior, such as substance use (Brown et al. 2008; W. D. Hall et al. 2016). Although experimentation with alcohol and nicotine may be considered developmentally nor-

The preparation of this manuscript was supported by National Institute on Alcohol Abuse and Alcoholism grant R01 AA023650 and National Institute on Drug Abuse grants R01 DA012237 and R21 DA043181.

3

mative, some adolescents progress to a more regular pattern of substance use, and to substance use disorders (SUDs). Among youth who report substance-related problems, some show a developmentally limited course, whereas others experience more chronic and severe substance-related problems that persist into adulthood (Zucker et al. 2016). In this chapter we review adolescence as a developmental period of peak risk for onset of substance use and substance-related problems, describe the prevalence and course of adolescent substance use, cover developmental considerations in the assessment of SUDs in adolescents, and summarize the literature on the prevalence and course of SUDs in youth.

Adolescence as a Critical Developmental Period for Initiation of Substance Involvement

Developmental contexts and transitions unique to adolescence influence the emergence and progression of substance involvement in youth (W. D. Hall et al. 2016). In particular, continuing brain development during adolescence, which involves synaptic pruning and continuing myelination, results in a developmentally normative delay in the maturation of behavioral inhibitory systems relative to neural systems associated with reward (e.g., sensation seeking) (Luna et al. 2013). This normative delay in the maturation of behavioral inhibition results in a greater propensity for reward seeking and risk-taking behavior in adolescents, compared with adults (Luna et al. 2013). The relative priority on reward-related behaviors during adolescence promotes the adoption of adult social roles (e.g., romantic relationships) and independence, but is also thought to underlie the adolescent increase in risk-taking behavior, such as substance use (Luna et al. 2013).

High-quantity consumption of a substance, in the context of continuing brain development through adolescence, may have adverse effects on neurodevelopment and increase the risk for addiction (Lisdahl et al. 2018). Specifically, heavy substance use during adolescence has been associated with neurocognitive deficits (Morin et al. 2019) and may alter the development of neural systems modulating reward and inhibitory behavior, as well as delay social maturation and disrupt the achievement of academic milestones (Anderson et al. 2010). Thus, initiation to substance use peaks at a time when the developing brain may be particularly vulnerable to substance dependence–related neuroadaptation, and possible neurotoxic effects of heavy, chronic substance use on brain development, highlighting the importance of early intervention in reducing risk for SUD in adolescence.

Prevalence of Substance Use in Adolescents

Substance involvement has been characterized along a continuum that spans abstinence, experimental use, emerging substance-related problems, and SUDs (i.e., abuse and dependence). Two national surveys, Monitoring the Future (MTF) and the National Survey on Drug Use and Health (NSDUH), provide estimates of the prevalence of adolescent substance use in the United States. The MTF collects substance use data annually from 8th, 10th, and 12th graders, and the NSDUH collects annual data on rates of substance use and SUDs from respondents age 12 years and older. These two national surveys provide complementary sources of information on the prevalence of adolescent substance use.

Patterns of Substance Use Onset

The prevalence of substance use increases steadily from age 12 to age 21 (Center for Behavioral Health Statistics and Quality 2017; Miech et al. 2017). The substances used most often by adolescents (ages 12–18) include alcohol, nicotine, and cannabis; rates of other illicit drug use (e.g., cocaine, opiates) are relatively low (Center for Behavioral Health Statistics and Quality 2017; Miech et al. 2017). Two primary periods of risk for substance use initiation are early adolescence (around ages 13–14, coincident with pubertal maturation) and the transition period from late adolescence to early adulthood (Degenhardt et al. 2016; W. D. Hall et al. 2016). The sequence of initiation to substance use ("gateway hypothesis") generally begins with use of alcohol and nicotine/tobacco, which is then typically followed by first use of cannabis prior to the first use of other illicit drugs (Degenhardt et al. 2016).

Alcohol, Nicotine, and Cannabis Use

Adolescents tend to engage in a risky pattern of alcohol use (e.g., heavy episodic drinking: consuming 5+ drinks in a row; high-intensity drinking: consuming 10+ or 15+ drinks in a row) that is associated with alcohol-related problems (see Chapter 7). Among 12- to 17-year-olds in the 2016 NSDUH, 4.9% reported episodic heavy drinking ("binge alcohol use") in the past month (Center for Behavioral Health Statistics and Quality 2017). Prevalence of episodic heavy drinking increased with school grade in the 2016 MTF, such that 3.4% of 8th graders, 9.7% of 10th graders, and 15.5% of 12th graders reported binge alcohol use in the past 2 weeks (Miech et al. 2017).

Nicotine use in the past month was reported by 5.3% of 12- to 17-year-olds in the 2016 NSDUH; 3.4% of adolescents reported use of cigarettes, the most popular form of nicotine delivery, and 1.4% reported using smokeless tobacco (Center for Behavioral Health Statistics and Quality 2017) (see Chapter 8). According to the 2016 MTF school-based survey, 2.6% of 8th graders, 4.9% of 10th graders, and 10.5% of 12th graders reported cigarette use in the past month (Miech et al. 2017).

Overall, cannabis was the illicit drug most commonly used by 12- to 17-year-olds in the NSDUH; however, the type of illicit drug most commonly used differed by age (Center for Behavioral Health Statistics and Quality 2017) (see Chapter 9). Specifically, among 12-year-olds in the 2016 NSDUH, a higher perecntage of youth reported any nonmedical use of prescription medication (e.g., pain relievers, tranquilizers, stimulants) in the past month than any cannabis use in the past month (0.5% vs. 0.2%) (Center for Behavioral Health Statistics and Quality 2017). In contrast, at ages 13–17 in the 2016 NSDUH, cannabis was generally the most commonly reported illicit drug used in the past month (with the percentage reporting such use increasing from 1.2% at age 13 to 15.5% at age 17) (Center for Behavioral Health Statistics and Quality 2017). In the 2016 MTF, cannabis was the illicit drug used most often in the past 30 days, with use reported by 5.4% of 8th graders, 14.0% of 10th graders, and 22.5% of 12th graders (Miech et al. 2017). Nonmedical use of prescription medication was the next most commonly reported substance use after cannabis, although the item was only asked of 12th graders (5.4% reported nonmedical use in the past 30 days) in the 2016 MTF. Although both the 2016 NSDUH and MTF surveys reported that cannabis is generally the illicit drug used most often by adolescents, NSDUH and MTF (12th grade) data both suggest that non–medically used prescription medication warrants careful assessment, since youth may have easy access to such medication (e.g., in their own homes, through their peers).

MTF data indicate that from 2006 to 2016, the prevalence of episodic heavy drinking (in the past 2 weeks) among adolescents showed an overall decreasing trend. Similar to alcohol use, the prevalence of cigarette use in the past month has shown an overall decline in the past decade. Illicit drug use overall has been steady in the last decade (Miech et al. 2017). Multiple factors may explain these trends, including increased public health and law enforcement efforts to curb substance use, media campaigns to reduce drunk driving and highlight tobacco-related harms to health, and increased perceptions of harm associated with episodic heavy drinking and tobacco use (Miech et al. 2017).

Trends in youth substance use that warrant attention include increasing state-level legalization of marijuana (medical and recreational), increasing potency of available cannabis, newer methods of substance use (e.g., vaping, dabbing, tinctures), and availability of emerging synthetic substances (e.g., synthetic cannabinoids, synthetic opioids such as fentanyl and U-47700, or "pink"). In particular, youth perceptions of health risks associated with marijuana use have shown an alarming decline, while prevalence of marijuana use has increased (Miech et al. 2018).

Differences in Substance Use Prevalence by Gender and Race/Ethnicity

In recent years, the gender gap in rates of adolescent substance use has narrowed, with females sometimes surpassing males in prevalence of use (Miech et al. 2017). For example, in the 2016 NSDUH, a slightly higher proportion of females, compared with males, reported binge drinking in the past month (5.4% vs. 4.4%), but males and females had similar prevalence of heavy alcohol use (i.e., binge drinking on 5 or more days in the past month: 0.9% vs. 0.6%) (Center for Behavioral Health Statistics and Quality 2017). Likewise, past-month prevalence of cigarette use was similar for 12- to 17-year-old males and females (3.8% vs. 3.1%, respectively) in the 2016 NSDUH (Center for Behavioral Health Statistics and Quality 2017). The narrowing gender gap in rates of substance use is even clearer in the MTF survey. For example, among 8th and 10th graders in the 2018 MTF, males and females had similar 30-day prevalence of cigarette use (8th graders: 2.5% vs. 2.6%; 10th graders: 5.0% vs. 4.6%; males vs. females), although among 12th graders, males continued to have slightly higher rates of cigarette smoking compared with females (12.7% vs. 8.1%) (Miech et al. 2017). The narrowing gender gap in rates of substance use, with rates in females catching up to or surpassing rates in males, at some ages, for certain substances, points to the need to identify and address gender-specific risk and protective factors when intervening with youth.

With regard to differences in race/ethnicity in substance use, 2016 MTF data indicate that among the three largest racial/ethnic groups (i.e., Caucasians, African Americans, Hispanics) in the survey, African American students, compared with their Caucasian peers, generally had lower rates of use for some substances, such as cigarette use and consuming five or more drinks in a row, but higher annual prevalence of marijuana use (e.g., among 8th graders, 12% vs. 8%) (Miech et al. 2017). Of some concern, among the three largest racial/ethnic groups, Hispanic 8th and 12th graders had some of the highest annual rates of use for many illicit drugs (e.g., among 12th graders: crack and crystal methamphetamine; Miech et al. 2017). These examples of differences in race/ethnicity in substance use suggest the potential benefit of culturally sensitive and tailored interventions to delay initiation of substance use and to prevent the escalation of substance involvement during adolescence (see, e.g., G. C. N. Hall et al. 2016).

Children of Substance-Using Parents

In the United States, roughly 12% of youth (age 17 or younger) live with a parent who has an SUD (Lipari and Van Horn 2017). Compared with children of non-substance-using parents (CNSUP), children of substance-using parents (CSUP) are more than twice as likely to have mental health conditions such as depression and conduct problems in adolescence (Solis et al. 2012). CSUP also tend to have earlier onset of substance use, accelerated trajectories of use, and higher rates of SUD (53% of CSUP have a SUD in young adulthood vs. 25% of CNSUP) (Solis et al. 2012). Greater risk for SUDs among CSUP likely represents an interaction of genetic and environmental (e.g., social learning, drug availability) influences. Regarding family environment, parents with SUDs may show deficits in parenting behavior, such as less warmth, harsher interaction styles, and less secure attachment to their child, possibly related to addiction's cycles of relapse and remission (Solis et al. 2012). As a consequence of possible exposure to a chaotic home environment associated with parental SUD, CSUP are at higher risk for maltreatment (e.g., parental emotional, physical, or sexual abuse; neglect) (Lipari and Van Horn 2017).

Parental substance use can have adverse effects on child development that begin as early as prenatal substance exposure (e.g., fetal alcohol syndrome). Other adverse effects on child development depend on a number of factors, such as the child's age (developmental maturation) at exposure and the severity of parental SUD (e.g., active use vs. in remission) (Solis et al. 2012). Greater risk for adverse outcomes has been associated with multiple parent-related problems, such as when the parent with SUD has a co-occurring mental health condition (e.g., depression, posttraumatic stress disorder), when the child lives with two parents with SUD, when there is active parental SUD, when the parental SUD is of longer duration and greater severity, and when the child is exposed to other types of family strain (e.g., poverty, family conflict) (Solis et al. 2012). In addition, protective factors, which support resilience (defined as the ability to adapt to adversity; American Psychological Association 2014), can buffer risk. Protective factors include, for example, at the individual level, coping and problem-solving skills, and self-control; at the family level, a caring non-substance-using adult (e.g., aunt, grandparent) who can provide a stable supportive relationship; and at the community level, support from non-substance-using peers and a positive bond with the school (Wlodarczyk et al. 2017).

For youth with a substance-using parent, prevention efforts and interventions to improve outcomes need to consider the whole family, identifying strengths and personalized service needs to enhance family functioning (Lipari and Van Horn 2017). Specifically, as an initial step, assessment can determine the specific types of evidence-based treatment to recommend for the parent (e.g., relapse prevention for substance use, behavioral parent training) and intervention, if indicated, for the adolescent (e.g., cognitive-behavioral therapy for depression) (Lipari and Van Horn 2017). Despite greater risk for adverse outcomes for CSUP, many of these youth show resilience, particularly in the presence of protective factors (Solis et al. 2012).

Trajectories of Substance Use During Adolescence

Cross-sectional prevalence data provide a snapshot of substance use at a given point in time but do not provide information on changes over time in an individual's pattern of substance use. Longitudinal studies beginning in adolescence and extending into young adulthood have identified prototypical trajectories of alcohol, cigarette, cannabis, and substance use more generally (e.g., Jackson and Sartor 2014). The most common trajectory types that have emerged in research based on community samples of youth are stable low, chronic high, developmentally limited, and later onset, increasing. In community samples, the developmentally normative and modal trajectory for alcohol, cigarette, and cannabis use involved light (i.e., experimental) to moderate use of alcohol and tobacco, and no use to light use of cannabis; the least-prevalent trajectory type generally involved heavy and chronic substance use (e.g., Jackson and Sartor 2014). Adolescents with trajectories involving low to no substance use through young adulthood tend to have the best outcomes, whereas individuals with more chronic and severe trajectories across substances, including trajectories of increasing use in the transition to adulthood, tend to have worse outcomes through young adulthood (e.g., Nelson et al. 2015).

Diagnosis of Substance Use Disorders

The *Diagnostic and Statistical Manual of Mental Disorders,* in both the fourth edition (DSM-IV; American Psychiatric Association 1994) and fifth edition (DSM-5; American Psychiatric Association 2013), define substance use disorders by a list of criteria, of which no single symptom is necessary or sufficient, and an algorithm that determines the presence or absence of a diagnosis. In addition, clinically significant impairment in functioning or subjective feelings of distress must be present for a SUD diagnosis to be made. Although DSM-5 is the current classification system, some national surveys (e.g., NSDUH) continue to use DSM-IV SUD criteria. There is support for the comparability of, as well as differences in, DSM-IV and DSM-5 SUD diagnoses (Chung et al. 2017).

DSM-IV recognized two aspects of SUDs: abuse and dependence. DSM-IV substance abuse required meeting at least one of four criteria representing certain recurrent psychosocial consequences related to substance use (e.g., drop in school grades due to substance use, interpersonal problems due to substance use, substance-related legal problems) and hazardous substance use (e.g., driving while intoxicated). DSM-IV substance dependence required meeting at least three of seven criteria within the same 1-year period. Dependence criteria included physical symptoms (i.e., a high level of tolerance, withdrawal), symptoms indicating high salience of substance use behavior (i.e., spending much time using, reducing activities in order to use a substance), and impaired control over substance use (i.e., using more or longer than intended, difficulty cutting down or abstaining from use, using despite adverse physical and psychological consequences of substance use). The seven dependence criteria were applied to all substances (except caffeine), with the exception that the withdrawal criterion did not apply to cannabis, hallucinogens, inhalants, and phencyclidine. Notably, the criteria used to diagnose substance abuse and dependence do not overlap, a diagnosis of nicotine "abuse" was not included in DSM-IV, and a diagnosis of dependence precluded the diagnosis of the milder disorder of abuse.

In contrast to DSM-IV, DSM-5 combines the DSM-IV abuse and dependence symptoms into a single SUD category, excludes substance-related legal problems (an abuse criterion) and adds a new craving criterion, based on empirical data and comprehensive reviews. Individuals whose use meets two or more criteria within a 12-month period pass the threshold for a DSM-5 SUD diagnosis. DSM-5 scales the severity of SUD based on the number of symptom criteria met: mild (2–3 symptoms), moderate (4–5 symptoms), and severe (6 or more symptoms). The scaling of SUD severity in DSM-5 represents an important contrast with DSM-IV's categorical approach to SUD diagnosis.

Notably, DSM-5's dimensional approach to SUD assessment is consistent with a parallel approach, Research Domain Criteria (RDoC; Cuthbert and Insel 2013). RDoC provides a dimensional alternative to DSM's categorical diagnoses and covers levels of analysis that span from genes through brain circuits to behavior. RDoC is represented by a matrix in which the columns are levels of analysis (e.g., genes, brain circuits, behavior) and the rows are specific domains (e.g., cognitive control, sensitivity to reward). Thus, each domain (e.g., cognitive control) is characterized across each level of analysis (e.g., genes). RDoC represents an important attempt to more parsimoniously characterize functioning along a continuum of severity, and in relation to biological markers to accelerate translation to empirically based treatment.

DSM-IV Prevalence of Substance Use Disorders in Adolescent Samples

In parallel with patterns of substance use, the most common SUDs among youth ages 12–17 involve alcohol, cannabis, and nicotine (Center for Behavioral Health Statistics and Quality 2017). Among adolescent substance users, a pattern of polysubstance use, which often involves alcohol, nicotine, and cannabis, is frequently observed (Winters et al. 2018). Cross-sectional survey data indicate that the prevalence of SUD increases with age through adolescence and peaks in young adulthood. In the 2016 NSDUH, prevalence of past-year DSM-IV SUD was 4.3% among 12- to 17-year-olds (2.0% had an alcohol diagnosis, 3.2% had an illicit drug diagnosis), increased to 15.1% among 18- to 25-year-olds, and declined to 6.9% among adults 26 years and older (Center for Behavioral Health Statistics and Quality 2017). Among past-month cigarette users ages 12–17, 29% were estimated to have nicotine dependence (Center for Behavioral Health Statistics and Quality 2017). For some adolescents, the transition from initial use to SUD may occur within 3 years of first use of a substance (Degenhardt et al. 2016), emphasizing the importance of early detection and intervention for substance-related problems.

In addition to adolescents whose use meets criteria for a DSM-IV SUD diagnosis, some youth report one or two dependence symptoms but their use does not meet the full criteria for a SUD. These subthreshold cases, known as "diagnostic orphans," represent up to an additional 17% of teens who report alcohol-related problems in community surveys (Chung et al. 2002). Youth with subthreshold symptoms of dependence are at higher risk for SUDs in young adulthood, highlighting the importance of early detection and intervention in adolescence to reduce SUDs in adulthood.

Differences in SUD Prevalence by Gender and Race/Ethnicity

Data from the 2016 NSDUH indicate similar rates of past-year DSM-IV illicit drug use disorder among 12- to 17-year-old males and females (3.2% for males and 3.1% for females), again pointing to a narrowing of the gender gap, particularly among adolescents, in rates of substance involvement (Center for Behavioral Health Statistics and Quality 2017). Likewise, the prevalence of DSM-IV nicotine dependence was similar for adolescent males and females in the 2016 NSDUH (1.1% vs. 0.9%, respectively; Center for Behavioral Health Statistics and Quality 2017). With regard to race/ethnicity, Caucasian, Hispanic, and African American youth ages 12–17 had similar prevalence rates of past-year illicit drug use disorder (3.2%, 3.4%, and 2.9%, respectively), but Caucasian and Hispanic youth had slightly higher prevalence rates of past-year alcohol use disorder compared with African American youth (2.1% and 2.3% vs. 1.0%, respectively; Center for Behavioral Health Statistics and Quality 2017). Caucasian youth also had higher rates of DSM-IV nicotine dependence compared with African American and Hispanic youth (1.4% vs. 0.5% and 0.3%, respectively) in the 2016 NSDUH (Center for Behavioral Health Statistics and Quality 2017).

SUD Diagnosis and Treatment Utilization

Very few adolescents whose use meets criteria for a DSM-IV SUD reported receiving treatment. Less than 1% of youth ages 12–17 reported receiving treatment for alcohol or other drugs in the past year, although 4.3% reported use that met criteria for a past-year DSM-IV SUD diagnosis (Center for Behavioral Health Statistics and Quality 2017). Among admissions to publicly funded substance use treatment, adolescents (ages 12–17) represented 3.9% of all admissions in 2016 (Substance Abuse and Mental Health Services Administration 2018). A majority (60.4%–71.1%) of adolescent admissions ages 12–17 years reported that cannabis was their primary substance on treatment admission (Substance Abuse and Mental Health Services Administration 2018). Among 12- to 17-year-olds in publicly funded addiction treatment, most were referred by the criminal justice system, with smaller proportions referred by schools or family (Substance Abuse and Mental Health Services Administration 2018). Treatment utilization statistics for adolescents suggest a high level of unmet treatment need, as well as the importance of increasing adolescents' readiness to change substance use behavior, because most youth do not refer themselves to treatment for substance use.

Developmentally Informed Substance Use Disorder Assessment

Given adolescent substance users' relatively short histories of use and developmental context (e.g., living with parents), there is a need to adapt SUD constructs and criteria in order to minimize false-positive and false-negative diagnostic and symptom assignments, and to increase overall validity of SUD diagnoses in adolescents (Kaminer and Winters 2015). Developmentally informed SUD symptom assessment involves consideration of how SUD constructs (e.g., tolerance) may manifest or be interpreted differently in adolescents and adults, identification of substance-related problems that are relevant to youth, and efforts to scale symptom and diagnostic thresholds to optimize performance in adolescents (Kaminer and Winters 2015). Comprehensive reviews of measures used to assess SUDs in adolescents are described in Chapter 3.

Certain SUD symptoms may manifest differently in adolescent and adults, or may be interpreted differently by adolescents, because of the developmental context in which a symptom occurs. For example, some adolescents endorsed "using more or longer than intended" because they drank more than the usual amount needed to become intoxicated, not because they had made a failed attempt to cut down on drinking (the intended meaning of the symptom). Some SUD criteria represent relatively abstract and complex constructs (e.g., a high level of tolerance to drug effects). As a way to improve the validity of assessment of relatively complex constructs, follow-up probes can help reduce false-positive symptom assignments (Kaminer and Winters 2015). For example, clarification can be obtained to determine whether much time spent obtaining alcohol reflects a compulsive pattern of use (the intended meaning of the criterion), or difficulties in obtaining alcohol due to minor status (possible false positive). Symptoms relevant to youth patterns of substance use, such as recurrent substance-related risky sexual behavior, repeated alcohol-related blackouts, and passing out from substance use, also warrant assessment. Developmentally based assessment can improve diagnostic validity.

Course of Adolescent-Onset Substance Use Disorders

Studies of clinical course, which document changes in severity as well as patterns of substance involvement over time, provide information on factors associated with the onset, maintenance, and remission of substance involvement. Multiple etiological models have been proposed to explain the onset and maintenance of SUD, including, for example, the use of substances to regulate affect (e.g., to "get high," to reduce negative mood), individual differences in sensitivity and response to drug effects, and deviance proneness (Zucker et al. 2016). In the following subsections we review research on the course of SUDs in community and treatment samples, and predictors of SUD course among treated adolescents.

SUD Course in Community Samples

Adolescents with alcohol use disorder (AUD) show heterogeneity in developmental course, represented by four main patterns (Zucker et al. 2016). One pathway involves limited course of AUD in adolescence or young adulthood, in which an individual "matures out" of alcohol-related problems (e.g., during the transition to adult roles of employment, parenthood, or marriage). Two trajectories represent more chronic AUD involving co-occurring externalizing (e.g., conduct problems) or internalizing (e.g., depression) psychopathology. Other patterns of adolescent-onset AUD continue into adulthood but do not involve co-occurring psychopathology and vary in chronicity (e.g., episodic vs. chronic).

Longitudinal studies of adolescent-onset cannabis use disorders, particularly in Europe and Australia, indicate that adolescent regular cannabis users tend to continue to use at a level that meets criteria for a cannabis use disorder through young adulthood (i.e., age 24; Swift et al. 2008), with rates of full remission from cannabis use disorder relatively low until at least the mid-30s (Farmer et al. 2015). Relative to other substances (e.g., opiates), however, cannabis has the highest rate of cessation of use (Calabria et al. 2010). Epidemiological studies suggest that risk for more chronic cannabis use disorder and AUD is concentrated primarily among individuals who establish more regular patterns of substance use during adolescence, although developmentally limited patterns of adolescent-onset cannabis use also have been observed. Given the concentration of substance-related problems in a high-risk subgroup of youth, we review, in the following subsection, the course of substance involvement among treated adolescents.

Posttreatment Course of Substance Involvement

Several models of substance use treatment for adolescents (e.g., group cognitive-behavioral therapy) are in use (National Institute on Drug Abuse 2014), and a meta-analysis of outpatient treatment outcomes indicated that no single "brand" of treatment for adolescent substance use is clearly superior to any others (Tanner-Smith et al. 2013). Treated adolescents generally show reductions in substance involvement compared with pretreatment levels, along with concurrent improvements in psychosocial functioning over the short- and longer-term (12-month) follow-up (Hogue et al. 2018; Tanner-Smith et al. 2013).

Risk for relapse is particularly high in the first few months after treatment, with roughly two out of three youth reporting a relapse to substance use within 6 months of completing outpatient treatment (Buckheit et al. 2018). Among adolescents, relapse is most often due to social pressure to engage in substance use or desire to increase positive feelings (Ramo and Brown 2008), suggesting the importance of an adolescent's social network in supporting recovery. Treatment gains may fade over time, underscoring the importance of continuing care to facilitate positive long-term outcomes (Buckheit et al. 2018).

Studies of short-term posttreatment course (i.e., ≤18-month follow-up) have identified multiple prototypical trajectories of substance involvement that include stable low and stable high levels of use, and increasing and decreasing patterns of use (e.g., Chung et al. 2008). Importantly, alcohol and marijuana use generally showed parallel reductions following treatment, rather than a pattern of substituting use of one substance for the other (Chung et al. 2008). The longer-term posttreatment trajectories most commonly identified across studies were stable abstinence, infrequent use, gradually decreasing substance involvement ("slow improvers"), and persistent high substance involvement. Although the actual proportion represented by each trajectory type differed across studies, the relative proportions were similar, with most youth classified as slow improvers or infrequent users, and smaller proportions in stable abstinence and persistent high substance involvement trajectories. The similarity in posttreatment patterns of change across drugs suggests that reductions in the use of one substance may be associated with parallel reductions in the use of other substances, rather than providing support for drug substitution effects, and that treatment has a general positive effect in reducing substance involvement for many youth.

Posttreatment Trajectories of Substance Involvement and Psychosocial Outcomes

As may be expected, adolescents in stable abstinence and low substance involvement trajectories following treatment generally have better emotional, interpersonal, and family functioning in young adulthood compared with those with chronic heavy substance involvement (Anderson et al. 2010). Changes in different areas of psychosocial functioning occur at different rates, with improvement in school functioning occurring within a year, and improvements in family functioning becoming evident only 2 years after treatment (Anderson et al. 2010). More chronic and severe trajectories of substance involvement also may reflect the impact of co-occurring psychopathology (e.g., conduct problems) in complicating the course of recovery from SUD. Despite significant reductions in substance involvement and improvements in areas of school performance, interpersonal relations, and other areas, treated teens continued to show greater problem severity compared with a community comparison sample (Anderson et al. 2010), and in one study, treated adolescent substance users were at higher risk for adverse outcomes (e.g., poverty, death) over 30-year follow-up (Hodgins et al. 2009). These studies show how adolescent-onset SUD can delay or disrupt the achievement of adolescent developmental milestones, with effects that persist into adulthood (Brown et al. 2008).

Predictors of SUD Course: Before, During, and After Treatment

The most robust pretreatment characteristics that have been associated with more persistent trajectories of substance involvement include temperament and co-occurring psychopathology (discussed in more detail in a later subsection). During treatment, factors associated with better outcomes include longer duration of treatment, greater readiness to change substance use behavior, and family involvement in treatment (for review, see Buckheit et al. 2018). Research suggests that at least 3 months of treatment is associated with better substance use outcomes, and that posttreatment factors generally account for more of the variance in outcome over 1-year follow-up than factors before and during treatment (Buckheit et al. 2018). Treatment may help to initially increase an adolescent's motivation to reduce substance use; however, the posttreatment environment (e.g., family, peers) is essential to maintaining treatment gains. Posttreatment factors associated with better outcomes include aftercare involvement, low levels of peer substance use, family support, and continued commitment to abstain (Buckheit et al. 2018). Dynamic models of posttreatment change in substance use and environmental context need to be investigated, because the importance of a course predictor may change with the transition from adolescence to young adulthood (e.g., shift in the importance of family vs. peer influence).

Mechanisms Underlying Intervention Effects

In response to meta-analyses indicating that no particular brand of treatment performs better than another (Tanner-Smith et al. 2013) and that treated youth generally show initial gains that fade over time (Buckheit et al. 2018), there has been a shift away from studying treatment outcomes to investigating "how" treatment works. A systematic review identified four adolescent studies that examined substance use treatment mechanisms, and found that social support, motivation to abstain, and positive parenting behaviors mediated treatment effects (Black and Chung 2014). Specifically, two community studies examined mechanisms of action for 12-step facilitation, finding evidence for social support as a mechanism of effect in one study (Chi et al. 2009), and motivation for abstinence in the other (Kelly et al. 2000). Two clinical studies found support for parenting behavior as a mediator of intervention effects (Henderson et al. 2009; Winters et al. 2014). Overall, however, research to date provides more evidence for "common" than for therapy-specific mechanisms of change. The lack of support for therapy-specific mechanisms of change may be due to the need for greater precision in defining and assessing relevant treatment processes (Black and Chung 2014).

Co-occurring Psychopathology and SUD Course

Co-occurring psychopathology refers to two or more psychiatric conditions that may occur simultaneously or sequentially in an individual. Comorbid conditions, such as conduct problems and depression, may affect the timing of SUD onset and its rate of development, severity, and duration (Winters et al. 2018). The conditions most commonly associated with adolescent substance involvement are conduct problems, mood disorders (e.g., depression), attention-deficit/hyperactivity disorder, and physical or sexual trauma (Winters et al. 2018). A majority (~60%) of adolescent substance users in community-based studies and treatment samples are estimated to have a co-occurring mental illness (Winters et al. 2018).

Dual diagnosis programs for adolescent substance users are in high demand, since youth in substance use treatment often indicate a need for intervention that addresses co-occurring psychiatric conditions (Substance Abuse and Mental Health Services Administration 2018). Youth with co-occurring conditions may benefit from stepped goals or a harm reduction approach that is discussed in the context of the adolescent's overall treatment priorities and personal short- and long-term goals (Bagot and Kaminer 2018). (See Part IV: Chapters 17–21 for more details about co-occurring disorders.)

Conclusion

The use of a developmental framework to assess adolescent substance involvement recognizes the unique features of adolescence, such as continuing brain development and a normative increase in risk-taking behavior, that may influence levels of substance involvement and the types of substance-related problems most often experienced by youth. Although there has been some decline in the prevalence of adolescent substance use in the past decade, cause for concern still exists with regard to the narrowing gender gap in substance use, particularly during adolescence, and perceptions of decreasing risk of harm from cannabis use along with increasing state-level legalization of cannabis. Multiple trajectories of substance involvement have been identified, with most youth showing no to low levels of use, or developmentally limited patterns of substance use and related problems. Developmentally informed assessment of adolescent substance involvement is essential to understanding etiology as well as the factors influencing clinical course. For many youth referred to substance use treatment, treatment generally results in some reduction in substance use compared to preintervention levels. However, multiple episodes of treatment may be needed for some adolescents, and co-occurring psychopathology complicates the course of recovery from adolescent-onset SUD. Research indicates that treatment for substance use may initially increase adolescents' readiness to change substance use behavior, but family, peers, and the larger community play important roles in supporting and maintaining stable recovery for adolescent substance users.

Key Points

- A developmental framework for adolescent substance use assessment incorporates unique features of adolescence, such as the continuing maturation of the brain into young adulthood, a normative increase in risk-taking behavior, and the increasing importance of peer relationships.

- Initiation to substance use peaks at a time when the developing brain may be particularly vulnerable to the neurotoxic effects of heavy substance use, highlighting the importance of efforts to prevent substance use.

- In recent years, the gender gap in rates of substance involvement has narrowed, with females catching up to, or surpassing, males in rates of use for certain substances, such as tobacco.

- Children of substance-using parents are at risk for adverse mental health outcomes, but many show resilience, especially in the presence of protective factors.

- On average, adolescents tend to show a reduction in use following treatment, but posttreatment course is variable, and aftercare helps to maintain treatment gains.

References

American Psychiatric Association: Diagnostic and Statistical Manual of Mental Disorders, 4th Edition. Washington, DC, American Psychiatric Association, 1994

American Psychiatric Association: Diagnostic and Statistical Manual of Mental Disorders, 5th Edition. Arlington, VA, American Psychiatric Association, 2013

American Psychological Association: The Road to Resilience. Washington, DC, American Psychological Association, 2014

Anderson KG, Ramo DE, Cummins KM, et al: Alcohol and drug involvement after adolescent treatment and functioning during emerging adulthood. Drug Alcohol Depend 107(2-3):171–181, 2010 19926231

Bagot K, Kaminer Y: Harm reduction for youth in treatment for substance use disorders: One size does not fit all. Current Addiction Reports 5(3):379–385, 2018

Black JJ, Chung T: Mechanisms of change in adolescent substance use treatment: how does treatment work? Subst Abus 35(4):344–351, 2014 24901750

Brown SA, McGue M, Maggs J, et al: A developmental perspective on alcohol and youths 16 to 20 years of age. Pediatrics 121 (suppl 4):S290–S310, 2008 18381495

Buckheit KA, Moskal D, Spinola S, et al: Clinical course and relapse among adolescents presenting for treatment of substance use risorders: recent findings. Current Addiction Reports 5(2):174–191, 2018

Calabria B, Degenhardt L, Briegleb C, et al: Systematic review of prospective studies investigating "remission" from amphetamine, cannabis, cocaine or opioid dependence. Addict Behav 35(8):741–749, 2010 20444552

Center for Behavioral Health Statistics and Quality: 2016 National Survey on Drug Use and Health: Detailed Tables. Rockville, MD, Center for Behavioral Health Statistics and Quality, Substance Abuse and Mental Health Services Administration, 2017

Chi FW, Kaskutas LA, Sterling S, et al: Twelve-step affiliation and 3-year substance use outcomes among adolescents: social support and religious service attendance as potential mediators. Addiction 104(6):927–939, 2009 19344442

Chung T, Martin CS, Armstrong TD, et al: Prevalence of DSM-IV alcohol diagnoses and symptoms in adolescent community and clinical samples. J Am Acad Child Adolesc Psychiatry 41(5):546–554, 2002 12014787

Chung T, Martin CS, Clark DB: Concurrent change in alcohol and drug problems among treated adolescents over three years. J Stud Alcohol Drugs 69(3):420–429, 2008 18432385

Chung T, Cornelius J, Clark D, et al: Greater prevalence of proposed ICD-11 alcohol and cannabis dependence compared to ICD-10, DSM-IV, and DSM-5 in treated adolescents. Alcohol Clin Exp Res 41(9):1584–1592, 2017 28667763

Cuthbert BN, Insel TR: Toward the future of psychiatric diagnosis: the seven pillars of RDoC. BMC Med 11:126, 2013 23672542

Degenhardt L, Stockings E, Patton G, et al: The increasing global health priority of substance use in young people. Lancet Psychiatry 3(3):251–264, 2016 26905480

Farmer RF, Kosty DB, Seeley JR, et al: Natural course of cannabis use disorders. Psychol Med 45(1):63–72, 2015 25066537

Hall GCN, Ibaraki AY, Huang ER, et al: A meta-analysis of cultural adaptations of psychological interventions. Behav Ther 47(6):993–1014, 2016 27993346

Hall WD, Patton G, Stockings E, et al: Why young people's substance use matters for global health. Lancet Psychiatry 3(3):265–279, 2016 26905482

Henderson CE, Rowe CL, Dakof GA, et al: Parenting practices as mediators of treatment effects in an early-intervention trial of multidimensional family therapy. Am J Drug Alcohol Abuse 35(4):220–226, 2009 20180674

Hodgins S, Larm P, Molero-Samuleson Y, et al: Multiple adverse outcomes over 30 years following adolescent substance misuse treatment. Acta Psychiatr Scand 119(6):484–493, 2009 19207133

Hogue A, Henderson CE, Becker SJ, et al: Evidence base on outpatient behavioral treatments for adolescent substance use, 2014-2017: outcomes, treatment delivery, and promising horizons. J Clin Child Adolesc Psychol 47(4):499–526, 2018 29893607

Jackson KM, Sartor CE: The natural course of substance use and dependence, in The Oxford Handbook of Substance Use Disorders. Edited by Sher K. New York, Oxford University Press, 2014, pp 67–131

Kaminer Y, Winters KC: DSM-5 criteria for youth substance use disorders: lost in translation? J Am Acad Child Adolesc Psychiatry 54(5):350–351, 2015 25901770

Kelly JF, Myers MG, Brown SA: A multivariate process model of adolescent 12-step attendance and substance use outcome following inpatient treatment. Psychol Addict Behav 14(4):376–389, 2000 11130156

Lipari RN, Van Horn SL: Children Living With Parents Who Have a Substance Use Disorder. Rockville, MD, Center for Behavioral Health Statistics and Quality, Substance Abuse and Mental Health Services Administration, 2017

Lisdahl KM, Shollenbarger S, Sagar KA, et al: The neurocognitive impact of alcohol and marijuana use on the developing adolescent and young adult brain, in Brief Interventions for Adolescent Alcohol and Substance Abuse. Edited by Monti PM, Colby SM, O'Leary Tevyaw T. New York, Guilford, 2018, pp 50–82

Luna B, Paulsen DJ, Padmanabhan A, Geier C: Cognitive control and motivation. Curr Dir Psychol Sci 22(2):94–100, 2013 25574074

Miech RA, Johnston LD, O'Malley PM, et al: Monitoring the Future: National Survey Results on Drug Use, 1975–2016: Volume I, Secondary School Students. Ann Arbor, MI, Institute for Social Research, The University of Michigan, 2017

Miech RA, Johnston LD, O'Malley PM, et al: Monitoring the Future: National Survey Results on Drug Use, 1975–2017: Volume I, Secondary School Students. Ann Arbor, MI, Institute for Social Research, The University of Michigan, 2018

Morin JG, Afzali MH, Bourque J, et al: A population-based analysis of the relationship between substance use and adolescent cognitive development. Am J Psychiatry 176(2):98–106, 2019 30278790

National Institute on Drug Abuse: Principles of Adolescent Substance Use Disorder Treatment: A Research-Based Guide (NIH Publ No 14-7953). Bethesda, MD, National Institute on Drug Abuse, 2014

Nelson SE, Van Ryzin MJ, Dishion TJ: Alcohol, marijuana, and tobacco use trajectories from age 12 to 24 years: demographic correlates and young adult substance use problems. Dev Psychopathol 27(1):253–277, 2015 25017089

Ramo DE, Brown SA: Classes of substance abuse relapse situations: a comparison of adolescents and adults. Psychol Addict Behav 22(3):372–379, 2008 18778130

Solis JM, Shadur JM, Burns AR, et al: Understanding the diverse needs of children whose parents abuse substances. Curr Drug Abuse Rev 5(2):135–147, 2012 22455509

Substance Abuse and Mental Health Services Administration: Treatment Episode Data Set (TEDS): 2016 Admissions to and Discharges From Publicly Funded Substance Use Treatment. Rockville, MD, Substance Abuse and Mental Health Services Administration, Center for Behavioral Health Statistics and Quality, 2018

Swift W, Coffey C, Carlin JB, et al: Adolescent cannabis users at 24 years: trajectories to regular weekly use and dependence in young adulthood. Addiction 103(8):1361–1370, 2008 18855826

Tanner-Smith EE, Wilson SJ, Lipsey MW: The comparative effectiveness of outpatient treatment for adolescent substance abuse: a meta-analysis. J Subst Abuse Treat 44(2):145–158, 2013 22763198

Winters KC, Lee S, Botzet A, et al: One-year outcomes and mediators of a brief intervention for drug abusing adolescents. Psychol Addict Behav 28(2):464–474, 2014 24955669

Winters KC, Botzet A, Lee S: Assessing adolescent substance use problems and other areas of functioning: state of the art, in Brief Interventions for Adolescent Alcohol and Substance Abuse. Edited by Monti PM, Colby SM, O'Leary Tevyaw T. New York, Guilford, 2018, pp 83–107

Wlodarczyk O, Schwarze M, Rumpf HJ, et al: Protective mental health factors in children of parents with alcohol and drug use disorders: a systematic review. PLoS One 12(6):e0179140, 2017 28609440

Zucker RA, Hicks B, Heitzeg M: Alcohol use and the alcohol use disorders over the life course: a cross-level developmental review, in Developmental Psychopathology. Edited by Cicchetti D. New York, Wiley, 2016, pp 1–40

2

Prevention of Substance Use and Substance Use Disorders

Lawrence M. Scheier, Ph.D.

Richard Catalano, Ph.D.

Ken C. Winters, Ph.D.

Although most young people who initiate the use of alcohol and other drugs (including tobacco) do not go on to develop a substance use disorder (SUD) (Lisdahl et al. 2018), the risk of developing a serious problem is greatly increased if drug use begins during adolescence (National Institute on Drug Abuse 2014). For example, adolescents that initiate substance use before age 14 years are at a significantly elevated risk to develop a SUD later in adolescence (Winters and Lee 2008) and have a 34% prevalence rate of a lifetime SUD (Substance Abuse and Mental Health Services Administration 2015). Yet delaying the onset of use can dramatically alter a youth's future risk; as a young person matures between 13 and 21 years, the likelihood of a lifetime

25

SUD drops approximately 4%–5% for each year that initiation of substance use is delayed (Substance Abuse and Mental Health Services Administration 2015). In this chapter, to facilitate a better understanding of the nature of vulnerability to drug use, we summarize individual and environmental risk and protective factors that place adolescents at risk for or protect them from initiating and maintaining drug use (National Research Council and Institute of Medicine 2009). We then provide an overview of evidence-based prevention approaches and discuss various challenges associated with implementing drug prevention programs as communities and schools seek to "scale up" a program and move it from "bench to trench."

Nature and Extent of the Problem

Preventing alcohol, tobacco, and other drug use among adolescents is a national priority (National Research Council and Institute of Medicine 2009). The estimated annual cost of abuse and dependence to U.S. society, including health care, law enforcement, crime, social, economic, and other costs, exceeds $530 billion (National Institute on Drug Abuse 2014). Although we cannot be certain who among those adolescents who try alcohol or other drugs or tobacco will develop a drug problem, longitudinal developmental studies that monitor the progression of drug use over time have identified a number of individual-level and environmental factors that are significantly associated with a higher likelihood of progressing from early experimental levels of drug use to a SUD. However, even with this knowledge, there is no silver bullet—or one causal factor that, if changed, would stop progression to a drug problem. There are many sources of increased risk, and many avenues lead to acquisition of substance abuse problems.

Background of Prevention Efforts

Very early efforts to prevent substance use and resulting consequences were largely ineffective, and both reviews and meta-analyses underscored the lack of rigorous evaluations. Thus, in the 1980s, when many drug prevention programs first became available, it was not clear whether substance abuse could be effectively prevented. In response, a number of prevention scholars advocated taking a public health approach (Catalano et al. 1998; DuPont et al. 2018).

The public health framework suggests that if you want to prevent a problem before it happens, you have to change the etiological factors associated with initiation and onset of drug use. In part as a response to the ineffectiveness of prevention efforts at the time, prevention researchers began to increasingly explore through longitudinal developmental studies the predictors of early stages of adolescent substance involvement. Through increasing investment in research, a set of longitudinal predictors of substance use—often called *risk factors* and *protective factors*—were identified at the individual, family, school, peer group, and community levels. The findings of this research began to be summarized in the 1980s and 1990s (National Research Council and Institute of Medicine 2009), and public health approaches were developed and tested using longitudinal research methods, leading eventually to the development of a wide range of effective prevention approaches (Hawkins et al. 2008).

Role of Risk and Protective Factors

Risk factors are those predictors associated with an increased likelihood of substance use and/or abuse or other behavioral disorders (National Research Council and Institute of Medicine 2009). Risk factors can encompass individual-level measures (e.g., genetic predisposition, personality, risk taking) and also the environments in which youth are socialized, including in the family (e.g., family conflict), at school (e.g., school failure), in peer group (e.g., friends who use), and in the community (e.g., neighborhood distress and availability of alcohol and drugs). Many risk factors for substance abuse are etiological risk factors for other problems, including delinquency, violence, teen pregnancy, dropping out of school, depression, and acting out and related behavior problems. Table 2–1 illustrates the predictive relationship between various risk factors and different types of problem behaviors. A check at the intersection of a row and column means there have been at least two longitudinal studies demonstrating that a particular risk factor predicts the specific health and behavior problems. As can be seen in the table, many of the same risk factors predict multiple problems. For example, the risk factor of "low neighborhood attachment and community disorganization" has been shown to predict youth substance abuse, delinquency, and violence. Because they predict future problem behaviors, malleable risk factors are potential targets for preventive action. Changing the risk factor of low neighborhood attachment and community disorganization has the potential to ameliorate all three undesirable outcomes.

Risk Factors

For many youth, the accumulation of risk begins early in childhood as they face numerous developmental challenges that without any offsetting protective influences become exacerbated as the youth are exposed to new environments (e.g., school and peers). This has been referred to as a "snowball" pattern of risk (Mitchell et al. 2001) to denote the rolling accumulation of risk. A variant of this pattern of risk develops when adolescents are exposed to risk by, for instance, affiliating with drug-using friends. Over time, continued exposure to peers through socialization and selection (different forms of risk), in the absence of any protective influences, can increase vulnerability to an accumulation (i.e., "snowstorm") of other risk factors (Toumbourou and Catalano 2005). Thus, for example, selection of drug-abusing friends might also be exacerbated by deviant attitudes and by opportunities for risky behavior that occur when socializing with drug-abusing friends. Below we provide brief descriptors of risk factors within four highly relevant domains: community, family, school, and individual.

Community Factors

Multiple factors at the community level have been associated with substance use and abuse. Perceived or actual availability of drugs, high levels of residential mobility, community laws or norms favorable to drug use, and community disorganization and low neighborhood attachment (i.e., cohesion among residents) are all associated with substance use (Beyers et al. 2004).

Family Factors

There is substantial evidence that children of alcoholics or addicts are at greater risk of developing abuse and dependence (see, e.g., Kendler et al. 2014). Some portion of this risk may be genetic, while a portion may reflect intergenerational transmission of poor coping skills, mental health problems, and family dysfunction (Prom-Wormley et al. 2014). There is also evidence that vulnerability to drug use is generalized across substances in adolescence (Young et al. 2006), and the developmental progression from initial experimentation through regular use to a SUD appears to be accompanied by a de-

Table 2–1. Risk factors for adolescent problem behaviors

Risk factors	Substance abuse	Delinquency	Teen pregnancy	School dropout	Violence	Depression and anxiety
Community						
Availability of drugs	✓				✓	
Availability of firearms		✓			✓	
Community laws and norms favorable toward drug use, firearms, and crime	✓	✓			✓	
Media portrayals of violence	✓				✓	
Transitions and mobility	✓	✓		✓		✓
Low neighborhood attachment and community disorganization	✓	✓			✓	
Extreme economic deprivation	✓	✓	✓	✓	✓	
Family						
Family history of the problem behavior	✓	✓	✓	✓	✓	✓
Family management problems	✓	✓	✓	✓	✓	✓

Table 2–1.   Risk factors for adolescent problem behaviors *(continued)*

Risk factors	Substance abuse	Delinquency	Teen pregnancy	School dropout	Violence	Depression and anxiety
Family *(continued)*						
Family conflict	✓	✓	✓	✓	✓	✓
Favorable parental attitudes and involvement in the problem behavior	✓	✓			✓	
School						
Academic failure beginning in late elementary school	✓	✓	✓	✓	✓	✓
Lack of commitment to school	✓	✓	✓	✓	✓	
Individual/peers						
Early and persistent antisocial behavior	✓	✓	✓	✓	✓	✓
Alienation and rebelliousness	✓	✓		✓		
Friends who engage in the problem behavior	✓	✓	✓	✓	✓	
Favorable attitudes toward the problem behavior	✓	✓	✓	✓		
Early initiation of the problem behavior	✓	✓	✓	✓	✓	
Constitutional factors	✓	✓			✓	✓

crease in the influence of shared environmental factors (family, peers) and a corresponding increase in the role of genetic and unique environmental vulnerability (Pagan et al. 2006).

Poor family management practices that elevate risk for substance use and problem behavior include parents' failure to set clear expectations for children's behavior; failure to supervise and monitor children; and excessively severe, harsh, or inconsistent punishment (Scheier and Hansen 2014). Children exposed to such poor family management practices are at increased risk for substance abuse and other problem behaviors (Brewer et al. 1995). Also, children who grow up exposed to high levels of family conflict— between their parents (i.e., marital distress) or between parent and child—are more likely to engage in drug use and exhibit problem behaviors than children raised in more harmonious families (National Research Council and Institute of Medicine 2009). In these instances, drug use may represent a form of coping with stress or finding ways to reduce anxiety that arises from feeling neglected by family members as well as being exposed to high levels of hostility among family members that can interfere with the acquisition of appropriate social-emotional regulation skills (Prom-Wormley et al. 2014). Parental attitudes favorable to drug use also play an important role in determining adolescent drug abuse (Peterson et al. 1994). This includes parental approval of drinking and drug use (National Research Council and Institute of Medicine 2009). Parents who tolerate deviance in the form of rebellious children, and who fail to monitor their activities (i.e., know where they are after school and know their playmates), tacitly support their children to violate norms and commit rules transgressions through permissive or inattentive parenting strategies.

School Factors

Academic failure increases the risk of later substance use as well as other problem behaviors (Centers for Disease Control and Prevention 2009). Young people experience school failure for a combination of reasons: they may lack stimulating teachers; they may have learning problems; they may feel neglected by their peers, have few friends, and withdraw from school; or they may experience low commitment to school. Low commitment to school often arises when youth no longer see the role of student as meaningful and rewarding. In many cases, students lack investment in learning; either they feel school is unsafe or they lack prosocial peer bonds and do not experience supportive encouragement from teachers and staff (Gottfredson and Gottfredson 2002; Karlamangla et al. 2006).

Individual and Peer Factors

Factors at the individual level include the individual's temperament, social preferences, and perceptions of harm associated with drug use. The greater the variety, frequency, and seriousness of antisocial behavior in childhood (Englund et al. 2008), as well as tolerance for deviance (e.g., Zucker 2008), the greater the likelihood for future substance abuse. Also, peer use of substances is a consistent predictor of substance use among youth (National Research Council and Institute of Medicine 2009).

Studies of peer influence on drug use have demonstrated that involvement with antisocial peers is a strong predictor of tobacco, alcohol, and other drug use, as well as criminality and risky sexual behavior (e.g., Oxford et al. 2001). The influence of peers perhaps captures a form of interactive continuity, in which deviant youth seek friendships that support their personality and behaviors. In addition, there is some evidence that peer influence may be moderated by youth perceptions of peers' attitudes toward academic achievement (Bryant and Zimmerman 2002).

Additional individual factors include favorable attitude toward substance use (Lipari et al. 2017; Spoth et al. 2008); disinhibitory traits (sensation seeking, low harm avoidance, risk taking, impulsivity, poor inhibitory control) (Byrne and Worthy 2019; King and Chassin 2008); low academic motivation and poor self-esteem (Scheier 2001); and onset of substance use during early adolescence (Zucker 2008).

Protective Factors

Protection is afforded to youth exposed to fewer risk factors and also occurs when specific developmental factors operate to buffer the effect of risk and reduce the likelihood of drug use (Dryfoos 1990). *Promotive factors* are etiological processes that have a direct negative relationship with substance use and abuse.

Social, Emotional, and Cognitive Competence

Competence encompasses a range of interpersonal skills that help youth integrate feelings, thinking, and actions to achieve specific social and interpersonal goals (Masten 2001). These skills include encoding relevant social cues, accurately interpreting those cues, generating effective solutions to interpersonal problems, making decisions, realistically anticipating consequences and potential obstacles to one's actions, and translating social decisions into effective behaviors (Consortium on the School-Based Promotion of Social Competence 1994). Randomized controlled drug prevention trials have demonstrated that enhancing competence (e.g., decision making, problem solving, self-management and anxiety reduction skills) protects youth from drug use (Botvin and Griffin 2004). Included in this domain is high intelligence; it may be that such youth have high-level social and emotional competence and are more able to take advantage of an enriched environment and to cope with high-risk situations and environments (Hawkins et al. 1992).

Resilient Temperament

Resilience represents an individual's adaptive capacity to manage change and stressful events in healthy and flexible ways. Resilience has been empirically identified as a characteristic of youth who when exposed to multiple risk factors or grow up facing adversity show successful responses to challenge. These youth are, in essence, able to transform adversity and find ways from what they have learned to achieve successful outcomes (Masten 2001). Pathways to substance abuse can often be traced back to the earliest years of life. For example, Williams and colleagues (2000) noted that a positive, sociable, and flexible temperament in early infancy and early childhood offered protection against later adolescent substance abuse. Wills and Ainette (2010) provide a comprehensive review of the temperament and drug use literatures.

Opportunities for and Recognition of Positive and Prosocial Experiences

Children who have developmentally appropriate opportunities to be meaningfully involved with the family, school, or community are less likely to develop problems (Darling and Steinberg 1993). For a child to acquire key interpersonal skills in early development, positive opportunities must be available (National Research Council and Institute of Medicine 2009). It is especially important for adolescents to interact with positively oriented peers and to be involved in roles in which they can make a contribution to their group, whether family, school, neighborhood, peer group, or larger community (Dryfoos 1990). Also, parents, teachers, and peers who provide recognition to the teenager for exhibiting skillful behavior and making healthy decisions can motivate the teenager to achieve prosocial goals (Guo et al. 2001). Various theories can be used to explain how association with prosocial figures produces conventional behavior, but the simplest learning explanation is that youth identify with and "introject" the values of the prosocial role models and benefit from this process through valued reward structures (e.g., parents reward their children for valued behavior).

Evidence-Based Programs

The 1980s witnessed a new generation of experimental studies evaluating drug prevention programs. This involved a slate of experimental studies that strategically focused on modifying predictors of a single problem, like substance use. These studies met with a modicum of success; however, they spawned discussion regarding the focus of prevention and whether it was best to focus on a single outcome (i.e., drug use), when youth engaged in many delinquent activities, with some using drugs and others engaging in related high-risk behaviors. Eventually, lively discussions among scientists, practitioners, and policy makers increasingly converged along a set of refined critiques and recommendations. Their recommendations suggested that prevention science should provide the research base supporting a focus on the intersection of the individual and his or her environment, and that, furthermore, these approaches should address the whole child and not be focused on a single problem behavior, with an emphasis on reducing developmentally salient risk and enhancing protective factors.

Randomized controlled trials conducted since the mid-1980s have demonstrated that a range of effective prevention approaches can reduce risk, increase protection, and reduce problem behaviors (National Research Council and Institute of Medicine 2009). Information detailing the various strategies underlying these programs is available at the website for the Campbell Collaboration (www.campbellcollaboration.org). We briefly review several of these programs and provide examples of their active ingredients and intervention modalities. However, we caution that the effectiveness of these programs will vary depending on numerous implementation factors, including their settings, compliance with study protocols (fidelity), and other factors (e.g., student receptivity, organizational climate) that influence program efficacy when implemented on a large-scale basis across communities.

School-Based Programs

School-based prevention approaches typically involve primary or "universal" prevention approaches that emphasize providing social and personal skills to all students in attendance regardless of their levels of risk. This should arguably provide the biggest bang for the dollar, as both low- and high-risk students present in school are exposed to the intervention. The intervention strategies include teaching social and assertiveness skills to help youth resist negative peer influences (e.g., offers to use drugs), and providing decision-making, self-management, and problem-solving skills to help them navigate the trials and tribulations of adolescent development. The same programs include teaching youth different ways to detect media influences that promote cigarette or alcohol use as well as providing normative education to help correct misperceptions regarding the social acceptability of drug use and also dispel the perceived benefits of drug use (Botvin and Griffin 2004). Additional programs emphasize enhancing instructional and classroom management skills and include classroom curricula to promote social, emotional and cognitive competence (Ialongo et al. 1999). There is also evidence that programs focusing on improving academic performance, increasing bonding to school, and reducing classroom management problems as early as elementary school produce reductions in early forms of aggressiveness including acting out, disruption, minor delinquency, and conduct problems later in life (Kellam and Anthony 1998).

Conrod (2016) tested a school-based program that is tailored based on an assessment of the student's personality risk. Self-reports were obtained from each student assessing their levels of hopelessness, anxiety-sensitivity, impulsivity, and sensation seeking, and this evaluation was used to assign students to an appropriate experimental condition. Compared with the control groups (no-intervention or a two-session group coping skills intervention targeting one of the four personality risk factors), the group in the tailored program had significantly lower drinking behaviors at 6-month follow-up, and some favorable effects were also apparent at 12 and 24 months postintervention. A replication study produced similar findings with a larger sample (Conrod 2016). Personality-tailored preventive interventions are a promising approach, one that is likely to have a significant presence in future applications of prevention research (Conrod 2016).

School-based brief selective interventions are an emerging trend to address students with substance use problems that are not yet severe (e.g., do not meet criteria for moderate to severe substance use disorder). Examples of evidence-based programs include brief strategic family therapy (Waldron and Turner 2008), MET/CBT5 (Godley et al. 2001), and Teen Intervene (Winters et al. 2012).

Parenting Programs

Programs that take a family-based or parenting-skills approach show significant though modest effects (Kelly and Connor 2012). Family-based prevention programs that emphasize malleable risk and protective factors, including boundaries, monitoring the adolescent's behaviors, frequent and effective parent-child communication, and attending to related family dynamics, produce long-term effects not only on substance abuse and dependence but on other problem behaviors as well (Kumpfer et al. 2018; Winters et al. 2014).

For example, the Nurse-Family Partnership program works with young, childless, single mothers during their first pregnancy until their child is 2 years old. The program focuses on teaching these mothers how to provide nurturing and supportive environments for their children and how to interact with their children in a way that promotes social and emotional competence (Olds et al. 1998). Another example is Guiding Good Choices (Hawkins and Catalano 1988). This five-session, 2-hour parent training program provides practical information for parents about the risks for and dangers of early initiation of substance use, and emphasizes a) creating opportunities for involvement and interaction in the family and rewarding children's participation in the family; b) establishing clear family rules about substance use, monitoring the behavior of children, and using consistent moderate discipline; c) teaching children skills needed to resist peer influences to use drugs; and d) reducing and managing family conflict (Hawkins and Catalano 1988). There is now considerable evidence for long-term effects of this program (Park et al. 2000).

Community Programs

Community-based prevention programs take a social systemic approach to prevention. Such programs bring together diverse stakeholders, and potentially combine human and financial resources, for more effective and sustainable community-based preventive efforts (see, e.g., Pentz et al. 2006). Communities That Care (CTC) is one of several exemplary community–based prevention programs. The program provides education and tools for community decision making in order to organize, assess, and prioritize prevention needs; match efficacious programs to prioritized needs; and provide training and technical assistance for implementing evidence-based programs with fidelity. Randomized control trials of CTC (involving 24 communities in the United States) that have followed students beginning at age 10 to 13 years showed reductions in the initiation of delinquency and alcohol use (past 30 days) during adolescence and durable program effects lasting into early adulthood (Hawkins et al. 2008; Oesterle et al. 2018). Reductions in cannabis use were not observed; however, the age of the CTC sample at follow-up was younger than the age at which cannabis use typically escalates among U.S. youth (16–17 years).

Environmental Strategies

Community-wide policies that seek to reduce supply (e.g., minimizing exposure to drugs and drug-using networks) and to change norms can also have a positive impact. For example, policies to restrict availability of tobacco to young people have resulted in decreased cigarette smoking among youth (Forster et al. 1998). Also, community-wide policy changes to reduce availability of alcohol to youth, including increasing the drinking age and restricting how alcohol is sold (Nelson et al. 2013), have decreased consumption and the frequency of alcohol-related traffic accidents and fatalities. Other examples include legislating a higher minimum age at which one may legally buy alcohol or cigarettes and modifying zoning ordinances that allow high density of liquor outlets in a neighborhood. For example, one law that has had a profound effect on alcohol-related mortality is raising the legal drinking age to 21. The research evidence supports that a legal drinking age of 21 years is associated with decreased alcohol-related motor vehicle fatalities (see Wagenaar and Toomey 2002 for review). On the other hand, more permissive laws that allow greater accessibility to alcohol or drugs are associated with increased use. For example, the recent changes in marijuana legislation, both legalizing and decriminalizing the drug in the United States, are associated with increased use of marijuana by adolescents and young adults (Johnston et al. 2018).

The media is also a tremendous influence in early-stage drug use. The intense attachment to social media by youth may be a risk factor for substance use. For example, alcohol-related Facebook activity (e.g., alcohol depictions by written postings or photos and images) was shown to be associated with binge drinking among college students (Marczinski et al. 2016), and the use of social media in general may promote binge drinking (Ceballos et al. 2018). Yet this intense attachment to social media by youth may itself provide an effective avenue for intervention (see Chapter 16 for further discussion).

Implementation of Prevention Programs

No matter how well conceived a drug prevention program, its efficacy hinges on the program being implemented well and with great care. Implementation addresses the issue of "the scientific study of methods to promote the systematic uptake of research findings and other evidence-based practices into routine practice, and, hence, to improve the quality and effectiveness of health services" (Eccles and Mittman 2006, p. 1). Regardless of venue (clinic, school, health care center, or service provider agency), the implementation process commences by introducing decision makers and key stakeholders to the basic concepts of a behavior change strategy. This process usually involves a presentation by the program developer's staff followed by an internal discussion among potential adopters. The discussion emphasizes the appropriateness of a specific program, whether there is sufficient empirical evidence supporting its use, economic factors that may come into play (cost and potential loss of economic productivity from down staff time during training), ease of implementation, and whether there are sufficient staff resources to shoulder the burden associated with implementation. Also, the agency (school or clinic) will want to know whether the program has long-term public health implications and whether it will address the needs of their population in a timely fashion. In short, practitioners have to feel that the program is desirable, compatible with their needs, cost-efficient, and easy to use and does not place too great a demand on their resources. It is this uptake of an "off the shelf" program that is the focus of implementation, and the entirety of the process is sometimes called "diffusion" or "technology transfer."

Organizations intent on implementing a behavior change program usually commence with an "in-service" training that targets practitioners (e.g., teachers or health educators) to optimize program delivery. As part of their training, staff work closely with the program developers to learn about factors that will boost fidelity (e.g., limiting adaptations). Practitioners should be knowledgeable about the theoretical framework that guides the intervention, its rationale, and the extent of its effectiveness. They must also have confidence they can efficaciously implement the program using the appropriate interactive techniques demonstrated to them during training. Fidelity to the core principles must be explained with an understanding that adherence to the lessons (structure and length) and quality teaching practices (interactive techniques) play a crucial role in program implementation and the success of the program on student outcomes.

Coaching has been shown to be fruitful in classroom-based interventions, including drug prevention programs (Ringwalt et al. 2009). Coaching helps to overcome certain barriers, which can include inadequate training and poor institutional support. Some drug prevention programs require the use of innovative interactive teaching strategies, a skill over which some implementers may show relatively little mastery. In a 3-year study of the All Stars prevention program, a drug prevention curriculum, Ringwalt and colleagues (2009) reported that students in classrooms with coached teachers reported lower rates of cigarette escalation (from non-use to use) compared with students exposed to the prevention curriculum delivered by noncoached teachers.

Other factors also come into play, including the program's sustainability and whether there is appropriate institutional buy-in to maintain the program beyond the initial thrust (i.e., continued financial support, dedication of personnel resources, a stable champion to reinforce buy-in, and related organizational climate factors that influence program institutionalization). Although many educators consider health promotion programs "extraneous to the core business of schools" (Bond et al. 2001), these efforts bear heavily on program sustainability from the point of adoption moving forward (Scheirer 2005).

Fidelity

Practitioners must implement a program as it was designed without deviations in delivery format or content. At its heart, fidelity consists of adherence, quality of delivery, and participant responsiveness (Dane and Schneider 1998). Programs characterized by high fidelity achieve better program outcomes (see, e.g., Flannery et al. 2014). Process evaluations can be used to assess program fidelity by gathering independent observational data (e.g., coding students and teachers during a live session), videotaping, completing provider-prepared checklists that determine coverage and levels of enthusiasm, and garnering feedback from those receiving and delivering the prevention program. Youth feedback is a crucial part of this process and can reveal their level of engagement in the program, whether they found the instructional methods and program content intriguing and also developmentally appropriate. Recent evidence reinforces the instrumental role in program outcomes played by student engagement (Hansen et al. 2019). There is also a growing literature documenting that teachers' attitudes toward the prevention program, reflecting their enthusiasm, support, and willingness to apply newly acquired instructional strategies, influence program outcomes (Aarons 2005). Practitioners must feel "motivated and inspired" to readily adopt a new innovation and believe that youth will benefit from the training, so they have added impetus to teach to the curriculum. Rohrbach et al. (2007) showed that trained and highly motivated teachers maintained adherence in program delivery and produced the same student outcomes in a drug prevention program that program specialists did.

School Fidelity

School-level factors may also influence fidelity and determine in part program outcomes. Key school-level factors that have been shown to influence program outcomes are leadership or the administration's voice to support the program (Kam et al. 2003), organizational readiness to maintain implementation at all costs (Beets et al. 2008), and quality of providers (Payne and Eckert 2010) and provider training (Hanley et al. 2009).

Adaptation

Frequently, practitioners waver in their fidelity and make modifications to both content and delivery format (Ringwalt et al. 2004). Indeed, there is never 100% compliance in real-world settings given the individualism associated with classroom-based teaching. No two teachers are alike in their delivery or even their expectation of student behavior. Some argue that flexibility should be built into implementation to ensure overall "fit" to the target population (Cohen et al. 2008). The demand for flexibility hinges partly on the need to modify the program delivery to address local needs of the population, emergent or otherwise. The absence of flexibility can produce dissent among practitioners responsible for the program's delivery or diminish enthusiasm among the target population who feel that with rigid adherence to a program their needs are not being met. In many cases practitioners feel they have their finger on the pulse of the participants because of their familiarity with them (working with the clientele day-to-day), and they institute changes to make the program more responsive to the target population. A teacher, for instance, can make subtle changes to the prescribed order of a program (i.e., sequence of intervention modules), incorporate personal anecdotes, utilize local community news to support relevant topics, or vary instructional modalities to teach a particular lesson. While all of these examples are well intentioned, they may go against the grain of the intervention, reducing the time on task and effectively leaving youth with less exposure to the core competencies contained in the curriculum.

There is considerable debate revolving around the latitude that is required for adaptation, particularly as it attends to "cultural adaptations." Resnicow et al. (2000) introduced the concept of "surface" versus "deep" structure changes to bring attention to the different levels of adaptation that can be instituted. Surface structure changes refer to food choices, cultural myths, mores, customs, and beliefs. Deep structure changes, on the other hand, refer to the core competencies and active ingredients of a program, which are by necessity tied to psychological factors that may in and of themselves reflect social, environmental and cultural influences. Most program developers are reluctant to allow deep structure changes because core competencies are theoretically tied to the program's rationale and active ingredients. There are, however, very good examples of where cultural adaptation to maintain relevance has worked favorably. The keepin' it REAL program is culturally grounded, with videotape materials for the curriculum created by Hispanic youth (Colby et al. 2013). Today, the program has achieved national dissemination as a part of the D.A.R.E. initiative (Day et al. 2017).

Future of Prevention Efforts

Despite their availability and federal government impetus to use evidence-based drug prevention programs, there are relatively low rates of adoption nationwide. One factor undermining the success of school-based interventions, according to Fixen et al. (2009), is the instrumental role played by practitioners (e.g., schoolteachers, health educators), who are the "intervention agent" and who function within unique systems that influence program outcomes. The plethora of moving parts and deviations introduced into each system produces an incredible volume of implementation differences, all veritably uncontrollable from an experimental point of view.

Perhaps a key piece toward improving adoption of evidence-based programs is to better understand if the actual methods used to teach drug prevention are developmentally sound and engaging to the students. Consider, for example, that role-plays are a formidable part of the interactive nature of drug prevention. Meta-analyses suggest that programs with interactive components produce better outcomes (Ennett et al. 2003; Tobler et al. 2000). However, the literature is rife with comparisons of the relative efficacy of core components (e.g., normative education vs. resistance training), rather than contrasting instructional methods (other than who delivers the program). Traditionally, meta-analyses coded "interactivity" dichotomously, indicating its presence or absence only, with no further dissection that could yield information on which instructional modality produced the largest effect. Moreover, the literature pays scant attention to whether youth enjoy role-plays, whether they like the curriculum and its delivery format, and to what extent they are receptive to the drug prevention messages (this is particularly noteworthy for media campaigns). Qualitative studies using formative evaluation techniques are an essential tool that can be used to help address this concern, but they are rarely applied (see, e.g., Boys et al. 1999).

There is little intersection between instructional methods for drug prevention and core subjects like math, English, or social sciences. Academic subjects rely heavily on rote memorization and finely tuned study habits. Drug prevention programs are more "experiential" and rely on cooperative learning involving candid discussion of family social interactions (boundaries, monitoring, and communication), peer influences and contexts that support deviant behavior, and application of critical thinking skills to achieve lifestyle congruence, to name just a few examples. The differences in teaching and learning strategies are best evidenced by the reliance in drug prevention on small group discussions and presentations accentuating relevant prevention themes, as well as competitive games that address normative misperception of drug use (e.g., Hansen 2015) or cognitive misperceptions and myths about drug use (e.g., Sussman 2015). The success of drug prevention programs should be measured in ways that demonstrate that students are learning new skills and are engaged in this learning process in an enthusiastic manner and that this combined instructional approach is reducing risk for maladaptive developmental outcomes.

This brings up the question whether alternative instructional technologies exist for teaching drug prevention. Using computer-mediated technology (i.e., personal computers or tablets accessing the Internet or smartphone and mobile devices) might reduce the stigma associated with having to discuss personal issues, family dynamics, and drug use in front of peers. These eHealth programs are self-paced, are accessible on demand, involve multimedia instructional technology, and capitalize on stealth learning principles. They also build on the principle of scaffolding, involving slow accretion of problem-solving skills, which is vital to student learning. A growing literature shows that many of the eHealth programs can achieve similar outcomes to classroom-based instructional programs, the latter of which are resource intensive and interfere with curricular instruction time (Champion et al. 2013). Overall, there has to be more work done to distinguish the relative merits of teaching and instructional strategies in drug prevention and more qualitative studies that are grounded in the lives of the target population.

Key Points

- Important prevention implications emerge from the research on risk and protection and the evaluation of prevention approaches.

- For maximum effect, prevention programs should address risk and protective factors early, for example, at the stage of development when the risk factor first emerges in the population, and they should address both individual and community-level factors.

- Numerous evidence-based preventive interventions are available to schools and communities.

- To optimize its effectiveness, a prevention program needs to be implemented by adhering to the basic principles of implementation fidelity, one of which centers on the need to administer the program as it was designed and closely deliver the intervention modalities.

- The challenge for prevention efforts in the early twenty-first century in the United States is to overcome the relatively low rates of adoption of widely available evidence-based drug prevention programs.

References

Aarons GA: Measuring provider attitudes toward evidence-based practice: consideration of organizational context and individual differences. Child Adolesc Psychiatr Clin N Am 14(2):255–271, viii, 2005 15694785

Beets MW, Flay BR, Vuchinich S, et al: School climate and teachers' beliefs and attitudes associated with implementation of the positive action program: a diffusion of innovations model. Prev Sci 9(4):264–275, 2008 18780182

Beyers JM, Toumbourou JW, Catalano RF, et al: A cross-national comparison of risk and protective factors for adolescent substance use: the United States and Australia. J Adolesc Health 35(1):3–16, 2004 15193569

Bond L, Glover S, Godfrey C, et al: Building capacity for system-level change in schools: lessons from the Gatehouse Project. Health Educ Behav 28(3):368–383, 2001 11380056

Botvin GJ, Griffin KW: Life skills training: Empirical findings and future directions. Journal of Primary Prevention 25(2):211–232, 2004

Boys A, Marsden J, Fountain J, et al: What influences young people's use of drugs? A qualitative study of decision-making. Drugs 6(3):373–387, 1999

Brewer DD, Hawkins JD, Catalano RF, et al: Preventing serious, violent, and chronic juvenile offending: a review of evaluations of selected strategies in childhood, adolescence, and the community, in A Sourcebook: Serious, Violent, and Chronic Juvenile Offenders. Edited by Howell JC, Krisberg B, Hawkins JD, et al. Thousand Oaks, CA, Sage, 1995, pp 61–141

Bryant AL, Zimmerman MA: Examining the effects of academic beliefs and behaviors on changes in substance use among urban adolescents. Journal of Educational Psychology 94(3):621–637, 2002

Byrne KA, Worthy DA: Examining the link between reward and response inhibition in individuals with substance abuse tendencies. Drug Alcohol Depend 194:518–525, 2019 30544087

Catalano RF, Arthur MW, Hawkins JD, et al: Comprehensive community and school-based interventions to prevent antisocial behavior, in Serious and Violent Juvenile Offenders: Risk Factors and Successful Interventions. Edited by Loeber R, Farrington DP. Thousand Oaks, CA, Sage, 1998, pp 248–283

Ceballos NA, Howard K, Dailey S, et al: Collegiate binge drinking and social media use among Hispanics and non-Hispanics. J Stud Alcohol Drugs 79(6):868–875, 2018 30573017

Centers for Disease Control and Prevention: Alcohol and other drug use and academic achievement. 2009. Available at: https://www.cdc.gov/healthyyouth/health_and_academics/pdf/alcohol_other_drug.pdf. Accessed April 24, 2019.

Champion KE, Newton NC, Barrett EL, et al: A systematic review of school-based alcohol and other drug prevention programs facilitated by computers or the Internet. Drug Alcohol Rev 32(2):115–123, 2013 23039085

Cohen DJ, Crabtree BF, Etz RS, et al: Fidelity versus flexibility: translating evidence-based research into practice. Am J Prev Med 35(5)(suppl):S381–S389, 2008 18929985

Colby M, Hecht ML, Miller-Day M, et al: Adapting school-based substance use prevention curriculum through cultural grounding: a review and exemplar of adaptation processes for rural schools. Am J Community Psychol 51(1–2):190–205, 2013 22961604

Conrod PJ: Personality-targeted interventions for substance use and misuse. Curr Addict Rep 3(4):426–436, 2016 27909645

Consortium on the School-Based Promotion of Social Competence: The school-based promotion of social competence: theory, research, practice, and policy, in Stress, Risk, and Resilience in Children and Adolescents: Processes, Mechanisms, and Interventions. Edited by Haggerty RJ, Sherrod LR, Garmezy N, et al. New York, Cambridge University Press, 1994, pp 268–316

Dane AV, Schneider BH: Program integrity in primary and early secondary prevention: are implementation effects out of control? Clin Psychol Rev 18(1):23–45, 1998 9455622

Darling N, Steinberg L: Parenting style as context: an integrative model. Psychological Bulletin 113(3):487–496, 1993

Day LE, Miller-Day M, Hecht ML, et al: Coming to the new D.A.R.E.: a preliminary test of the officer-taught elementary keepin' it REAL curriculum. Addict Behav 74:67–73, 2017 28595059

Dryfoos JG: Adolescents at Risk: Prevalence and Prevention. New York, Oxford University Press, 1990

DuPont RL, Han B, Shea CL, et al: Drug use among youth: national survey data support a common liability of all drug use. Prev Med 113:67–73, 2018 29758306

Eccles MP, Mittman BS: Welcome to Implementation Science. Implement Sci 1:1, 2006 1436009

Englund MM, Egeland B, Oliva EM, et al: Childhood and adolescent predictors of heavy drinking and alcohol use disorders in early adulthood: a longitudinal developmental analysis. Addiction 103 (suppl 1):23–35, 2008 18426538

Ennett ST, Ringwalt CL, Thorne J, et al: A comparison of current practice in school-based substance use prevention programs with meta-analysis findings. Prev Sci 4(1):1–14, 2003 12611415

Fixen DL, Blasé KA, Naoom SF, et al: Core implementation components. Research on Social Work and Practice 19(5):531–540, 2009

Flannery KB, Fenning P, Kato MM, et al: Effects of school-wide positive behavioral interventions and supports and fidelity of implementation on problem behavior in high schools. Sch Psychol Q 29(2):111–124, 2014 24188290

Forster JL, Murray DM, Wolfson M, et al: The effects of community policies to reduce youth access to tobacco. Am J Public Health 88(8):1193–1198, 1998 9702146

Godley SH, Meyers RJ, Smith JE, et al: The Adolescent Community Reinforcement Approach for Adolescent Cannabis Users: Cannabis Youth Treatment (CYT) Series, Vol 4 (DHHS Publ No 01-3489). Rockville, MD, Center for Substance Abuse Treatment, Substance Abuse and Mental Health Services Administration, 2001

Gottfredson DC, Gottfredson GD: Quality of school-based prevention programs: results from a national study. Journal of Research in Crime and Delinquency 39(1):3–35, 2002

Guo J, Hawkins JD, Hill KG, et al: Childhood and adolescent predictors of alcohol abuse and dependence in young adulthood. J Stud Alcohol 62(6):754–762, 2001 11838912

Hanley S, Ringwalt C, Vincus AA, et al: Implementing evidence-based substance use prevention curricula with fidelity: the role of teacher training. J Drug Educ 39(1):39–58, 2009 19886161

Hansen WB: All Star: a conceptual history, in Handbook of Adolescent Drug Prevention: Research, Intervention Strategies, and Practice. Edited by Scheier LM. Washington, DC, American Psychological Association, 2015, pp 197–216

Hansen WB, Fleming CB, Scheier LM: Self-reported engagement in a drug prevention program: individual and classroom effects on proximal and behavioral outcomes. J Prim Prev 40(1):5–34, 2019 30631997

Hawkins JD, Catalano RF: Preparing for the Drug Free Years: Family Guide. South Deerfield, MA, Channing Bete, 1988

Hawkins JD, Catalano RF, Miller JY: Risk and protective factors for alcohol and other drug problems in adolescence and early adulthood: implications for substance abuse prevention. Psychol Bull 112(1):64–105, 1992 1529040

Hawkins JD, Kosterman R, Catalano RF, et al: Effects of social development intervention in childhood 15 years later. Arch Pediatr Adolesc Med 162(12):1133–1141, 2008 19047540

Ialongo NS, Werthamer L, Kellam SG, et al: Proximal impact of two first-grade preventive interventions on the early risk behaviors for later substance abuse, depression, and antisocial behavior. Am J Community Psychol 27(5):599–641, 1999 10676542

Johnston LD, Miech RA, O'Malley PM, et al: Monitoring the Future: National Survey Results on Drug Use: 1975–2017: Overview, Key Findings on Adolescent Drug Use. Ann Arbor, MI, Institute for Social Research, The University of Michigan, 2018

Kam C-M, Greenberg MT, Walls CT: Examining the role of implementation quality in school-based prevention using the PATHS curriculum. Promoting Alternative THinking Skills curriculum. Prev Sci 4(1):55–63, 2003 12611419

Karlamangla A, Zhou K, Reuben D, et al: Longitudinal trajectories of heavy drinking in adults in the United States of America. Addiction 101(1):91–99, 2006 16393195

Kellam SG, Anthony JC: Targeting early antecedents to prevent tobacco smoking: findings from an epidemiologically based randomized field trial. Am J Public Health 88(10):1490–1495, 1998 9772850

Kelly AB, Connor JP: Review: some universal family-based prevention programmes provide small reductions in alcohol use in youths in the short and long term. Evid Based Ment Health 15(1):16, 2012 22140219

Kendler KS, Maes HH, Sundquist K, et al: Genetic and family and community environmental effects on drug abuse in adolescence: a Swedish national twin and sibling study. Am J Psychiatry 171(2):209–217, 2014 24077613

King KM, Chassin L: Adolescent stressors, psychopathology, and young adult substance dependence: a prospective study. J Stud Alcohol Drugs 69(5):629–638, 2008 18781237

Kumpfer KL, Scheier LM, Brown J: Strategies to avoid replication failure with evidence-based prevention interventions: case examples from the Strengthening Families Program. Eval Health Prof January 1, 2018 [Epub ahead of print] 29719987

Lipari RN, Ahrnsbrak RD, Pemberton MR, et al: Risk and protective factors and estimates of substance use initiation: results from the 2016 National Survey on Drug Use and Health. NSDUH Data Review, September 2017. Available at: https://www.samhsa.gov/data/sites/default/files/NSDUH-DR-FFR3-2016/NSDUH-DR-FFR3-2016.htm. Accessed April 24, 2019.

Lisdahl KM, Shollenberger S, Sagar KA, et al: The neurocognitive impact of alcohol and marijuana use on the developing adolescent and young adult brain, in Brief Interventions for Adolescent Alcohol and Substance Abuse. Edited by Monti PM, Colby SM, O'Leary Tevyaw T. New York, Guilford, 2018, pp 50–82

Marczinski CA, Hertzenberg H, Goddard P, et al: Alcohol-related Facebook activity predicts alcohol use patterns in college students. Addict Res Theory 24(5):398–405, 2016 28138317

Masten AS: Ordinary magic: resilience processes in development. Am Psychol 56(3):227–238, 2001 11315249

Mitchell P, Spooner C, Copeland J, et al: The Role of Families in the Development, Identification, Prevention and Treatment of Illicit Drug Problems. Canberra, Australian National Health and Medical Research Council, 2001. Available at: https://trove.nla.gov.au/work/32927292?q&online=true. Accessed April 24, 2019.

National Institute on Drug Abuse: Principles of Adolescent Substance Use Disorder Treatment: A Research-Based Guide (NIH Publ No 14-7953). Bethesda, MD, National Institute on Drug Abuse, 2014

National Research Council and Institute of Medicine: Preventing Mental, Emotional, and Behavioral Disorders Among Young People: Progress and Possibilities. Washington, DC, The National Academies Press, 2009

Nelson TF, Xuan Z, Babor TF, et al: Efficacy and the strength of evidence of U.S. alcohol control policies. Am J Prev Med 45(1):19–28, 2013 23790985

Oesterle S, Kuklinski MR, Hawkins JD, et al: Long-term effects of the Communities That Care trial on substance use, antisocial behavior, and violence through age 21 years. Am J Public Health 108(5):659–665, 2018 29565666

Olds D, Henderson CR Jr, Cole R, et al: Long-term effects of nurse home visitation on children's criminal and antisocial behavior: 15-year follow-up of a randomized controlled trial. JAMA 280(14):1238–1244, 1998 9786373

Oxford ML, Harachi TW, Catalano RF, et al: Preadolescent predictors of substance initiation: a test of both the direct and mediated effect of family social control factors on deviant peer associations and substance initiation. Am J Drug Alcohol Abuse 27(4):599–616, 2001 11727879

Pagan JL, Rose RJ, Viken RJ, et al: Genetic and environmental influences on stages of alcohol use across adolescence and into young adulthood. Behav Genet 36(4):483–497, 2006 16586152

Park J, Kosterman R, Hawkins JD, et al: Effects of the "Preparing for the Drug Free Years" curriculum on growth in alcohol use and risk for alcohol use in early adolescence. Prev Sci 1(3):125–138, 2000 11525344

Payne AA, Eckert R: The relative importance of provider, program, school, and community predictors of the implementation quality of school-based prevention programs. Prev Sci 11(2):126–141, 2010 19902357

Pentz MA, Jasuja GK, Rohrbach LA, et al: Translation in tobacco and drug abuse prevention research. Eval Health Prof 29(2):246–271, 2006 16645186

Peterson PL, Hawkins JD, Abbott RD, et al: Disentangling the effects of parental drinking, family management, and parental alcohol norms on current drinking by Black and White adolescents. Journal of Research on Adolescence 4:203–227, 1994

Prom-Wormley E, Maes HH, Scheier LM: Parental influence on adolescent drug use, in Parenting and Teen Drug Use: The Most Recent Findings From Research, Prevention, and Treatment. Edited by Scheier LM, Hansen WB. New York, Oxford University Press, 2014, pp 15–36

Resnicow K, Soler R, Brathwaite RL, et al: Cultural sensitivity in substance use prevention. Journal of Community Psychology 28(3):271–290, 2000

Ringwalt CL, Vincus A, Ennett S, et al: Reasons for teachers' adaptation of substance use prevention curricula in schools with non-white student populations. Prev Sci 5(1):61–67, 2004 15058914

Ringwalt CL, Pankratz MM, Hansen WB, et al: The potential of coaching as a strategy to improve the effectiveness of school-based substance use prevention curricula. Health Educ Behav 36(4):696–710, 2009 17652615

Rohrbach LA, Dent CW, Skara S, et al: Fidelity of implementation in Project Towards No Drug Abuse (TND): a comparison of classroom teachers and program specialists. Prev Sci 8(2):125–132, 2007 17180722

Scheier LM: Etiologic studies of adolescent drug use: a compendium of data resources and their implications for prevention. Journal of Primary Prevention 22(2):125–168, 2001

Scheier LM, Hansen WB (eds): Parenting and Teen Drug Use: The Most Recent Findings From Research, Prevention, and Treatment. New York, Oxford University Press, 2014

Scheirer MA: Is sustainability possible? A review and commentary on empirical studies of program sustainability. American Journal of Evaluation 26(3):320–347, 2005

Spoth R, Greenberg M, Turrisi R: Preventive interventions addressing underage drinking: state of the evidence and steps toward public health impact. Pediatrics 121 (suppl 4):S311–S336, 2008 18381496

Substance Abuse and Mental Health Services Administration: Behavioral Health Trends in the United States: Results From the 2014 National Survey on Drug Use and Health. NSDUH Series H-50. HHS Publ No SMA 15-4927. Rockville, MD, Substance Abuse and Mental Health Services Administration, Center for Behavioral Health Statistics and Quality, 2015. Available at: https://www.samhsa.gov/data/sites/default/files/NSDUH-FRR1-2014/NSDUH-FRR1-2014.pdf. Accessed April 24, 2019.

Sussman SY: Evaluating the efficacy of Project TND: evidence from seven research trials, in Handbook of Adolescent Drug Prevention: Research, Intervention Strategies, and Practice. Edited by Scheier LM. Washington, DC, American Psychological Association, 2015, pp 159–176

Tobler NS, Roona MR, Ochshorn P, et al: School-based adolescent drug prevention programs: 1998 meta-analysis. Journal of Primary Prevention 20(4):275–336, 2000

Toumbourou JW, Catalano RF: Predicting developmentally harmful substance use, in Preventing Harmful Substance Use: The Evidence Base for Policy and Practice. Edited by Stockwell T, Gruenewald PJ, Toumbourou JW, et al. London, Wiley, 2005, pp 53–65

Wagenaar AC, Toomey TL: Effects of minimum drinking age laws: review and analyses of the literature from 1960 to 2000. J Stud Alcohol Suppl 14(14):206–225, 2002 12022726

Waldron HB, Turner CW: Evidence-based psychosocial treatments for adolescent substance abuse. J Clin Child Adolesc Psychol 37(1):238–261, 2008 18444060

Williams B, Sanson A, Toumbourou J, et al: Patterns and Predictors of Teenagers' Use of Licit and Illicit Substances in the Australian Temperament Project Cohort. Melbourne, Australia, The Ross Trust, 2000

Wills TA, Ainette MG: Temperament, self-control, and adolescent substance use: a two-factor model of etiological processes, in Handbook of Drug Use Etiology: Theory, Methods, and Empirical Findings. Edited by Scheier LM. Washington, DC, American Psychological Association, 2010, pp 127–146

Winters KC, Lee CY: Likelihood of developing an alcohol and cannabis use disorder during youth: association with recent use and age. Drug Alcohol Depend 92(1–3):239–247, 2008 17888588

Winters KC, Fahnhorst T, Botzet A, et al: Brief intervention for drug-abusing adolescents in a school setting: outcomes and mediating factors. J Subst Abuse Treat 42(3):279–288, 2012 22000326

Winters KC, Botzet A, Fahnhorst T: Adolescent drug abuse treatment: family and related approaches, in Parenting and Teen Drug Use: The Most Recent Findings From Research, Prevention, and Treatment. Edited by Scheier LM, Hansen WB. New York, Oxford University Press, 2014, pp 193–213

Young SE, Rhee SH, Stallings MC, et al: Genetic and environmental vulnerabilities underlying adolescent substance use and problem use: general or specific? Behav Genet 36(4):603–615, 2006 16619135

Zucker RA: Anticipating problem alcohol use developmentally from childhood into middle adulthood: what have we learned? Addiction 103 (suppl 1):100–108, 2008 18426543

3

Screening and Assessing Youth With Substance Use Disorder

Ken C. Winters, Ph.D.

Randy Stinchfield, Ph.D.

Andria M. Botzet, M.A.

Adolescent use of alcohol and other drugs (hereafter, referred to as "drugs") significantly elevates a person's risk for developing a substance use disorder (SUD) and experiencing a variety of other negative consequences, including delinquency, emotional distress, school failure, risky sexual behavior, motor vehicle injuries or fatalities, and possible disruption in brain development (Chung and Martin 2010).

The preparation of this manuscript was partially supported by National Institute on Drug Abuse grant DA029795. The authors wish to extend their gratitude to Tamara Fahnhorst and Ali Stockness (Nicholson) for their research contributions to this chapter.

51

Accurate and developmentally specific measurement of adolescent drug use, and of related co-occurring disorders and risk and protective variables, is essential to providing a precise understanding of the nature and extent of a teenager's drug use and to assist in determining his or her treatment needs. The assessment plan also needs to consider the developmental periods of those being assessed. In this chapter we focus on practical measurement and evaluation issues faced by those in clinical or research settings. Specifically, we discuss the following issues: principles of assessment, self-report and its validity, alternatives to self-report, core clinical content for assessment, assessment instruments, treatment outcome assessment, and the clinical interview.

Principles of Assessment

The initial step in identifying whether an adolescent may be involved with drugs involves a screening. The results from a screening are relevant for deciding the need (or not) for a comprehensive assessment (although in some clinical instances, a screening is used to determine the need for a brief intervention). The comprehensive assessment is used to explore in depth the extent and nature of the drug use, co-occurring problems, and treatment needs. It is imperative that a treatment program use at least one of the adolescent-specific and psychometrically sound tools as part of intake and treatment planning.

Screening

A screening should be relatively brief and consist of straightforward questions, such as recent history of drug use (e.g., "How often did you use the following drugs in the past 6 months?") and situations in which drug use is common (Winters et al. 2018). It is also advisable to ask the adolescent the benefits and negatives of using (decisional balance exercise). These latter questions can be helpful in gauging the functional value of drug use and establishing if the youth has experienced any drug-related negative consequences.

Comprehensive Assessment

When the screening results suggest that a possible drug use problem exists, a comprehensive assessment is indicated. This process involves a detailed assessment of the numerous content areas: drug use history, including age at onset and frequency and quantity of use; criteria for SUDs; other negative consequences not part of the SUD criteria (e.g., school difficulties, social and physical problems); circumstances and context of drug use, including affiliation with drug-using peers; internal and external triggers associated with drug use; criteria for other behavioral and mental co-occurring problems; family relationships and home life; and problem recognition and readiness for treatment.

Self-Report Method

Self-report is a hallmark of screening and comprehensive assessment, given its convenience, relative low cost, and the view that the client is the most knowledgeable reporter. Formats typically used in clinical settings are the self-administered questionnaire (SAQ; either paper-and-pencil or computer administered) and the interview. Other self-report methods, and ones more commonly used by researchers, are the timeline follow-back (TLFB) and the computer-assisted interview (CAI). Whereas research on the concordance of all of these formats suggests that, for the most part, they are comparable in terms of accuracy of disclosing (Winters et al. 2018), they each have their specific strengths. For example, standardized SAQs minimize bias from the influence of the assessor, and many SAQs include scales designed to assess response bias. Yet the clinical interview can promote the validity of self-report by virtue of the interviewer expressing empathy about the client's situation, which may improve the respondent's willingness to self-disclose. Also, information may be gained by observing nonverbal clues such as emotional characteristics, and follow-up questioning may elicit information that could not have been obtained using a SAQ.

The validity of adolescent self-report method is a long-standing question in the research literature (Allen and Wilson 2003). Sources of invalid self-report include purposeful distortion of the truth, lack of insight, inattentiveness, or misunderstanding of the question. Developmental factors may mediate variability in the validity of self-report. Adolescence is a developmental period characterized by unique cognitive, social, and ego functioning (Masten et al. 2008; Noam and Houlihan 1990), all which may impact the adolescent's perception and reporting of personal problems and his or her environment.

Alternatives to Self-Report

Although we view self-report method as a necessary component of the assessment process, it is advisable to supplement it with other sources of information. Self-report is not infallible, and other sources provide unique information not available from self-report. A brief overview of three non-self-report methods follows.

Biologically Based Drug Testing

Examples of drug testing to detect that the person has been exposed to drugs are urinalysis, hair analysis, saliva testing, and sweat testing (Allen et al. 2003; Dolan et al. 2004). Details of drug testing are provided in Chapter 5.

Parent Report

Parents are usually willing participants in the assessment process, but there are limits to what can be expected. A meta-analysis of the association between youth and parent reports of psychopathology revealed low to moderate correlations (De Los Reyes et al. 2015). Parents can be a good source of information about some mental health problems experienced by their son or daughter, particularly externalizing disorders such as attention-deficit/hyperactivity disorder and conduct problems (Ivens and Rehm 1988; Rey et al. 1992). Yet parents typically do not know details about their teenager's drug use (Waters et al. 2003). For example, Edelbrock and colleagues (1986) found that the agreement for SUD symptoms between mother and child reports averaged only 63%; Weissman and colleagues (1987) reported just a 17% average agreement between mother and son reports. (It is likely that peers are a more accurate source of drug use about a teenager, although it is not realistic to expect a friend to participate in an assessment.)

Clinical Observation

Direct observation of behavioral indicators of drug use can supplement the assessment process. Indicators include needle marks, slurred or incoherent speech, shaking of hands or twitching of eyelids, and unsteady gate. The Simple Screening Instrument for Alcohol and Other Drugs (Center for Substance Abuse Treatment 1994) includes a 14-item checklist of observable signs that may indicate drug use.

Core Clinical Content of a Comprehensive Assessment

As noted in the opening to this chapter, a thorough assessment of an adolescent suspected of drug involvement involves a review of a diverse range of variables. In this section we discuss three main content domains: drug abuse problem severity, biopsychosocial factors, and cognitive factors.

Drug Abuse Problem Severity

This domain pertains to the details of an adolescent's drug involvement and resulting diagnostic symptoms. Specific variables that come under this domain are age at onset of first use of individual drugs; age at onset of regular (e.g., weekly or daily) use of drugs; lifetime and more recent (e.g., prior 6 months) pattern of use for each drug; the specific drug or drugs that are preferred; the social and psychological motives or benefits of drug use (e.g., use for fun; use to be with friends; use to deal with anxiety); and the presence of DSM-based symptoms of a substance use disorder. The last-mentioned component merits further discussion.

When an adolescent's drug use escalates from experimentation to regular and heavy use, then the criteria for a SUD may be met. The differential diagnosis of adolescent SUDs requires consideration that the symptoms of drug use not be due to premorbid or concurrent problems, such as conduct disorder or family issues. Given the frequent comorbidity of SUDs and other psychiatric disorders (Grella et al. 2001), it is important that the assessor comprehensively review, via a timeline, the past and present history of psychiatric symptoms. This type of detailed interview can help sort out the course of the onset of SUD symptoms and symptoms related to a mental or behavior illness.

The DSM-5 criteria have the following key features: none of the criteria directly refer to onset, quantity, or frequency variables; a single SUD for each substance class is used, using a set of 11 symptoms for most substances; and a SUD diagnosis is assigned on the basis of how many symptoms are met: no disorder (0–1), mild SUD (2–3), moderate SUD (4–5), or severe SUD (6 or more) (American Psychiatric Association 2013).

The DSM-5 criteria for SUD include changes from DSM-IV relevant to adolescents that are supported by research: removal of the distinction between abuse and dependence criteria; elimination of the "legal problems" symptom;

and addition of the symptom pertaining to craving and a strong desire to use (see Chapter 1 of this manual). Recent commentary pieces have discussed the pros and cons of the DSM-5 criteria for adolescents (Kaminer and Winters 2012; Winters et al. 2011a).

The general view is that some criteria have questionable validity for adolescents. For example, the two physiological symptoms, tolerance and withdrawal, are not highly relevant to young people who are going through neurodevelopmental changes and are not yet chronic users. In addition, the meaning of some symptoms for adolescents, who are relatively inexperienced with the effects of drugs, may lead to higher rates of false-positive endorsements, and the definition of mild SUD (2–3 symptoms) may identify too many youth that do not have a problem given that some criteria may be developmentally normative for adolescents and could be easily labeled as a symptom.

Biopsychosocial Factors

The biopsychosocial domain is defined as the personal and environmental factors that are presumed to contribute to the onset, maintenance, and progression of the adolescent's drug involvement. Assessing these factors provides valuable information for treatment planning (Shoham and Insel 2011). Underlying risk factors (i.e., predictors associated with an increased likelihood of drug use) need to be addressed because they may be triggers of drug use; protective factors (i.e., promotive factors that have a direct negative relationship with drug use) can be harnessed to help with behavior change strategies. And the likelihood that an adolescent may use drugs in the future has been shown to be positively related to the presence of risk factors (National Institute on Drug Abuse 2014). Chapter 2 in this manual provides a description of prominent risk and protective factors that research has identified as being associated with adolescent drug use. We provide an overview of clinically oriented psychosocial assessment instruments later in this chapter.

Cognitive Factors

The third major content area of interest involves the group of cognitive variables that affect the adolescent's problem recognition and readiness to change. Adolescence is a developmental period during which brain maturation is occurring in significant ways. Research with animals and with humans supports the view that the adolescent brain does not fully develop until early adulthood (Giedd 2004). These changes can impact cognitive and behavioral functioning (Masten et al. 2008) and shape the adolescent's perception of personal problems and how these problems are self-reported. From structural and functional neuroimaging studies we know that neural circuitry undergoes major reorganization during adolescence, particularly in those regions of the brain relating to decision making, working toward goals, critical thinking, adaptability, and being aware of one's own emotions as well as those of others (Dayan et al. 2010). How does brain development affect the assessment process? We note two ways:

1. Assessing risk behavior needs to consider the situation and context in which the risk behaviors occur. Adolescent behavior can be greatly influenced by the emotion of the moment, including peer influences (Clark and Winters 2002); understanding if risk behavior also occurs in the absence of context influenced is important. In addition, some adolescents are the "ringleaders" of their peer groups, and they initiate social pressures on others.
2. Adolescence is a developmental period in which egocentric perceptions may have an impact on insight and contribute to biased views about one's behavior (Winters and Arria 2011). Such poor insight can contribute to low problem recognition, even in the face of obvious objective facts. For example, adolescents may over-ascribe the source of personal behavior to an external source (e.g., parents, unfair rules).

It is advisable to use standardized instruments and structured interviews that have been specifically developed for and psychometrically validated on youth in clinical settings. These instruments can minimize response biases due to multiple sources (e.g., context of the assessment; adolescent insight issues). Also, some standardized tests contain validity scales that provide information about possible faking tendencies, such as faking bad and faking good, and other types of invalid responding (e.g., inattention, random responding).

Assessment Instruments

The development and evaluation of clinically relevant assessment instruments to address adolescent drug involvement has been significant since the mid-

1980s (Winters et al. 2018). These instruments include screening and comprehensive tools and interview and self-administered formats. Several reviews and summaries of this vast instrumentation field are available. They include the following: *Screening and Assessing Adolescents for Substance Use Disorders* (Center for Substance Abuse Treatment 1999); *Assessing Alcohol Problems: A Guide for Clinicians and Researchers* (Allen and Wilson 2003); journal articles (e.g., Leccese and Waldron 1994; Winters and Kaminer 2008); and book chapters (e.g., Winters et al. 2018). Another resource, the PhenX Toolkit (Hamilton et al. 2011), provides detailed descriptions of public domain, standardized measures for up to 15 complex diseases and disorders, behavioral and personality traits, and environmental exposures. The toolkit's substance abuse instruments, which were selected by experts, consist of adult and adolescent measures for tobacco, alcohol, and other substance use and for assessing SUDs.

In what follows we provide an overview of the major groups of instruments in the field (screens, interviews, and questionnaires). We only include those instruments for which there are published favorable psychometric data on reliability and validity (see also Chapter 4 in this manual).

Screening Tools

Four categories of screening instruments are described below: alcohol, all substances (including alcohol), non-alcohol drugs, and multiproblem screens (Table 3–1).

Alcohol Screens

The Adolescent Drinking Inventory (Harrell and Wirtz 1989) is a 24-item screener that measures psychological symptoms, physical symptoms, social symptoms, and loss of control due to drinking. Scoring to the Adolescent Drinking Inventory provides a single score with cutoffs and two research subscale scores (self-medicating drinking and rebellious drinking). The 23-item Rutgers Alcohol Problem Index (White and Labouvie 1989) measures alcohol use problems in multiple areas of functioning—family life, social relations, psychological adjustment, delinquency, physical problems, and neuropsychological adjustment. The third tool in this category is the Alcohol Screening and Brief Intervention for Youth (National Institute on Alcohol Abuse and Alcoholism 2011). The tool consists of just two questions; one focuses on drinking frequency and the other on drinking frequency by the adolescent's peers.

Table 3–1. Screening instruments

Instrument	Purpose	Source	Examples group used	Norms	Normed groups	Format	Time (minutes)
Adolescent Alcohol and Drug Involvement Scale (AADIS)	Screen for drug abuse problem severity	Moberg 2003	Adolescents referred for emotional or behavioral disorders	Yes	Substance abusers	14 items	5
Adolescent Drinking Inventory (ADI)	Screen for alcohol use problem severity	Harrell and Wirtz 1989	Adolescents suspected of alcohol use problems	Yes	Nonclinical sample; substance abusers	24 items	5
CRAFFT	Screen for drug use problem severity	Knight et al. 2003	Adolescents referred for emotional or behavioral disorders	Yes	Nonclinical sample; substance abusers	6 items	5
Drug Abuse Screening Test for Adolescents (DAST-A)	Screen for drug use problem severity	Martino et al. 2000	Adolescents referred for emotional or behavioral disorders	Yes	Substance abusers	27 items	5

Table 3–1. Screening instruments *(continued)*

Instrument	Purpose	Source	Examples group used	Norms	Normed groups	Format	Time (minutes)
Drug Use Screening Inventory—Revised (DUSI-R)	Screen for substance use problem severity and related problems	Tarter et al. 1992	Adolescents referred for emotional or behavioral disorders	Yes	Substance abusers	159 items	20
Global Appraisal of Individual Needs (GAIN)–Short Screener (GAIN-SS)	Screen for drug use problem severity and related problems	Dennis et al. 2006	Adolescents referred for emotional or behavioral disorders	Yes	Substance abusers	20 items	3–5
Personal Experience Screening Questionnaire (PESQ)	Screen for substance use problem severity	Winters 1992	Adolescents referred for emotional or behavioral disorders	Yes	Nonclinical sample; substance abusers	40 items	10

Table 3–1. Screening instruments (*continued*)

Instrument	Purpose	Source	Examples group used	Norms	Normed groups	Format	Time (minutes)
Problem Oriented Screening Instrument for Teenagers (POSIT)	Multiproblem screen for substance use problem severity and related problems	Latimer et al. 1997; Rahdert 1991	Adolescents referred for emotional or behavioral disorders	Yes	Nonclinical sample; substance abusers	139 items	20–25
Rutgers Alcohol Problem Index (RAPI)	Screen for alcohol use problem severity	White and Labouvie 1989	Adolescents at risk for alcohol use problems	Yes	Nonclinical sample; substance abusers	23 items	10
Substance Abuse Subtle Screening Inventory— Adolescents (SASSI-A)	Screen for substance use problem severity and related problems	Miller 2002	Adolescents referred for emotional or behavioral disorders	Yes	Nonclinical sample; substance abusers	81 items	10–15

Note. Contact instrument author for any non-English translations.

Two other tools that were developed for adults, the TWEAK and the Alcohol Use Disorders Identification Test (AUDIT), have been used with young adults and found to be psychometrically favorable (Winters et al. 2011b).

Screens for All Substances

The 14-item Adolescent Alcohol and Drug Involvement Scale (AADIS; Moberg 2003) generically screens for drug abuse problem severity scale. The CRAFFT 2.0 (Knight et al. 2002) begins with three drug use frequency items, followed by six items that screen for drug-related problems and consequences. Screening to Brief Intervention (S2BI), which consists of three to seven items, depending on responses, asks the respondent whether he or she has used tobacco, alcohol, marijuana, and other drugs (Levy et al. 2014). The Global Appraisal of Individual Needs (GAIN)–Short Screener (GAIN-SS; Dennis et al. 2006) is a 3- to 5-minute screener that can be used to quickly identify those who would likely have a disorder based on the full companion instrument, the Global Appraisal of Individual Needs (GAIN; Dennis 1999). The 40-item Personal Experience Screening Questionnaire (PESQ; Winters 1992) consists of a problem severity scale, drug use history, questions about select psychosocial problems, and response distortion tendencies (faking good and faking bad). The 81-item adolescent version of the Substance Abuse Subtle Screening Inventory–2 (Miller 2002) yields scores for several scales, including face-valid alcohol, face-valid other drug, obvious attributes, subtle attributes, and defensiveness.

Screens for Non-alcohol Drugs

Only one screen is available for non-alcohol drugs—the 27-item Drug Abuse Screening Test for Adolescents (Martino et al. 2000). This tool was adapted from Skinner's (1982) adult tool, the Drug Abuse Screening Test.

Multiproblem Screens

Two multiproblem screen instruments are available. The 139-item Problem Oriented Screening Instrument for Teenagers (POSIT; Rahdert 1991) covers 10 functional adolescent problem areas: substance use, physical health, mental health, family relations, peer relationships, educational status, vocational status, social skills, leisure and recreation, and aggressive behavior/delinquency. Cut scores for determining the need for further assessment have been rationally established, and some have been confirmed with empirical procedures (Latimer et al. 1997). The Drug Use Screening Inventory—Revised (Tarter et al. 1992) is a 159-item instrument that measures drug use problem severity and related problems. It produces scores on 10 subscales and one lie scale.

Comparisons of Screens

Empirical comparisons of screens have been conducted. D'Amico and colleagues (2016) compared NIAAA's 2-item screen (Alcohol Screening and Brief Intervention for Youth), the AUDIT, the CRAFFT, and the PESQ. CRAFFT and PESQ performed equally as the best in predicting a SUD. Knight and colleagues (2003) compared the criterion validity of AUDIT, POSIT, CAGE (a 4-item screen for alcohol problems), and CRAFFT in an adolescent sample. Three—AUDIT, POSIT, and CRAFFT—were found to have acceptable validity data.

Comprehensive Assessment Instruments

There are numerous tools—diagnostic interviews, problem-focused interviews, and multiscale questionnaires—to choose from when the clinical situation calls for a comprehensive assessment. These tools provide information to confirm a SUD diagnosis and identify coexisting problems, as well as provide information to assist with treatment planning.

Diagnostic Interviews

Diagnostic interviews provide a means to assess DSM-based criteria, including SUDs and other psychiatric disorders (Table 3–2). The majority of interviews are highly structured; the interviewer reads verbatim a series of questions in a decision-tree format, and the answers to these questions are restricted to a few predefined alternatives. The interviewer has no or minimal responsibility for interpreting the respondent's reply. Well-researched structured interviews that assess all psychiatric disorders are the Diagnostic Interview for Children and Adolescents—Revised (DICA-R; Reich et al. 1992) and the Diagnostic Interview Schedule for Children (DISC; Shaffer et al. 1996). Both of these interviews have parent and youth versions.

There are three comprehensive diagnostic interviews that focus on adolescent diagnostic criteria for SUDs. The Adolescent Diagnostic Interview (Winters and Henly 1993) assesses DSM-5 diagnostic symptoms associated with SUDs, as well as history of drug use and screens for several adolescent psychiatric disorders. The Customary Drinking and Drug Use Record (Brown et al.

Table 3–2. Comprehensive assessment instruments: diagnostic interviews

Instrument	Purpose	Source	Examples group used	Norms	Normed groups	Format	Time (minutes)
Adolescent Diagnostic Interview (ADI)	Assess DSM-IV substance use disorders and problems	Winters and Henly 1993	Adolescents suspected of drug use problems	NA	NA	Structured interview	45–60
Customary Drinking and Drug Use Record (CDDR)	Assess DSM-IV substance use disorders and problems	Brown et al. 1998	Adolescents suspected of drug use problems	NA	NA	Structured interview	10–30
Diagnostic Interview for Children and Adolescents—Revised (DICA-R)	Assess DSM-IV child/adolescent disorders	Reich et al. 1992	Youth suspected of mental or behavioral problems	NA	NA	Structured interview	45–60
Diagnostic Interview Schedule for Children—Revised (DISC-R)	Assess DSM-IV child/adolescent disorders	Shaffer et al. 1996	Youth suspected of mental or behavioral problems	NA	NA	Structured interview	45–60
Global Appraisal of Individual Needs (GAIN)	Assess DSM-IV substance use disorders and problems	Dennis 1999	Adolescents suspected of drug use problems	NA	NA	Structured interview	60–90

Note. Contact instrument author for any non-English translations. NA = not available.

1998) measures alcohol and other drug use consumption, DSM-IV substance dependence symptoms (including a detailed assessment of withdrawal symptoms), and several types of consequences of drug involvement. The third instrument in this subgroup is the widely used GAIN (Dennis 1999; Dennis et al. 2004). The GAIN has eight core sections: Background, Substance Use, Physical Health, Risk Behaviors and Disease Prevention, Mental and Emotional Health, Environment and Living Situation, Legal, and Vocational.

Problem-Focused Interviews

These interviews measure several problem areas associated with adolescent drug involvement, including details of the adolescent's drug use history, and signs of a drug problem (e.g., negative personal consequences, loss of control, and psychosocial risk factors) (Table 3–3). But these tools do not have items that allow one to make a formal diagnosis of an SUD. The Comprehensive Adolescent Severity Inventory (Meyers et al. 2006) measures education, substance use, use of free time, leisure activities, peer relationships, family life, psychiatric status, and legal history. The assessor makes severity ratings for each major section based on the respondent's answers. The Teen Addiction Severity Index (Kaminer et al. 1993) consists of seven content areas: chemical use, school status, employment-support status, family relationships, legal status, peer-social relationships, and psychiatric status. A medical status section was not included because it was deemed to be less relevant to adolescent drug abusers. Adolescent and interviewer severity ratings are elicited on a 5-point scale for each of the content areas. A companion tool, the Teen Treatment Services Review (Kaminer et al. 1998), measures the type and number of services that the youth received during the treatment episode.

Multiscale Questionnaires

There is a large group of multiscale questionnaires (Table 3–4). Examples in this set are self-administered (either paper-and-pencil or computer administered) and typically provide via computer scoring reports with normed scale scores and interpretation narratives. In addition to scales for drug use problem severity and psychosocial risk factors, some of the questionnaires include measures of response distortion tendencies (e.g., faking bad, faking good). The Adolescent Self-Assessment Profile–II (Wanberg 1998) is a 225-item instrument that measures in-depth drug involvement, including drug use frequency,

Table 3–3.   Comprehensive assessment instruments: problem-focused interviews

Instrument	Purpose	Source	Examples group used	Norms	Normed groups	Format	Time (minutes)
Comprehensive Adolescent Severity Inventory (CASI)	Assess drug use and other life problems	Meyers et al. 2006	Adolescents suspected of drug use problems	NA	NA	Semistructured interview	45–55
Teen Addiction Severity Index (T-ASI)	Assess drug use and other life problems	Kaminer et al. 1993	Adolescents at risk for drug use problems	NA	NA	Semistructured interview	20–45

Note.   Contact instrument author for any non-English translations. NA = not available.

drug use consequences and benefits, and major risk factors (e.g., deviance, peer influence). Supplemental scales based on common factors are also scored. The Hilson Adolescent Profile (Inwald et al. 1986; Streeter and Franklin 1991) consists of 310 items (true/false) and 16 scales, two of which measure alcohol and other drug use. The other content scales assess psychiatric-based domains (e.g., antisocial behavior, depression) and psychosocial problems (e.g., family conflicts). The 108-item, computer-assisted Juvenile Automated Substance Abuse Evaluation (Ellis 1987) produces a five-category score, ranging from no use to drug abuse (including a suggested classification of a SUD), as well as a summary of drug use history, a measure of life stress, and a scale for test-taking attitude. The Personal Experience Inventory (Winters and Henly 1994) consists of 276 items across several scales that measure substance use involvement (including drug use history), psychosocial risk, and response distortion tendencies. Supplemental problem screens measure eating disorders, suicide potential, physical/sexual abuse, and parental history of drug abuse.

Treatment Outcome Assessment

The evaluation of treatment outcome requires, at minimum, an intake assessment tool that is comprehensive and a parallel, follow-up version that provides the basis for comparing baseline and posttreatment functioning. In this light, a good intake instrument to accommodate assessing change after treatment should include measures of drug use problem severity (e.g., drug use history, diagnostic symptoms), psychosocial functioning (e.g., school, family), and co-occurring behavioral disorders. Also relevant are the assets that the youth and family can utilize to promote recovery and what obstacles exist related to participation in primary treatment and aftercare. Follow-up tools provide a measure of treatment effectiveness; common features are adjustments in the time frame (e.g., "since you were discharged from the treatment program") and content (e.g., "How have you made changes in your social life to promote recovery?") of the intake questionnaire. In addition to the core questions that follow-up the questions asked on the intake tool, questions unique to the follow-up period may include use for aftercare services, progress with goals, plans for the future, and other variables of interest that the treatment approach targeted (e.g., change in readiness to change; change in coping with drug use triggers).

Table 3–4.   Comprehensive assessment instruments: multiscale questionnaires

Instrument	Purpose	Source	Examples group used	Norms	Normed groups	Format	Time (minutes)
Adolescent Self-Assessment Profile–II (ASAP-II)	Multiscale measure of drug use and related problems	Wanberg 1998	Adolescents suspected of substance use problems	Yes	Nonclinical sample; substance abusers	225 items	45–60
Hilson Adolescent Profile (HAP)	Multiscale measure of alcohol and drug use and related problems	Inwald et al. 1986	Adolescents suspected of substance use and related problems	Yes	Nonclinical sample; substance abusers	310 items	45
Juvenile Automated Substance Abuse Evaluation (JASAE)	Multiscale measure of drug use and related problems	Ellis 1987	Adolescents suspected of substance use problems	Yes	Nonclinical sample; substance abusers	108 items	20
Personal Experience Inventory (PEI)	Multiscale measure of drug use and related problems	Winters and Henly 1994	Adolescents suspected of substance use problems	Yes	Nonclinical sample; substance abusers	276 items	45–60

Note.   Contact instrument author for any non-English translations. NA=not available.

The Clinical Interview

The initial clinical interview with the adolescent is an important part of the assessment process. Below are key clinical guidelines for conducting an initial clinical interview with an adolescent client.

1. Even a fact-gathering interview can be based on motivational interviewing principles. Expressing empathy and avoiding argumentation can go a long way in building rapport with the adolescent and promoting self-disclosure. Begin with small talk and focus early in the interview on the current situation and pressing issues. The comprehensive interviews reviewed above have introductory sections with suggested questions along these lines.
2. Communicate that you are an advocate for the teenager, with limits. This involves highlighting the adolescent's strengths and steering goal setting along realistic lines. When appropriate, offer constructive criticism and use light confronting if merited.
3. It is advisable to split the initial session into two parts: the first part with the teenager alone and the second part with the parent(s) alone. Do not sit behind a desk.
4. Acknowledge to the adolescent that you understand that she or he is dealing with a difficult situation, but also that the course of action will require some steps that involve her or him.
5. Explore the functional value of the adolescent's drug use (e.g., drugs may be serving a social and psychological purpose). This does not mean you are approving drug use. The value of this information is to help increase the adolescent's insight about what are sources of his or her drug cravings.

Key Points

- The assessment process includes both a screening (brief and limited in scope) and a comprehensive assessment (detailed, diagnostically oriented, and a source for treatment referral decisions).

- Despite limitations with self-report, obtaining assessment information directly from the adolescent is necessary; parents typically can only provide limited information about their teenager's substance use.

- Numerous psychometrically sound screening and comprehensive tools have been developed specifically for use with adolescents.

- The clinical interview is a valuable vehicle for obtaining assessment information.

References

Allen JP, Wilson VB (eds): Assessing Alcohol Problems: A Guide for Clinicians and Researchers, 2nd Edition. Rockville, MD, National Institute on Alcohol Abuse and Alcoholism, 2003. Available at: https://pubs.niaaa.nih.gov/publications/assessingalcohol/index.htm. Accessed April 25, 2019.

Allen JP, Sillanaukee P, Strid N, et al: Biomarkers of heavy drinking, in Assessing Alcohol Problems: A Guide for Clinicians and Researchers, 2nd Edition. Edited by Allen JP, Wilson VB. Rockville, MD, National Institute on Alcohol Abuse and Alcoholism, 2003, pp 37–53

American Psychiatric Association: Diagnostic and Statistical Manual of Mental Disorders, 5th Edition. Arlington, VA, American Psychiatric Association, 2013

Brown SA, Myers MG, Lippke L, et al: Psychometric evaluation of the Customary Drinking and Drug Use Record (CDDR): a measure of adolescent alcohol and drug involvement. J Stud Alcohol 59(4):427–438, 1998 9647425

Center for Substance Abuse Treatment: Simple Screening Instruments for Outreach for Alcohol and Other Drug Abuse and Infectious Diseases: Treatment Improvement Protocol (TIP) Series No 11 (DHHS Publ No SMA 94-2094). Rockville, MD, Substance Abuse and Mental Health Services Administration, Center for Substance Abuse Treatment, 1994

Center for Substance Abuse Treatment: Screening and Assessing Adolescents for Substance Use Disorders: Treatment Improvement Protocol (TIP) Series No 31 (HHS Publ No SMA 12-4079). Rockville, MD, Substance Abuse and Mental Health Services Administration, 1999

Chung T, Martin CS: Prevalence and clinical course of adolescent substance use and substance use disorders, in Clinical Manual of Adolescent Substance Abuse Treatment. Edited by Kaminer Y, Winters KC. Washington, DC, American Psychiatric Association, 2010, pp 1–23

Clark DB, Winters KC: Measuring risks and outcomes in substance use disorders prevention research. J Consult Clin Psychol 70(6):1207–1223, 2002 12472298

D'Amico EJ, Parast L, Meredith LS, et al.: Screening in primary care: what is the best way to identify at-risk youth for substance use? Pediatrics 138(6):e20161717, 2016

Dayan J, Bernard A, Olliac B, et al: Adolescent brain development, risk-taking and vulnerability to addiction. J Physiol Paris 104(5):279–286, 2010 20816768

De Los Reyes A, Augenstein TM, Wang M, et al: The validity of the multi-informant approach to assessing child and adolescent mental health. Psychol Bull 141(4):858–900, 2015 25915035

Dennis ML: Global Appraisal of Individual Needs (GAIN): Administration Guide for the GAIN and Related Measures. Normal, IL, Chestnut Health Systems, 1999

Dennis ML, Funk R, Godley SH, et al: Cross-validation of the alcohol and cannabis use measures in the Global Appraisal of Individual Needs (GAIN) and Timeline Followback (TLFB; Form 90) among adolescents in substance abuse treatment. Addiction 99 (suppl 2):120–128, 2004 15488110

Dennis ML, Chan YF, Funk RR: Development and validation of the GAIN Short Screener (GSS) for internalizing, externalizing and substance use disorders and crime/violence problems among adolescents and adults. Am J Addict 15 (suppl 1):80–91, 2006 17182423

Dolan K, Rouen D, Kimber J: An overview of the use of urine, hair, sweat and saliva to detect drug use. Drug Alcohol Rev 23(2):213–217, 2004 15370028

Edelbrock C, Costello AJ, Dulcan MK, et al: Parent-child agreement on child psychiatric symptoms assessed via structured interview. J Child Psychol Psychiatry 27(2):181–190, 1986 3958075

Ellis BR: Juvenile Automated Substance Abuse Evaluation (JASAE). Clarkston, MI, ADE Inc., 1987

Giedd JN: Structural magnetic resonance imaging of the adolescent brain. Ann N Y Acad Sci 1021:77–85, 2004 15251877

Grella CE, Hser Y-I, Joshi V, et al: Drug treatment outcomes for adolescents with co-morbid mental and substance use disorders. J Nerv Ment Dis 189(6):384–392, 2001 11434639

Hamilton CM, Strader LC, Pratt JG, et al: The PhenX Toolkit: get the most from your measures. Am J Epidemiol 174(3):253–260, 2011 21749974

Harrell A, Wirtz PM: Screening for adolescent problem drinking: validation of a multidimensional instrument for case identification. Psychological Assessment 1:61–63, 1989

Inwald RE, Brobst MA, Morissey RF: Identifying and predicting adolescent behavioral problems by using a new profile. Juvenile Justice Digest 14:1–9, 1986

Ivens C, Rehm LP: Assessment of childhood depression: correspondence between reports by child, mother, and father. J Am Acad Child Adolesc Psychiatry 27(6):738–747, 1988 3198560

Kaminer Y, Winters KC: Proposed DSM-5 substance use disorders for adolescents: if you build it, will they come? Am J Addict 21(3):280–281, author reply 282, 2012 22494232

Kaminer Y, Wagner E, Plummer B, et al: Validation of the Teen Addiction Severity Index (T-ASI): preliminary findings. Am J Addict 2(3):250–254, 1993

Kaminer Y, Blitz C, Burleson JA, et al: The Teen Treatment Services Review (T-TSR). J Subst Abuse Treat 15(4):291–300, 1998 9650137

Knight JR, Sherritt L, Shrier LA, et al: Validity of the CRAFFT substance abuse screening test among adolescent clinic patients. Arch Pediatr Adolesc Med 156(6):607–614, 2002 12038895

Knight JR, Sherritt L, Harris SK, et al: Validity of brief alcohol screening tests among adolescents: a comparison of the AUDIT, POSIT, CAGE, and CRAFFT. Alcohol Clin Exp Res 27(1):67–73, 2003 12544008

Latimer WW, Winters KC, Stinchfield RD: Screening for drug abuse among adolescents in clinical and correctional settings using the Problem-Oriented Screening Instrument for Teenagers. Am J Drug Alcohol Abuse 23(1):79–98, 1997 9048149

Leccese M, Waldron HB: Assessing adolescent substance use: a critique of current measurement instruments. J Subst Abuse Treat 11(6):553–563, 1994 7884839

Levy S, Weiss R, Sherritt L, et al: An electronic screen for triaging adolescent substance use by risk levels. JAMA Pediatr 168(9):822–828, 2014 25070067

Martino S, Grilo CM, Fehon DC: Development of the Drug Abuse Screening Test for Adolescents (DAST-A). Addict Behav 25(1):57–70, 2000 10708319

Masten AS, Faden VB, Zucker RA, et al: Underage drinking: a developmental framework. Pediatrics 121 (suppl 4):S235–S251, 2008 18381492

Meyers K, Hagan TA, McDermott P, et al: Factor structure of the Comprehensive Adolescent Severity Inventory (CASI): results of reliability, validity, and generalizability analyses. Am J Drug Alcohol Abuse 32(3):287–310, 2006 16864465

Miller G: Adolescent Substance Abuse Subtle Screening Inventory–2. Springville, IN, SASSI Institute, 2002

Moberg DP: Screening for alcohol and other drug problems using the Adolescent Alcohol and Drug Involvement Scale (AADIS). Madison, Center for Health Policy and Program Evaluation, University of Wisconsin–Madison, 2003

National Institute on Alcohol Abuse and Alcoholism: Alcohol Screening and Brief Intervention for Youth: A Practitioner's Guide (NIH Publ No 11-7805). National Institute on Alcohol Abuse and Alcoholism, 2011. Available at: http://pubs.niaaa.nih.gov/publications/Practitioner/YouthGuide/YouthGuide.pdf. Accessed April 26, 2019.

National Institute on Drug Abuse: Principles of Adolescent Substance Use Disorder Treatment: A Research-Based Guide (NIH Publ No 14-7953). Bethesda, MD, National Institute on Drug Abuse, 2014

Noam GG, Houlihan J: Developmental dimensions of DSM-III diagnoses in adolescent psychiatric patients. Am J Orthopsychiatry 60(3):371–378, 1990 2382690

Rahdert E (ed): The Adolescent Assessment/Referral System Manual (DHHS Publ No ADM 91-1735). Rockville, MD, National Institute on Drug Abuse, 1991

Reich W, Shayla JJ, Taibelson C: The Diagnostic Interview for Children and Adolescents—Revised (DICA-R). St. Louis, MO, Washington University, 1992

Rey JM, Schrader E, Morris-Yates A: Parent-child agreement on children's behaviours reported by the Child Behaviour Checklist (CBCL). J Adolesc 15(3):219–230, 1992 1447409

Shaffer D, Fisher P, Dulcan MK, et al: The NIMH Diagnostic Interview Schedule for Children Version 2.3 (DISC-2.3): description, acceptability, prevalence rates, and performance in the MECA Study. Methods for the Epidemiology of Child and Adolescent Mental Disorders Study. J Am Acad Child Adolesc Psychiatry 35(7):865–877, 1996 8768346

Shoham V, Insel TR: Rebooting for whom? Portfolios, technology, and personalized intervention. Perspect Psychol Sci 6(5):478–482, 2011 26168199

Skinner H: Development and Validation of a Lifetime Alcohol Consumption Assessment Procedure: Substudy No 1248. Toronto, ON, Canada, Addiction Research Foundation, 1982

Streeter CL, Franklin C: Psychological and family differences between middle class and low income dropouts: a discriminant analysis. The High School Journal 74(4):211–219, 1991

Tarter RE, Laird SB, Bukstein O, et al: Validation of the adolescent drug use screening inventory: preliminary findings. Psychology of Addictive Behaviors 6:322–236, 1992

Wanberg K: User's Guide to the Adolescent Self-Assessment Profile–II (ASAP-II). Arvada, CO, Center for Addictions Research and Evaluation, 1998

Waters E, Stewart-Brown S, Fitzpatrick R: Agreement between adolescent self-report and parent reports of health and well-being: results of an epidemiological study. Child Care Health Dev 29(6):501–509, 2003 14616908

Weissman MM, Wickramaratne P, Warner V, et al: Assessing psychiatric disorders in children. Discrepancies between mothers' and children's reports. Arch Gen Psychiatry 44(8):747–753, 1987 3632247

White HR, Labouvie EW: Towards the assessment of adolescent problem drinking. J Stud Alcohol 50(1):30–37, 1989 2927120

Winters KC: Development of an adolescent alcohol and other drug abuse screening scale: Personal Experience Screening Questionnaire. Addict Behav 17(5):479–490, 1992 1332434

Winters KC, Arria A: Adolescent brain development and drugs. Prev Res 18(2):21–24, 2011 22822298

Winters KC, Henly GA: Adolescent Diagnostic Interview Schedule and Manual. Los Angeles, CA, Western Psychological Services, 1993

Winters KC, Henly GA: Personal Experience Inventory and Manual. Los Angeles, CA, Western Psychological Services, 1994

Winters KC, Kaminer Y: Screening and assessing adolescent substance use disorders in clinical populations. J Am Acad Child Adolesc Psychiatry 47(7):740–744, 2008 18574399

Winters KC, Martin CS, Chung T: Substance use disorders in DSM-V when applied to adolescents. Addiction 106(5):882–884, discussion 895–897, 2011a 21477236

Winters KC, Toomey T, Nelson TF, et al: Screening for alcohol problems among 4-year colleges and universities. J Am Coll Health 59(5):350–357, 2011b 21500052

Winters KC, Botzet A, Lee S: Assessing adolescent substance use problems and other areas of functioning: state of the art, in Brief Interventions for Adolescent Alcohol and Substance Abuse. Edited by Monti PM, Colby SM, O'Leary Tevyaw T. New York, Guilford, 2018, pp 83–107

4

Primary Care and Pediatric Settings

Screening, Brief Intervention, and Referral to Treatment (SBIRT)

Areej Hassan, M.D., M.P.H.

Sion K. Harris, Ph.D.

John Rogers Knight, M.D.

Substance use among adolescents is a serious public health problem associated with significant morbidity and mortality. Alcohol and other drug use is strongly linked to the leading causes of death (motor vehicle crashes, falls, suicide, overdoses, and homicide) in this age group. Substance-abusing adolescents are also at higher risk for other health and social consequences, including assaults and violence, teen pregnancy, sexually transmitted infections, depression, and school failure and dropout (Adrian and Barry 2003; Berg et al. 2013;

Brook et al. 2012; DuRant et al. 1999; Levy et al. 2009). Harm occurs at all levels of consumption—no amount of use is "safe." The younger an adolescent initiates substance use, the more likely it is that drug dependence or addiction will develop in adulthood (Hingson et al. 2006); moreover, the earlier within adolescence that use starts, the greater the likelihood that a substance use disorder (SUD) will emerge during adolescence (Winters and Lee 2008). These concerns are reflected in the Healthy People 2020 objectives, which call for reducing adolescent substance use (U.S. Department of Health and Human Services 2019).

According to the 2017 Youth Risk Behavior Survey, nearly two-thirds (60.4%) of high school students have tried alcohol and over one-third (35.6%) have tried marijuana by senior year of high school; 29.8% reported current (past 30 days) alcohol use, with smaller numbers reporting current binge drinking (13.0%) and current marijuana use (19.8%) (Centers for Disease Control and Prevention 2017). Among the 64.5% of students who drove a car or other vehicle during the 30 days prior to the survey, 13% had used marijuana at least once prior to driving, and 5.5% had drank alcohol; 16.5% had ridden in a car with a driver who had been drinking alcohol (Centers for Disease Control and Prevention 2017).

There have been some changing trends to note in recent years. First, although cannabis remains the illicit drug most commonly used by adolescents in the United States, numbers had been declining until 2014. Concerns about adolescent cannabis use have correlated with changing policies that may contribute to changes in availability and/or perceived risk of use. To date, 33 states have legalized cannabis for "medical" use, and 11 states allow recreational use (Berke and Gould 2019). Since the mid-2000s, perceived risk of cannabis use has fallen markedly among students in 8th, 10th, and 12th grades, and these declines have continued (Johnston et al. 2018). Second, electronic or "e-vapor" products, which deliver nicotine via vapor, continue to attract adolescents using flavored nicotine. Almost half (42.2%) of students have ever tried vaping, and 13.2% currently vape (Centers for Disease Control and Prevention 2017). Finally, misuse of prescription pain medications continues to remain a significant concern; 14% of students reported they had taken prescription pain medicine without a doctor's prescription or differently than how a doctor told them to use it one or more times during their life (Centers for Disease Control and Prevention 2017). Deaths from opioid overdose have increased in recent years and have been identified as a significant public health burden in the United States.

Prevention and early intervention are critical strategies for reducing adolescent substance use and associated negative outcomes. With more than 80% of adolescents seeing a primary care provider (PCPs) yearly, PCPs are uniquely positioned to provide an opportunity for adolescents to have a private conversation and teachable moment about sensitive topics with a trusted adult (McCarty et al. 2019; National Center for Health Statistics 2016). Research has found that adolescents consider physicians to be an authoritative source of knowledge about alcohol and other drugs and are receptive to discussing substance use (Harris et al. 2009).

Over the past decade, there has been growing interest and research in an integrated approach called Screening, Brief Intervention, and Referral to Treatment (SBIRT) as a means of addressing adolescent substance use (Babor et al. 2007; Ozechowski et al. 2016; Substance Abuse and Mental Health Services Administration 2011). By using rapid screening and assessment tools, clinicians can quickly screen (S) adolescents for use and assess the extent of their use, provide an immediate brief intervention (BI), and determine need for follow-up or referral to treatment (RT). Although specific SBIRT screening tools and intervention strategies have well-documented efficacy for adult alcohol use, fewer studies of SBIRT efficacy have been conducted in the adolescent age group (Bertholet et al. 2005; Jonas et al. 2012; Kaner et al. 2018; O'Donnell et al. 2014). However, given ongoing emerging research and the minimal cost and potential benefit of this approach, standards for adolescent health care continue to incorporate SBIRT (Levy 2014).

Despite recommendations from the American Academy of Pediatrics (AAP) and the National Institute on Alcohol Abuse and Alcoholism (NIAAA) to use SBIRT as part of health supervision visits, actual practices are inconsistent (Committee on Substance Use and Prevention 2016; National Institute on Alcohol Abuse and Alcoholism 2011). The most frequently cited barriers to screening are lack of time, insufficient training, and lack of familiarity with standardized tools (Van Hook et al. 2007). To address these barriers, screening must be easy to administer and accurately distinguish between risk groups so that a clinician can quickly determine the appropriate level of intervention. Similarly, a simplified, practical approach to brief intervention is critical to support widespread implementation. This chapter serves as a research-informed guide for providers to incorporate the SBIRT framework during adolescent health visits.

Screening and Screening Tools

The primary goal of screening is to identify adolescents at high risk for an SUD, leading to a rapid assessment that places the adolescent on a spectrum of substance use experience from abstinence to SUD in order to administer an appropriate clinical intervention ranging from positive reinforcement to treatment program referrals. Using a validated developmentally appropriate screening tool is critical to accurate assessment of use, given that even experienced health care providers often underestimate level of use when relying on clinical impressions alone (Stevens et al. 2008; Wilson et al. 2004).

Although current recommendations from professional organizations recommend screening at health maintenance visits, there is research to show that 1) positive screens for problematic use are higher among patients presenting for urgent care and follow-up visits and 2) providers are more likely to engage in an active intervention during a sick or follow-up visit in comparison to a routine well visit (Hassan et al. 2009; Knight et al. 2007b). Adolescents with problematic use may miss their routine visits and instead present with acute problems (such as sexually transmitted infections or injuries), suggesting that providers may miss opportunities to provide appropriate substance use interventions if screening is limited only to well visits. Providers should strongly consider incorporating screening when seeing adolescents with concerns that may be related to alcohol (e.g., injuries, sexually transmitted infections, gastrointestinal problems, chronic pain), concerns related to change in behavior (e.g., change in grades, increased oppositional behavior, missed school), and concerns related to mental health (e.g., depression, anxiety).

Screening can be done face-to-face between provider and patient or via self-administered screens (computer or paper). Adolescents prefer self-administered screens and report greater honesty when completing the screen on their own even when they know that their provider will have access to results (Knight et al. 2007a). Self-administered screening prior to the appointment also adds an additional benefit of more time available during the visit for focused counseling and intervention between the provider and patient.

Whatever the route of administration, adolescents should be assured of confidentiality, which has been shown to improve accuracy of reported risk behaviors (Ford et al. 1997). If the screening is taking place in person, providers should have the parent (or guardian or friend) leave the room for the confidential part of the visit. Similarly, if the adolescent is filling out the screen on paper or on a computer, he or she should be in a private area of the office without a parent present.

The best screening tools are usually those that consist of the fewest number of validated questions that can elicit accurate and reliable responses. There are several validated, developmentally appropriate substance use screening tools that can be used in the adolescent population as part of a primary care visit. An overview of recommended tools is presented in Table 4–1 (see Chapter 3 for a listing of additional screening tools).

CRAFFT 2.0

CRAFFT 2.0 is a revised, updated, and recently revalidated version of the original CRAFFT screen that has been validated in a number of research studies and found to have good sensitivity and specificity for identifying adolescents with symptoms that may meet DSM-5 criteria for an SUD (Cummins et al. 2003; Knight et al. 2002; Mitchell et al. 2014; Subramaniam et al. 2010). CRAFFT is a mnemonic for the key words in the six screening questions: CAR, RELAX, ALONE, FORGET, FAMILY/FRIENDS, and TROUBLE. This updated version begins with three past-12-month frequency-of-use questions regarding alcohol, marijuana, and other drugs. The answers that patients provide to these three questions determine which of the six original CRAFFT questions should be asked. These opening questions help to shorten the screening process if there is no prior use of substances, by employing a skip pattern: patients who have no past-12-month use answer the CAR question only. Patients who provide an answer of 1 or more days to any of the opening questions are asked all six CRAFFT questions. Each "yes" response to the CRAFFT questions is scored 1 point. Responses to the six-item screen are totaled to determine a final CRAFFT score to determine low, medium, or high risk levels.

Regardless of previous alcohol or drug use, all patients should be asked the CAR question ("Have you ever ridden in a CAR driven by someone [including yourself] who was 'high' or had been using alcohol or drugs?") Alcohol-

Table 4–1. Screening tools for adolescent substance use

Screen	Questions	Scoring
CRAFFT (alcohol/drug)	*Introductory quick screen for ANY use:* During the past 12 months did you… 1. Drink any alcohol (more than a few sips)? (Do not count sips of alcohol taken during family or religious events.) 2. Smoke any marijuana or hashish? 3. Use anything else to get high? (anything else includes illegal, over-the-counter, and prescription drugs, and things that you sniff or "huff") *Questions for ALL regardless of use:* 1. Have you ever ridden in a CAR driven by someone (including yourself) who was "high" or had been using alcohol or drugs? *Follow-up questions for those with ANY use:* 2. Do you ever use alcohol or drugs to RELAX, feel better about yourself, or fit in? 3. Do you ever use alcohol or drugs while you are by yourself, or ALONE? 4. Do you ever FORGET things you did while using alcohol or drugs? 5. Do your FAMILY or FRIENDS ever tell you that you should cut down on your drinking or drug use? 6. Have you ever gotten into TROUBLE while you were using alcohol or drugs?	Each "yes" = 1 point on C, R, A, F, T items. *Low risk:* No use in past 12 months, score of 0 *Medium risk:* No use in past 12 months and "yes" to CAR question OR Positive use in past 12 months and score 2 *High risk:* Positive use in past 12 months and score ≥2

Table 4–1. Screening tools for adolescent substance use *(continued)*

Screen	Questions	Scoring
NIAAA screen (alcohol)	*Elementary school age (9–11 years):* 1. Do you have any friends who drank beer, wine, or any drink containing alcohol in the past year? 2. How about you—have you ever had more than a few sips of beer, wine, or any drink containing alcohol? *Middle school age (11–14 years):* 1. Do you have any friends who drank beer, wine, or any drink containing alcohol in the past year? 2. How about you—in the past year, on how many days have you had more than a few sips of beer, wine, or any drink containing alcohol? *High school age (14–18 years):* 1. In the past year, on how many days have you had more than a few sips of beer, wine, or any drink containing alcohol? 2. If your friends drink, how many drinks do they usually drink on an occasion?	*If age is ≤11:* High risk: any drinking *If age is 12–15:* Moderate risk: 1–5 days High risk: ≥6 days *If age is 16:* Low risk: 1–5 days Moderate risk: 6–11 days High risk: ≥12 days *If age is 17:* Low risk: 1–5 days Moderate risk: 6–23 days High risk: ≥24 days *If age is 18:* Low risk: 1–12 days Moderate risk: 12–51 days High risk: ≥52 days

Table 4–1.   Screening tools for adolescent substance use (*continued*)

Screen	Questions	Scoring
AUDIT (alcohol)	1. How often do you have a drink containing alcohol?	Score for each question ranges from 0 to 4, with 4 being highest risk.
	2. How many drinks containing alcohol do you have on a typical day when you are drinking?	*Age is 18 or younger:*
	3. How often do you have 5 or more drinks on one occasion?	Alcohol problem use: 2
	4. How often during the last year have you found that you were not able to stop drinking once you had started?	Alcohol abuse or dependence: ≥3
	5. How often during the last year have you failed to do what was normally expected of you because of drinking?	
	6. How often during the last year have you needed a first drink in the morning to get yourself going after a heavy drinking session?	
	7. How often during the last year have you had a feeling of guilt or remorse after drinking?	
	8. How often during the last year have you been unable to remember what happened the night before because of your drinking?	
	9. Have you or someone else been injured because of your drinking?	
	10. Has a relative, friend, doctor, or other health care worker been concerned about your drinking or suggested you cut down?	

Table 4–1. Screening tools for adolescent substance use *(continued)*

Screen	Questions	Scoring
S2BI (alcohol/drug)	In the past year, how many times (never; once or twice; monthly; weekly or more) have you used: Tobacco? Alcohol? Marijuana? **STOP if answers to all previous questions are "never"** In the past year, how many times (never; once or twice; monthly; weekly or more) have you used: Prescription drugs that were not prescribed for you (such as pain medication or Adderall)? Illegal drugs (such as cocaine or ecstasy)? Inhalants (such as nitrous oxide)? Herbs or synthetic drugs (such as salvia, "K2," or bath salts)?	*No use:* "never" *No SUD:* "once or twice" *Mild or moderate SUD:* "monthly" *Severe SUD:* "weekly or more"

Note. AUDIT = Alcohol Use Disorders Identification Test; NIAAA = National Institute on Alcohol Abuse and Alcoholism; S2BI = Screening to Brief Intervention Tool; SUD = substance use disorder.

associated motor vehicle crashes are a leading cause of death among adolescents (Gonzales et al. 2014; National Center for Injury Prevention and Control 2016). Therefore, addressing riding risk is an important point of intervention that has the potential to save many young lives.

NIAAA Screen

The NIAAA has developed a two-item screening guide with two age-specific questions related to friends' drinking and personal drinking (National Institute on Alcohol Abuse and Alcoholism 2011). The versions of the scale for ages 9–11 and ages 11–14 start by first asking questions about friends' use to introduce the topic in a less threatening way before asking about personal use; in older adolescents this order is reversed. The questions differ slightly based on target age group. Any drinking by friends should increase concern about the patient's personal drinking, but ultimately the adolescent's risk level (low, moderate, high) is assessed by age-sensitive cutoff points of personal use.

AUDIT

The Alcohol Use Disorders Identification Test (AUDIT) is a 10-question instrument that explores alcohol-related behaviors (Babor et al. 2001). Although the AUDIT was originally designed for adults, research has supported its use in adolescents using a lower threshold to identify problematic alcohol use. Each item has a score ranging from 0 to 4; responses are summed, and the total score correlates with risk. A score of 2 raises concern for alcohol problem use, and score of 3 or more raises concern for alcohol abuse or dependence.

S2BI (Screening to Brief Intervention Tool)

The Screening to Brief Intervention Tool (S2BI) is a brief screening tool that can be used to identify adolescents with severe substance use (Levy et al. 2014). Adolescents answer three initial screening questions, and those with *any* previous use of tobacco, alcohol, or marijuana complete four additional questions about use of other substances. Frequency of use has been found to correspond with DSM-5 diagnoses; adolescents who report monthly use may meet criteria for mild or moderate SUD, and those reporting weekly or more frequent use may meet criteria for severe SUD.

* * *

It is important to note that regardless of the screen used during the visit, providers should further probe adolescents, especially those in moderate and highest risk categories, to gather more history regarding specific behaviors, risks taken, patterns of use, and associated consequences. The screening tools themselves are not formal diagnostic instruments. DSM-5 remains the gold standard for diagnosis based on evidence of impaired control, social impairment, risky use, and pharmacological criteria (Box 4–1) (American Psychiatric Association 2013). The severity of the SUD (mild, moderate, severe) is determined on the basis of 11 criteria. Although providers may choose to obtain laboratory drug testing as part of their assessment, it is a scientifically complex and intrusive procedure that provides very limited information in the diagnosis of a SUD.

Box 4–1.   DSM-5 Criteria for Alcohol Use Disorder

A. A problematic pattern of alcohol use leading to clinically significant impairment or distress, as manifested by at least two of the following, occurring within a 12-month period:

1. Alcohol is often taken in larger amounts or over a longer period than was intended.
2. There is a persistent desire or unsuccessful efforts to cut down or control alcohol use.
3. A great deal of time is spent in activities necessary to obtain alcohol, use alcohol, or recover from its effects.
4. Craving, or a strong desire or urge to use alcohol.
5. Recurrent alcohol use resulting in a failure to fulfill major role obligations at work, school, or home.
6. Continued alcohol use despite having persistent or recurrent social or interpersonal problems caused or exacerbated by the effects of alcohol.
7. Important social, occupational, or recreational activities are given up or reduced because of alcohol use.
8. Recurrent alcohol use in situations in which it is physically hazardous.
9. Alcohol use is continued despite knowledge of having a persistent or recurrent physical or psychological problem that is likely to have been caused or exacerbated by alcohol.
10. Tolerance, as defined by either of the following:

a. A need for markedly increased amounts of alcohol to achieve intoxication or desired effect.

b. A markedly diminished effect with continued use of the same amount of alcohol.

11. Withdrawal, as manifested by either of the following:

a. The characteristic withdrawal syndrome for alcohol (refer to Criteria A and B of the criteria set for alcohol withdrawal).

b. Alcohol (or a closely related substance, such as a benzodiazepine) is taken to relieve or avoid withdrawal symptoms.

Specify if:

In early remission: After full criteria for alcohol use disorder were previously met, none of the criteria for alcohol use disorder have been met for at least 3 months but for less than 12 months (with the exception that Criterion A4, "Craving, or a strong desire or urge to use alcohol," may be met).

In sustained remission: After full criteria for alcohol use disorder were previously met, none of the criteria for alcohol use disorder have been met at any time during a period of 12 months or longer (with the exception that Criterion A4, "Craving, or a strong desire or urge to use alcohol," may be met).

Specify if:

In a controlled environment: This additional specifier is used if the individual is in an environment where access to alcohol is restricted.

Specify current severity:

Mild: Presence of 2–3 symptoms.

Moderate: Presence of 4–5 symptoms.

Severe: Presence of 6 or more symptoms.

Source.   Adapted from American Psychiatric Association: *Diagnostic and Statistical Manual of Mental Disorders,* 5th Edition, Arlington, VA, American Psychiatric Association, 2013. Copyright © 2013 American Psychiatric Association. Used with permission.

Brief Interventions

All adolescents may benefit from brief counseling focused on substance use, even those who have never tried alcohol or other drugs, as any delay in initiation allows for further brain development and neuronal maturation and reduces risk for an SUD later in life (Hingson et al. 2006). Brief interventions are dialogues initiated by providers encouraging patients to make healthy choices and prevent, reduce, or stop risk behaviors. Interventions should be tailored by the provider on the basis of individual screening results.

While intervention components vary in published studies, principles of motivational interviewing have been found to be helpful. For more information on motivational interviewing and brief interventions, see Chapter 13.

Results of systematic reviews examining the impact of brief interventions on adolescent substance use are mixed mainly because of differing study objectives, medical settings, context of delivery, intervention features, and outcome measures. There has been evidence to show that brief interventions can delay or reduce adolescent substance use when used in primary care settings. In a study of more than 2,000 adolescent primary care patients with no previous substance use, Harris et al. (2012) found that a brief computer-facilitated screening and brief advice protocol addressing substance use risk had a significant impact on initiation of substance use, compared with adolescents receiving usual care. Those who received the intervention had a 44% and 53% lower rate of initiating drinking by 1-year follow-up in the United States and the Czech Republic, respectively (Harris et al. 2012). In Brazil, adolescent primary care patients who received 2–3 minutes of brief physician advice along with printed information had significantly less increase in substance use and associated problems at 6-month follow-up (De Micheli et al. 2004). Similarly, a U.S.-based study found that adolescents receiving a computerized motivational intervention addressing cannabis use had a lower initiation rate (among previous nonusers) and lower frequency of use (among previous users) at both 3- and 6-month follow-up visits (Walton et al. 2014). Finally, Newton et al. (2018) completed a systematic review of 11 brief alcohol interventions aimed at adolescents in primary care settings, some with targeted intervention approach and others done universally. The authors found that brief interventions using both approaches can result in positive changes in alcohol-related outcomes, although this was not a consistent finding in all studies (Newton et al. 2018).

Although there is no established gold standard intervention, there are existing algorithms that providers can use to guide intervention after adolescents have been screened and assessed for substance use. The two most commonly used algorithms come from the AAP and the NIAAA (Committee on Substance

Use and Prevention 2016; National Institute on Alcohol Abuse and Alcoholism 2011). Regardless of which screening tool is used, the brief intervention strategy used remains consistent as it correlates to reported substance use severity. Interventions range from giving praise and encouragement for those with no substance use, promoting patient strengths while providing clear advice and education about risks for adolescents with previous use, and implementing brief interventions using motivational interviewing elements and possible referral to treatment for those with high-risk use.

Case Vignettes

Low Risk

Adolescents who report no use of alcohol or drugs in the previous year and have never ridden with an impaired driver are considered at "low risk." It is recommended that providers give positive reinforcement, including praise and encouragement for making a good decision regarding their health. Providers can also use this opportunity to discuss risks of driving and riding risks and help adolescents develop a safe plan to get home ahead of time, such as outlined in the Contract for Life (Students Against Destructive Decisions; https://crafft.org/contract). Providers should inform the adolescents that they can return at any time if they initiate use or have further questions. Confidentiality should be emphasized prior to discussion.

> Neela is a 16-year-old girl who comes in for her annual physical examination in order to participate on the tennis team. She has a history of mild intermittent asthma. She denies all previous substance use—she denies that she has ever drunk alcohol, denies ever smoking marijuana, and denies that she has used any other drugs to get high. She has never ridden in a car with an impaired driver. She has attended two parties in the last year where other students had been drinking.
>
> Her PCP begins: "I wanted to begin by telling you that part of your visit with me is always considered confidential. That means that anything you tell me will not be shared with others unless I think there is a risk to your safety or someone else's safety. Should that happen, I will let you know, and we will figure out a plan together of what the next steps will be.
>
> I'm glad to hear that you are not drinking or using any drugs. I think that's a smart decision and hope that you will continue to make good choices re-

garding your health. I do want to talk to you about car safety. For your own safety, never get in a car with someone who has been drinking or using drugs, even if that person doesn't seem drunk or high. Always try to make arrangements ahead of time for a safe ride home. Some of my patients identify a friend or another adult they can call for backup. Others have talked to their parents and have agreed that they can always call for a ride with no questions or discussion until the next day. Think about what you would do and try to make a plan for safe rides home.

I want you to know if things ever change, you can always come back and ask me more questions. I'm here to keep you healthy, not to pass judgment."

Medium (or Moderate) Risk

Adolescents who have ridden with an impaired driver or those who have tried substances in the past but whose use is infrequent and constitutes a low likelihood of an SUD are considered at "medium risk" (or "moderate risk"). For these adolescents, providers should discuss risks of substance use, along with brief advice to avoid further use. A succinct message to stop substance use because of negative health risks may lead to decreased use or abstinence among adolescents. Brief motivational interviewing aimed at having the adolescent recognize problems secondary to substance use can be helpful, with a plan to follow up in 1 month.

Marcus is a 16-year-old boy who comes into the office after injuring his ankle the night before the visit. He has had various sports-related injuries in the past but no other diagnoses. On further questioning, he admits he has been high on several occasions, although not at time of injury. He admits to trying alcohol in the past, but denies that he has ever "gotten drunk." He has never used any other drugs other than marijuana, which he began to use about 6 months ago. He denies any substance use in the last 3 months, which coincides with the start of the football season. He admits that he thinks he does not play as well when he is using marijuana.

His PCP says: "Thank you for being honest about trying alcohol and marijuana in the past. I'm glad to see that you haven't used substances in the past 3 months. As your doctor, my recommendation is to not use alcohol, marijuana, or other drugs because it can harm your developing brain, it can interfere with your learning at school, and, as you have recognized, it can be especially detrimental to your athletic ability and eligibility. You have the potential to be a great player, and I would hate to see alcohol or drugs get in the way of this goal. Would you be willing to try not using for the remainder of the season and then check in again with me?"

High Risk

If initial screening results correlate to "high risk," providers should always probe further to gain additional history. Example questions include "How much do you usually use—can you estimate the number of drinking days per month, and the number of drinks in a day?" Providers can use positive responses to screening questions as a way to gather more information—for example, "Can you tell me more about times that you have gotten into trouble when using substances?" Additional history can help the provider identify factors that can then be used as part of the brief intervention to enhance the adolescent's motivation to change behavior.

Brief interventions should combine personalized feedback and advice based on screening and assessment, discussion of the concerns or problems that adolescents have experienced as a result of their substance use, and motivational interviewing strategies aimed at helping the adolescent recognize that the benefits of behavior change outweigh benefits of continued use with concrete plan for behavior change. All patients should at a minimum be encouraged to follow up with their PCP, and, depending on level of risk, additional steps may include referrals, discussion with parents, and immediate interventions for acute care.

Katie is a 17-year-old girl who comes to the office to discuss emergency contraception. She reports that she was drunk at a party last night and had sex with a new male partner. She cannot remember if they used a condom. She is not currently on contraception; she used Plan B once in the past, about 6 months ago. She is otherwise healthy with no significant past medical history. She is a senior in high school, plays soccer, and is planning to attend college. She lives at home with her parents. She denies symptoms of depression or anxiety.

On screening, she reports that she drinks alcohol and has tried marijuana but has never used other drugs. On the CRAFFT, she answered yes to the RELAX, FORGET, and TROUBLE questions, giving her a score of 3. On follow-up assessment questions, Katie admits that there were several occasions when she has drunk in excess and been "wasted." She was suspended for 2 days because she brought a bottle of vodka to a school football game. Her parents found out after notification from the school and grounded her. She says that she drinks less than her friends and does not think that her drinking is a problem. She has never tried to quit drinking. After being asked whether she has any concerns about continued drinking, Katie pauses and then says that she is worried that her early acceptance to college may be revoked.

Her PCP responds: "Thank you for answering questions honestly. I'm concerned about your alcohol use. You told me that you have drunk in excess several times, which can lead to other risky situations, such as unprotected sex last night; this puts you at risk for sexually transmitted infections and/or unplanned pregnancy. You were recently suspended. Your parents have been concerned about your drinking. You have been so excited to move to New York for college, and I share your concern that alcohol use could get in the way of you achieving this and other things you care about. How would you feel about not drinking for a while?"

Katie says that she is not interested in quitting. She cannot imagine being the only one at a party with her friends not drinking. She does agree to limit herself to no more than two drinks and will make sure she has someone she can rely on for safe transportation among her friends. She agrees to return for follow-up in 2 weeks.

Referral to Treatment

Many adolescents who screen positive for substance use can be managed effectively in the primary care office. Adolescents who are found to have alcohol or drug dependence and those who repeatedly engage in substance-related high-risk behaviors that threaten their or other's safety (e.g., repeated driving while intoxicated) require referral to more intensive substance abuse treatment. See Chapter 6 for more information on treatment placement.

If more intensive treatment is needed, the provider must determine whether to involve parents in treatment planning. Many adolescents who seek care may request that their parents not be notified of their substance use. Extensive research documents the importance of confidentiality in promoting adolescent's access to health care, particularly for issues such as substance use (Ford et al. 1997, 1999; Reddy et al. 2002). Most professional medical organizations support confidential care for adolescents for a broad range of services, including pertaining to substance use (American College of Obstetricians and Gynecologists 1998; Confidential Health Services for Adolescents 1993; Ford et al. 2004). Laws differ in each state and define the extent of confidentiality. In many states, adolescents are allowed to seek treatment for substance use without parental consent. However, if adolescents are covered by their parents' health insurance, accessing treatment may still breach their confidentiality. With each patient, the provider must carefully weigh the risks of breaking confidentiality (i.e., losing therapeutic alliance with their patient) with the risks of maintaining it (i.e., continued high-risk behavior and failure to engage in treatment). If confidentiality is upheld, adolescents still may be able to access services through the school or community.

If there is concern about the imminent safety of an adolescent because of current substance use, this must be addressed directly and honestly both with the adolescent and with the parent. Providers should empathize with the adolescent but ultimately decide what is in the best interest of ensuring patient safety. Oftentimes, it is possible to reach an agreement with the adolescent about involving parents by offering to meet with both the parent and adolescent together and coming to an agreement on what details will be disclosed (Dakof et al. 2001).

Troubleshooting

Providers should have a safety protocol—that is, a list of signs of clinical deterioration (significant negative change in any aspect of functioning; "no show") and a safety plan if the adolescent shows indications of suicide risk and thus may require a more intensive intervention. Parents will need to be instructed to contact the provider for assistance and directions according to specific communication information included in the protocol.

Key Points

- Screening with evidence-based tools such as the CRAFFT test can identify youth at high risk for substance use disorder (SUD).

- Practical screening, brief intervention, and referral to treatment algorithms are available to guide primary care providers in addressing varied levels of substance use in adolescents.

- Providers must use their clinical judgment to weigh the risks and benefits of maintaining confidentiality when concerned about the adolescent's health and safety.

- Providers should familiarize themselves with substance use and SUD assessment and treatment resources in their community to ensure appropriate referrals and continuity of care.

References

Adrian M, Barry SJ: Physical and mental health problems associated with the use of alcohol and drugs. Subst Use Misuse 38(11–13):1575–1614, 2003 14582571

American College of Obstetricians and Gynecologists: ACOG educational bulletin. Confidentiality in adolescent health care. Number 249, August 1998. Int J Gynaecol Obstet 63(3):295–300, 1998 9989903

American Psychiatric Association: Diagnostic and Statistical Manual of Mental Disorders, 5th Edition. Arlington, VA. American Psychiatric Association, 2013

Babor TF, Higgins-Biddle JC, Saunders J, et al: AUDIT: The Alcohol Use Disorders Identification Test: Guidelines for Use in Primary Health Care, 2nd Edition. Geneva, World Health Organization, 2001

Babor TF, McRee BG, Kassebaum PA, et al: Screening, Brief Intervention, and Referral to Treatment (SBIRT): toward a public health approach to the management of substance abuse. Subst Abus 28(3):7–30, 2007 18077300

Berg N, Kiviruusu O, Karvonen S, et al: A 26-year follow-up study of heavy drinking trajectories from adolescence to mid-adulthood and adult disadvantage. Alcohol Alcohol 48(4):452–457, 2013 23531717

Berke J, Gould S: States where marijuana is legal. Business Insider, 2019. Available at: https://www.businessinsider.com/legal-marijuana-states-2018-1. Accessed April 26, 2019.

Bertholet N, Daeppen JB, Wietlisbach V, et al: Reduction of alcohol consumption by brief alcohol intervention in primary care: systematic review and meta-analysis. Arch Intern Med 165(9):986–995, 2005 15883236

Brook JS, Lee JY, Brown EN, et al: Comorbid trajectories of tobacco and marijuana use as related to psychological outcomes. Subst Abus 33(2):156–167, 2012 22489588

Centers for Disease Control and Prevention: Youth Risk Behavior Survey System. 2017. Available at: www.cdc.gov/yrbs. Accessed on April 26, 2019.

Committee on Substance Use and Prevention: Substance use screening, brief intervention, and referral to treatment (policy statement). Pediatrics 138(1):e20161210, 2016 27325638

Confidential Health Services for Adolescents: Confidential health services for adolescents. Council on Scientific Affairs, American Medical Association. JAMA 269(11):1420–1424, 1993 8441220

Cummins LH, Chan KK, Burns KM, et al: Validity of the CRAFFT in American-Indian and Alaska-Native adolescents: screening for drug and alcohol risk. J Stud Alcohol 64(5):727–732, 2003 14572196

Dakof GA, Tejeda M, Liddle HA: Predictors of engagement in adolescent drug abuse treatment. J Am Acad Child Adolesc Psychiatry 40(3):274–281, 2001 11288768

De Micheli D, Fisberg M, Formigoni ML: Study on the effectiveness of brief intervention for alcohol and other drug use directed to adolescents in a primary health care unit (in Portuguese). Rev Assoc Med Bras (1992) 50(3):305–313, 2004 15499485

DuRant RH, Smith JA, Kreiter SR, et al: The relationship between early age of onset of initial substance use and engaging in multiple health risk behaviors among young adolescents. Arch Pediatr Adolesc Med 153(3):286–291, 1999 10086407

Ford CA, Millstein SG, Halpern-Felsher BL, et al: Influence of physician confidentiality assurances on adolescents' willingness to disclose information and seek future health care: a randomized controlled trial. JAMA 278(12):1029–1034, 1997 9307357

Ford CA, Bearman PS, Moody J: Foregone health care among adolescents. JAMA 282(23):2227–2234, 1999 10605974

Ford CA, English A, Sigman G: Confidential Health Care for Adolescents: position paper for the Society for Adolescent Medicine. J Adolesc Health 35(2):160–167, 2004 15298005

Gonzales K, Roeber J, Kanny D, et al; Centers for Disease Control and Prevention (CDC): Alcohol-attributable deaths and years of potential life lost—11 States, 2006–2010. MMWR Morb Mortal Wkly Rep 63(10):213–216, 2014 24622285

Harris SK, Woods ER, Sherritt L, et al: A youth-provider connectedness measure for use in clinical intervention studies. J Adolesc Health 44 (2 suppl):S35–S36, 2009

Harris SK, Csémy L, Sherritt L, et al: Computer-facilitated substance use screening and brief advice for teens in primary care: an international trial. Pediatrics 129(6):1072–1082, 2012 22566420

Hassan A, Harris SK, Sherritt L, et al: Primary care follow-up plans for adolescents with substance use problems. Pediatrics 124(1):144–150, 2009 19564294

Hingson RW, Heeren T, Winter MR: Age at drinking onset and alcohol dependence: age at onset, duration, and severity. Arch Pediatr Adolesc Med 160(7):739–746, 2006 16818840

Johnston LD, Miech RA, O'Malley PM, et al: Monitoring the Future: National Survey Results on Drug Use: 1975–2017: Overview, Key Findings on Adolescent Drug Use. Ann Arbor, MI, Institute for Social Research, The University of Michigan, 2018

Jonas DE, Garbutt JC, Amick HR, et al: Behavioral counseling after screening for alcohol misuse in primary care: a systematic review and meta-analysis for the U.S. Preventive Services Task Force. Ann Intern Med 157(9):645–654, 2012 23007881

Kaner EF, Beyer FR, Muirhead C, et al: Effectiveness of brief alcohol interventions in primary care populations. Cochrane Database Syst Rev 2:CD004148, 2018 29476653

Knight JR, Sherritt L, Shrier LA, et al: Validity of the CRAFFT substance abuse screening test among adolescent clinic patients. Arch Pediatr Adolesc Med 156(6):607–614, 2002 12038895

Knight JR, Harris SK, Sherritt L, et al: Adolescents' preference for substance abuse screening in primary care practice. Subst Abus 28(4):107–117, 2007a 18077307

Knight JR, Harris SK, Sherritt L, et al: Prevalence of positive substance abuse screen results among adolescent primary care patients. Arch Pediatr Adolesc Med 161(11):1035–1041, 2007b 17984404

Levy S: Brief interventions for substance use in adolescents: still promising, still unproven. CMAJ 186(8):565–566, 2014 24733767

Levy S, Sherritt L, Gabrielli J, et al: Screening adolescents for substance use-related high-risk sexual behaviors. J Adolesc Health 45(5):473–477, 2009 19837353

Levy S, Weiss R, Sherritt L, et al: An electronic screen for triaging adolescent substance use by risk levels. JAMA Pediatr 168(9):822–828, 2014 25070067

McCarty CA, Levy S, Harris SK: Alcohol use screening and behavioral counseling with adolescents in primary care: a call to action. JAMA Pediatr 173(1):12–14, 2019 30422269

Mitchell SG, Kelly SM, Gryczynski J, et al: The CRAFFT cut-points and DSM-5 criteria for alcohol and other drugs: a reevaluation and reexamination. Subst Abus 35(4):376–380, 2014 25036144

National Center for Health Statistics: Health, United States, 2015: With Special Feature on Racial and Ethnic Health Disparities. National Center for Health Statistics, May 2016. Available from: https://www.ncbi.nlm.nih.gov/books/NBK367640/. Accessed April 26, 2019.

National Center for Injury Prevention and Control: Ten leading causes of injury deaths by age group highlighting unintentional injury deaths, United States—2016. 2016. Available at: https://www.cdc.gov/injury/images/lc-charts/leading_causes_of_death_highlighting_unintentional_2016_1040w800h.gif. Accessed April 26, 2019.

National Institute on Alcohol Abuse and Alcoholism: Alcohol Screening and Brief Intervention for Youth: A Practitioner's Guide (NIH Publ No 11-7805). National Institute on Alcohol Abuse and Alcoholism, 2011. Available at: http://pubs.niaaa.nih.gov/publications/Practitioner/YouthGuide/YouthGuide.pdf. Accessed April 26, 2019.

Newton AS, Mushquash C, Krank M, et al: When and how do brief alcohol interventions in primary care reduce alcohol use and alcohol-related consequences among adolescents? J Pediatr 197:221.e2–232.e2, 2018 29656865

O'Donnell A, Anderson P, Newbury-Birch D, et al: The impact of brief alcohol interventions in primary healthcare: a systematic review of reviews. Alcohol Alcohol 49(1):66–78, 2014 24232177

Ozechowski TJ, Becker SJ, Hogue A: SBIRT-A: Adapting SBIRT to maximize developmental fit for adolescents in primary care. J Subst Abuse Treat 62:28–37, 2016 26742723

Reddy DM, Fleming R, Swain C: Effect of mandatory parental notification on adolescent girls' use of sexual health care services. JAMA 288(6):710–714, 2002 12169074

Stevens J, Kelleher KJ, Gardner W, et al: Trial of computerized screening for adolescent behavioral concerns. Pediatrics 121(6):1099–1105, 2008 18519478

Students Against Destructive Decisions: The contract for life. Available at: https://crafft.org/contract. Accessed July 23, 2019.

Subramaniam M, Cheok C, Verma S, et al: Validity of a brief screening instrument-CRAFFT in a multiethnic Asian population. Addict Behav 35(12):1102–1104, 2010 20805016

Substance Abuse and Mental Health Services Administration: Screening, Brief Intervention and Referral to Treatment (SBIRT) in Behavioral Healthcare, 2011. Available at: https://www.samhsa.gov/sites/default/files/sbirtwhitepaper_0.pdf.

U.S. Department of Health and Human Services: Healthy People 2020: Substance abuse objectives. 2019. Available at https://www.healthypeople.gov/2020/topics-objectives/topic/substance-abuse/objectives. Accessed April 26, 2019.

Van Hook S, Harris SK, Brooks T, et al; New England Partnership for Substance Abuse Research: The "Six T's": barriers to screening teens for substance abuse in primary care. J Adolesc Health 40(5):456–461, 2007 17448404

Walton MA, Resko S, Barry KL, et al: A randomized controlled trial testing the efficacy of a brief cannabis universal prevention program among adolescents in primary care. Addiction 109(5):786–797, 2014 24372937

Wilson CR, Sherritt L, Gates E, et al: Are clinical impressions of adolescent substance use accurate? Pediatrics 114(5):e536–e540, 2004 15520086

Winters KC, Lee CY: Likelihood of developing an alcohol and cannabis use disorder during youth: association with recent use and age. Drug Alcohol Depend 92(1–3):239–247, 2008 17888588

Bioassays and Detection of Substances of Abuse in Youth

Albert J. Arias, M.D.

Wendy Welch, M.D., C.P.E.

Yifrah Kaminer, M.D., M.B.A.

The detection and confirmation of alcohol and other substances of abuse in adolescents has been challenging. There are two general classes of assessments: a) a subjective one based on self-report and/or collateral information with or without the use of specific rating scales (see Chapter 3 for more information on measurements), and b) laboratory or objective indicators of substance use such as drug urinalysis and body tissue (i.e., hair, skin, blood) testing. Relying on self-report of drug use in the adolescent population has been problematic. Youth in community, school, and justice system–related settings may either deny use or underreport the amounts, frequency, and latency of drug used (Buchan et al. 2002). Underreporting may be for legal reasons or may be due to family response, impact on social desirability, or other perceived consequences.

In contrast to self-report only, drug testing generates objective information about drug use.

In addition to chemically screening samples of patient fluids or tissue for drugs of abuse (or their metabolites), the clinician may gain information about the patient's status by testing other biological markers that correspond to drug and alcohol use. A *biomarker* is any material or substance used as an indicator of a biological state. Biomarkers may range from those that directly detect the substance and/or its metabolites to those that signal end-organ damage from chronic substance use. Biomarkers can be useful in working with adolescent clinical populations by contributing to screening and diagnostic efforts, and by identifying relapse, continued use, and occult use of substances in patients who have already been identified as having substance use disorders (SUDs).

Biomarkers, in conjunction with collateral history, clinical assessment and rating scales, aid in the screening and diagnosis of SUDs (Center for Substance Abuse Treatment 2006). Additionally, biomarker tests can be used in the home setting by parents and are available over the counter. In this chapter, we review ethical, legal, and practical considerations of drug testing for youth in school, home, and clinical settings.

Social Context of Youth Drug Testing

Illegal drug use commonly begins during the teenage years. Some adolescents are drinking alcohol while under the legal age (21 years in the United States or 18 and even 16 years in European countries, respectively). Parents are not usually aware of the extent and details of their teenagers' drug use. School and home drug testing in the United States has been in use for more than a decade. Parents, schools, and the legal system have been struggling with the following questions: What is the purpose of drug testing for youth? Is it legal to conduct drug testing for adolescents? How can testing be done effectively and confidentially? Can the results be utilized in ways that foster access to appropriate clinical assessments, triage, and referral?

School Drug Testing

The purpose of random student drug testing (RSDT) is preventive in nature and aims to keep U.S. youth safe, healthy, and drug free. More specifically,

RSDT programs have four primary goals: to deter and prevent use, to reinforce all other prevention efforts, to identify students who need help getting and staying drug free, and to prepare students for workplace drug testing (DuPont et al. 2013). One study estimated that about 14% of all U.S. school districts use RSDT in at least one of their high schools (Ringwalt et al. 2008). The use of RSDT in schools faced two important legal challenges. In 1995, the Supreme Court ruled that drug testing for athletes is constitutional (Knight and Levy 2007). Then in 2002, the Supreme Court ruled that schools can test any students involved in any extracurricular activities because, according to the majority opinion, it "is a reasonably effective means of addressing the School District's legitimate concerns in preventing, deterring, and detecting drug use" and does not violate the Fourth Amendment" (Knight and Levy 2007, p. 419). However, RSDT programs remain controversial, and the American Academy of Pediatrics' position is that there is not sufficient reason to justify these programs (Levy et al. 2014).

A recent review of the literature points out the mixed evidence supporting RSDT programs, which can be beneficial under certain circumstances. The review highlights the overall lack of rigorous evaluations of the effectiveness of RSDT programs, and also that they are most likely to be useful in preventing the development of SUDs when used in conjunction with a broad-based program that includes student assistance services in a nonpunitive fashion (DuPont et al. 2013).

Home Drug Testing

Parents usually resort to home drug testing after a child has repeatedly violated trust by continued drug use despite promises to quit. Findings of drugs and drug paraphernalia, and physical signs of drug use, signal to parents the need to take active measures. Clarifying and enforcing the expectation that adolescents are not permitted to use nicotine, alcohol, and other psychoactive drugs is essential. If the adolescent is in treatment for an SUD, the counselor, parent, and consenting youth should contract for home drug testing. An effective contract includes respectfully negotiating negative and positive consequences for drug use or non-use. These consequences might include curfew hours and restrictions on car use or social and entertainment opportunities. Refusal to give urine for analysis is considered a positive sample, which should activate the contracted consequences. Parents should be consistent and stand firm in light of expected manipulations, acting-out behaviors, or any effort to test their will. If they face difficulties, further consultation opportunities with the counselor and members of the treatment team should be available.

Concordance Among Reports

A common perception in assessing adolescents with SUDs is that relying solely on adolescent self-report is certain to result in data with limited reliability. Most adolescents are at least somewhat coerced into screening or assessment of their substance use. The majority of these youth do not perceive their levels of use as severe enough to warrant an intervention and consequently are reluctant to cooperate fully (Kaminer 1994). Self-reports may, however, provide reliable and valid information, *particularly when no legal contingencies for drug use are pending* (Barnea et al. 1987; Buchan et al. 2002; Burleson and Kaminer 2006). A study by Burleson and Kaminer (2006) examined the parent-child subjective agreement, as well as agreement with objective results (i.e., drug urinalysis), for adolescents with SUDs in an outpatient program. The agreement between urinalysis and youth self-report, while moderate, was higher than any agreement with parental assessments. Associations between urinalysis and self-report for cannabis use were highest ($r=0.64$ at a 3-month assessment, 0.69 at 9 months), followed by self-report and collateral informant's report ($r=0.49$ at 3 months, 0.55 at 9 months), and finally urinalysis and collateral informant's report ($r=0.28$ at 3 months, 0.43 at 9 months). Under these conditions, self-reports produce accurate information in at least 95% of adolescent alcohol and other substance abuse. Presumably, for these disorders, parents' reports identify very few additional cases (Cantwell et al. 1997).

Available Biomarkers

Biomarkers may be found in urine, hair, saliva, sweat, and blood. Traditionally, the most common drug test panel is the NIDA-5 panel used to identify the five drugs (opiates, phencyclidine [PCP], tetrahydrocannabinol [THC], cocaine, and amphetamines) mandated in federal workplace testing guidelines. However, over the last decade there has been a dramatic increase in the availability of more advanced and comprehensive point-of-care (POC) and laboratory-based drug testing. These panels can be tested in each of the aforementioned fluids. Screening urine tests consist of immunoassays using monoclonal antibodies against the specific drug or drug metabolite. Immunoassay tests have high sensitivity but lower specificity due to occasional cross-reactivity. Such qualitative tests are often all that is needed in a clinical setting.

Drug-use biomarker tests vary in their sensitivity and specificity depending on the method used and the sample source. Confirmation testing of a positive result is performed with gas or liquid chromatography and mass spectrometry, which detect the specific substance or its metabolite with high specificity. Screening tests available for office use tend to be reasonably sensitive and specific.

In-office screening is cost-effective, with most 5- to 12-panel tests costing less than $10. Although these qualitative screening tests will detect the presence of the substance above a threshold cutoff, they do not give quantitative information. In general, POC screening kits, combined with occasional use of regional laboratories for confirmatory testing, are all that is needed for most cases involving clinical management. Sending samples to a regional commercial laboratory is considerably more expensive (often costing between $100 and $1,000 for a 5- to 10-panel test) and results in a report of quantitative levels of substances and metabolites. This testing might be necessary for legal cases, as well as to resolve the discrepancy between self-report and on-site qualitative urine testing by confirming a continued decrease in drug levels for a heavy cannabis user. In forensic cases, the clinician should consult a medical review officer or a medical toxicologist. Many regional commercial toxicology laboratories offer free consultation with one of their toxicologists for clinical purposes.

Overview of Testing by Sample Source

Urine tests are the most cost-effective and widely available tests for substance use. They can detect a wide range of substances and can be done in the office or at home. However, falsification of urine tests is possible, especially when sample collection is unobserved (DuPont and Selavka 2008). When clinical information suggests tampering or adulteration, the clinician should order an observed test. Urine samples can be retained for about 1 year and can be retested if original results are disputed. The Internet has become a source of providing information about obtaining adulterants and urine substitutes to produce false-negative results (Greenfield and Hennessy 2008). The period of detection of most substances and their metabolites in urine is relatively short, often only 1–3 days, depending on substance type and acute versus chronic use. The level of the substance or of its metabolite in the urine is influenced by fluid consumption, enabling patients to obscure drug use through abrupt drinking of large amounts of fluids to dilute the urine sample (DuPont and Selavka 2008). Parents can easily obtain urine drug screening kits for in-home use at their local drug store or via the Internet. Some of these tests include indicators for urine tampering by testing for changes in pH, specific gravity, and creatinine. Measurement of temperature is another commonly used method of testing for urine tampering (i.e., the cup should feel warm when filled with fresh urine).

Saliva tests can be performed in the office. Saliva collection is easy and adulteration is difficult, but there is only a short window of detection (6–12 hours). Drugs are present in lower concentrations in saliva than in other fluids, except for blood, in which concentrations are equal to those in saliva (DuPont and Selavka 2008).

Hair testing accounts for the 90 days prior to when the hair sample is taken, with the exception of the 7 days that the hair requires to grow out of the follicle (hair grows approximately 1 cm per month). Usually the proximal 1.5 cm of hair strand is tested, accounting for approximately the last 90 days of drug use beginning about 7 days prior to the date the hair sample was taken. Hair testing can discriminate between the amount of substance used and the chronicity of use (DuPont and Selavka 2008). Hair testing is more resistant to tampering and falsification, and despite an alleged racial and hair color bias, none has been scientifically detected (Mieczkowski and Lersh 2002; Mieczkowski and Newel 2000). Perming, bleaching, and straightening treatments may alter drug levels in the hair. Hair testing is more expensive than other means, cannot be completed on site, is done by relatively few laboratories, and reveals only a limited number of substances. Home kits that test hair samples for cocaine, marijuana, opiates, ecstasy, amphetamine, and PCP are available.

For sweat testing, a patch is applied to a patient to prospectively test for substance use over a 1- to 3-week period. Substances enter the sweat from the bloodstream via passive diffusion (Cone 1997). As the water, oxygen, and carbon dioxide evaporate from the patch, traces of substance remain. The amount of the substance is not affected by fluid consumption. If the patch is removed or tampered with, it will pucker (De Giovanni and Fucci 2013). The patch's adhesive film also changes color when removed. The sweat patch is available from PharmChem, Inc. (www.pharmchek.com), which tests for cocaine, marijuana, opiates, amphetamines, methamphetamines, and PCP. Unlike urine testing, the patch can detect both the parent drug and its metabolite. An immunoassay screening test is followed by confirmation of any positive results via gas chromatography–mass spectrometry (GC-MS). The test is more expensive than urine or saliva testing, but less expensive than hair testing.

Direct testing of many substances can be performed on blood samples via immunoassay or GC-MS (Kerrigan and Phillips 2001). Testing blood samples may be a useful method for avoiding tampering (as can occur with urine samples) but is more costly. Substances in the blood are usually cleared within 12 hours (DuPont and Selavka 2008).

In the adolescent population, screening tests for episodic drug use (e.g., binge drinking during the weekends) would be particularly useful, as would a biomarker that could indicate low-level but chronic drug use. Because sensitivity and specificity data are calculated from an adult population, the results discussed are indicative of that population, and results must be extrapolated to the adolescent population until more studies are conducted.

Testing for Specific Drugs of Abuse

The properties of common biomarker tests for drug and alcohol use are described in Table 5–1.

Alcohol

For detecting alcohol consumption, breath analysis is a highly sensitive test with low cost, yet it is only effective for minutes to hours after drinking based on the amount consumed and the individual's metabolism (Greenfield and Hennessy 2008). Its best purpose is to determine use at a specific point in time rather than as a measure of chronic use.

Biomarkers for detecting use and relapse in alcohol use disorders are numerous, but there are specific limitations to their use. Alcohol biomarkers include serum γ-glutamyltransferase (GGT), aspartate transaminase (AST), alanine transaminase (ALT), mean corpuscular volume (MCV), carbohydrate-deficient transferrin (CDT), ethyl glucuronide (EtG), ethyl sulfate (EtS), and phosphatidylethanol (PEth).

Table 5–1. Properties of common drug screens

Drug of abuse	Sample type	Method of detection[a]	Approximate sensitivity (%)	Approximate specificity (%)	Common detection cutoff (ng/L)	Approximate window of detection for use
Alcohol	Blood	GGT	40–73	63–91		4 weeks
	Urine	CDT	40–63	80–93		3 weeks
		EtG	80.5	78.7		3–5 days
Cannabis	Urine	IA screen	73–97	83–99	50	72–96 hours
		CHRM	77.2	100		
Heavy chronic use						Up to about 5 weeks
Nicotine						
Cotinine	Urine	IA screen	98	97		3–4 days
	Saliva		93	95	10	3–4 days
Carbon monoxide	Breath (exhaled)					4–5 hours

Table 5–1. Properties of common drug screens *(continued)*

Drug of abuse	Sample type	Method of detection[a]	Approximate sensitivity (%)	Approximate specificity (%)	Common detection cutoff (ng/L)	Approximate window of detection for use
Benzodiazepines	Urine	IA screen	77–91	87–97	1,000	Varies based on half-life (often ≥24 hours)
		CHRM	8–23	97–100		
Opioids	Urine					
6-monoacetylmorphine		GC-MS				4–6 hours[b]
Morphine		IA screen	84–95	89.4–99	300	24 hours
		CHRM	41–73	96–100		
Buprenorphine		IA screen	88–100	91–100	2.5–10	48–56 hours
Norbuprenorphine						
Oxycodone		IA screen	75	92	1,000	1–3 days
Cocaine (via benzoylecgonine)	Urine	IA screen	72–98	88–99	300	8 hours
		CHRM	50–84	99–100	300	48–72 hours

Table 5–1. Properties of common drug screens *(continued)*

Drug of abuse	Sample type	Method of detection[a]	Approximate sensitivity (%)	Approximate specificity (%)	Common detection cutoff (ng/L)	Approximate window of detection for use
Amphetamines	Urine	IA screen	44–94	84–99	1,000	48 hours
		CHRM	54–71	98–99	500	48–72 hours
MDMA (ecstasy)[c]	Urine	IA screen	99.4[d]	97.8[d]	500	1–3 days

Note.   CDT =carbohydrate-deficient transferrin; CEDIA=cloned enzyme donor immunoassay; CHRM=chromatography methods other than GC-MS; EtG=ethyl glucuronide; GC-MS=gas chromatography–mass spectrometry; GGT=γ-glutamyl transferase; IA screen=immunoassay-based screening systems; MDMA=3,4-methylenedioxymethamphetamine.

[a]GC-MS is the gold standard for identifying substances and is usually assumed to be near 100% sensitive and 100% specific because it can detect and differentiate trace amounts of most substances. However, errors are possible because of sample mishandling or improper operation or maintenance of the GC-MS machines.

[b]Because of its very short half-life, heroin is usually not tested in blood or urine, but its metabolites 6-monoacetylmorphine and morphine can be detected for a brief window of time, allowing heroin use to be differentiated from morphine and codeine use.

[c]MDMA will cross-react as amphetamines with a number of in-office screening kits (Crouch et al. 2002).

[d]From Loor et al. 2002, using CEDIA multiplex assay.

Source.   Adapted and compiled from Benowitz 1996; Cooke et al. 2008; Ferrara et al. 1994; Korzec et al. 2005; Leino and Loo 2007; Manchikanti et al. 2011; Miller et al. 2006; Niemelä 2016; Substance Abuse and Mental Health Services Administration 2012; Verstraete 2004; Verstraete and Heyden 2005; Wolff et al. 1999; Wurst et al. 2004.

The most commonly used biomarker is serum GGT. This biomarker is elevated in individuals who have been drinking at least five drinks per day for several weeks, and it has moderate sensitivity and specificity (Center for Substance Abuse Treatment 2006). It is not increased in individuals who occasionally binge on alcohol. In individuals who consume 40 g/day of alcohol, elevated GGT levels are found in 20% of males and 15% of females. In individuals who drink more than 60 g/day of alcohol, elevated GGT levels are found in 40%–50% of males and 30% of females. GGT level returns to normal after 4–5 weeks of abstinence from excessive alcohol intake (the half-life of GGT is between 14 and 26 days) (Sharpe 2001). The test has been found to perform best in adults ages 30–60 years because GGT levels are rarely elevated in subjects under age 30 (Whitfield et al. 1978). GGT level elevation reflects liver damage secondary to alcoholism, but GGT levels can also be elevated as a result of liver and biliary disease, nicotine use, obesity, and microsomal enzyme–inducing medications.

Increased AST and ALT levels indicate heavy alcohol use over several weeks, with moderate sensitivity and specificity. AST and ALT reflect liver damage secondary to alcohol use, with AST being more sensitive than ALT. These tests have been found to perform best in adults ages 30–70. Elevations in levels of AST and ALT due to non-alcohol-related causes are similar to those of GGT, and excessive coffee consumption can lower values (Center for Substance Abuse Treatment 2006).

MCV can be used to detect heavy drinking that lasts at least a few months. MCV may be elevated after a month of drinking 60 g/day of alcohol, and MCV returns to baseline after several months of abstinence (Whitehead et al. 1978). It has low sensitivity and moderate-to-high specificity, without gender effect (Center for Substance Abuse Treatment 2006), although studies have found that measuring MCV in women may be more sensitive than measuring CDT or GGT (Sillanaukee et al. 1998). Liver diseases, hemolysis, anemia, folate deficiency, bleeding disorders, and medications reducing folate may also cause elevated MCV.

CDT was the first biomarker to receive U.S. Food and Drug Administration approval (Center for Medicare and Medicaid Services 2001). CDT is elevated when an individual has been drinking five drinks per day for about 2 weeks (Center for Substance Abuse Treatment 2006). Another study showed that CDT levels were elevated in subjects consuming 50–80 g/day of alcohol for at least 1 week; CDT's half-life is 15 days for a decrease in the level (Stibler 1991). Its sensitivity is moderate and specificity is high. CDT is less sensitive for women and younger individuals, but it is good at detecting relapse to drinking. CDT has been found to perform better at detecting alcohol dependence than at detecting high alcohol consumption without dependence (Mikkelsen et al. 1998). False positives may be caused by carbohydrate-deficient glycoprotein syndrome, fulminant hepatitis C, iron deficiency, and hormonal status in women (Center for Substance Abuse Treatment 2006).

EtG is a direct metabolite of ethanol that is formed by enzymatic conjugation of ethanol with glucuronic acid. Alcohol in the urine is normally detected for only a few hours, whereas EtG can be detected for several days. Ethyl sulfate (EtS) is formed by the direct conjugation of ethanol with a sulfate group. The two tests are often done simultaneously, because EtG is sensitive to degradation by other factors, such as infection, but EtS is not easily degraded by bacterial contaminants. Urine EtG sensitivity and specificity for differentiating nondrinkers and light drinkers from heavy drinkers have been estimated at 80.5% and 78.7%, respectively, at a cutoff level of 0.445 mg/L (Wurst et al. 2004). Differences in ethnicity, gender, and age do not affect the test results. The test is inexpensive. Incidental exposure to alcohol contained in foods, cosmetics, hygiene products, and medications may cause false-positive results (Substance Abuse and Mental Health Services Administration 2012).

False positives can occur, and the interpretation of positive tests requires the clinician to be knowledgeable in the related causes. Therefore, negative results may be more meaningful than positive results. However, it may be possible for patients to dilute urine EtG with excessive water intake (Wojcik and Hawthorne 2007).

By raising the cutoff point for metabolite detection with EtG, false positives can be reduced. Many laboratories offering the EtG test now offer a variety of cutoff points, which they suggest may eliminate false positives. Further independent investigation into the use of EtG is warranted. The EtG test is most useful in clinical or legal settings that require abstinence. EtG can also be tested in hair samples, with high sensitivity (0.92) and specificity (0.96) for detecting heavy drinking (>60 g/day alcohol) at a cutoff level of 27 pg/mg (Morini et al. 2009).

PEth is a phospholipid formed only in the presence of ethanol (Aradottir et al. 2006). PEth is raised when a person has had three or four drinks per day for a few days. It has high sensitivity and unknown specificity. There are no known sources of false positives (Substance Abuse and Mental Health Services Administration 2012). In a study of adults with alcohol dependence, the sensitivity of PEth was 99% among all patients despite quantity of alcohol use, whereas the sensitivity of CDT and GGT was related to the amount of ethanol intake (Aradottir et al. 2006).

Cannabis

THC and its metabolite 11-nor-9-carboxy-THC (THC-COOH) both have a terminal half-life of 48 hours or longer (Gustafson et al. 2004). Testing for THC-COOH is usually done in urine and serum. THC-COOH is more abundant than THC in these fluids (Johansson and Halldin 1989). A urine level of 20–200 ng/mL of THC-COOH corresponds with 10–50 mg of cannabis use (Wall et al. 1983). A urine screen may be positive for 1–3 days. With chronic cannabis use, the range of detection estimated varies from 1 to 11 weeks because of the lipophilic nature of THC, which is stored in fatty tissues and released back into blood over time (Hall and Degenhardt 2005). It can be clinically useful to consider the use of "creatinine-corrected" cannabinoid levels (Musshoff and Madea 2006), which are obtained by measuring the urine creatinine concentration and contrasting the levels as a ratio. Over time, in a now-abstinent previously chronic user, the ratio of urine cannabinoid to creatinine should follow a general linear trend downward.

Cannabis also can be detected in the blood, ranging from 0 to 500 ng/mL. Levels of more than 10–15 ng/mL indicate recent use. The ratio of THC to THC-COOH can be used to extrapolate time since last use. Saliva testing of cannabis is not sensitive. Cannabis can be detected in hair if use is twice per week for the 90-day period prior to sampling (DuPont and Selavka 2008). Some evidence suggests that pubic hair may contain higher concentrations. Sweat patches can be used to test for cannabis but, as in saliva, concentrations tend to be lower in sweat than in urine (Hall and Degenhardt 2005).

Recently, with the legalization of recreational cannabis, there has been renewed interest in new and alternative ways to assess acute cannabis intoxication and differentiate acute use from recent past use, especially since THC is detectable in the urine for very long periods of time. This is important both clinically to assess progress in treatment and forensically to assess whether or not someone was intoxicated at the time of breaking the law (e.g., while driving). A promising new approach is to measure breath levels much as in the testing for alcohol. This THC breath concentration device is investigational and still under development (Himes et al. 2013). In the latest testing, the device can sensitively measure breath THC for up to 3 hours after drug use and can distinguish between acute use and recent use.

Nicotine

Cotinine, a metabolite of nicotine, is the preferred biomarker to test for cigarette smoking, and can be found in saliva, urine, and blood (Florescu et al. 2009). Although a number of other biomarkers can be used for detecting cigarette smoking, cotinine is the most commonly tested because it has the most ideal window of detection, at around 3–4 days. Hair testing for nicotine is a promising new method for measuring cigarette smoking and exposure to cigarette smoke. To gather information regarding the recency of smoking, particularly for research purposes, one can measure carbon monoxide quantitative level by having the individual breathe into a specific instrument. The instrument costs approximately $1,500.

Sedatives, Hypnotics, and Anxiolytics

Immunoassay screens for benzodiazepines are readily available; however, the sensitivity and window of detection vary for the different compounds. Because of the variability in cross-reactivity for different benzodiazepines and the large proportion of conjugated benzodiazepines excreted in the urine (which are often not cross-reactive with immunoassays aimed at detecting the actual benzodiazepine molecules), urine drug screening by immunoassay can be difficult to interpret. For example, some screening assays are much less sensitive to detecting clonazepam than alprazolam (DeRienz et al. 2008). By adding β-glucuronidase enzyme to urine samples and hydrolyzing the conjugates, sensitivity to benzodiazepines can be improved considerably.

Opiates

Urine tests for opiates detect morphine (the main metabolite of heroin), which can usually be detected 12–36 hours after use. Poppy seed consumption can yield a positive urine test; however, fentanyl may not be detected on standard panels. In hair sampling, poppy seed use does not lead to positive results for opiates (DuPont and Selavka 2008). Longer-acting opiates may be detected in the urine for up to 4 days. Saliva testing has about the same sensitivity as urine testing (Jaffe and Strain 2005). Regular opioid immunoassay screens are less sensitive for synthetic and semisynthetic opioids, with variable cross-reactivity (Haller et al. 2006). Specific immunoassays must be ordered to detect fentanyl and related compounds. Oxycodone also should be tested for specifically, because many regular opioid screens detect only high levels of oxycodone in the urine, leading to false negatives. Methadone and buprenorphine are not detected by standard opioid screens, so specific immunoassay screens must be used to detect their presence in urine.

For patients taking buprenorphine or buprenorphine/naloxone, immunoassay testing will identify the presence or absence of buprenorphine in the urine. If a patient is suspected of diverting buprenorphine, yet positive results are obtained on immunoassay, sending the specimen for definitive testing of the metabolite norbuprenorphine can provide clarity. A negative norbuprenorphine confirmatory test following a positive buprenorphine immunoassay test indicates that the patient is placing buprenorphine products in the urine sample in an attempt to mask nonadherence and, possibly, diversion. Observed urine testing for such patients is recommended (Hurford et al. 2017). Additionally, the ratio of norbuprenorphine to buprenorphine can be clinically usefully in approximating the patient's regularity of administration and degree of adherence to the medication regime. Anecdotally, whether strict ratios should be used to confirm adherence is controversial, and many clinicians use it as a rough guide. That is to say, there may be substantial variability in norbuprenorphine-to-buprenorphine blood and urine level ratios even among generally adherent patients, so to accuse patients of nonadherence if they have less than about a 10:1 ratio may be unrealistic and clinically inappropriate.

Dextromethorphan

Dextromethorphan is an ingredient in commonly abused over-the-counter cough suppressant medications. It has a complex pharmacological mechanism of action, acting as a noncompetitive *N*-methyl-D-aspartate (NMDA) antagonist, a σ_1 receptor agonist, and a voltage-gated calcium channel blocker (Werling et al. 2007). Although antitussive effects are thought to be mediated by dextromethorphan's effects on sigma receptors, the psychotropic properties of dextromethorphan are usually attributed to its ability to antagonize NMDA receptors (Boyer 2004; Brown et al. 2004). Dextromethorphan is often abused by adolescents because it is readily available in cough syrups and in over-the-counter cough and cold preparations. Overdose and severe toxicity with dextromethorphan can cause death, probably through respiratory depression (Logan et al. 2009).

Direct urine testing of dextromethorphan appears to have limited accessibility in the United States. Kim et al. (2006) reported a standardization of a method for the analysis of dextromethorphan and its metabolite dextrorphan in urine but stated that further experimentation would be needed to generalize results to monitoring illegal use. In our own research into the local availability of such tests, we found that local commercial and hospital laboratories only offer serum levels, making serial monitoring more cumbersome for the patient. Dextromethorphan may yield a false-positive result on a urine screen for opiates and/or PCP because of its molecular basis and mode of action, respectively, although this is more likely to occur when large dosages are used.

Cocaine

Cocaine use can be tested using urine, blood, hair, perspiration, and saliva. Cocaine has a short elimination half-life of 1 hour. Benzoylecgonine is a cocaine metabolite with a half-life of 6 hours and is thus used in testing biological fluids for cocaine use (Warner 1993). Acute cocaine use can be monitored in the urine 1–2 days after recent use, and prolonged positive results (up to weeks) may be present in chronic, heavy users (>0.5 g/day) (Burke et al. 1990). False-positive results may be caused by high dosages of prilocaine (Baselt and Baselt 1987) and coca tea (Mazor et al. 2006). False-negative results may be caused by the addition of drain cleaner (e.g., Drano), bleach, or sodium chloride solution (Mikkelsen and Ash 1988).

A study examining the monitoring of cocaine use via sweat patches in an adult outpatient sample found a sensitivity of 95.0% and a specificity of 92.6% based on comparison with urine test results and self-reports over a 1-week period (Chawarski et al. 2007). Hair analysis has been used to probe for chronic use, because the hair matrix absorbs and traps cocaine. Measuring the distance of cocaine concentrations from the hair root can be used to approximate time elapsed since drug use (Mercolini et al. 2008). Other research has found that cocaine and benzoylecgonine can be measured in the hair as early as 1 day after intranasal use, and therefore hair analysis is able to differentiate between chronic and episodic cocaine use (Ursitti et al. 2001).

Amphetamine and Methamphetamine

Methamphetamine undergoes *N*-demethylation to its metabolite amphetamine. A considerable portion of the parent compound is excreted into the urine unchanged, with the exact amount varying based on urinary pH level (Hsu et al. 2003; Schepers et al. 2003). Metabolites of amphetamine may be detected in blood, urine, saliva, sweat, and hair. Screening for amphetamine should also include testing for methamphetamine, methylenedioxyamphetamine (MDA), methylenedioxyethylamphetamine (MDEA), and methylenedioxymethyl-amphetamine (MDMA). Hsu et al. (2003) described monoclonal antibody tests to differentiate among amphetamine, methamphetamine, and MDMA, because MDMA may require higher concentrations to yield a positive result on amphetamine immunoassays. The Division of Workplace Programs of the Substance Abuse and Mental Health Services Administration (2004) specifies an initial immunoassay-positive drug test for amphetamine at a level ≥1,000 ng/mL and confirmatory tests for amphetamine and methamphetamine via GC-MS at a level ≥500 ng/mL. If the methamphetamine test is positive, the result must also contain amphetamine at a concentration ≥200 ng/mL. A study by Verstraete and Heyden (2005) comparing urine immunoassays found that fewer false positives or false negatives can be obtained if the cutoff for detection of amphetamine and MDMA is optimized based on each laboratory's validation and not set at 500 ng/mL.

The amphetamine assay is perhaps the most difficult test to interpret clinically because of the large numbers of false-positive results due to medications containing amphetamine and medication with similar structures. Some prescribed and over-the-counter medications that can trigger a false positive include amantadine, benzphetamine, bupropion, chlorpromazine, clobenzorex, L-deprenyl, desipramine, dextroamphetamine, ephedrine, fenproporex, isometheptene, isoxsuprine, labetalol, methamphetamine, L-methamphetamine, methylphenidate, phentermine, phenylephrine, phenylpropanolamine, promethazine, pseudoephedrine, ranitidine, ritodrine, selegiline, thioridazine, trazodone, trimethobenzamide, and trimipramine (Moeller et al. 2008). Some commonly used immunoassay-based testing kits have fewer false positives (Hsu et al. 2003).

Methods of differentiating illicit amphetamine use versus legal use of amphetamine medications based on the enantiomeric ratio of amphetamine have been proposed, but the clinical usefulness of such methods is questionable (Kraemer and Maurer 2002). Diagnostix developed a commercially available enzyme-linked immunosorbent assay (ELISA) for methylphenidate and ritalinic acid in urine, but it is expensive and nonquantitative. Lewis et al. (2003) developed an "in-house" quantitative, rapid, and direct ELISA for methylphenidate equivalents in urine that has acceptable performance, allowing its routine use in the laboratory. This test may be helpful in identifying those who are abusing others' prescription drugs and in cutting down on adolescent trafficking of prescription methylphenidate to peers for profit.

Clinically, confirmation of methamphetamine in the urine indicates the use of methamphetamine. Selegiline, a monoamine oxidase A inhibitor, is metabolized to methamphetamine in the body. The only other available approved prescription drug in the United States that is metabolized to methamphetamine is benzphetamine, which is used for weight loss. For a patient with attention-deficit/hyperactivity disorder who requires pharmacotherapy, medications other than amphetamine (e.g., atomoxetine, bupropion, modafinil) should be considered when there is a concern about possible stimulant abuse, because this may allow for easier detection of illicit amphetamine or designer drug abuse.

Hallucinogens

Most hallucinogens, such as lysergic acid diethylamide (LSD), can be tested in the blood or urine using GC-MS methods (Burnley and George 2003). Psilocybin and its metabolite psilocin are psychoactive alkaloids found in certain species of mushrooms. Levels can be detected in the serum, with a half-life of psilocin at 163 minutes when given as pure psilocybin by mouth (Passie et al. 2002). Mescaline, a ring-substituted phenethylamine, is a hallucinogenic alkaloid found in peyote cactus. It can be detected in urine and serum via GC-MS (Habrdova et al. 2005).

Phencyclidine and Phencyclidine-Like Substances

Biomarkers for PCP use are thought to be somewhat unreliable because observed individuals with acute psychotic reactions can have an undetectable serum level due to PCP's long duration of action, lipophilicity, and pKa (Javitt and Zukin 2005). Sweat patches may be used for the detection of PCP. Rapid screening tests are not readily available for ketamine, which reacts unreliably with urine immunoassays for PCP (Javitt and Zukin 2005).

Inhalants

Most inhalants are difficult to track via biomarkers in bodily fluids. Toluene can be measured directly in the serum. Industry maximum exposure is 100 parts per million, which yields a blood level of 0.5 μg/g, whereas blood levels during intoxication range from 0.8 to 8.0 μg/g. Blood levels can normalize 4–10 hours after exposure. Hippuric acid, a direct metabolite, can be measured in urine. Recent intoxication can be assumed given a ratio of 1 g or more of hippurate to 1 g of creatinine in the urine. False-positive results may occur with concomitant intake of benzoic acid food preservatives (Crowley and Sakai 2005). Red and white blood cell counts, as well as kidney and liver functioning, may be altered because of toxic reactions (Schuckit 2000). Testing for volatile inhalant use must be performed on blood samples using headspace gas chromatography (Broussard 2000).

Anabolic-Androgenic Steroids

The range of normal plasma testosterone levels in men is from 300 to 1,000 ng/dL. The following anabolic steroid compounds can be measured in the urine via gas chromatography–thermionic specific detection and gas chromatography–flame ionization detection: testosterone, 19-noretiocholanolone, oxymetholone, dehydroepiandrosterone, 10-norestosterone, 11-β-hydroxyandrosterone, metandienone, 19-norandrosterone, 16-α-hydroxyetiocholanolone, 17-α-epitestosterone, and stanozolol. Hair can also be tested for anabolic steroids. Changes in liver function, cholesterol, and endocrine measures can occur in adolescents who use these substances to enhance athletic performance (Pope and Brower 2009).

Conclusion

Although experts disagree regarding the usefulness of routine drug screening (Gold et al. 2006; Levy et al. 2006), biomarker testing can provide useful objective information that can strengthen clinical evaluations and serve as a launching point for further evaluations and diagnostic clarity. Clinicians should consider drug testing in patients with a history of substance misuse or SUD who are receiving controlled substances for co-occurring disorders or other indications (e.g., dextroamphetamine for attention-deficit/hyperactivity disorder). Since prescribed medications can have potentially lethal interactions with drugs of abuse, drug testing can serve as an objective means of identifying potential risks. Testing can also be used to ascertain adherence to the treatment regimen and can potentially help identify diversion when part of a comprehensive diversion process. Biomarker testing is clinically useful for the assessment, screening, and monitoring of adolescent substance use in conjunction with comprehensive clinical interviews, rating scales, and corollary information. Biomarker testing can be used as a tool for outreach testing in settings other than the doctor's office, such as at home and at school. Urine, blood, sweat, hair, and saliva can all be used to test for multiple drugs of abuse. Choosing the most appropriate sample source and test depends on the specific substance(s) of interest, suspected pattern of drug use, and intent or purpose of testing.

Key Points

- Use of objective biomarkers for the detection of drug use is important and is legal in the adolescent population in the appropriate clinical contexts.

- Qualitative screening kits for use with saliva and urine samples are widely available, rapid, and a convenient form of testing for clinical and legal management.

- The choice between qualitative and quantitative tests depends on the purpose of the test and what will be done with the results.

- It is important to be aware of the cutoff point (for cannabis in particular), sensitivity, and specificity of the test used for a specific drug.

Relevant Websites

American Association of Medical Review Officers Registry: www.aamro.com

Institute for Behavior and Health: Guide to Responsible Family Drug Testing and Alcohol Testing and Smarter Student Drug Testing: www.ibhinc.org

Substance Abuse and Mental Health Services Administration Certified Lab List: www.samhsa.gov/workplace/resources/drug-testing/certified-lab-list

References

Aradottir S, Asanovska G, Gjerss S, et al: PHosphatidylethanol (PEth) concentrations in blood are correlated to reported alcohol intake in alcohol-dependent patients. Alcohol Alcohol 41(4):431–437, 2006 16624837

Barnea Z, Rahav G, Teichman M: The reliability and consistency of self-reports on substance use in a longitudinal study. Br J Addict 82(8):891–898, 1987 3479170

Baselt RC, Baselt DR: Little cross reactivity of local anesthetics with Abuscreen, EMIT d.a.u., and TDX immunoassays for cocaine metabolite (letter). Clin Chem 33(5):747, 1987 3568392

Benowitz NL: Pharmacology of nicotine: addiction and therapeutics. Annu Rev Pharmacol Toxicol 36:597–613, 1996 8725403

Boyer EW: Dextromethorphan abuse. Pediatr Emerg Care 20(12):858–863, 2004 15572980

Broussard LA: The role of the laboratory in detecting inhalant abuse. Clin Lab Sci 13:205–209, 2000 11586505

Brown C, Fezoui M, Selig WM, et al: Antitussive activity of sigma-1 receptor agonists in the guinea-pig. Br J Pharmacol 141(2):233–240, 2004 14691051

Buchan BJ, L Dennis M, Tims FM, et al: Cannabis use: consistency and validity of self-report, on-site urine testing and laboratory testing. Addiction 97 (suppl 1):98–108, 2002 12460132

Burke WM, Ravi NV, Dhopesh V, et al: Prolonged presence of metabolite in urine after compulsive cocaine use. J Clin Psychiatry 51(4):145–148, 1990 2182612

Burleson J, Kaminer Y: Adolescent alcohol and marijuana use: concordance among objective-, self-, and collateral-reports. J Child Adolesc Subst Abuse 16(1):53–68, 2006

Burnley BT, George S: The development and application of a gas chromatography-mass spectrometric (GC-MS) assay to determine the presence of 2-oxo-3-hydroxy-LSD in urine. J Anal Toxicol 27(4):249–252, 2003 12820748

Cantwell DP, Lewinsohn PM, Rohde P, et al: Correspondence between adolescent report and parent report of psychiatric diagnostic data. J Am Acad Child Adolesc Psychiatry 36(5):610–619, 1997 9136495

Center for Medicare and Medicaid Services: Medicare program; negotiated rulemaking: coverage and administrative policies for clinical diagnostic laboratory services. Final rule. Fed Regist 66(226):58788–58890, 2001 11780624

Center for Substance Abuse Treatment: The Role of Biomarkers in the Treatment of Alcohol Use Disorders (DHHS Publ No SMA-06-4223). Rockville, MD, Center for Substance Abuse Treatment, Substance Abuse and Mental Health Services Administration, 2006

Chawarski MC, Fiellin DA, O'Connor PG, et al: Utility of sweat patch testing for drug use monitoring in outpatient treatment for opiate dependence. J Subst Abuse Treat 33(4):411–415, 2007 17512157

Cone EJ: New developments in biological measures of drug prevalence. NIDA Res Monogr 167:108–129, 1997 9243559

Cooke F, Bullen C, Whittaker R, et al: Diagnostic accuracy of NicAlert cotinine test strips in saliva for verifying smoking status. Nicotine Tob Res 10(4):607–612, 2008 18418783

Crouch DJ, Hersch RK, Cook RF, et al: A field evaluation of five on-site drug-testing devices. J Anal Toxicol 26(7):493–499, 2002 12423006

Crowley TJ, Sakai J: Inhalant related disorders, in Kaplan and Sadock's Comprehensive Textbook of Psychiatry, 8th Edition, Vol 1. Edited by Sadock B, Sadock V. Philadelphia, PA, Lippincott Williams & Wilkins, 2005 pp 1247–1257

De Giovanni N, Fucci N: The current status of sweat testing for drugs of abuse: a review. Curr Med Chem 20(4):545–561, 2013 23244520

DeRienz RT, Holler JM, Manos ME, et al: Evaluation of four immunoassay screening kits for the detection of benzodiazepines in urine. J Anal Toxicol 32(6):433–437, 2008 18652750

DuPont RL, Selavka CM: Testing to identify recent drug use, in The American Psychiatric Publishing Textbook of Substance Abuse Treatment, 4th Edition. Edited by Galanter M, Kleber HD. Washington, DC, American Psychiatric Publishing, 2008 pp 655–664

DuPont RL, Merlo LJ, Arria AM, et al: Random student drug testing as a school-based drug prevention strategy. Addiction 108(5):839–845, 2013 22906236

Ferrara SD, Tedeschi L, Frison G, et al: Drugs-of-abuse testing in urine: statistical approach and experimental comparison of immunochemical and chromatographic techniques. J Anal Toxicol 18(5):278–291, 1994 7990448

Florescu A, Ferrence R, Einarson T, et al: Methods for quantification of exposure to cigarette smoking and environmental tobacco smoke: focus on developmental toxicology. Ther Drug Monit 31(1):14–30, 2009 19125149

Gold MS, Frost-Pineda K, Goldberger BA, DuPont RL: Physicians and drug screening. J Adolesc Health 39(2):154–155, 2006 16857524

Greenfield SF, Hennessy G: Assessment of the patient, in The American Psychiatric Publishing Textbook of Substance Abuse Treatment, 4th Edition. Edited by Galanter M, Kleber HD. Washington, DC, American Psychiatric Publishing, 2008, pp 55–78

Gustafson RA, Kim I, Stout PR, et al: Urinary pharmacokinetics of 11-nor-9-carboxy-delta9-tetrahydrocannabinol after controlled oral delta9-tetrahydrocannabinol administration. J Anal Toxicol 28(3):160–167, 2004 15107145

Habrdova V, Peters FT, Theobald DS, et al: Screening for and validated quantification of phenethylamine-type designer drugs and mescaline in human blood plasma by gas chromatography/mass spectrometry. J Mass Spectrom 40(6):785–795, 2005 15827969

Hall W, Degenhardt L: Cannabis-related disorders, in Kaplan and Sadock's Comprehensive Textbook of Psychiatry, 8th Edition, Vol 2. Edited by Sadock B, Sadock V. Philadelphia, PA, Lippincott Williams & Wilkins, 2005, pp 1211–1220

Haller CA, Stone J, Burke V, et al: Comparison of an automated and point-of-care immunoassay to GC-MS for urine oxycodone testing in the clinical laboratory. J Anal Toxicol 30(2):106–111, 2006 16620541

Himes SK, Scheidweiler KB, Beck O, et al: Cannabinoids in exhaled breath following controlled administration of smoked cannabis. Clin Chem 59(12):1780–1789, 2013 24046200

Hsu J, Liu C, Liu CP, et al: Performance characteristics of selected immunoassays for preliminary test of 3,4-methylenedioxymethamphetamine, methamphetamine, and related drugs in urine specimens. J Anal Toxicol 27(7):471–478, 2003 14607002

Hurford M, Baxter L, Brown L, et al: Consensus Statement: Appropriate Use of Drug Testing in Clinical Addiction Medicine. Rockville, MD, American Society of Addiction Medicine 2017. Available at: https://www.asam.org/docs/default-source/quality-science/appropriate_use_of_drug_testing_in_clinical-1-(7).pdf?sfvrsn=2. Accessed May 9, 2019.

Jaffe JH, Strain EC: Opioid-related disorders, in Kaplan and Sadock's Comprehensive Textbook of Psychiatry, 8th Edition. Edited by Sadock B, Sadock V. Philadelphia, PA, Lippincott Williams & Wilkins, 2005, pp 1265–1290

Javitt D, Zukin SR: Phencyclidine (or phencyclidine-like)-related disorders, in Kaplan and Sadock's Comprehensive Textbook of Psychiatry, 8th Edition. Edited by Sadock B, Sadock V. Philadelphia, PA, Lippincott Williams & Wilkins, 2005, pp 1291–1300

Johansson E, Halldin MM: Urinary excretion half-life of delta 1-tetrahydrocannabinol-7-oic acid in heavy marijuana users after smoking. J Anal Toxicol 13(4):218–223, 1989 2550702

Kaminer Y: Adolescent Substance Abuse: A Comprehensive Guide to Theory and Practice. New York, Plenum, 1994

Kerrigan S, Phillips WH Jr: Comparison of ELISAs for opiates, methamphetamine, cocaine metabolite, benzodiazepines, phencyclidine, and cannabinoids in whole blood and urine. Clin Chem 47(3):540–547, 2001 11238309

Kim EM, Lee JS, Park MJ, et al: Standardization of method for the analysis of dextromethorphan in urine. Forensic Sci Int 161(2–3):198–201, 2006 16837153

Knight JR, Levy S; The national debate on drug testing in schools (editorial). J Adolesc Health 41(5):419–420, 2007 17950160

Korzec A, de Bruijn C, van Lambalgen M: The Bayesian Alcoholism Test had better diagnostic properties for confirming diagnosis of hazardous and harmful alcohol use. J Clin Epidemiol 58(10):1024–1032, 2005 16168348

Kraemer T, Maurer HH: Toxicokinetics of amphetamines: metabolism and toxicokinetic data of designer drugs, amphetamine, methamphetamine, and their N-alkyl derivatives. Ther Drug Monit 24(2):277–289, 2002 11897973

Leino A, Loo BM: Comparison of three commercial tests for buprenorphine screening in urine. Ann Clin Biochem 44(Pt 6):563–565, 2007 17961313

Levy S, Harris SK, Sherrit L, et al: Drug testing of adolescents in general medical clinics, in school and at home: physician attitudes and practices. J Adolesc Health 38(4):336–342, 2006 16549293

Levy S, Siqueira LM, Ammerman SD, et al; Committee on Substance Abuse: Testing for drugs of abuse in children and adolescents. Pediatrics 133(6):e1798–e1807, 2014 24864184

Lewis MG, Lewis JG, Elder PA, et al: An enzyme-linked immunosorbent assay (ELISA) for methylphenidate (Ritalin) in urine. J Anal Toxicol 27(6):342–345, 2003 14516486

Logan BK, Goldfogel G, Hamilton R, et al: Five deaths resulting from abuse of dextromethorphan sold over the Internet. J Anal Toxicol 33(2):99–103, 2009 19239735

Loor R, Lingenfelter C, Wason PP, et al: Multiplex assay of amphetamine, methamphetamine, and ecstasy drug using CEDIA technology. J Anal Toxicol 26(5):267–273, 2002 12166813

Manchikanti L, Malla Y, Wargo BW, et al: Comparative evaluation of the accuracy of immunoassay with liquid chromatography tandem mass spectrometry (LC/MS/MS) of urine drug testing (UDT) opioids and illicit drugs in chronic pain patients. Pain Physician 14(2):175–187, 2011 21412372

Mazor SS, Mycyk MB, Wills BK, et al: Coca tea consumption causes positive urine cocaine assay. Eur J Emerg Med 13(6):340–341, 2006 17091055

Mercolini L, Mandrioli R, Saladini B, et al: Quantitative analysis of cocaine in human hair by HPLC with fluorescence detection. J Pharm Biomed Anal 48(2):456–461, 2008 18394843

Mieczkowski T, Lersh K: Drug testing police officers and police recruits: the outcome of hair analysis and urinalysis compared. Policing 25(3):581–601, 2002

Mieczkowski T, Newel R: Statistical examination of hair color as a potential biasing factor in hair analysis. Forensic Sci Int 107(1–3):13–38, 2000 10689560

Mikkelsen SL, Ash KO: Adulterants causing false negatives in illicit drug testing. Clin Chem 34(11):2333–2336, 1988 3052928

Mikkelsen IM, Kanitz RD, Nilssen O, et al: Carbohydrate-deficient transferrin: marker of actual alcohol consumption or chronic alcohol misuse? Alcohol Alcohol 33(6):646–650, 1998 9872354

Miller EI, Wylie FM, Oliver JS: Detection of benzodiazepines in hair using ELISA and LC-ESI-MS-MS. J Anal Toxicol 30(7):441–448, 2006 16959136

Moeller KE, Lee KC, Kissack JC: Urine drug screening: practical guide for clinicians. Mayo Clin Proc 83(1):66–76, 2008 18174009

Morini L, Politi L, Polettini A: Ethyl glucuronide in hair. A sensitive and specific marker of chronic heavy drinking. Addiction 104(6):915–920, 2009 19392911

Musshoff F, Madea B: Review of biologic matrices (urine, blood, hair) as indicators of recent or ongoing cannabis use. Ther Drug Monit 28(2):155–163, 2006 16628124

Niemelä O: Biomarker-based approaches for assessing alcohol use disorders. Int J Environ Res Public Health 13(2):166, 2016 26828506

Passie T, Seifert J, Schneider U, et al: The pharmacology of psilocybin. Addict Biol 7(4):357–364, 2002 14578010

Pope HG, Brower KJ: Anabolic-androgenic steroid-related disorders, in Kaplan and Sadock's Comprehensive Textbook of Psychiatry, 9th Edition, Vol 1. Edited by Sadock B, Sadock V. Philadelphia, PA, Lippincott Williams & Wilkins, 2009, pp 1419–1431

Ringwalt C, Vincus AA, Ennett ST, et al: Random drug testing in US public school districts. Am J Public Health 98(5):826–828, 2008 18381986

Schepers RJ, Oyler JM, Joseph RE Jr, et al: Methamphetamine and amphetamine pharmacokinetics in oral fluid and plasma after controlled oral methamphetamine administration to human volunteers. Clin Chem 49(1):121–132, 2003 12507968

Schuckit MA: Glues, inhalants, and aerosols, in Drug and Alcohol Abuse: Critical Issues in Psychiatry. Boston, MA, Springer, 2000, pp 221–230

Sharpe PC: Biochemical detection and monitoring of alcohol abuse and abstinence. Ann Clin Biochem 38(Pt 6):652–664, 2001 11732647

Sillanaukee P, Aalto M, Seppä K: Carbohydrate-deficient transferrin and conventional alcohol markers as indicators for brief intervention among heavy drinkers in primary health care. Alcohol Clin Exp Res 22(4):892–896, 1998 9660318

Stibler H: Carbohydrate-deficient transferrin in serum: a new marker of potentially harmful alcohol consumption reviewed. Clin Chem 37(12):2029–2037, 1991 1764777

Substance Abuse and Mental Health Services Administration: Mandatory guidelines for federal workplace drug testing programs. Federal Register 69(19644–19673):249–259, 2004

Substance Abuse and Mental Health Services: The role of biomarkers in the treatment of alcohol use disorders, 2012 Revision (HHS Publ No SMA 12-4686). Advisory 11(2):2012. Available at: http://adaiclearinghouse.org/downloads/Advisory-The-Role-of-Biomarkers-in-the-Treatment-of-Alcohol-Use-Disorders-434.pdf. Accessed April 26, 2019.

Ursitti F, Klein J, Koren G: Confirmation of cocaine use during pregnancy: a critical review. Ther Drug Monit 23(4):347–353, 2001 11477315

Verstraete AG: Detection times of drugs of abuse in blood, urine, and oral fluid. Ther Drug Monit 26(2):200–205, 2004 15228165

Verstraete AG, Heyden FV: Comparison of the sensitivity and specificity of six immunoassays for the detection of amphetamines in urine. J Anal Toxicol 29(5):359–364, 2005 16105261

Wall ME, Sadler BM, Brine D, et al: Metabolism, disposition, and kinetics of delta-9-tetrahydrocannabinol in men and women. Clin Pharmacol Ther 34(3):352–363, 1983 6309462

Warner EA: Cocaine abuse. Ann Intern Med 119(3):226–235, 1993 8323092

Werling LL, Lauterbach EC, Calef U: Dextromethorphan as a potential neuroprotective agent with unique mechanisms of action. Neurologist 13(5):272–293, 2007 17848867

Whitehead TP, Clarke CA, Whitfield AG: Biochemical and haematological markers of alcohol intake. Lancet 1(8071):978–981, 1978 76902

Whitfield JB, Hensley WJ, Bryden D, et al: Effects of age and sex on biochemical responses to drinking habits. Med J Aust 2(14):629–632, 1978 32469

Wojcik MH, Hawthorne JS: Sensitivity of commercial ethyl glucuronide (ETG) testing in screening for alcohol abstinence. Alcohol Alcohol 42(4):317–320, 2007 17376784

Wolff K, Farrell M, Marsden J, et al: A review of biological indicators of illicit drug use, practical considerations and clinical usefulness. Addiction 94(9):1279–1298, 1999 10615715

Wurst FM, Wiesbeck GA, Metzger JW, et al: On sensitivity, specificity, and the influence of various parameters on ethyl glucuronide levels in urine—results from the WHO/ISBRA study. Alcohol Clin Exp Res 28(8):1220–1228, 2004 15318121

Placement Criteria and Integrated Treatment Services for Youth With Substance Use Disorders

Marc Fishman, M.D.

Treatment planning for adolescents with substance use disorders (SUDs) begins with a comprehensive assessment and case formulation that informs the appropriate selection of treatment setting, objectives, and curriculum, including length of stay, intervention modalities, and intensity (i.e., dosage and frequency) of the interventions provided. Placement decisions require determination of treatment needs, and consideration of where and how those services should be effectively and safely delivered (Fishman 2008).

The *ASAM Criteria: Treatment Criteria for Addictive, Substance-Related, and Co-Occurring Conditions*, 3rd Edition (Mee-Lee et al. 2013), referred to as the ASAM Criteria, has become the standard in the field for standardized treatment matching guidelines, with the goal of finding the optimal fit between patient needs and available treatment. In addition to its function as an algorithm for level-of-care placement decisions, it is also a guideline for treatment matching and treatment planning in general. Its overall approach is to guide the clinician by organizing assessment data into six broad categories of assessment dimensions that serve to focus the assessment on key practical domains with central treatment implications. The six ASAM Criteria assessment dimensions are listed and described in Table 6–1.

ASAM Criteria describes various adolescent levels of care as detailed in Table 6–2. The criteria serve as a prescription for the adolescent continuum of care by describing the broad range of service components expected in each level of care. Such a prescription should not be construed rigidly, because flexibility and innovation are encouraged, particularly because not all services or levels of care are available in all communities (e.g., rural areas).

General Principles of Treatment Planning and Placement

An important general principle of treatment planning is the need to account for the continuity of care and coordination of treatment across episodes of care. Although some adolescents with mild to moderate severity do achieve abstinence after receiving time-limited, discrete interventions, many do not. Moreover, the higher the severity, the less likely this response is. Much more typical is a waxing-waning, remitting-relapsing course over a prolonged period of time and across several episodes of care at different levels and services of care. The optimal continuity of care is based on a treatment system that includes step-up and step-down levels of care to match the adolescents' changing needs based on their response at different levels of care. Poor responders to initial treatment may need longer-term continuing care, extended monitoring phases, and repeated booster doses (for more details, see Chapter 12).

Barriers

Barriers to treatment planning include the availability of adequate resources and feasibility and acceptability by meeting the expectations of the youth and family. Considerations include availability of local services, financial costs of care, difficulties navigating complex systems, transportation, and language bar-

Table 6–1.   ASAM Criteria assessment dimensions

Dimension	Description
1. Acute intoxication and/ or withdrawal potential	Relating to the potential for acute and subacute intoxication and withdrawal and ensuing treatment needs
2. Biomedical conditions and complications	Relating to medical symptoms and comorbidity—preexisting, substance-induced, and substance-exacerbated conditions—and ensuing treatment needs
3. Emotional, behavioral, or cognitive conditions and complications	Relating to psychiatric symptoms and comorbidity—preexisting, substance-induced, and substance-exacerbated conditions—and ensuing treatment needs
4. Readiness to change	Relating to treatment engagement, motivation, resistance, and stages of change
5. Relapse, continued use, or continued problem potential	Relating to the likelihood of relapse and continuation of substance use and associated problems, along with potential consequences and ensuing treatment needs
6. Recovery/living environment	Relating to the family, peers, living situation, and home setting

riers. Clinicians need to appreciate the burden of treatment on both adolescents and families.

Particularly challenging is matching youth with high baseline severity and impairment to treatment settings that can provide high-intensity services (e.g., frequency, dosage, versatile treatment approaches). In such instances, lower levels of care may not be as effective (Dasinger et al. 2004) or may not even be able to engage or "capture" (as in the case of a runaway who does not show up for a partial hospitalization program) adolescents with higher severity. Increased intensity, however, can sometimes be counterproductive if it increases resistance by the youth or family. In these circumstances, it is useful to enhance motivation for change and increased engagement (see the discussion of Dimension 4 below). Nonetheless, the ASAM Criteria describes a full range of treatment services appropriate to the needs of all substance-involved ado-

Table 6–2.   ASAM Criteria adolescent levels of care

Level 0.5: Early intervention

Level 1: Outpatient services

Level 2: Intensive outpatient/partial hospitalization services

  2.1: Intensive outpatient (IOP)

  2.5: Partial hospitalization (partial hospital/day program)

Level 3: Residential/inpatient services

  3.1: Clinically managed low-intensity residential

  3.5: Clinically managed medium-intensity residential

  3.7: Medically monitored high-intensity inpatient

Level 4: Medically managed intensive inpatient services (hospital)

lescents, whether they are privately insured, publicly insured, underinsured, or uninsured. Although they may not have access to it, many indigent adolescents may need an even broader continuum of services than those with greater resources. In general, adolescents with fewer supports, less resiliency, and lower levels of baseline functioning may need a higher intensity of services and longer lengths of service at all levels of care than do those with economic advantage and better social supports.

Adolescents generally need an array of services that are broader than SUD counseling alone for the multiple problems they face. Provision of services should be coordinated, taking into consideration that even when services are available, they might be fragmented and/or only partially effective. Examples of frequently needed linkages include psychiatric, medical, family, social welfare, special education, school support, and juvenile justice. Case management, integration of services by a single provider, co-location within a single institution ("one-stop shopping"), interdisciplinary teams, cross-training and broadening of disciplinary focus, active coordination of service linkages among separate providers, and primary provider team leadership are all approaches that are attempted, but unfortunately integration is rare. Generally, the higher the severity of the adolescent's SUD, the higher the need for multidimensional integration of services.

Decision Rules for Adolescent Placement

ASAM Criteria contains decision rules for adolescent placement that are distinct from those for adults because of the special developmental needs of adolescents. Although payers or regulators may sometimes choose to apply a definition based on a rigid application of an age cutoff, such as age 18, there are many cases in which individual variation and the functional immaturity of a particular patient dictate that the adolescent criteria would be more appropriate for a young adult than the adult criteria. (Young adults [18–25 years] require a special approach. Some providers have begun to develop specialized programming for this group and its unique clinical needs.)

Dimensional Assessment and Treatment Planning Using the ASAM Criteria

In this section, clinical considerations are reviewed for treatment planning and matching by each of the six ASAM Criteria assessment dimensions.

Dimension 1: Acute Intoxication and Withdrawal Potential

One consideration in Dimension 1 is the need for withdrawal management (also known as "detoxification") services when there is potential for withdrawal. Intensive management of withdrawal is most frequently needed in adolescents with opioid dependence, with the current modern opioid crisis. The trend for treatment of severe opioid withdrawal in adolescents, as in adults, is the use of tapering doses of the partial agonist buprenorphine, which replaces or is added to more indirect symptom reduction agents such as clonidine (Marsch et al. 2005). Opioid dependence is generally an indicator of increased psychosocial impairment (Clemmey et al. 2004), with increased severity in all of the assessment dimensions. In particular, the presence of withdrawal symptoms of sufficient severity to require pharmacological intervention is considered a marker for very high risk of relapse, with resultant need for higher levels of monitoring and treatment intensity, including environmental control to decrease access to substances and to increase likelihood of initiation of the next phase of treatment and continuing care. This same principle applies to withdrawal management from benzodiazepines, other sedative-hypnotics, and alcohol (use of which is common in adolescents, but only infrequently with full physiological dependence requiring medical withdrawal management). Medical withdrawal management in adolescents should be conducted with residential support.

Another Dimension 1 consideration is the persistence of subacute psychiatric intoxication and withdrawal symptoms and syndromes. These issues overlap considerably with those involved in the assessment for Dimension 3 and are especially salient because of potential direct links to the toxic effects of substances and the frequent confusion in diagnosis and treatment. In patients in whom substance toxicity has caused serious psychiatric morbidity (e.g., cannabis-induced psychosis), the emphasis should be on detoxification and the need to ensure abstinence, possibly by confinement if necessary. When there are difficult diagnostic dilemmas in distinguishing substance-induced symptoms from autonomous syndromes (e.g., major depressive disorder vs. stimulant withdrawal depression), there is a need for increased intensity of monitoring, and often a period of short-term residential abstinence is required to clarify diagnosis and treatment.

Dimension 2: Biomedical Conditions and Complications

Dimension 2 includes treatment services for the wide variety of medical conditions commonly associated with adolescent substance use, some of which may be a marker for overall severity and progression of SUDs. Severe medical complications of substance use include traumatic injuries (either accidental or due to victimization) associated with any substance intoxication, respiratory depression caused by opioid overdose, sudden inhalant death syndrome (from cardiac arrhythmia and hypoxia), and seizures caused by either stimulant or inhalant intoxication. Acute alcohol poisoning is a severe medical complication that is more typical of adolescents than adults. The sequelae of injection drug use are well known and include soft-tissue infections, HIV, endocarditis, hepatitis B, and especially hepatitis C.

There is a need for assessment and treatment of the sexually transmitted infections associated with high-risk sexual behaviors in substance-involved adolescents (e.g., chlamydial, gonococcal, and human papillomavirus (HPV); and syphilis). These are too often overlooked because individuals are frequently asymptomatic. Access to contraception and education regarding barrier methods for prevention of sexually transmitted infections are essential. When treatment services are being selected, the special needs and medical vulnerabilities of pregnant substance-using teenagers require particular care. The need for education, prevention, and treatment services related to sexual behaviors cannot be overemphasized.

The involvement of primary care medicine (pediatrics and family medicine) in SUD treatment can make a valuable contribution but unfortunately occurs infrequently. Primary care settings are essential for delivering prevention and early intervention services, as well as providing longitudinal and coordinated continuity of specialty care.

Increasing interest is being shown in stepped-care models, such as the Screening, Brief Intervention, and Referral to Treatment (SBIRT) model (see Chapter 4 for more information). Such models would be especially applicable in the emergency department and in the general medical setting, where patients with lower-severity cases might respond to briefer, time-limited interventions. More complex or refractory cases (e.g., chronic medical conditions such as diabetes; chronic pain) would be linked to specialty care.

Dimension 3: Emotional, Behavioral, or Cognitive Conditions and Complications

Psychiatric comorbidity is the rule rather than the exception among adolescents with SUDs. Please refer to Part IV, "Co-occurring Disorders in Youth," in this manual (Chapters 17–21).

Adolescents who have not been diagnosed with a psychiatric disorder because a formal psychiatric evaluation has not been conducted or their symptoms are subsyndromal may still experience Dimension 3 problems and need treatment decisions. Examples include hyperactivity or distractibility without a diagnosis of attention-deficit/hyperactivity disorder, mood lability and explosive temper without a diagnosis of bipolar disorder, dysphoric mood and loss of interests without a diagnosis of depression, and various nonspecific symptoms (e.g., problems with anger management; social withdrawal induced or exacerbated by substance use).

An important aspect of the Dimension 3 assessment that features prominently in early triage for treatment matching is the assessment for dangerousness—that is, whether the adolescent needs placement or urgent services for suicidality, assaultiveness, risk of victimization, acute psychosis, or other issues related to safety of self or others. Another indicator of this dimension is the extent to which emotional or behavioral symptoms interfere with or distract from treatment and recovery efforts. Examples include difficulty attending to treatment sessions because of problems with attention and concentration, and difficulty in completing recovery assignments or absorbing treatment material because of problems with memory or comprehension. Another useful metric is the impact of emotional or behavioral problems on social functioning and difficulties in meeting role responsibilities in the major arenas of family, school, work, and personal relationships. Examples include problems in managing peer or family conflict, home rules, legal and conduct problems, truancy, school performance, and loneliness. The acquisition of self-regulation skills is an essential goal of treatment for substance users, and particularly for adolescents in neurocognitive impairment and/or developmental immaturity. Another consideration is the extent to which ability for self-care or management of daily living activities, physical and sexual safety, nutrition, and hygiene has been affected.

There is a great need for program development and cross-training of counselors and youth workers regarding co-occurring disorders and treatments (Fishman 2016). This nomenclature refers not only to the intensity of available professional services (e.g., psychiatry, psychology, nursing, occupational therapy) but also to the ability of the staff and the overall milieu to tolerate or to provide meaningful interventions for potentially provocative or disruptive psychiatric symptoms and behaviors (e.g., aggression, oppositionality, suicidal thoughts, psychosis, self-induced vomiting, self-injurious behaviors such as cutting).

Dimension 4: Readiness to Change

The key considerations in Dimension 4 are motivation and engagement, which involve the ability and willingness to attend and participate in treatment, an attitude of help seeking, and the actual track record of treatment utilization. Assessments of and interventions for motivation and engagement are important both for the adolescent and for the family or caregiver, and are often different for each.

Because of their developmental immaturity, adolescents tend to present at earlier stages of readiness to change than do adults. Also contributing to poor readiness to change are the low perceptions of harm of substance use. For example, the attitude that marijuana is "no problem" is increasingly prominent in the current medicalization and legalization environment of decreased societal stigma against and decreased restrictions on access to cannabis. Thus, it is uncommon for adolescents to be ready for treatment at first presentation, and role induction is critical. Use of the concepts and strategies of motivational interviewing and motivational enhancement therapy is vital in order to appreciate the adolescents' current goals and his order level of motivation to change.

External pressures to seek treatment tend to be more effective for adolescents than adults (Deas et al. 2000). Common externally oriented goals and contingencies that tend to motivate adolescents include parental and other caregiver pressures and influences (e.g., approval, privileges, rewards, disciplinary consequences); legal mandates and sanctions; peer pressures, influences, and affiliations; and contingencies related to school (e.g., suspension, participation in athletic teams and other extracurricular activities). Manipulations of such external contingencies are often effective, even in the absence of subjective internal motivation. Emphasis on juvenile justice involvement, use of court mandates and monitoring, and application of legal contingencies can be extremely helpful. It is sometimes difficult, but nevertheless vital, to achieve effective cooperation and coordination between treatment providers and the juvenile justice system. Specific approaches that emphasize juvenile justice integration have been developed and may provide a good match for adolescents with low levels of treatment engagement in the context of delinquency and adjudication. One example is juvenile drug courts, which utilize a specified set of graduated sanctions and rewards, and which have staff whose training and goals cross between the justice and treatment systems. (For more information, see Chapter 22 of this manual.)

A variety of practical strategies may be effective in promoting engagement. These can include assertive outreach, such as use of texting, phone calls, social media, or even home visits, for adolescents or families who are more difficult to engage. School-based services are an increasingly widespread method for improving engagement by co-locating treatment in convenient community settings (Onrust et al. 2016). Also appropriate in some circumstances are strategies that target typical practical engagement barriers. These strategies could include providing transportation, assisting with public benefits (e.g., Medicaid), and developing advances and flexibility in reimbursement structures that increase access. Because many adolescents may perceive traditional treatment as boring, treatment providers have adopted approaches that emphasize active rather than passive learning and using experiential and fun activities that can be energetic while preserving serious therapeutic content.

Finally, treatment alliance may be the most powerful tool for engagement (Brown 2001). Treatment engagement is probably as much about the messenger as the message. Attention and expression of interest and concern are potent motivators for adolescents in general. Additionally, many substance-involved adolescents have had few connections with benevolent adults, or few prosocial adult role models. Adolescents who are rewarded and engaged by a relationship with an adult may benefit from individual (rather than group) counseling or from mentoring over a longer duration. The subjective sense of a positive helping relationship with a provider (an individual or even an institution) also often helps with reengagement following dropout or relapse. Engagement may also be enhanced by the adult's acknowledgment and even partial endorsement of adolescent culture, including its typical stance of nonconformity with adult and mainstream norms. Culturally and/or ethnically specific programming can also serve as an engagement tool.

Dimension 5: Relapse, Continued Use, or Continued Problem Potential

Important goals in Dimension 5 are to predict the risk of further substance use (either relapse or continuing use), to assess potential dangerousness, and to choose appropriate interventions in response to risk. An adolescent's historical patterns of use and of change are often likely to predict future course of illness, including relapse potential. For example, some adolescents are more likely to have a rapid course of full reinstatement of substance dependence with severe impairment following a single lapse episode, whereas others are likely to have a more indolent course, with only gradual escalation of substance use. Knowledge of the individual's response to past treatment also may serve as a guide to placement. On the one hand, if a particular treatment intervention or modality, dose of treatment, or level of care led to a significant period of improvement for an adolescent in the past, then it may be appropriate to repeat that treatment following a relapse or exacerbation. These recommendations apply not only to professional treatment but also to other interventions and circumstances, such as parental involvement and juvenile justice contingencies. This approach is one way of informing treatment and placement matching decisions on an individualized basis.

Although there may be some enduring effectiveness of time-limited interventions (Dennis et al. 2004; Hser et al. 2001; Muck et al. 2001), many adolescents are refractory (at least initially) to treatment, and many adolescents have partial posttreatment improvements that are short of abstinence or "full" recovery. Furthermore, the course for many adolescents, especially those with higher severity, is characterized by remission and relapse, with multiple episodes of treatment over time. Dimension 5 assessment guides practitioners in planning longitudinal treatment that supports incremental improvements, accommodates shifting priorities, and responds to periodic relapse and/or exacerbation. It is sometimes difficult for parents, policy critics, and other stakeholders to accept and characterize partial improvements as successes; however, the substantial increases in psychosocial functioning that usually accompany partial decreases in substance use are an important measure of treatment effectiveness, and also a critical part of what shapes ongoing treatment planning in Dimension 5. The unrealistic expectation of "cure" sometimes contributes to the view that high-severity or refractory cases are "chronic" and not worthy of additional efforts or resources. This view is contrary to the more appropriate view of therapeutic optimism and problem management common to other health care arenas.

One area of particular interest related to Dimension 5 is that of continuing care. Ongoing treatment at less intensive levels of care (step-down, aftercare, or continuing care), with the intent of consolidating and sustaining gains initiated at more intensive levels of care, should be an expected feature of successful treatment across a continuum of care. Because enduring treatment effectiveness may be tempered by the attenuation of treatment effect over time, the need for ongoing reinforcement or periodic booster doses of treatment and/or monitoring checkups should be anticipated. Rates of utilization of continuing care are alarmingly low following index episodes of residential (Fishman et al. 2005; Godley et al. 2007) and outpatient (Kaminer et al. 2008) treatment. Assertive continuing care approaches have been successful using home delivery of counseling following episodes of residential treatment (Godley et al. 2003) and telephone-based care following episodes of outpatient treatment (Kaminer and Napolitano 2010). Another assertive continuing care approach used treatment engagement outreach by telephone and text, family involvement (intersection with Dimension 6), and home delivery of relapse prevention medications following acute residential treatment for opioid addiction (Vo et al. 2018). The development of pharmacological strategies for management of relapse potential, involving the use of primary anti-addiction medications (sometimes referred to as anti-craving agents, or medication-assisted recovery), holds exciting new promise, especially for patients with opioid use disorder (Borodovsky et al. 2018). (See Chapter 12 for more information on continuity of care.)

Dimension 6: Recovery/Living Environment

In Dimension 6, the keys include the influences of the parents and other caretakers, the home environment, peers, and the community. During assessment, families are necessary collateral informants. Furthermore, given the tendency of adolescents to minimize impairment, collateral informants usually present a more accurate account of psychosocial function. Adolescents' history should also be considered in a family system context. Despite their developmentally appropriate bravado of independence, adolescents continue to rely heavily on the supports and influences of adults. It is important to try to understand how the home environment, especially the family, shapes an adolescent's behavior. In turn, such an understanding can provide a basis for informing interventions and treatment. A wide range of family-based intervention strategies are available. These include family education, individual family counseling and therapy, multifamily groups, parenting interventions, enhancement of mutual family support, and others. Some interventions have the goal of improving parents' knowledge, because parents are often underinformed about substance use, access to substances, the course and treatment of SUDs, normative and deviant aspects of adolescent culture, and availability of treatment resources. Some interventions have the goal of using the family's influence to support the adolescent's engagement and involvement in treatment.

Some interventions have the goal of helping the family to improve its approach to monitoring, supervision, and home interventions. These interventions are based on the concept that the adolescents themselves may not be the initial or most important locus of change. Rather, it may be more effective to expect that the family as the primary locus of change will in turn change the adolescent. Parents often need help with setting consistent limits, providing effective discipline, and modeling prosocial behaviors.

By the time of presentation to treatment, many parents are often stuck in an embattled and ineffective mode of monitoring and supervision that alternates unpredictably between overreactive, punitive responses and abdication of the parenting role. These families need encouragement and refereeing for both sides to find common ground for positive reengagement. Many parents need help with the unrealistic hope that their adolescents will somehow change through a fundamental self-change in worldview, or with the expectation of self-maturation. These parents are understandably weary of the unending battles but are also overwhelmed by the amount of work required day in and day out to effectively reshape behaviors. Many parents need guidance for use of behavioral contingencies, especially rewards, to reinforce desired behaviors. Families may be helped by instruction and practice in how to conduct effective negotiations. Various skills-based interventions target communication skills, problem-solving skills, or home behavior management skills for adolescents or for caretakers or for both together. Although such family-based interventions may be arrayed with or added on to other treatment approaches, some approaches are committed to a primary role for family-based treatments (see Chapter 14 for more information about family therapy).

Other Dimension 6 interventions include efforts to make the recovery environment safer by attenuating toxic environmental influences, such as substance abuse, maltreatment, criminal behaviors, and antisocial attitudes in the home. Some adolescents have a social network composed primarily or even exclusively of those who use substances, a social context that may portray substance use as normative. Some adolescents have no role models of abstinence or the experience of living in an environment that fosters healthy prosocial development and functioning.

In severe situations, the best action may be temporary removal of adolescents from toxic home environments and placement in residential treatment to provide reprieve or counterbalancing interventions. Some preliminary work has suggested that adolescents with significant levels of acute traumatic stress may be more responsive to residential than to outpatient levels of care (Funk et al. 2003; National Institute on Drug Abuse, 2014), given that the former provides temporary removal from sources of stress. For especially severe cases, efforts may be necessary to remove adolescents more definitively from toxic environments and find long-term residential treatment or alternative living arrangements (e.g., placement with other family members).

Treatment Matching and Placement

Once treatment service needs and approaches have been determined, the next goal is to create the opportunity for their implementation through placement referral recommendations. Researchers and clinicians are just beginning to untangle the heterogeneity of adolescent SUDs and to gain some broader understanding about staging and subgroups, as well as the treatment response patterns of those subgroups. As understanding develops, it will become more realistic to propose more specific and operationalized treatment matching guidelines, which will eventually lead to specific practice guidelines that recommend specific treatment interventions, modalities, doses, lengths of treatment, and so on. While work is ongoing to expand the underdeveloped continuum, practitioners have to adapt realistically to the resources at hand. Often, when a given level of care is not practicably available, a more intensive level of care that is available is the best substitute. Another approach that is sometimes successful is to creatively weave together a multidimensional array of services from a variety of sources that approximates the intensity of the unavailable level of care. An example of the former approach is the common practice of using inpatient psychiatric hospitalization as a setting for stabilization of substance-related crises when no medically monitored high-intensity residential program is available. Another example is the use of brief residential placement for daily support and monitoring when no Level 2.5 PHP/day program is available. An example of the latter "patchwork" approach is substituting increased frequency of Level 1 outpatient sessions (say, two or three per week) for an unavailable Level 2.1 intensive outpatient program. Another example might be combining a Level 2.5 PHP/day program with an alternative, temporary living situation (e.g., with a relative) that is less problematic than the home environment as a substitution for an unavailable Level 3.5 residential placement.

Issues regarding longitudinal follow-up are critical, especially for adolescents because they are so dynamic in their developmental changes and needs. Long-term relationships with youth and families, with the expectation of accommodating dropping in and dropping out, with changing needs over time, should be standard. Facilitation of continuity between linked episodes of care at different levels of care based on need is vital and includes coordination, assertive outreach, and overlapping levels of care. ASAM Criteria was developed as a consensus-based guide to best practices by committees of experts and diverse stakeholders. As such, the application of the criteria is not concretely operationalized or based on standardized assessment instruments, and their use clearly relies on the utilization of sound clinical interpretation and judgment. The ongoing process of further operationalizing the adult ASAM Criteria through its computer version (CONTINUUM) shows one possible future direction for increased reliability. Work is beginning on developing a computerized version of the adolescent ASAM Criteria as well.

Key Points

- ASAM Criteria provides a standard approach and practical organization for treatment planning that includes assessment of severity in each dimension; determination of treatment service needs in each assessment dimension; and selection of setting, program, and placement in an integrated treatment plan.

- The field is accumulating knowledge about specific strategies for matching heterogeneous subtypes of youth with substance use disorders, based on their clinical characteristics, to different treatment interventions, modalities, doses, and levels of care.

- The treatment service delivery system is being improved by broadening the continuum of care to more fully include continuing care, longitudinal monitoring, and coordinating between episodes of treatment at different levels of care.

References

Borodovsky JT, Levy S, Fishman M, et al: Buprenorphine treatment for adolescents and young adults with opioid use disorders: a narrative review. J Addict Med 12(3):170–183, 2018 29432333

Brown S: Facilitating change for adolescent alcohol problems: a multiple options approach, in Innovations in Adolescent Substance Abuse Interventions. Edited by Wagner E, Waldron H. New York, Elselvier Science, 2001, pp 169–187

Clemmey P, Payne L, Fishman M: Clinical characteristics and treatment outcomes of adolescent heroin users. J Psychoactive Drugs 36(1):85–94, 2004 15152712

Dasinger LK, Shane PA, Martinovich Z: Assessing the effectiveness of community-based substance abuse treatment for adolescents. J Psychoactive Drugs 36(1):27–33, 2004 15152707

Deas D, Riggs P, Langenbucher J, et al: Adolescents are not adults: developmental considerations in alcohol users. Alcohol Clin Exp Res 24(2):232–237, 2000 10698377

Dennis M, Godley SH, Diamond G, et al: The Cannabis Youth Treatment (CYT) Study: main findings from two randomized trials. J Subst Abuse Treat 27(3):197–213, 2004 15501373

Fishman M: Treatment planning, matching, and placement for adolescents with substance use disorders, in Adolescent Substance Abuse: Psychiatric Comorbidity and High-Risk Behaviors. Edited by Kaminer Y, Bukstein OG. New York, Routledge/Taylor & Francis, 2008, pp 87–110

Fishman M: The relationship between substance use disorders and psychiatric comorbidity: implications for integrated health services, in Youth Substance Abuse and Co-Occurring Disorders. Edited by Kaminer Y. Arlington, VA, American Psychiatric Association Publishing, 2016, pp 21–48

Fishman M, Payne L, Clemmey P: Engagement in adolescent continuing care. Presentation at the Joint Meeting on Adolescent Treatment Effectiveness, Washington, DC, March 21, 2005

Funk RR, McDermeit M, Godley SH, et al: Maltreatment issues by level of adolescent substance abuse treatment: the extent of the problem at intake and relationship to early outcomes. Child Maltreat 8(1):36–45, 2003 12568503

Godley S, Godley M, Karvinen T, et al: The assertive continuing care protocol: a case manager's manual for working with adolescents after residential treatment for alcohol and other substance use disorders. 2003. Available at: https://www.researchgate.net/publication/279719617_The_Assertive_Aftercare_Protocol_for_Adolescent_Substance_Abusers. Accessed April 29, 2019.

Godley MD, Godley SH, Dennis MI: The effect of assertive continuing care on continuing care linkage, adherence and abstinence following residential treatment for adolescents with substance use disorders. Addiction 102(1):81–93, 2007 17207126

Hser YI, Grella CE, Hubbard RL, et al: An evaluation of drug treatments for adolescents in 4 US cities. Arch Gen Psychiatry 58(7):689–695, 2001 11448377

Kaminer Y, Napolitano C: Telephone Continuing Care Therapy for Adolescents. Center City, MN, Hazelden, 2010

Kaminer Y, Burleson JA, Burke RH: Efficacy of outpatient aftercare for adolescents with alcohol use disorders: a randomized controlled study. J Am Acad Child Adolesc Psychiatry 47(12):1405–1412, 2008 18978635

Marsch LA, Bickel WK, Badger GJ, et al: Comparison of pharmacological treatments for opioid-dependent adolescents: a randomized controlled trial. Arch Gen Psychiatry 62(10):1157–1164, 2005 16203961

Mee-Lee D, Shulman GD, Fishman M, et al: The ASAM Criteria: Treatment Criteria for Addictive, Substance-Related, and Co-occurring Conditions, 3rd Edition. Chevy Chase, MD, American Society of Addiction Medicine, 2013

Muck R, Zempolich K, Titus J, et al: An overview of the effectiveness of adolescent substance abuse treatment models. Youth and Society 33(2):143–168, 2001

National Institute on Drug Abuse: Principles of Adolescent Substance Use Disorder Treatment: A Research-Based Guide (NIH Publ No 14-7953). Bethesda, MD, National Institute on Drug Abuse, 2014

Onrust SA, Otten R, Lammers J, et al: School-based programmes to reduce and prevent substance use in different age groups: what works for whom? Systematic review and meta-regression analysis. Clin Psychol Rev 44:45–59, 2016 26722708

Vo HT, Burgower R, Rozenberg I, et al: Home-based delivery of XR-NTX in youth with opioid addiction. J Subst Abuse Treat 85:84–89, 2018 28867062

PART II

Description, Diagnosis, and Interventions for Specific Substances of Abuse

7

Youth Alcohol Use

Robert Miranda Jr., Ph.D.

Ryan W. Carpenter, Ph.D.

Each year in the United States, an estimated 623,000 adolescents ages 12–17 develop a sufficient spectrum of alcohol-related problems to warrant a diagnosis of alcohol use disorder (AUD) (Substance Abuse and Mental Health Services Administration 2016), and alcohol misuse remains a major impetus for substance abuse treatment admissions among teenagers. According to the World Health Organization (WHO), worldwide, more than a quarter of all 15- to 19-years-olds are current drinkers. Prevalence rates of current drinking are highest in Europe (44%), followed by the Americas and the Western Pacific Region (38%). Drinking peaks between 20–24 years, when rates of use become higher than in the total population. Prevalence of episodic heavy drinking is common between the ages of 15–24 years, particularly in males.

The authors acknowledge the National Institute on Alcohol Abuse and Alcoholism for its support of this work (K24 AA026326, T32 AA07459).

Until 2025, total alcohol consumption per capita in persons age 15 years and older is projected to increase worldwide.

Youth whose use meets the DSM-5 criteria for an AUD report symptoms that reflect loss of control, preoccupation and personal negative consequences, and, in some cases, tolerance and withdrawal. As summarized in Chapter 1 of this manual, youth whose use meets two or more criteria within a 12-month period pass the threshold for a DSM-5 AUD diagnosis; subgroups of severity are based on the number of symptom criteria met: mild (2–3 criteria), moderate (4–5 criteria), and severe (6 or more criteria). Also noteworthy is the developmental course of adolescents with an AUD. Chapter 1 provides more details on this issue, but suffice it to indicate that the developmental course of AUD shows heterogeneity that ranges from the individual maturing out of alcohol-related problems to the disorder remaining chronic. Prevention of substance use disorders is reviewed in Chapter 2.

The treatment of adolescents with AUD remains challenging (for detailed discussion of specific psychosocial interventions, see Part 3 of this manual). Clinical trials and meta-analyses show that psychosocial interventions, including family, cognitive-behavioral, and motivational enhancement therapies, yield only modest short-term benefit. Less than one-third of youth experience sustained benefit from existing treatments; the majority of treated youth return to drinking within 6 months posttreatment. One potential way to advance treatment options for youth who struggle to reduce their alcohol use is to augment the best available psychosocial interventions with pharmacotherapy.

Pharmacological Treatment of Adolescent Alcohol Misuse

The U.S. Food and Drug Administration (FDA) has approved three medications to treat AUD in adults, which we review in this chapter, and researchers have identified additional promising compounds. Whereas on the whole medication development research has improved the quality of care for adults, our understanding of whether and how medications might advance treatment options for adolescents with AUD is at a nascent stage. In this light, we review the state of science on pharmacotherapy for adults with AUD and then discuss the relevance of this literature on adolescents who struggle to reduce their alcohol use. Specifically, we start with an overview of what is known about medications for treating AUD in *adults* based on over three decades of research.

This involves reviews of the mechanisms by which medications are thought to exert their beneficial effects and the medications used to treat AUD in adults, including those approved by the FDA and promising new medications. We then provide a comprehensive review of existing research on whether and how these medications affect *adolescent* alcohol use. Shortcomings of this work are discussed. Although we focus on randomized controlled trials that studied alcohol misuse as the primary treatment target, open-label studies and case reports are also reviewed.

Treatment Targets: Mechanisms of Action

Medications for AUD target myriad neuropharmacological mechanisms, including, but not limited to, modulation of opioid, glutamatergic, and γ-aminobutyric acid (GABA) neurotransmission. Despite this range, pharmacotherapies are thought to affect alcohol use through one or more common biobehavioral mechanisms that are central to the relapse process (Heilig and Egli 2006). These mechanisms include blunting alcohol craving; altering subjective responses to alcohol consumption, either by blunting pleasurable rewarding effects or producing strong adverse reactions; and mitigating negative affect associated with withdrawal during protracted abstinence. By intervening on these mechanisms, medications exert beneficial effects by reducing the likelihood of initiating alcohol use (i.e., increasing abstinence) or attenuating the amount of alcohol consumed during a drinking episode (i.e., reducing heavy drinking).

Blunting Alcohol Craving

Empirical evidence that craving is a valuable target for pharmacotherapy comes from several sources. Craving is a strong predictor of alcohol use in the human laboratory and the natural environment, and medications that decrease cue-elicited craving in the laboratory also blunt craving in clinical trials (Mason et al. 2014; Miranda et al. 2014b). Cue-elicited craving involves systematic exposure to alcohol cues under controlled experimental conditions in the human laboratory while subjective and physiological reactivity (i.e., heart rate, blood pressure, salivation) is assessed. The premise is that exposure to alcohol cues simulates high-risk situations for relapse and therefore affords a useful paradigm for screening medications and understanding how efficacious pharmacotherapies reduce drinking.

Human studies and preclinical models suggest that individuals for whom alcohol and other drug cues attain incentive motivational value or incentive salience are those most likely to exhibit relapse. Retrospective studies show that stronger cue reactivity is associated with past instances of relapse (Erblich and Bovbjerg 2004). In addition, craving in response to alcohol cues in abstinent alcoholics is predictive of subsequent drinking outcomes, including relapse (Spagnolo et al. 2014); albeit a few studies did not find this association (Witteman et al. 2015). Given the clinical relevance of craving and the utility of the cue reactivity paradigm, the National Institute on Alcohol Abuse and Alcoholism (NIAAA) is leveraging this paradigm to screen novel compounds within its broader medication development pipeline.

Altering Subjective Responses to Alcohol Consumption

The acute reinforcing properties of alcohol are chief determinants of drinking in all contemporary theoretical models of AUD, and there is strong evidence that certain individuals are uniquely sensitive to these effects in ways that confer heightened liability for hazardous drinking. It is therefore not surprising that clinical scientists have characterized the subjective effects of alcohol consumption and examined if and how medications alter these responses in the human laboratory and, more recently, real-world settings (Miranda et al. 2016). The guiding hypothesis for this work is that medications reduce drinking, at least in part, by dampening the pleasurable and stimulatory effects of alcohol ingestion or enhancing its unpleasant effects.

Empirical support for this contention stems from research that shows subjective alcohol effects predict subsequent volumes of alcohol consumption, such that stimulatory effects are associated with more alcohol use and dysphoric effects predict less use in adolescents and adults. Therefore, medications that dull the pleasurable effects of alcohol or boost its unpleasant effects may decrease the quantity of alcohol consumed, particularly from harmful levels. A variety of medications (i.e., baclofen, naltrexone, ondansetron, sertraline, and topiramate) affect the intoxicating properties of alcohol.

Mitigating Negative Affect Associated With Withdrawal During Protracted Abstinence

The unpleasantness of protracted abstinence and withdrawal is considered a contributor to relapse in adults, and therefore an important target of pharmacotherapy. As individuals progress in AUD pathology, neurobiological reward functions become compromised while the stress reactivity system becomes hypersensitive. This confluence of downregulated sensitivity to rewards and upregulated reactivity to stressors confers heightened liability to seek and consume alcohol for negative reinforcement purposes. Yet, despite a strong theoretical foundation, medication development research largely neglected this treatment target until the past decade (Koob and Mason 2016). Although alcohol withdrawal is uncommon among youth, even those with AUD, several medications shown to treat AUD in adults have actions that can be considered relevant for treating the withdrawal/negative affect, including acamprosate and varenicline (Koob and Mason 2016).

FDA-Approved Medications for Adults

A considerable empirical literature on the clinical use of medications to treat AUD has mounted since the late 1980s. Numerous pharmacotherapy trials were funded by the NIAAA, three medications received FDA approval, and additional promising compounds were identified. Although these efforts improved treatment for adults, no medication is approved to treat adolescents with AUD. Although the FDA does not prohibit prescribing medications for off-label indications if the health care provider judges it is medically appropriate, it is important to consider the scientific rationale and empirical evidence (including safety) when evaluating the appropriateness of such unapproved use.

The following is a description of FDA-approved medications for treating AUD in adults, along with an overview of the evidence for their use and information about their side effect profiles. It is important to consider, however, that evidence from several branches of medicine highlights problems with inferring the safety and efficacy of medication use with adolescents from adult data. Moreover, there is reason to believe that such inferences may present particular issues in the context of addiction treatment due to several clinically relevant differences between adolescents and adults. Adolescents exhibit AUD symptom presentations and associated features that are distinct from adults. In addition, preclinical and emerging human evidence shows that adolescents experience the acute effects of alcohol consumption in unique ways (Miranda et al. 2014a; Spear 2014). These differences, which appear attributable to the substantial neuronal remodeling that occurs during adolescence, are thought to heighten vulnerability to heavy drinking and AUD pathology and may impact how youth respond to medications. Consequently, as with prescribing practices for all medications, documentation of the rationale for the use of medication, discussion of the risk-benefit ratio with the adolescent and family, and patient education regarding the dosing schedule and scope and time course of anticipated effects must be provided by the health care provider prior to initiating pharmacotherapy.

Disulfiram

Disulfiram is an aldehyde dehydrogenase inhibitor approved by the FDA more than 60 years ago to treat alcoholism among adults. By inhibiting aldehyde dehydrogenase, disulfiram potentiates accumulation of acetaldehyde, a toxic metabolite of alcohol, and causes a host of adverse reactions, such as nausea, vomiting, diarrhea, flushing, sweating, tachycardia, and hypotension. Although the frequency of these symptoms is not well characterized, onset typically occurs within 15 minutes of alcohol ingestion and lasts up to several hours. The presumed mechanism of action is the patient's awareness that consuming alcohol while taking disulfiram will result in this adverse reaction.

Empirical evidence for the clinical efficacy of disulfiram in adults is mixed. A meta-analysis of 22 randomized controlled trials with 2,414 participants showed that disulfiram demonstrated beneficial effects, such as abstinence, reduced days of alcohol use, and longer duration to the first heavy drinking day, in open-label studies, but not in double-blind clinical trials unless administration of the medication was supervised (Skinner et al. 2014). The side effect profile of disulfiram, beyond events associated with the disulfiram-alcohol interaction, is generally considered minimal and mainly includes drowsiness. More serious but rare reactions, such as cardiovascular collapse, hepatitis, neuropathy, optic neuritis, psychosis, and confusion, can also occur, and this calls into question the appropriateness of this medication for patients with harm reduction goals rather than abstinence (Kranzler and Soyka 2018).

Naltrexone

Naltrexone is a μ-, κ-, and δ-opioid receptor antagonist and a frontline medication for treating AUD in adults. By attenuating opioidergic activity, this medication is thought to blunt dopaminergic transmission in mesolimbic reward pathways (Benjamin et al. 1993) and reduce craving and the reinforcing effects of alcohol (Valenta et al. 2013). More than 20 randomized controlled trials of oral naltrexone for alcohol misuse in adults have been published, and results of meta-analyses show that it reduces the quantity and frequency of alcohol use as well as relapse rates in heavy drinking adults, with modest magnitude effect sizes (Jonas et al. 2014; Maisel et al. 2013). There is considerable variability in patient responsiveness to naltrexone, however, with approximately only 1 of every 12 people treated with naltrexone showing reductions in heavy drinking (Jonas et al. 2014). Given this considerable person-to-person variability, a growing focus of clinical research is to identify patient characteristics that predict naltrexone treatment responsiveness. The predictive value of previously studied moderators (e.g., sex, pretreatment drinking), however, is low (Garbutt et al. 2014).

Support for the hypothesis that naltrexone affects drinking by blunting alcohol craving comes from clinical trials that show it reduced the frequency and intensity of weekly craving ratings (Maisel et al. 2013). A meta-analysis of laboratory studies found that naltrexone blunts craving caused by exposure to alcohol cues (Hendershot et al. 2017). The magnitude of this effect was modest, however, and there is considerable variability in craving response that warrants further attention in subgroup analyses.

Both daily and targeted oral dosing show beneficial effects on alcohol use, and an FDA-approved injectable formulation with long-acting effects is also available for patients able to abstain from alcohol in an outpatient setting before treatment initiation. Findings from a multicenter 24-week randomized controlled trial with 624 adults showed that the injectable formulation, compared with placebo, significantly reduced the median frequency of binge drinking from 19.3 days per month pretreatment to 3.1 days per month (Garbutt et al. 2005). Only one small study, to our knowledge, directly compared the effects of the oral (50 mg/day) and injectable (380 mg) formulations on alcohol use. They found that patients in both conditions were less likely to engage in binge drinking during the 45-day monitoring period (Busch et al. 2017). The likelihood of no binge drinking increased from 13.6% pretreatment to 75.0% posttreatment in patients taking the oral dose, while it increased from 13.6% to 77.8% in those administered the injectable formulation. However, the small sample size precluded a direct statistical comparison between the two conditions.

Pooled side effect data from clinical trials show that the commonly reported adverse effects of oral naltrexone, as compared with placebo, include somnolence, nausea, decreased appetite, vomiting, insomnia, abdominal pain, and dizziness (Rösner et al. 2010). Long-acting naltrexone can cause the same adverse events as oral naltrexone and also injection-site reactions. It is important to note that naltrexone blocks the therapeutic effects of opioid analgesics and can precipitate opioid withdrawal in a patient who is physically dependent on opioids.

Acamprosate

Acamprosate was first marketed to treat alcohol dependence in Europe nearly 30 years ago. In 2004, the FDA approved acamprosate for maintaining alcohol abstinence for patients already abstinent at the start of medication treatment. Although the precise neuropharmacological mechanisms by which acamprosate affects alcohol use remain unknown, preclinical studies point to glutamatergic modulation and consequent counteraction of alcohol-induced hyperactivation and dopamine release in the nucleus accumbens.

Several meta-analyses examined the efficacy of acamprosate on alcohol use outcomes and concluded it yields small-to-moderate magnitude effect sizes (Jonas et al. 2014; Maisel et al. 2013). For example, a recent meta-analysis of 16 controlled trials comprising 4,349 adults showed that acamprosate, compared with placebo, produced greater reductions in the risk of drinking among abstinent patients (Maisel et al. 2013). It had no effect on the likelihood of binge drinking. In terms of its safety profile, acamprosate has no known interactions with other psychotropic medications, and the only adverse event that occurs more frequently with acamprosate than placebo is diarrhea.

Other Medications for Treating AUD in Adults

Many putative pharmacotherapies beyond those approved by the FDA have been studied for potential efficacy for treating AUD. Of these medications, the following agents show promise.

Topiramate and Gabapentin

Two anticonvulsant medications show promise for treating AUD. Topiramate is a mixed GABA agonist and AMPA/kainate glutamate receptor antagonist approved by the FDA to treat seizure disorder, migraine headaches, and obesity. Since the first evidence emerged supporting its efficacy for reducing alcohol use (Johnson et al. 2003), it has received considerable attention as a promising pharmacotherapy for AUD. Meta-analyses have found that topiramate increases abstinence, reduces heavy drinking, and lowers liver enzyme levels, with small to moderate magnitude effect sizes (Arbaizar et al. 2010; Blodgett et al. 2014). Other positive findings suggest that topiramate reduces adverse consequences from drinking, improves quality of life, and exhibits larger magnitude effect sizes than other pharmacotherapies (Arbaizar et al. 2010; Johnson et al. 2004). Many patients cannot tolerate its adverse side effect profile, however, which includes (but is not limited to) paresthesia, dysgeusia, word-finding difficulties, and difficulty with concentration or attention.

Gabapentin is another FDA-approved medication for treating epilepsy (as well as neuropathic pain) that shows promise for reducing alcohol use. It is thought to modulate GABA activity by indirectly interacting with voltage-gated calcium channels (Sills 2006). Three randomized controlled trials are published to date, and on the whole, gabapentin improved abstinence rates and reduced heavy drinking (Brower et al. 2008; Furieri and Nakamura-Palacios 2007; Mason et al. 2014). One study had high (43%) dropout rates (Mason et al. 2014), however, and there is evidence that some patients, and especially those with co-occurring opioid misuse, abuse gabapentin, which highlights the need to carefully assess for co-occurring opioid use when considering this medication for AUD (Smith et al. 2016). Common adverse events associated with gabapentin treatment include dizziness, somnolence, ataxia or gait disorder, and peripheral edema.

Nalmefene

Nalmefene is a μ- and δ-opioid receptor antagonist and a κ-opioid receptor partial agonist approved in Europe to treat AUD. A meta-analysis showed that nalmefene reduced overall alcohol use and binge drinking in clinical trials (Palpacuer et al. 2015). However, some researchers have raised questions about the quality of evidence supporting the efficacy of nalmefene (Fitzgerald et al. 2016). Common side effects include nausea, dizziness, insomnia, headache, vomiting, fatigue, and somnolence.

Baclofen

Baclofen is a GABA agonist approved by the FDA to reduce spasticity associated with neurological disorders. Although preclinical studies showed promise for reducing alcohol use, randomized controlled trials have shown mixed findings. While baclofen increases overall abstinence rates compared with placebo, it does not increase the number of days abstinent or reduce heavy drinking. Findings from two recent meta-analyses showed that baclofen, relative to placebo, increased the likelihood of abstinence during treatment and lengthened the duration to first relapse, especially among patients who had heavy pretreatment drinking levels (Pierce et al. 2018; Rose and Jones 2018). In terms of common side effects, baclofen is associated with sedation and drowsiness, dizziness, headache, confusion, muscle stiffness, excessive perspiration, itching or pruritus, abnormal muscle movements, numbness, and slurred speech.

Indications for Adolescent Use

No medication is approved by the FDA to treat AUD among adolescents. Randomized controlled trials are the gold standard for evaluating the efficacy of interventions, including pharmacotherapies. In terms of adolescent AUD, however, many published reports are case studies or open-label trials, and all bear substantial limitations that preclude inferences about the efficacy of the medication studied. According to the FDA (21 CFR 814.3; April 1, 2018), pediatric patients include individuals younger than 22 years, with adolescents defined as youth ages 12 through 21 years. This window is generally consistent with neurodevelopmental evidence that adolescence extends to the early to mid-20s. In this review, we focus on clinical trials that targeted youth younger than 25 years. Adult trials that employed a minimum age requirement of 18 years but did not specifically evaluate the efficacy of the study medication on the subset of patients younger than 25 years are not discussed.

Case Studies

Myers et al. (1994) reported on the use of disulfiram in two teenagers with alcohol dependence; one remained abstinent and the other experienced early relapse. Wold and Kaminer (1997) reported on a 17-year old with alcohol dependence and conduct disorder and a family history of alcoholism. He received naltrexone as adjunct to an outpatient partial hospital program, remained abstinent for 30 days, and reported a decrease in craving. Lifrak et al. (1997) reported on two adolescents, ages 16 and 18 years, treated with naltrexone for 12 weeks; one remained abstinent for 26 weeks, the other decreased the number of drinking days and quantity of alcohol consumed, and both reported reductions in craving.

Open-Label Trials

Cornelius et al. (2001) conducted a 12-week study of fluoxetine (as an adjunct to supportive psychotherapy) in 13 adolescents with depression and alcohol abuse or dependence. Results indicated a significant reduction in drinks per drinking day and a trend toward reduced drinking days per week, and 7 of 13 participants showed improvement in AUD symptoms. At 1-year follow-up (n = 10), the decrease in AUD symptoms was sustained, but no additional reduction in drinking was found (Cornelius et al. 2004). At 3-year follow-up (n = 10), 4 of 10 patients had symptoms that met AUD criteria, and although they were drinking less than at baseline, they continued to binge drink at high rates (Cornelius et al. 2005). Dawes et al. (2005) reported that ondansetron reduced drinking and craving in 12 adolescents with alcohol dependence. But because participants received weekly psychotherapy during the 8-week open-label trial, it was not possible to evaluate the efficacy of ondansetron. Lastly, in a 6-week study of naltrexone, 5 adolescents with alcohol dependence reported fewer drinks per drinking day, reduced craving, and a low occurrence of side effects (Deas et al. 2005).

Randomized Controlled Trials

Niederhofer and colleagues, in three 90-day randomized trials with adolescents in Austria, found that 1) seven adolescents treated with disulfiram were continuously abstinent throughout the trial, compared with two receiving placebo (N = 26) (Niederhofer and Staffen 2003); 2) teenagers (N = 26) treated with cyanamide, an aldehyde dehydrogenase inhibitor, had a greater number of days of continuous abstinence and a longer duration of cumulative abstinences than those on placebo (Niederhofer et al. 2003a); and 3) 20 adolescents treated with naltrexone were continuously abstinent throughout the trial, compared with 10 randomly assigned to placebo (Neiderhofer et al. 2003b). Although findings from the Niederhofer studies show promise, discrepancies in some of the described sample sizes, the ages of participants, and the doses studied cloud the results.

More recently, Miranda and colleagues (2014b) examined the efficacy and mechanisms of naltrexone (50 mg/day) among adolescents ages 15–19 years, using a double-blind, placebo-controlled, within-subjects crossover design. Naltrexone treatment reduced the likelihood of drinking and heavy drinking and blunted alcohol craving. Finally, a randomized controlled clinical trial with young adults ages 18–25 years showed that naltrexone (25 mg daily + 25 mg targeted) plus a brief motivational intervention reduced the number of drinks per drinking day by the end of the 8-week treatment period (O'Malley et al. 2015). At the 12-month follow-up assessment, there were no differences between conditions, but drinking reductions observed during the active treatment phase were maintained (DeMartini et al. 2014).

Conclusion

Adolescence is a key developmental stage for the onset and progression of AUD. The profile of available interventions for youth, however, is limited in scope because of reliance on psychosocial treatments that yield modest and often only short-term effectiveness. Although clinical scientists have leveraged pharmacotherapy to advance treatment options for adults, double-blind, placebo-controlled clinical trials with adolescents are few. Optimizing treatment options for youth requires closing this important gap while combining evidence-based pharmacotherapy with psychosocial interventions.

Key Points

- Mounting evidence suggests that pharmacotherapy can augment behavioral intervention effects for adolescents with alcohol use disorder (AUD).

- Adolescents with AUD may benefit from the same types of medications shown to reduce alcohol use in adults, although caution must be exercised when one is relying on adult data to inform adolescent treatment.

- Pharmacotherapy studies for adolescent alcohol misuse suggest that naltrexone is well tolerated and may help adolescents reduce alcohol use.

- Given the dearth of robust pharmacotherapy research for treating adolescents with AUD, medication should *not* be the first-line treatment option for adolescents.

References

Arbaizar B, Diersen-Sotos T, Gómez-Acebo I, et al: Topiramate in the treatment of alcohol dependence: a meta-analysis. Actas Esp Psiquiatr 38(1):8–12, 2010 20931405

Benjamin D, Grant ER, Pohorecky LA: Naltrexone reverses ethanol-induced dopamine release in the nucleus accumbens in awake, freely moving rats. Brain Res 621(1):137–140, 1993 7693299

Blodgett JC, Del Re AC, Maisel NC, et al: A meta-analysis of topiramate's effects for individuals with alcohol use disorders. Alcohol Clin Exp Res 38(6):1481–1488, 2014 24796492

Brower KJ, Myra Kim H, Strobbe S, et al: A randomized double-blind pilot trial of gabapentin versus placebo to treat alcohol dependence and comorbid insomnia. Alcohol Clin Exp Res 32(8):1429–1438, 2008 18540923

Busch AC, Denduluri M, Glass J, et al: Predischarge injectable versus oral naltrexone to improve postdischarge treatment engagement among hospitalized veterans with alcohol use disorder: a randomized pilot proof-of-concept study. Alcohol Clin Exp Res 41(7):1352–1360, 2017 28605827

Cornelius JR, Bukstein OG, Birmaher B, et al: Fluoxetine in adolescents with major depression and an alcohol use disorder: an open-label trial. Addict Behav 26(5):735–739, 2001 11676382

Cornelius JR, Bukstein OG, Salloum IM, et al: Fluoxetine in depressed AUD adolescents: a 1-year follow-up evaluation. J Child Adolesc Psychopharmacol 14(1):33–38, 2004 15142389

Cornelius JR, Clark DB, Bukstein OG, et al: Fluoxetine in adolescents with comorbid major depression and an alcohol use disorder: a 3-year follow-up study. Addict Behav 30(4):807–814, 2005 15833583

Dawes MA, Johnson BA, Ma JZ, et al: Reductions in and relations between "craving" and drinking in a prospective, open-label trial of ondansetron in adolescents with alcohol dependence. Addict Behav 30(9):1630–1637, 2005 16084024

Deas D, May MP, Randall C, et al: Naltrexone treatment of adolescent alcoholics: an open-label pilot study. J Child Adolesc Psychopharmacol 15(5):723–728, 2005 16262589

DeMartini KS, Gueorguiva R, Leeman RF, et al: Naltrexone for non-treatment seeking young adult drinkers: one-year outcomes. Alcohol Clin Exp Res 38 (suppl 1):212A, 2014

Erblich J, Bovbjerg DH: In vivo versus imaginal smoking cue exposures: is seeing believing? Exp Clin Psychopharmacol 12(3):208–215, 2004 15301638

Fitzgerald N, Angus K, Elders A, et al: Weak evidence on nalmefene creates dilemmas for clinicians and poses questions for regulators and researchers. Addiction 111(8):1477–1487, 2016 27262594

Furieri FA, Nakamura-Palacios EM: Gabapentin reduces alcohol consumption and craving: a randomized, double-blind, placebo-controlled trial. J Clin Psychiatry 68(11):1691–1700, 2007 18052562

Garbutt JC, Kranzler HR, O'Malley SS, et al; Vivitrex Study Group: Efficacy and tolerability of long-acting injectable naltrexone for alcohol dependence: a randomized controlled trial. JAMA 293(13):1617–1625, 2005 15811981

Garbutt JC, Greenblatt AM, West SL, et al: Clinical and biological moderators of response to naltrexone in alcohol dependence: a systematic review of the evidence. Addiction 109(8):1274–1284, 2014 24661324

Heilig M, Egli M: Pharmacological treatment of alcohol dependence: target symptoms and target mechanisms. Pharmacol Ther 111(3):855–876, 2006 16545872

Hendershot CS, Wardell JD, Samokhvalov AV, et al: Effects of naltrexone on alcohol self-administration and craving: meta-analysis of human laboratory studies. Addict Biol 22(6):1515–1527, 2017 27411969

Johnson BA, Ait-Daoud N, Bowden CL, et al: Oral topiramate for treatment of alcohol dependence: a randomised controlled trial. Lancet 361(9370):1677–1685, 2003 12767733

Johnson BA, Ait-Daoud N, Akhtar FZ, et al: Oral topiramate reduces the consequences of drinking and improves the quality of life of alcohol-dependent individuals: a randomized controlled trial. Arch Gen Psychiatry 61(9):905–912, 2004 15351769

Jonas DE, Amick HR, Feltner C, et al: Pharmacotherapy for adults with alcohol use disorders in outpatient settings: a systematic review and meta-analysis. JAMA 311(18):1889–1900, 2014 24825644

Koob GF, Mason BJ: Existing and future drugs for the treatment of the dark side of addiction. Annu Rev Pharmacol Toxicol 56:299–322, 2016 26514207

Kranzler HR, Soyka M: Diagnosis and pharmacotherapy of alcohol use disorder: a review. JAMA 320(8):815–824, 2018 30167705

Lifrak PD, Alterman AI, O'Brien CP, Volpicelli JR: Naltrexone for alcoholic adolescents. Am J Psychiatry 154(3):439–441, 1997 9054806

Maisel NC, Blodgett JC, Wilbourne PL, et al: Meta-analysis of naltrexone and acamprosate for treating alcohol use disorders: when are these medications most helpful? Addiction 108(2):275–293, 2013 23075288

Mason BJ, Quello S, Goodell V, et al: Gabapentin treatment for alcohol dependence: a randomized clinical trial. JAMA Intern Med 174(1):70–77, 2014 24190578

Miranda RJr, Monti PM, Ray L, et al: Characterizing subjective responses to alcohol among adolescent problem drinkers. J Abnorm Psychol 123(1):117–129, 2014a 24661164

Miranda R, Ray L, Blanchard A, et al: Effects of naltrexone on adolescent alcohol cue reactivity and sensitivity: an initial randomized trial. Addict Biol 19(5):941–954, 2014b 23489253

Miranda RJr, MacKillop J, Treloar H, et al: Biobehavioral mechanisms of topiramate's effects on alcohol use: an investigation pairing laboratory and ecological momentary assessments. Addict Biol 21(1):171–182, 2016 25353306

Myers WC, Donahue JE, Goldstein MR: Disulfiram for alcohol use disorders in adolescents. J Am Acad Child Adolesc Psychiatry 33(4):484–489, 1994 8005901

Niederhofer H, Staffen W: Comparison of disulfiram and placebo in treatment of alcohol dependence of adolescents. Drug Alcohol Rev 22(3):295–297, 2003 15385223

Niederhofer H, Staffen W, Mair A: Comparison of cyanamide and placebo in the treatment of alcohol dependence of adolescents. Alcohol Alcohol 38(1):50–53, 2003a 12554608

Neiderhofer H, Staffen W, Mair A: Comparison of naltrexone and placebo in treatment of alcohol dependence of adolescents. Alcoholism Treatment Quarterly 21(2):87–95, 2003b

O'Malley SS, Corbin WR, Leeman RF, et al: Reduction of alcohol drinking in young adults by naltrexone: a double-blind, placebo-controlled, randomized clinical trial of efficacy and safety. J Clin Psychiatry 76(2):e207–e213, 2015 25742208

Palpacuer C, Laviolle B, Boussageon R, et al: Risks and benefits of nalmefene in the treatment of adult alcohol dependence: a systematic literature review and meta-analysis of published and unpublished double-blind randomized controlled trials. PLoS Med 12(12):e1001924, 2015 26694529

Pierce M, Sutterland A, Beraha EM, et al: Efficacy, tolerability, and safety of low-dose and high-dose baclofen in the treatment of alcohol dependence: a systematic review and meta-analysis. Eur Neuropsychopharmacol 28(7):795–806, 2018 29934090

Rose AK, Jones A: Baclofen: its effectiveness in reducing harmful drinking, craving, and negative mood. A meta-analysis. Addiction 113(8):1396–1406, 2018 29479827

Rösner S, Hackl-Herrwerth A, Leucht S, et al: Opioid antagonists for alcohol dependence. Cochrane Database Syst Rev (12):CD001867, 2010 21154349

Sills GJ: The mechanisms of action of gabapentin and pregabalin. Curr Opin Pharmacol 6(1):108–113, 2006 16376147

Skinner MD, Lahmek P, Pham H, et al: Disulfiram efficacy in the treatment of alcohol dependence: a meta-analysis. PLoS One 9(2):e87366, 2014 24520330

Smith RV, Havens JR, Walsh SL: Gabapentin misuse, abuse and diversion: a systematic review. Addiction 111(7):1160–1174, 2016 27265421

Spagnolo PA, Ramchandani VA, Schwandt ML, et al: Effects of naltrexone on neural and subjective response to alcohol in treatment-seeking alcohol-dependent patients. Alcohol Clin Exp Res 38(12):3024–3032, 2014 25581657

Spear LP: Adolescents and alcohol: acute sensitivities, enhanced intake, and later consequences. Neurotoxicol Teratol 41:51–59, 2014 24291291

Substance Abuse and Mental Health Services Administration (SAMHSA): 2015 National Survey on Drug Use and Health (NSDUH). Table 5.5A: Substance use disorder in past year among persons aged 12–17, by demographic characteristics: numbers in thousands, 2014 and 2015. September 2016. Available at: https://www.samhsa.gov/data/sites/default/files/NSDUH-DetTabs-2015/NSDUH-DetTabs-2015/NSDUH-DetTabs-2015.htm#tab5-5a. Accessed April 29, 2019.

Valenta JP, Job MO, Mangieri RA, et al: μ-Opioid receptors in the stimulation of mesolimbic dopamine activity by ethanol and morphine in Long-Evans rats: a delayed effect of ethanol. Psychopharmacology (Berl) 228(3):389–400, 2013 23503684

Witteman J, Post H, Tarvainen M, et al: Cue reactivity and its relation to craving and relapse in alcohol dependence: a combined laboratory and field study. Psychopharmacology (Berl) 232(20):3685–3696, 2015 26257163

Wold M, Kaminer Y: Naltrexone for alcohol abuse. J Am Acad Child Adolesc Psychiatry 36(1):6–7, 1997 9000774

8

Youth Tobacco Use

Grace Kong, Ph.D.
Suchitra Krishnan-Sarin, Ph.D.

Tobacco use remains the leading cause of preventable disease and death worldwide (World Health Organization 2017). To prevent morbidity and mortality related to tobacco use, tobacco prevention must focus on youth because tobacco use is initiated during adolescence. Nicotine, a key active constituent in tobacco products, has more powerful rewarding effects in youth than in adults, and even occasional use of tobacco use can lead to nicotine dependence among youth (National Center for Chronic Disease Prevention and Health Promotion 2014). Initiation of tobacco/nicotine use during adolescence often marks the start of an addiction that lasts a lifetime. Furthermore, although serious health burden from tobacco use, such as emergence of cancers and cardiovascular, oral, and respiratory diseases, may only occur in adulthood and after long-term tobacco use, youth can experience a variety of negative health effects due to tobacco use, including disruption of the normal brain development, impaired lung growth, and other respiratory symptoms (e.g., asthma) (National Center for Chronic Disease Prevention and Health Promotion 2014).

Comprehensive tobacco control efforts have dramatically reduced the rates of cigarette smoking among youth in the past few decades; however, 8.1% of U.S. high school students still report current use of cigarettes (i.e., in the past 30 days) (Gentzke et al. 2019), indicating the need for continuous efforts to prevent tobacco use and treat nicotine dependence among youth.

Noncigarette Tobacco/Nicotine Products

A significant challenge in preventing and treating tobacco use among youth in recent years is the rapidly changing tobacco use landscape among youth. Cigarettes are no longer the most commonly used tobacco product among high school students; use of noncombustible products like e-cigarettes is highest (20.8%), followed by cigarettes (8.1%), cigars (including little cigars, cigarillos; 7.6%), smokeless tobacco (5.9%), and hookah (4.1%) (Gentzke et al. 2019). Furthermore, use of multiple tobacco products (or polytobacco use) is common; 11.3% of high school students report using more than one tobacco product. The most common combinations of tobacco product use are cigarettes with e-cigarettes and cigarettes with cigars (Kowitt et al. 2015). Polytobacco use can place youth at greater risk for nicotine dependence and exposure to harm. Given the changing tobacco use patterns, clinicians need to understand the appeal and use of both noncombustible and combustible tobacco products among youth.

E-Cigarettes

E-cigarettes are battery-powered devices that heat a liquid (i.e., e-liquid), which usually contains nicotine, propylene glycol (PG), vegetable glycerin (VG), and other additives, such as flavor chemicals. A serious concern is the growing popularity of e-cigarettes among youth. Since 2011, use of e-cigarettes has surpassed cigarette smoking among high school students (Gentzke et al. 2019). Youth endorse e-cigarettes as the first tobacco product tried, and many youth initiate with e-cigarettes that do not contain nicotine and then switch to nicotine-containing e-cigarettes (Krishnan-Sarin et al. 2015). Thus, understanding the youth appeal of e-cigarettes is important to inform youth e-cigarette prevention.

E-cigarettes have many components that appeal to youth. For instance, youth are drawn to the presence of diverse flavors (Kong et al. 2015). E-cigarettes come in many sweet flavors (e.g., bubble gum, gummy bear) and unique flavor names (e.g., unicorn milk) that are attractive to youth. The appeal of e-cigarettes may also be related to innovations in e-cigarette devices. Recent evidence suggests that youth use a wide variety of e-cigarette devices: disposable e-cigarettes that resemble cigarettes (e.g., cigalikes); advanced-generation models, such as rechargeable penlike devices, devices that use tanks or cartridges, or box-shaped mechanical mods (mech-mods); and, more recently, pod devices that resemble a USB stick (e.g., JUUL is a popular pod brand) (Krishnan-Sarin et al. 2019). The most popular devices used among youth are mod and pod devices.

The underlying appeal of advanced-generation devices may also be related to their customizable features, such as a variety of nicotine levels, flavors, and PG/VG ratio (Camenga et al. 2018), and the fact that they can be used for alternative behaviors like dripping (i.e., applying drops of e-liquid directly on heated atomizer to intensify throat hit and flavors, and to produce large amount of vapor) or conducting vape tricks/"cloud chasing" (i.e., creating shapes or large volumes of "clouds" using exhaled aerosol) (Krishnan-Sarin et al. 2017; Pepper et al. 2017).

The use of pod devices, such as JUUL, among youth is concerning. JUUL was first introduced in the U.S. market in 2015, and by 2017, it had become the largest retail e-cigarette brand in the United States (Huang et al. 2019). JUUL devices produce little vapor, have high levels of nicotine, and are easy to conceal and use discreetly in schools because of their small size. The rapid popularity of JUUL may be responsible for the increase in e-cigarette use among youth according to the most recent national data; among 12th graders, "any vaping" in the past 12 months increased from 27.8% in 2017 to 37.3% in 2018, and nicotine use doubled during this time period as well (11.0%–20.9%) (Johnston et al. 2019).

Another concern with e-cigarette devices is that they can be used to vaporize cannabis. The smell of cannabis is significantly reduced when it is vaped versus when it is combusted, which makes vaping cannabis easy to conceal from authority and to use in public areas (e.g., schools, concerts, home). An alarming finding is that vaping cannabis is common among youth. Among high school students who have ever tried e-cigarettes, 26.5% reported vaping cannabis (Morean et al. 2015). Recent national data indicate that vaping marijuana among youth increased from 9.5% in 2017 to 13.1% in 2018 (Johnston et al. 2019). These findings suggest that e-cigarettes provide another means for youth to use substances other than nicotine, such as cannabis, and thus may further place youth at risk for developing addictions to other substances.

Cigars

Cigars are different from cigarettes in that cigars are tobacco that is wrapped in tobacco leaf or a substance containing tobacco, whereas cigarettes are tobacco wrapped in paper. Cigars are a diverse tobacco product; they include 1) cheap, flavored little cigars that resemble standard cigarettes; 2) cigarillos, which are also cheap and flavored but are bigger than little cigars and which may come with a plastic or wooden mouth tip; and 3) premium large cigars.

The prevalence of current cigar use (including little cigars and cigarillos) among U.S. youth is double the rate observed among U.S. adults (7.6% vs. 3.8%) (Gentzke et al. 2019; Wang et al. 2018). Cigar use among youth is concerning because cigar use is not a safe alternative to cigarette use. Cigar use is more toxic than cigarette use, and continued use causes cancers of the lung and upper aerodigestive tract (Baker et al. 2000)

Cigars have several characteristics that appeal to youth: 1) they are available in appealing flavors (King et al. 2014); 2) they cost less than cigarettes (Delnevo et al. 2017)—some flavored little cigars are sold in a single or a double unit packs for very low prices (e.g., $.99); and 3) cigarillos can be manipulated to create blunts (i.e., cigars are hollowed out and tobacco is replaced with marijuana) (Kong et al. 2017; Schauer et al. 2017). The concurrent use of both marijuana and nicotine through blunt use may expose youth to greater harm and addiction to both substances. Another concern is that the sale of cheap cigars are concentrated disproportionally in predominantly black communities (Richardson et al. 2013).

Accumulating epidemiological studies, which indicate high prevalence of cigar use among youth (Gentzke et al. 2019), coupled with adverse health consequences of cigar smoking (Baker et al. 2000) and many youth-appealing components, demonstrate a strong need to develop comprehensive tobacco control policies and interventions aimed at preventing youth cigar use.

Hookah

Hookah, also known as "water pipe," has been used to smoke tobacco in the Middle East and in parts of Asia for centuries. Hookah has become a popular novel form of tobacco use among youth in other parts of the world in recent years. Youth view hookah use as a trendy, popular social activity, and perceive the product to have lower harm and addictiveness than cigarettes because tobacco smoke is passed through the water, which is believed to reduce toxicants (Smith et al. 2011). Such positive but faulty perceptions are concerning because hookah use is not a safer alternative to cigarette use and health risks that are comparable to those of cigarettes (Cobb et al. 2010).

Smokeless Tobacco

Smokeless tobacco use, which includes chewing tobacco, snuff, dip, and snus, is disproportionately high among young white males in rural areas in the United States and among youth in Southeast Asian countries (Rani et al. 2017). In many of these subpopulations, smokeless tobacco use is culturally ingrained because males typically use these products as a rite of passage or during participating in sports or other activities (Couch et al. 2017). Although smokeless tobacco is not combusted, its use is not safe. Smokeless tobacco use can cause dental diseases such as gum disease, tooth decay, and tooth loss, as well as cancers of the mouth, esophagus, and pancreas (World Health Organization 2007).

Summary of Noncigarette Tobacco/Nicotine Products

An overarching common theme across all tobacco products is that there is no safe level of nicotine exposure for youth. While different tobacco products may range in harm, use of any tobacco product places youth at risk for developing nicotine dependence and other adverse health outcomes. Thus, youth-based prevention/cessation strategies for these disparate tobacco products are needed.

A robust body of literature indicates that a comprehensive tobacco prevention and control approach that combines educational, clinical, regulatory, economic, and social strategies is required to reduce tobacco use among youth (National Center for Chronic Disease Prevention and Health Promotion 2014). At the macro level, policies can restrict youth access to tobacco products, advertising content, and product features (e.g., ban appealing flavors). These regulations should apply not only to cigarettes but also to all tobacco products, including e-cigarettes. An example of a regulation of e-cigarettes could involve limiting the levels of nicotine and prohibiting the use of ingredients other than nicotine. More than 30 other countries have already applied regulations like this to reduce youth e-cigarette use (Institute for Global Tobacco Control 2018). The United States has not taken such measures, and they should follow suit to take additional measures to protect youth from initiating tobacco/nicotine products.

In addition to the macro-level tobacco control approaches, micro-level approaches are also a necessary component of comprehensive tobacco control efforts. A critical micro-level tobacco control approach is developing and implementing effective youth-based tobacco prevention/cessation interventions that address the changing tobacco use landscape among youth. However, much of the research to date on diagnosis and tobacco prevention/cessation interventions has focused on cigarettes, and there is a significant lack of tobacco interventions addressing other tobacco products. Clinicians can still draw from the existing strategies to diagnose and treat noncigarette tobacco use behaviors and nicotine dependence among youth. In the following sections, we summarize the existing literature on the diagnosis and treatment of cigarettes among youth to inform clinician on these strategies.

Diagnosis

The first step to preventing tobacco use and treating nicotine dependence among youth is to conduct appropriate assessment of the types of tobacco product used; severity of use behaviors, including nicotine dependence; and willingness to quit. Clinicians should be aware of different terminology used to refer to various tobacco products. Tobacco products are often referred to by their brand names. For example, youth may use words such as "JUULing" or "vaping" to refer to e-cigarette use or "Black and Milds" to refer to cigarillos. Clinicians should consider the use of pictures of tobacco products to identify the products being used. Also, given that tobacco products are used to vape or smoke other substances such as marijuana, it is important to clarify what substance is being smoked or vaped.

Adolescents are sensitive to nicotine effects and experience symptoms of nicotine dependence soon after tobacco use initiation (DiFranza et al. 2002). Thus, it is important to assess nicotine dependence among youth who use tobacco product at any level. Commonly used measures of dependence that have been validated among youth are the modified Fagerström Tolerance Questionnaire (mFTQ; Prokhorov et al. 2017) and Hooked on Nicotine Checklist (HONC; DiFranza et al. 2002). The mFTQ's 7 items focus on frequency of smoking, inhalation, and difficulty refraining from smoking. HONC's 10 items focus on the loss of autonomy over tobacco.

It is important to note that these nicotine dependence assessments were developed to assess nicotine dependence in the context of cigarette smoking. Given the changing landscape of tobacco use among youth, there is a strong need to develop and validate effective nicotine dependence measures that consider nuances of unique tobacco products. To date, one such measure, the 4-item Patient-Reported Outcomes Measurement Information System Nicotine Dependence Item Bank for e-cigarettes (PROMIS-E), has been psychometrically validated for assessing nicotine dependence in adolescent e-cigarette users (Morean et al. 2018). More specific measures on nicotine dependence in the context of other types of tobacco product use are needed.

Identification of motivations to quit among tobacco users is helpful to identify appropriate interventions. Youth willing to quit tobacco should be provided with effective treatments, and youth unwilling to quit should be provided with a brief intervention designed to increase their motivations to quit (see subsection "Cessation Interventions" later in this chapter).

Prevention

Tobacco prevention interventions reduce the risk of smoking initiation among youth. These interventions include behavioral counseling interventions delivered face-to-face or via phone, print materials, or computer applications (U.S. Preventive Services Task Force 2013). Clinicians who have direct contact with youth could tailor interventions to each patient and educate them on the harms of various tobacco products. Prevention messages should be delivered to all youth, especially those who have not initiated tobacco product use but who are susceptible to use or who are curious about using, because any form of tobacco experimentation is not safe.

Prevention messages should be clear, personally relevant, and age appropriate. Tobacco prevention messages that resonate with youth include emphasis on the negative effect of tobacco use on their health and appearance, cognition, and sports performance, as well as focus on the monetary cost, and how the tobacco industry deceives them (National Center for Chronic Disease Prevention and Health Promotion 2014). Prevention messages that focus on how nicotine dependence hijacks decision-making abilities and independence also seem to resonate with youth (Roditis et al. 2019). These themes have been incorporated by the U.S. Food and Drug Administration (FDA) in its The Real Cost campaign, which is a national cigarette prevention campaign targeting youth on social media websites and television. The FDA's media prevention campaigns have also begun to address noncigarette tobacco products, such as relaying the risks of e-cigarette use to youth and targeting efforts to educate rural youth on the harms of smokeless tobacco. Mass media prevention campaigns are effective because of their wide reach and use of themes that resonate with youth. Continued efforts to develop media prevention campaigns targeting noncigarette tobacco products are needed to prevent all tobacco use among youth.

Cessation Interventions

A low-intensity intervention such as the "5As" approach is recommended for all health professionals working with youth (U.S. Department of Health and Human Services 2012). The 5As approach to preventing tobacco use includes the following:

- Ask about tobacco use.
- Advise the tobacco user to stop using tobacco products.
- Assess willingness to quit.
- Assist the tobacco user to formulate a quit plan.
- Arrange for follow-up to assess the need for further advising and encouragement.

The brief advice and information should motivate a behavior change and prompt a discussion with youth about tobacco use (e.g., expectations regarding tobacco use). This brief intervention, which takes 3–10 minutes, has been shown to be as effective as other psychosocial interventions in motivating youth to quit smoking (Audrain-McGovern et al. 2011).

In addition to the 5As, many other types of smoking cessation interventions have been developed for youth. These interventions are largely grounded in psychosocial theories using social and cognitive approaches, and some are based on pharmacological principles (Simon et al. 2015). Psychosocial interventions use cognitive-behavioral therapy (CBT), motivational approaches, contingency management (CM), or transtheoretical model of change (TTM). It is important to note that these approaches are rarely offered as a stand-alone treatment in clinical and in research settings. Rather, different approaches are combined. While the combination of the approaches is varied, each approach has shown to be effective in achieving short-term abstinence among adolescent smokers.

Cognitive-Behavioral Therapy

CBT for smoking cessation includes a variety of components, including goal setting, self-monitoring, development of problem-solving and coping skills to build self-efficacy, and cognitive reframing. Goal setting includes setting a quit date. Self-monitoring includes identifying cravings, withdrawal symptoms, and high-risk situations for smoking. Coping skills could be developed to cope with withdrawal symptoms and scenarios that trigger smoking. Stress/anger management skills could be developed to manage negative emotions to prevent relapse. Cognitive reframing refers to identifying negative maladaptive thoughts about one's ability to quit and developing new ways to think about the situations. For example, maladaptive thoughts after a relapse (e.g., "Quitting is so hard, I'll never be able to quit smoking") could be challenged, and new, more adaptive thoughts (e.g., "I can try again. It's hard to quit smoking but I can do it.") could be developed and practiced until they become automatic.

The most studied CBT intervention for youth is the American Lung Association's Not On Tobacco, or N-O-T, intervention. This intervention is conducted in 10 group sessions, separated by gender, in school settings. The intervention involves providing support, guidance, instructions on how to quit, and problem-solving and coping skills development to prevent and deal with relapse. This intervention has been tested in various locations with refinement and has shown modest short-term abstinence rates (Horn et al. 2005).

Motivational Interviewing (Motivational Enhancement)

Motivational interviewing (MI, or motivational enhancement [ME]) strategies involve strengthening a tobacco user's desire for quitting and reducing ambivalence about quitting through expressing empathy, addressing resistance without confrontation, and supporting individual self-efficacy (Miller and Rollnick 2002). Specific strategies include using open-ended questions, using reflective listening, summarizing, developing discrepancy between current behaviors and important goals/beliefs, and affirming and eliciting "change talk."

A large trial randomly assigned 355 adolescent smokers to participate in five sessions of MI (three 45-minute office sessions and two 30-minute phone sessions) or five sessions of 5As. This study did not observe any differences in the abstinence rates between the two groups, but MI produced greater reduction in cigarettes smoked per day, and both groups showed a modest quit rate at the end of the study (Audrain-McGovern et al. 2011).

Contingency Management

Based on operant behavior-reshaping concepts, CM interventions follow two simple principles: first, that tobacco use is maintained by the reinforcing effects of the drug (i.e., nicotine), and second, that tobacco use can be reduced by the availability of alternative, nondrug reinforcers. CM interventions can be adapted in clinical settings by following the basic tenets: 1) selecting a target behavior that can be quantified objectively (e.g., reduction in number of days smoked, abstinence, treatment attendance), 2) monitoring the behavior frequently using biological markers when possible (e.g., breath carbon monoxide [CO]; nicotine or cotinine levels), 3) providing tangible reinforcers (e.g., incentives, prizes, privileges) when the target behavior occurs, and 4) withholding incentives when the target behavior is not met (Petry 2000).

The largest study assessing CM among youth randomly assigned 82 adolescent smokers to participate in a 4-week treatment in which adolescents received one of three interventions: daily CM for abstinence, weekly CBT without CM, or a combination of weekly CBT and daily CM for abstinence (Krishnan-Sarin et al. 2013). The results showed that CM and the combination of CM and CBT yielded higher abstinence rates at the end of treatment than CBT alone.

Transtheoretical Model of Change

TTM indicates the level of readiness to make a behavioral change, such as quitting tobacco use (Prochaska and DiClemente 1983). It assumes that behavior change occurs in five stages: 1) precontemplation (not planning to quit in the next 6 months), 2) contemplation (thinking about quitting in the next

6 months, but not next month), 3) preparation (intending to quit next month), 4) action (have been attempting to quit for less than 6 months), and 5) maintenance (have quit for at least 6 months). Clinicians can identify youth's stage of change and attempt to facilitate behavior change through the stages of change using the ME strategies described earlier.

An example of an intervention assessing TTM is a study that randomly assigned 755 adolescent smokers to participate in either a 3-month TTM intervention delivered using text messaging on mobile phones or an assessment-only control group (Haug et al. 2013). The content of the text messaging feedback was tailored based on the responses to stage of behavior change, intention to quit, and smoking status. For example, adolescent smokers in the precontemplation stage received text messages that were designed to increase motivations to change, such as messages that emphasized the risks of smoking, monetary costs of smoking, or social norms of smoking. Participants in the action stage received text messages that motivated them to continue trying to quit by rewarding themselves for staying abstinent or providing strategies to cope with cravings. This study did not observe differences in abstinence rates between the two groups at the end of treatment, but adolescents in the TTM condition reported greater reduction in cigarettes smoked per day than adolescents in the control condition.

Pharmacological Interventions

Available pharmacological interventions for tobacco dependence are nicotine replacement therapy (NRT), bupropion, and varenicline. NRT works by supplying low doses of nicotine, thereby easing the symptoms of nicotine withdrawal and reducing cravings for nicotine. NRT comes in many different forms: patch, gum lozenge, inhaler, and nasal spray. NRT is the first proven effective medication for assisting adult smokers to quit and remains the first line of pharmacotherapy in helping adult smokers quit smoking (Fiore et al. 2008). Varenicline (trade name Chantix), which is a partial nicotinic agonist, and bupropion (Zyban, for smoking cessation), which is a norepinephrine-dopamine reuptake inhibitor, are also commonly used pharmacological treatments for smoking cessation among adult smokers.

Evidence on the efficacy of pharmacological interventions for smoking cessation among youth remains uncertain given the lack of studies in this topic area. The small number of existing studies on this topic do not have sufficient sample sizes to accurately assess their efficacy (Fanshawe et al. 2017). Currently, no pharmacological treatments are approved for youth under 18 years of age. However, the American Academy of Pediatrics recommends pharmacological interventions to be offered to youth who want treatment given the efficacy of these intervention in adults and the serious harm of nicotine dependence (Jenssen and Wilson 2017).

Treatment Modality and Setting

In general, tobacco cessation interventions can be delivered individually or in a group in schools or hospital settings, or remotely using mobile phones or computers. The most recent Cochrane review of tobacco cessation interventions for youth suggests that group counseling is the most effective method of delivering smoking cessation interventions to youth (Fanshawe et al. 2017). Group counseling can be a viable option for school and clinical settings to help youth to quit tobacco use. We outline the evidence on the most common tobacco cessation treatment setting and modality.

Schools

The advantage of school-based tobacco prevention programs is the ability to reach a captive audience. Although the interventions that have been delivered in schools are heterogeneous, they often focus on social influence models that teach students how to resist social pressures to use tobacco products. School-based programs have shown promising short-term efficacy (Wiehe et al. 2005). There is some evidence that multimodal interventions that use relevant social context and involve school- and community-based components, such as mass media tobacco prevention campaigns, can be effective (Backinger and Leischow 2001).

Health Care Settings

Health care settings provide a unique opportunity to facilitate the delivery of tobacco interventions to youth who are not receiving treatment. The majority of the studies in medical settings provided brief advice interventions to adults, but the hospital is also a feasible setting to reach youth smokers (Colby et al. 1998), and evidence suggests that brief advice smoking cessation interventions in medical settings have a small effect on smoking cessation (Stead et al. 2018).

Web and Mobile Phones

Web- and mobile phone–based interventions have a wide reach potential, can be provided at a relatively low cost, and can be tailored and automated to motivate quit behaviors. Most existing studies of such interventions for youth are based on psychosocial theories (e.g., motivational messages), and often combine this approach with other treatment modalities (e.g., in-person brief advice sessions) (Hutton et al. 2011; Kong et al. 2014). Currently, there is insufficient evidence of the effectiveness of web-based interventions because there is too much heterogeneity in the content, format, and outcomes (Hutton et al. 2011).

Mobile phones are also extremely popular among adolescents and can be used to deliver tailored smoking cessation interventions in real time. Although the reviews on the efficacy of this modality have focused on adults, it appears to be a promising mode of intervention delivery to youth (Kong et al. 2014). Currently, the National Cancer Institute sponsors a free mobile phone–based text message–based intervention (SmokefreeTXT for Teens) specifically tailored for youth that offers motivational messages to quit, quit tips, and skills to deal with cravings, withdrawal symptoms, and relapses. Clinicians can refer youth to this program and inform them to simply text the word QUIT to 47848 from a mobile phone to enroll.

Conclusion

Cigarettes are no longer the most common tobacco product used by youth. The growing popularity of noncigarette tobacco products among youth presents a new challenge in preventing youth tobacco use. Use of any form of tobacco is unsafe and is not recommended for youth. Despite the evolving tobacco use landscape among youth, diagnosis and treatment of use of noncigarette tobacco products are extremely limited and need more research. However, clinicians who work directly with youth can still have an impact by educating youth about the effects and consequences of all tobacco use and motivating them to stop using these products. Clinicians should first assess the type of tobacco product used, the severity of use, and youth's willingness to quit. Although prevention and cessation interventions have not been assessed for noncigarette tobacco products and future research is needed, clinicians can choose and adapt from a variety of prevention/treatment strategies and treatment modalities that exist for youth cigarette smoking.

Key Points

- E-cigarette use is rapidly reversing progress in reducing tobacco use in youth

- Clinicians need to understand the appeal, use patterns, and terminology of new tobacco/nicotine products and delivery systems among youth.

- Appropriate diagnosis of tobacco use involves assessing the types of product used; severity of use behavior, including nicotine dependence; and willingness to quit.

- There is a lack of noncigarette tobacco/nicotine prevention/cessation interventions for youth. However, clinicians can choose among and adapt a variety of prevention/treatment strategies and treatment modalities that exist for youth cigarette smoking,

References

Audrain-McGovern J, Stevens S, Murray PJ, et al: The efficacy of motivational interviewing versus brief advice for adolescent smoking behavior change. Pediatrics 128(1):e101–e111, 2011 21690120

Backinger CL, Leischow SJ: Advancing the science of adolescent tobacco use cessation. Am J Health Behav 25(3):183–190, 2001 11322616

Baker F, Ainsworth SR, Dye JT, et al: Health risks associated with cigar smoking. JAMA 284(6):735–740, 2000 10927783

Camenga DR, Morean ME, Kong G, et al: Appeal and use of customizable e-cigarette product features in adolescents. Tobacco Regulatory Science 4(2):51–60, 2018

Cobb C, Ward KD, Maziak W, et al: Waterpipe tobacco smoking: an emerging health crisis in the United States. Am J Health Behav 34(3):275–285, 2010 20001185

Colby SM, Monti PM, Barnett NP, et al: Brief motivational interviewing in a hospital setting for adolescent smoking: a preliminary study. J Consult Clin Psychol 66(3):574–578, 1998 9642898

Couch ET, Darius E, Walsh MM, et al: Smokeless tobacco decision-making among rural adolescent males in California. J Community Health 42(3):544–550, 2017 27796632

Delnevo CD, Hrywna M, Giovenco DP, et al: Close, but no cigar: certain cigars are pseudo-cigarettes designed to evade regulation. Tob Control 26(3):349–354, 2017 27220622

DiFranza JR, Savageau JA, Fletcher K, et al: Measuring the loss of autonomy over nicotine use in adolescents: the DANDY (Development and Assessment of Nicotine Dependence in Youths) study. Arch Pediatr Adolesc Med 156(4):397–403, 2002 11929376

Fanshawe TR, Halliwell W, Lindson N, et al: Tobacco cessation interventions for young people. Cochrane Database Syst Rev 11:CD003289, 2017 29148565

Fiore MC, Jaén C, Baker TB, et al: Treating Tobacco Use and Dependence: 2008 Update. Rockville, MD, US Department of Health and Human Services, Public Health Service, 2008

Gentzke AS, Creamer M, Cullen KA, et al: Vital Signs: Tobacco product use among middle and high school students—United States, 2011–2018. MMWR Morb Mortal Wkly Rep 68(6):157–164, 2019 30763302

Haug S, Schaub MP, Venzin V, et al: Efficacy of a text message-based smoking cessation intervention for young people: a cluster randomized controlled trial. J Med Internet Res 15(8):e171, 2013 23956024

Horn KH, Dino G, Kalsekar I, et al: The impact of Not on Tobacco on teen smoking cessation: end-of-program evaluation results, 1998 to 2003. J Adolesc Res 20:640–661, 2005

Huang J, Duan Z, Kwok J, et al: Vaping versus JUULing: how the extraordinary growth and marketing of JUUL transformed the US retail e-cigarette market. Tob Control 28:146–151, 2019 29853561

Hutton HE, Wilson LM, Apelberg BJ, et al: A systematic review of randomized controlled trials: Web-based interventions for smoking cessation among adolescents, college students, and adults. Nicotine Tob Res 13(4):227–238, 2011 21350042

Institute for Global Tobacco Control: Country laws regulating e-cigarettes: a policy scan. 2018. Available at: https://www.globaltobaccocontrol.org/e-cigarette_policyscan. Accessed May 1, 2019.

Jenssen BP, Wilson KM: Tobacco control and treatment for the pediatric clinician: Practice, policy, and research updates. Acad Pediatr 17(3):233–242, 2017 28069410

Johnston LD, Miech RA, O'Malley PM, et al: Monitoring the Future National Survey Results on Drug Use, 1975–2018: Overview, Key Findings on Adolescent Drug Use. Ann Arbor, MI, Institute for Social Research, The University of Michigan, 2019

King BA, Tynan MA, Dube SR, et al: Flavored-little-cigar and flavored-cigarette use among U.S. middle and high school students. J Adolesc Health 54(1):40–46, 2014 24161587

Kong G, Ells D, Camenga D, et al: Text messaging-based smoking cessation intervention: a narrative review. Addict Behav 39(5):907–917, 2014 24462528

Kong G, Morean ME, Cavallo DA, et al: Reasons for electronic cigarette experimentation and discontinuation among adolescents and young adults. Nicotine Tob Res 17(7):847–854, 2015 25481917

Kong G, Bold KW, Simon P, et al: Reasons for cigarillo initiation and cigarillo manipulation methods among adolescents. Tob Regul Sci 3(2) (suppl 1):S48–S58, 2017 29085867

Kowitt SD, Patel T, Ranney LM, et al: Poly-tobacco use among high school students. Int J Environ Res Public Health 12(11):14477–14489, 2015 26580636

Krishnan-Sarin S, Cavallo DA, Cooney JL, et al: An exploratory randomized controlled trial of a novel high-school-based smoking cessation intervention for adolescent smokers using abstinence-contingent incentives and cognitive behavioral therapy. Drug Alcohol Depend 132(1–2):346–351, 2013 23523130

Krishnan-Sarin S, Morean ME, Camenga DR, et al: E-cigarette use among high school and middle school students. Nic Tob Res 17:810–818, 2015 25385873

Krishnan-Sarin S, Morean M, Kong G, et al: E-cigarette and "dripping" among high-school youth. Pediatrics 139(3):e20163224, 2017 28167512

Krishnan-Sarin S, Jackson A, Morean M, et al: E-cigarette devices used by high-school youth. Drug Alcohol Depend 194:395–400, 2019 30497057

Miller WR, Rollnick S: Motivational Interviewing: Preparing People for Change, 2nd Edition. New York, Guilford, 2002

Morean ME, Kong G, Camenga DR, et al: High school students' use of electronic cigarettes to vaporize cannabis. Pediatrics 136(4):611–616, 2015 26347431

Morean ME, Krishnan-Sarin S, Sussman S, et al: Psychometric evaluation of the Patient-Reported Outcomes Measurement Information System (PROMIS) nicotine dependence item bank for use with electronic cigarettes. Nicotine Tob Res January 2, 2018 [Epub ahead of print] 29301008

National Center for Chronic Disease Prevention and Health Promotion, Office on Smoking and Health: The Health Consequences of Smoking—50 Years of Progress. A Report of the Surgeon General. Atlanta, GA, Centers for Disease Control and Prevention, 2014

Pepper JK, Lee YO, Watson KA, et al: Risk factors for youth e-cigarette "vape trick" behavior. J Adolesc Health 61(5):599–605, 2017 28712592

Petry NM: A comprehensive guide to the application of contingency management procedures in clinical settings. Drug Alcohol Depend 58(1-2):9–25, 2000 10669051

Prochaska JO, DiClemente CC: Stages and processes of self-change of smoking: toward an integrative model of change. J Consult Clin Psychol 51(3):390–395, 1983 6863699

Prokhorov AV, Khalil GE, Foster DW, et al: Testing the nicotine dependence measure mFTQ for adolescent smokers: a multinational investigation. Am J Addict 26(7):689–696, 2017 28708935

Rani M, Thamarangsi T, Agarwal N: Youth tobacco use in South-East Asia: implications for tobacco epidemic and options for its control in the region. Indian J Public Health 61(suppl):S12–S17, 2017 28928313

Richardson A, Rath J, Ganz O, et al: Primary and dual users of little cigars/cigarillos and large cigars: demographic and tobacco use profiles. Nicotine Tob Res 15(10):1729–1736, 2013 23645607

Roditis ML, Jones C, Dineva AP, et al: Lessons on addiction messages from "The Real Cost" campaign. Am J Prev Med 56(2S1):S24–S30, 2019 30661522

Schauer GL, Rosenberry ZR, Peters EN: Marijuana and tobacco co-administration in blunts, spliffs, and mulled cigarettes: a systematic literature review. Addict Behav 64:200–211, 2017 27654966

Simon P, Kong G, Cavallo DA, et al: Update of adolescent smoking cessation interventions: 2009–2014. Curr Addict Rep 2(1):15–23, 2015 26295017

Smith JR, Novotny TE, Edland SD, et al: Determinants of hookah use among high school students. Nicotine Tob Res 13(7):565–572, 2011 21454909

Stead LF, Bergson G, Lancaster T: Physician advice for smoking cessation. Cochrane Database Syst Rev 11:CD000165, 2018 18425860

U.S. Department of Health and Human Services: Surgeon General's Report—Preventing Tobacco Use among Youth and Young Adults. Atlanta, GA, U.S. Department of Health and Human Services, 2012

U.S. Preventive Services Task Force: Tobacco use in children and adolescents: primary care intervention. August 2013. Available at: https://www.uspreventiveservicestaskforce.org/Page/Document/UpdateSummaryFinal/tobacco-use-in-children-and-adolescents-primary-care-interventions. Accessed May 1, 2019.

Wang TW, Asman K, Gentzke AS, et al: Tobacco use among adults—United States, 2017. MMWR Morb Mortal Wkly Rep 67(44):1225–1232, 2018 30408019

Wiehe SE, Garrison MM, Christakis DA, et al: A systematic review of school-based smoking prevention trials with long-term follow-up. J Adolesc Health 36(3):162–169, 2005 15737770

World Health Organization: IARC Monographs on the Evaluation of Carcinogenic Risks to Humans. Lyon, France, World Health Organization, International Agency for Research on Cancer, 2007

World Health Organization: WHO Report on the Global Tobacco Epidemic, 2017. Geneva, World Health Organization, 2017

9

Youth Cannabis Use

Christian Thurstone, M.D.
Yifrah Kaminer, M.D., M.B.A.

Cannabis use and cannabis use disorder (CUD) among youth continue to present significant public health concerns. In the United States, 76% of all youth in substance use treatment report cannabis as their primary substance. Cannabis use peaks during college years, and nearly 10% of first-year students have use that meets diagnostic criteria for CUD. Although difficult to demonstrate causality, research across multiple domains highlights the short and long-term deleterious effects associated with adolescent cannabis use. These include but are not limited to dependence on cannabis and potential transition to other drugs of abuse, including opioids; increased risk of motor vehicle crashes; early onset of psychosis; increased suicidal behavior liability; diminished cognitive and scholastic performance; school dropout; and cardiovascular effects (Ammerman and Tau 2016; Hall 2015; Singh et al. 2018).

In this chapter we focus on the harmful effects on youth and public health of Δ-9-tetrahydrocannabinol (THC), the primary psychoactive cannabinoid, and how to address them in the era of a shifting legal status of cannabis. We review the endocannabinoid system; describe cannabis products; and discuss cannabis interactions with other drugs (including medications), prevalence and epidemiology of cannabis use, negative consequences of cannabis use on youth, specific health concerns, interventions pertaining to prevention and treatment, the legalization conundrum, and recommendations for public health policies.

The Endocannabinoid System

Cannabis targets the endocannabinoid system, which contributes to organogenesis, neurogenesis, and gliogenesis of the central nervous system (CNS). The endocannabinoid system controls neuronal hardwiring during prenatal ontogeny relevant to the development of neural pathways, such as the cortico-striato-thalamic circuit, that are implicated in addiction and psychiatric disorders. Cannabinoid$_1$ (CB1) receptor (CB1R) is the most abundant G protein–coupled receptor in the adult brain and mediates neurobehavioral effects of THC. CB1Rs are abundant in brain areas involved in learning and memory (e.g., hippocampus), cognitive and emotional processes (e.g., striatum, amygdala, prefrontal cortex), motor function (e.g., basal ganglia, cerebellum), and regulation of feeding and stress response via the hypothalamic-pituitary axis (HPA) and gonadal axis. Despite its low abundance in the brain, modulation of CNS cannabinoid$_2$ receptors (CB2Rs) have been implicated in addictive disorders. Both CB1R and CB2R are present in peripheral tissues, including the immune and reproductive systems (Szutorisz and Hurd 2016).

Definitions and Description of Cannabis Products

Cannabis sativa and *Cannabis indica* are two common variants of a plant whose buds and leaves are smoked (burning cannabis), vaporized (inhaled aerosolized cannabis), cooked for edibles such as candies and gummy bears, used oro-mucosally (lollipops, lozenges), administered sublingually, and/or liquefied for drinking such as sodas (Ammerman and Tau 2016). In the 1960s and 1970s the concentration of THC in smokable cannabis was 2%–4%. Continued cloning of plants and improved growing methods have led to increased potency. Presently the concentration of THC in street cannabis is as high as 16%–20%, and in "concentrates" such as marijuana wax THC concentrations reach about 25% by weight and are likely to increase further (Rocky Mountain High Intensity Drug Trafficking Area 2018). Commercial cannabis oil for topical use (resin, concentrates) has reached 60%–90% THC, and there are alarming reports in the media that these potent products have been used in nontopical forms. For example, *dabbing* is the process of burning concentrated cannabis, usually in the form of wax or resin, by placing it on a heated piece of metal and inhaling the vapors.

Other delivery methods that appeal to young users include e-cigarettes and vaping devices (e.g., JUUL), which are the size of a flash drive. Similarly to nicotine vaping reviewed in Chapter 8 of this manual, the rapid increase in vaping cannabis by ordinary e-cigarettes and JUUL has been alarming (Johnston et al. 2018; Morean et al. 2015). E-cigarette use predicts subsequent cannabis use among youth, with a stronger association among younger (12- to 14-year-old) adolescents (Dai et al. 2018). Vaping results in a higher exposure of concentration of THC (compared with just smoking "weed"). Vaping is less detectable than smoking and has become endemic in American schools. The prevalence of cannabis smoking surpassed tobacco smoking in 2011. The combination of nicotine and cannabis in e-cigarettes is likely to increase the prevalence of nicotine use in this generation of youth.

These products are available illegally as well as legally at dispensaries of "medical" cannabis and/or "smoke" shops in countries (e.g., Uruguay, Canada) and U.S. states that have legalized sales of cannabis for medical or recreational purposes. There are several hundred known chemicals present in different ratios and compositions in multiple diverse strains of cannabis. In addition to THC, the primary psychoactive cannabinoid, there are nonpsychoactive cannabinoids such as terpenes and cannabidiol (CBD) that have been reported to have potential medicinal effect on several disorders. However, precise medical use remains elusive because of difficulties in identifying optimal compositions and ratios to impact anti-inflammatory and cytotoxic activities. Furthermore, the "entourage" or synergistic effects of different compounds in marijuana have been challenging for the development of medical-grade products. CBD has not been approved for use in a "natural" herblike nonpharmacological form by the U.S. Food and Drug Administration (FDA). Presently, CBD products advertised or available commercially have not been regulated for quality, concentration, CBD/THC ratio, potential harmful or useless additives, fungi contamination, mold growth, or even toxic pesticides used for cultivating the cannabis plants.

Butane hash oil (BHO) and K2 are dangerous cannabis-based or cannabis-like products, respectively. BHO, honey oil, wax, and Shatter are potent cannabis concentrates. Some are called the "crack of pot." The significant adverse effects of BHO and K2 are reviewed later in this chapter in the section "Specific Health Concerns."

Cannabis Drug and Medication Interactions

Legal cannabis products in the United States include legal FDA-approved synthetic forms of THC-based cannabinoids. Dronabinol is an oral medication. Marinol (Schedule III) is the product in a capsule, while Syndros (Schedule II) is a liquid form. Nabilone (Cesamet) is an oral capsule with possibly higher abuse potential registered as Schedule II. Nabiximols (Sativex), which contains equal amounts of THC and CBD, has been approved in Canada, Spain, Australia, and the United Kingdom only. It is awaiting FDA approval. In 2018 Epidiolex (oral CBD with less than 1% THC) was approved for rare, intractable, treatment-resistant pediatric epilepsy such as Lennox-Gastaut syndrome and Dravet syndrome. Minors are able to obtain medical marijuana with parents' written permission and in some cases other restrictions (Ammerman and Tau 2016). A systematic review of reports to identify the evidence base of cannabinoids as a medical treatment in children and adolescents found evidence for benefit in epilepsy and chemotherapy-induced nausea and vomiting (Wong and Wilens 2017). There is insufficient evidence at present to support use for spasticity, neuropathic pain, posttraumatic stress disorder, and Tourette's syndrome.

Clinicians need to be aware of potential interactions between cannabis and other illegal drugs and medications. With regard to medications, an adjustment of dosage might be necessary when cannabis is being used by a patient. Cannabis has additive CNS depressant effects with alcohol, barbiturates, and benzodiazepines. Also, alcohol may increase THC levels. The potential interaction with opiates, particularly as it pertains to pain management, will be addressed in Chapter 10 of this manual.

THC and CBD are metabolized by cytochrome P450 (CYP) enzymes (3A4 and 2C9). CBD is also metabolized by CYP2C19. Consequently, compounds (including, for practical reasons, medications) that inhibit or induce the production of these enzymes would have an effect on THC and CBD concentration. THC is a CYP1A2 inducer; therefore, it might decrease serum levels of clozapine, duloxetine, naproxen, cyclobenzaprine, olanzapine, haloperidol, and chlorpromazine.

CBD is a potent inhibitor of CYP2D6 and CYP3A4 and may increase serum concentration of drugs metabolized by these enzymes. CYP2D6 metabolizes selective serotonin reuptake inhibitors, tricyclic antidepressants, antipsychotics, beta-blockers and opioids (including codeine and oxycodone). CYP3A4 metabolizes about a quarter of all drugs, including (but not limited to) benzodiazepines, haloperidol, antihistamines, and calcium channel blockers (District of Columbia, Department of Health 2015).

Prevalence and Epidemiology of Cannabis Use

The prevalence of cannabis use worldwide is alarming. Cannabis is available for adolescents from several sources: purchased in the street or stolen or diverted from relatives or others who are legal medical cannabis users or from adults in states where cannabis use is legal for recreational purpose. Cannabis is not a harmless compound. However, the changes in cannabis legal status and use of terms such as "medical cannabis" have contributed to the already biased perception of youth that marijuana use is safe. This perception has been correlated with an increase in the prevalence of marijuana use and decrease in age at first onset. In Canada, among youth ages 15–19 years, the rate of past year use was 20.6%. In Australia, 4% of the same age group used cannabis weekly. In the United Kingdom, 4% of younger adolescents ages 11–15 years used cannabis in the past month, while in the United States, almost 7% of high school seniors are daily users (Gobbi et al. 2019).

A school-based survey in the United States, known as Monitoring the Future (MTF; Johnston et al. 2018), has been conducted since 1975. Data are collected from 8th, 10th, and 12th graders. The 2018 MTF survey found the following rates of cannabis use: among 8th graders, past year 10.5%, past month 5.6%, and daily 0.7%; among 10th graders, past year 27.5%, past month 16.7%, and daily 3.4%; and among 12th graders, past year 35.9%, past month 22.2%, and daily 5.8%. According to 2018 survey data, the past-month prevalence of marijuana use is similar for males and females. However, among 12th graders, males compared with females are twice as likely to have past-month daily use (7.8% vs. 3.6%). Knapp et al. (2019) reported that the most frequent route of use is still smoking, with substantial numbers of youth reporting vaping and edible use. Prevalence of cannabis vaping in the last 12-month report in the 2018 MTF was 4.4%, 12.4%, and 13.1% of 8th, 10th, and 12th graders respectively.

Compared with other age groups, marijuana is disproportionately used by adolescents and young adults. Also, adolescents who use multiple administration routes tend to report high frequency of other substances tried. According to the National Survey on Drug Use and Health (Center for Behavioral Health Statistics and Quality 2017), past-month prevalence of marijuana use peaks at ages 19–21 years (Figure 9–1). Rates of new use of cannabis have also been reported by the 2017 National Survey on Drug Use and Health surveys; 2.4 million individuals report being a new user of marijuana every year, and 58.5% are under the age of 18 years.

Negative Consequences of Cannabis on Youth

Research across multiple domains highlights the short- and long-term deleterious effects associated with youth cannabis use. A pivotal concern is that the early onset and high prevalence of youth cannabis use, as well as the continued increase of cannabis potency, affect macro and micro brain structures and neurodevelopmental processes (Pierre 2017; Reece 2019). These findings are associated with negative cognitive and psychobehavioral consequences, addictive disorders, and adverse consequences of risk-taking behaviors (Hall 2015).

Potential Multigenerational Effects of Cannabis Use

Epigenetic typically refers to mechanisms that modulate gene expression without altering the genetic code and protracted effects on behavior (Szutorisz and Hurd 2016). The growing use of cannabis and THC concentration has led to increased attention on not only the impact of direct exposure on the developing brain and behavior later in life, but also the potential cross-generational consequences of parental THC exposure before mating transmitted in sperm and oocytes. Germline exposure studies in animal models show that at the

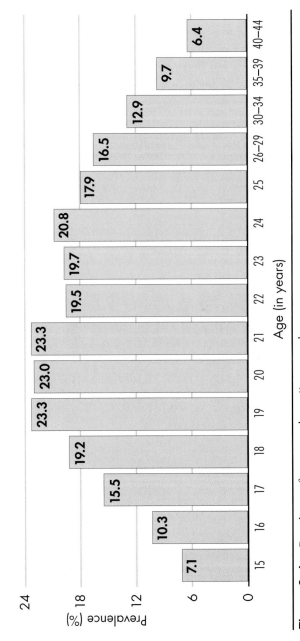

Figure 9–1. Prevalence of past-month marijuana use by age.
Source. Data from 2017 National Survey on Drug Use and Health (Center for Behavioral Health Statistics and Quality 2017).

molecular level, parental THC exposure is associated with changes in mRNA expression of cannabinoid, dopamine, and glutamatergic receptor genes in the striatum and altered synaptic plasticity in neurophysiological measures (for review, see Szutorisz and Hurd 2016). These effects may predispose future generations to vulnerability to psychiatric and addictive disorders. In animal studies, increased heroin self-administration in adult offspring with germline THC exposure was reported. Also, adolescent females treated with a cannabinoid agonist before mating had progeny that exhibited increased morphine sensitivity (for review, see Szutorisz and Hurd 2016).

Our knowledge of the teratogenic effects of cannabis is incomplete but likely to rapidly grow given increased use. Increased THC concentration and entry into the food chain may have epigenetic "footprints" via binding proteins transmissible through the sperm for several generations (Reece 2019). Furthermore, additional studies addressing quantitative aspects of cannabis use (i.e., increased THC concentration, dosage, and frequency) are necessary to clarify the association and causation of type, severity, and maintenance of negative consequences as well as the potential recovery trajectories following abstinence.

It is noteworthy that pregnant adolescents are about 1.8 times more likely to report past-month marijuana use than nonpregnant adolescents (Salas-Wright et al. 2015). Maternal use of cannabis and other psychoactive drugs during pregnancy and its impact on the developing brain of the fetus, newborn, and infant are reviewed in Chapter 23 of this manual.

Structural Brain Changes

In order to improve the efficacy of signal conduction during the transition from childhood to adulthood, the developing adolescent brain is characterized by two important processes: axonal myelination and synaptic pruning. At the molecular level, repeated THC exposure disrupts endocannabinoid signaling with CB1Rs. THC alters axonal morphology, and this affects computational power of neural circuitries and induces neurodegeneration at all developmental stages from in utero to adulthood (Reece 2019; Tortoriello et al. 2014). Consequently, youth up to age 25 years (when the brain prefrontal cortex, which is responsible for reward inhibition and the operation of highly executive functions, reaches maturity) are vulnerable to the effects of cannabis on psychosocial and cognitive development. A number of studies have determined an association between cannabis use and brain changes involving structures governing memory, higher-order cognition, complex attention, and emotional processing in animals and humans (Pierre 2017). These include reduced volume of the hippocampus, temporal cortex, insula, and orbitofrontal cortex. Frequent use of high-potency cannabis is associated with disturbed corpus callosum microstructural white matter organization in individuals with and without psychosis (Rigucci et al. 2015). Some changes appear to be dose related. It is not yet clear how to quantify the brain changes and the associated functional cognitive and behavioral deficits. However, there is no "safe" amount of cannabis that can be used to prevent these neuroanatomical changes.

Specific Health Concerns

Cannabis Use and Cognition

Marijuana use causes impairments in attention, concentration, decision making, impulsivity, and working memory. In daily users, this impairment may last for up to 4 weeks after cessation of use (Levine et al. 2017). Meier et al. (2012) reported that adolescent-onset, long-term use of at least 4 days per week predicts an 8-point decline in IQ on average. This decline was not reversible with a year of abstinence. Frequency of marijuana use predicts decreased executive functioning and learning, especially for adolescents with initiation of use by age 14 (Castellanos-Ryan et al. 2017). Furthermore, weekly use compared with no marijuana use predicts deficits in executive functioning and verbal IQ for up to 30 days (Scott et al. 2018). Loss of synapses following adolescent cannabis exposure was directly related to memory formation and forgetfulness (Szutorisz and Hurd 2016). There is strong evidence that marijuana users on average have less academic success than non-users (Fergusson et al. 2003; Silins et al. 2015). In a 10-year longitudinal study of 1,265 youth in New Zealand, those who used marijuana by age 15 were 3.6 times less likely to graduate from high school, 2.3 times less likely to enroll in college, and 3.7 times less likely to get a college degree than non-users (Fergusson et al. 2003). Furthermore, youth who use marijuana at least weekly are 60% more likely to drop out of high school compared with non-users (Silins et al. 2015). Another important indicator of adolescent use is school suspensions and expulsions for substance use. The Colorado Department of Education reported a 40% increase in school suspensions and expulsions for substances since 2009, the year cannabis was commercialized (through dispensaries).

Marijuana Use and Psychosis

One of the first gene-by-environment epigenetic associations described with cannabis use relevant to psychiatric vulnerability involved the catechol O-methyltransferase (COMT) gene and schizophrenia risk. COMT, which metabolizes catecholamine neurotransmitters such as dopamine, has long been implicated in substance use. The Val/Met COMT polymorphism increases COMT activity and, thus, levels of dopamine, which plays a critical role in reward, motivation, cognition and other behaviors linked to addiction. Given that the status of COMT DNA methylation depended on the frequency of cannabis use, it remains unanswered whether such epigenetic alterations persist long after drug use cessation.

Marijuana intoxication may cause acute psychosis (D'Souza et al. 2004). This effect may depend on the potency and amount of ingestion. Time to maximum blood concentration by consuming marijuana edibles is about 2 hours (Borgelt et al. 2013). Therefore, people may consume edibles and not feel any immediate effects. As a result, they may continue consuming and ultimately experience extreme paranoia and psychosis (Vo et al. 2018). Adolescent exposure to marijuana predicts up to a twofold increased risk of psychosis and schizophrenia in adulthood (Levine et al. 2017). This dose-dependent finding has been replicated at least nine times in large cohort studies controlling for multiple variables, including family history, psychosis preceding marijuana use, and intoxication at the time of final assessment. A review by Bagot and colleagues (2015) concluded that early age at initiation of cannabis use is associated with increased prevalence of early-onset psychosis. Among young adults with first break psychosis, adolescent marijuana exposure predicts up to a 6-year earlier onset (Di Forti et al. 2014). This finding also appears to be dose dependent and especially robust for young people who use concentrated products. Bonny-Noach and Sagiv-Alayoff (2017) studied trends among emerging adult travelers who developed a first-time psychosis after visiting known "drug-party" world destinations such as Goa, India, or South America and concluded that the majority of them consumed had hashish or ganja. There is no known safe amount of marijuana exposure in adolescents to avoid the development of psychosis. Among adults with schizophrenia, marijuana use predicts a worse course of the disorder with more hospitalizations and more days of hospitalization over time (Manrique-Garcia et al. 2014). For more information and treatment implications on co-occurring psychotic disorders, see Chapter 19.

Cannabis Use, Depression, Anxiety, and Suicide

A recent systematic review and meta-analysis of cannabis and co-occurring disorders suggests that the high prevalence of cannabis use in adolescents, and perhaps the growing potency of THC, might contribute to the development of depression (odds ratio [OR] = 1.37) and suicidality (ideation OR = 1.50; attempt OR = 3.46), but not anxiety disorders, later during young adulthood (Gobbi et al. 2019). Another meta-analysis did not find a relationship between acute marijuana use and suicidal ideation or behavior but did find associations between chronic or heavy marijuana use and death by suicide (OR = 2.56), suicidal ideation (OR = 2.53), and suicide attempt (OR = 3.2) (Borges et al. 2016). The different outcomes are the result of differences in research methodologies. A recent study of 7,805 dizygotic and 6,181 monozygotic twins showed that among twins discordant for using 100 or more times in their life, the twin with marijuana use was 2.1 times as likely to have a lifetime history of major depressive disorder, 2.6 times more likely to have a lifetime history of suicidal ideation, and 4.4 times more likely to have a lifetime history of a suicide attempt (Agrawal et al. 2017). Of note, youth with onset of depression, suicidal ideation, or suicide attempt before marijuana use were not included in these analyses. For more information on co-occurring suicidal behavior and its treatment, see Chapter 18.

Cannabis Use and Addictive Disorders

About 1 in 6 youth who use marijuana develop a CUD within 12 months of first use (Forman-Hoffman et al. 2017) as compared with 1 in 11 adults (Hall and Degenhardt 2009). In DSM-5 (American Psychiatric Association 2013), a diagnosis of CUD relies on a set of 11 symptoms similarly to those for other substance use disorders (SUDs). Meeting a threshold of 2 of 11 criteria suffices to meet diagnosis (mild, 2–3; moderate, 4–5; severe, ≥6). Physical dependence on cannabis is formally recognized in DSM-5. About two-thirds of youth who present for substance treatment report physical dependence, including tolerance to and withdrawal from the drug (Vandrey et al. 2005). Symptoms of marijuana withdrawal include anxiety, hot and cold spells, insomnia, irritability, mild tremor, restlessness, strange "marijuana" dreams, and weight loss. Symptoms start within a day of cessation of use, peak around days 2–4, and last about 2 weeks. Early onset of marijuana use by about age 16 years compared with later predicts a 2.7-fold increased risk of developing a CUD (Swift et al. 2008). Adolescents with moderate to high cannabis use followed from age 14 to 32 years showed increased likelihood for tobacco dependence compared with the no or low cannabis use trajectory. Marijuana cessation programs should include tobacco use strategies (Brook et al. 2015). Adolescent marijuana use also predicts a two- to threefold increased risk of using other substances (Levine et al. 2017). The reason for this "gateway effect" is not clear. It could be that marijuana primes the brain to respond more favorably to other substances or that youth who use marijuana have a propensity to have risky behaviors in general (Levine et al. 2017). It is also possible that some youth simply chase a "better high" than the one achieved by cannabis use and consequently abuse prescription opiates, heroin, and cocaine.

An 8-year longitudinal study of 260 youth in substance treatment and matched control subjects showed that for every year the onset of marijuana use was delayed, there was a 27% decrease in the risk of developing injection drug use (Thurstone et al. 2013). A recent independent study conducted in Connecticut (A. C. Swindell, unpublished report, 2016) has received little attention despite its important conclusion that there is a relationship between marijuana use and the abuse of opioid pain medications and heroin. This study included a control group and is based on data from a total of 6,000 Connecticut high school students over a period of 12 years. Marijuana users were 14 times more likely to abuse pain medications and more than 4 times more likely to use heroin, compared with non–marijuana users. To put these numbers in context, according to the Connecticut medical examiner report, 75 youth up to the age of 25 years died from opioid overdose in 2015. This is most likely a conservative number. Furthermore, the current use of an additional illicit drug is about five times higher among marijuana users. Swindell's report concludes that "these correlations are about the same in towns across

Connecticut, regardless of socioeconomic and demographics and have been stable since at least 2008."

Finally, additional public health issues pertaining to the cannabis-opiates "connection," such as cannabis's controversial role in the desperate effort to slow and reverse the opioid epidemic and cannabis replacement of or addition to opiate treatment for pain management, are reviewed in Chapter 10.

Cannabis-Related Emergencies

A recent study of adults referrals to the emergency department (ED) showed that inhaled cannabis was more likely than ingested cannabis to cause hyperemesis syndrome (18% vs. 8%), while consumption of edible cannabis was more likely than smoking to result in psychiatric presentation (18% vs. 11%), intoxication (48% vs. 28%), and cardiovascular effects (8% vs. 3%), and more ED visits than expected by the amount of edibles sales compared with smoked/vaped cannabis (Monte et al. 2019).

A review of ED visits by children and adolescents reported an array of cannabis-related symptoms from acute use (smoking and particularly ingestion of edibles) or exposure (Chen and Klig 2019). Common presentations include acute intoxication, hyperemesis, and physical injuries from impaired psychomotor function. Uncommon presentations include cardiorespiratory effects, hyperkinesis, and coma in young children (Chen and Klig 2019).

A study conducted at Children's Hospital Colorado reported a significant increase in ED visits related to ingestion of cannabis-infused products and edibles by young children (Wang et al. 2013). About two-thirds of children presenting with a marijuana ingestion required medical hospitalization for lethargy. Some children required admission to an intensive care unit. Therefore, ingestion of marijuana by children should be considered a medical emergency.

Cannabis Effects on the Cardiovascular System

Recent reports suggest causation of cardiac arrhythmias (Robinson et al. 2018), myocardial infarction in youth and adults (Singh et al. 2018; Tocs et al. 2019), and stroke (Wolff and Jouanjus 2017). The increase in the amount of THC in various cannabis products might be a contributing factor to the cardiovascular effects. THC has been known to have a vasodilatation effect on blood vessels. Consequently, its use is contraindicated in those with cardiac ailments, including angina pectoris and post–myocardial infarction.

Cannabis Use and Other Medical Effects

Cannabis has been associated with potential harmful effects on other bodily systems. These include potential carcinogenic effects on testicles (nonseminoma type) and lungs (Hall 2015). Smoked cannabis is associated with bronchitis. Burning cannabis to its combustion point releases not only THC but also tar, carbon monoxide, ammonia, acetaldehyde, and other potentially hazardous compounds. Cannabis does not appear to increase lung cancer or chronic obstructive pulmonary disease. It is not clear if cannabis is associated with increased risk of pneumonia, although THC suppresses alveolar macrophage function.

Reproductive effects have been reported in cannabis users, including poor sperm quality and higher risk of anovulation due to poor-quality oocytes in females. These have been attributed to interruption of CB1R expression necessary for controlling chromatin condensation in the cells.

Driving Under the Influence

Similarly to alcohol, cannabis alters perception and psychomotor performance, and this may contribute to an increased risk for car crashes. Unfortunately, more than 50% of cannabis users in Colorado believe that it is safe to drive under the influence. A similar percentage reported driving high on average 12 times in the last 30 days. Although the legal limit is 5 ng/mL, in many fatalities the level was 30 ng/mL or higher (Rocky Mountain High Intensity Drug Trafficking Area 2018). Salomonsen-Sautel et al. (2014) examined the proportion of traffic fatalities nationally in which the driver tested positive for marijuana and found significant increases in Colorado compared with non–medical marijuana states starting in 2009, which corresponds to the commercialization of marijuana in the state. One limitation of the study is a lack of information on the amount of intoxication at the time of the crash. Percentage of total fatalities of drivers testing positive for cannabis increased by 30% (8.8%–11.4%) during the commercialization of medical cannabis (2009–2012) and since the legalization of cannabis for recreational use (2013–2017) by approximately 90% (11.4%–21.3%). The National Highway Traffic Safety Administration recommends not driving for at least 3 hours after smoking marijuana. Drivers who consume marijuana edibles may need to wait longer (Rocky Mountain High Intensity Drug Trafficking Area 2018).

Butane Hash Oil and K2 Effects

Dabbing of concentrated BHO comes with potent health concerns, including that the illegal process of cooking it with the flammable gas butane (known as "blasting") may cause a fiery explosion resulting in severe burns or death reminiscent of methamphetamine labs accidents. Also, inhalation of butane and the ingestion of contaminants in the cannabis like pesticides and fungi can be harmful.

K2, or "Spice," and "bath salts" represent a group of different synthetic (clandestine lab–produced) cannabinoids or cathinones that are smoked recreationally. These synthetic drugs bind to CB1 receptors much more strongly than does THC. K2 has stimulant-like effects associated with unpredictable adverse effects, including anxiety, agitation, paranoia, heart palpitations, seizures, high blood pressure and bleeding, and it can cause death. It cannot be detected using standard urine toxicology screens. Overdose threshold is unpredictable.

Prevention and Treatment

Adolescence is characterized by neuropsychological processes in which dopamine-related overvaluation of reward in the limbic system, underestimation of risk, and immature regulatory inhibitory functions in the prefrontal cortex can explain the high level of sensation-seeking behaviors, including cannabis use (Ammerman and Tau 2016).

The two main reasons for using cannabis for the first time are the erroneous perception of its diminishing harmfulness and its legal/medical status. Between 10% and 20% of young adolescents in states that have not legalized cannabis stated that a change in its legal status would be a reason for them to use it (Palamar et al. 2014). Furthermore, a large international study concluded that any change in cannabis legal status starting with decriminalization would lead to, first, an increase in number of first-time users for 5 years until it would plateau and, second, a decrease in age at first use (Williams and Bretteville-Jensen 2014). A U.S. study provided evidence to support concerns that decriminalization may be a risk factor for future increases in youth marijuana use and acceptance (Miech et al. 2015).

Consequently, it is imperative to restore the evidence-based knowledge on the harmfulness of marijuana. More challenging is the task of curbing access to cannabis by minors. A substantial number of adolescents do not use cannabis. The low-risk characteristics are better relationships with parents and beliefs that drug use is problematic (Burdzovic Andreas et al. 2016). In addition, the likelihood of receiving cannabis use offers is higher for adolescents with externalizing disorders (including low-level delinquency) and those with cannabis-using friends. These results may have implications for novel preventive strategies targeting cannabis-exposed adolescents. High school seniors with cannabis abstinence 1 year after last use indicated losing enjoyment of its use. Those who have never smoked cannabis reported concerns about getting addicted, use being against their beliefs, not liking cannabis users, and not having friends who use cannabis (Martz et al. 2018). Parental education level is pivotal in prevention efforts. Eight-graders whose parents did not complete high school were more likely (10% vs. 3%) to have used cannabis in the past month compared with those whose parents completed college.

Prevention efforts can be divided into universal or selective prevention. Whereas the effect size of universal prevention programs is generally low, selective programs are becoming more popular in schools as a means to address youth who are already starting to use or are showing a high-risk personality profile (Conrod 2016). For more information on prevention, see Chapter 2.

An important aspect of prevention should focus on driving under the influence of cannabis. While most teens agree that driving under the influence of alcohol is dangerous, unfortunately 34% of high school juniors and seniors believe that cannabis improves their driving abilities. Also, 41% believe that cannabis has no effect on their driving skills (Students Against Destructive Decisions 2012). Initial data on the legalization of marijuana raise concerns about its potential impact on "kids and cars." Moving forward, additional protections are likely needed to prevent marijuana use and make treatment for adolescents with CUD more accessible. In terms of driving, public education around the dangers of driving under the influence is needed. Data and clear policy around measurements of intoxication and driving impairment are also needed.

Psychosocial Interventions

A Cochrane systematic review of psychosocial interventions concluded that intensive intervention provided over more than four weekly sessions of motivational enhancement therapy (MET) and cognitive-behavioral therapy (CBT) with abstinence-based incentives was most consistently supported for treatment of CUD (Gates et al. 2016). Outcome measures included frequency of use and severity of dependence. For more information about psychosocial interventions, see Part III (Chapters 12–16) in this manual.

The four-site Cannabis Youth Treatment (CYT) study of 600 youth with CUD has been the benchmark for psychosocial treatment of CUD (Dennis et al. 2004) (see Chapter 13 for a review of the study.)

In an effort to improve outcomes, one study randomly assigned 153 youth with CUD to receive either CBT or CBT plus contingency management (CM). The study found that CM increased the proportion of youth achieving a month of abstinence by the end of treatment from 31% to 53% (Stanger et al. 2015). See Chapter 13 for more details on CM.

Recently, harm reduction perspectives have been reported to be common among college students (Bravo et al. 2017a). A study of protective behavioral strategies (PBS) among students who have been using cannabis reported that PBS may buffer risk factors and enhance protective factors among users. Furthermore, PBS constitute a mechanism by which cannabis users may moderate their use and attenuate their risk of experiencing cannabis-related consequences (Bravo et al. 2017b). In terms of therapists' shifting attitude and acceptance of harm reduction as an outcome goal, students enrolled in addiction studies training programs appear to be more accepting of clients who decide to pursue nonabstinence either as an intermediate step on the way to abstinence or as a final goal. Thurstone et al. (2017) have developed a motivational interviewing/acceptance and commitment therapy model. For more information on harm reduction, see Chapter 12.

Pharmacological Interventions

A comprehensive review of pharmacological treatment of cannabis-related disorders showed that only gabapentin for cannabis was somewhat effective in a single adult study for withdrawal, while dronabinol (synthetic THC) was not. Other trials of antidepressants, anticonvulsants, and antianxiety agents in adults were not effective (Gorelick 2016). N-acetylcysteine (NAC) has been hypothesized to reduce the reinstatement of drug seeking in animal models. In a placebo-controlled trial for adolescents with CUD, the NAC group (1,200 mg bid) were twice as likely to submit a negative urine specimen and to achieve end-of-treatment abstinence as the placebo group (Gray et al. 2012). However, a similar adult-based trial could not replicate these findings.

Tomko et al. (2018) examined the role of depressive symptoms in treatment of adolescent CUD with NAC in a placebo-controlled trial. Results did not support NAC's effect on depressive symptoms or as a mediator of cannabis cessation. NAC was more effective at promoting abstinence among adolescents with heightened baseline depressive symptoms. A placebo-controlled trial of atomoxetine for CUD with comorbid attention-deficit/hyperactivity disorder (ADHD) did not show efficacy for CUD or for ADHD (Thurstone et al. 2010). Further pharmacological research is necessary to complement the psychosocial interventions.

An important issue in adolescent substance treatment is co-occurring psychiatric disorders. For example, the CYT study found that about 80% of youth had a co-occurring psychiatric disorder and 60% had a history of emotional, physical, or sexual abuse (Dennis et al. 2004). These prevalences were found even with exclusion criteria that excluded youth with severe psychiatric disorders and SUD. Despite the prevalence of co-occurring psychiatric disorders, few youth receive care for both (Hawkins 2009). For more information on co-occurring disorders, see Part 4 (Chapters 17–21), and on integrated systems of care, see Chapter 6.

A pivotal problem in adolescent substance treatment is access to care. According to the National Survey on Drug Use and Health, only 6.3% of adolescents who need substance treatment access care. According to the Treatment Episode Data Set, about two-thirds of adolescents in substance treatment access care through juvenile justice department involvement. Access is even worse for African American and Latino youth, who, compared with Caucasian youth, are more likely to access treatment through juvenile justice involvement (Alegria et al. 2011). Providing treatment in nontraditional, community settings, such as afterschool clubs and schools, might be a way to improve access to care. See Chapter 22 for treatment of youth with SUDs in the juvenile justice system.

Impact of Liberalization of Cannabis Policies on Youth

Various states and countries are reviewing their policies around liberalization of marijuana use. Options include depenalization, decriminalization, and legalization. In depenalized and decriminalized settings, marijuana remains illegal. *Depenalization* refers to reducing criminal penalties associated with marijuana possession or distribution. *Decriminalization* is a step further, with criminal penalties removed and replaced with civil penalties such as a fine or mandatory treatment. The Netherlands and Portugal have a history of marijuana depenalization and decriminalization, not legalization as many erroneously believe. *Legalization* refers to removing all penalties and sanctions against marijuana use. Legalization in the United States presents certain challenges because legal actions are protected by the First Amendment guaranteeing free speech. Free speech, in turn, allows for commercialization, marketing, and lobbying efforts to promote sales and use.

Another change is the medicalization of marijuana. In medicalized systems, marijuana use for recreational purposes remains illegal. However, there is a process for people to attain marijuana for medical use. Addressing the full gamut of the limitations of medical cannabis dispensaries is beyond the scope of this chapter. However, we shall briefly mention the lack of professional knowledge and training among staffers ("budtenders"). An example of a serious lack of professionalism is found in a recent survey in Colorado, in which 69% of budtenders recommended marijuana to pregnant women who were wondering if it would help with first-trimester morning sickness (Dickson et al. 2018). Additional problems include a lack of supervision of quality and safety of the products and the ease of getting a medical cannabis card by many who do not meet the criteria. There are also ample opportunities for diversion of cannabis to minors and adults. Reports from Colorado and a secondary analysis of the MTF study reveal that many adolescents are using diverted medical marijuana (Boyd et al. 2015; Salomonsen-Sautel et al. 2012).

It is important to note that no medicine in a smokable form exists in the United States. In the state of Minnesota, for example, smokable medical cannabis is not allowed.

Finally, another important concept is the commercialization of marijuana. *Commercialization* refers to allowing businesses to cultivate, market, and sell marijuana. An example of noncommercialized legalization is Uruguay, which has state-run marijuana stores. Examples of commercialized markets are California, Colorado, and Washington, and most recently Canada.

Compared with older age groups (over 25 years of age), youth disproportionately use more marijuana and are more vulnerable to negative consequences because of the developmental stage of their brain. The legal alcohol and tobacco industries have targeted youth with their marketing to develop early-onset use, which makes youth more likely to progress to regular use and dependence. Regular users, in turn, provide the bulk of profits to the alcohol and tobacco industries. The emerging marijuana industry and JUUL are following suit, regardless of empty denials. Figure 9–2 shows the change in past-month marijuana use for adolescents and young adults in Colorado compared with national data over time using data from the National Survey on Drug Use and Health. In summary, trend data indicate that marijuana use among both adolescents and young adults, as well as negative consequences of use, has increased in Colorado and other legalized cannabis use states over the last decade compared with the rest of the country. For updated details regarding traffic fatalities, public health and ED data, poison control, school negative consequences, social impact, and so forth, see the Rocky Mountain High Intensity Drug Trafficking Area website (https://rmhidta.org).

Recommendations for Public Health Policies

Policy makers and the public need real-time data on both the consequences of legalization and the related monetary costs. Meanwhile, the industry's influence on policy should be significantly curtailed. Smart Approaches to Marijuana (SAM), a not-for-profit organization, recommends that research efforts and data collection focus on the following categories that are relevant to youth prevention and intervention:

- Emergency room and hospital admissions related to marijuana
- Marijuana potency and price trends in the legal and illegal markets
- School incidents related to marijuana, including representative data sets
- Extent of marijuana advertising toward youth and its impact
- Marijuana-related car crashes, including THC levels even when testing positive for alcohol
- Mental health effects of marijuana
- Admissions to treatment and counseling intervention programs
- Cost of mental health and addiction treatment related to increased marijuana use
- Cost of needing but not receiving treatment
- Effect on the market for alcohol and other drugs

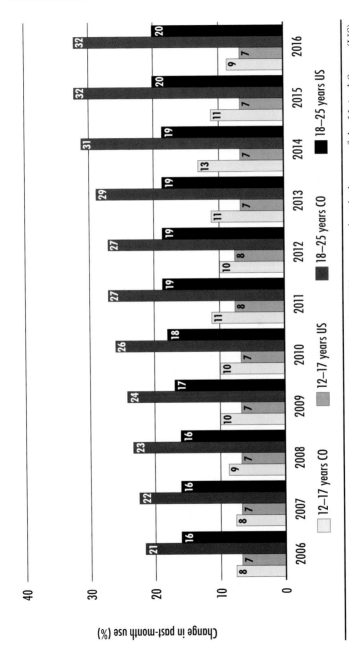

Figure 9–2. Past-month marijuana use by youth in Colorado (CO) compared with the rest of the United States (US).
Source. Data from Azofeifa et al. 2016a, 2016b; Substance Abuse and Mental Health Services Administration 2019.

Key Points

- Exposure to cannabis in adolescence predicts cognitive impairment and decreased school achievement.

- Cannabis may cause an addictive disorder in one of six adolescents within 1 year of use and may increase the likelihood of other psychoactive drug use.

- Cannabis use increases the likelihood of developing early-onset psychosis, schizophrenia, suicidal behavior, depression, and cardiovascular problems.

- Driving under the influence of cannabis is hazardous.

- Cannabis may have cross-generational epigenetic effects at the molecular level.

References

Agrawal A, Nelson EC, Bucholz KK, et al: Major depressive disorder, suicidal thoughts and behaviours, and cannabis involvement in discordant twins: a retrospective cohort study. Lancet Psychiatry 4(9):706–714, 2017 28750823

Alegria M, Carson NJ, Goncalves M, et al: Disparities in treatment for substance use disorders and co-occurring disorders for ethnic/racial minority youth. J Am Acad Child Adolesc Psychiatry 50(1):22–31, 2011 21156267

American Psychiatric Association: Diagnostic and Statistical Manual of Mental Disorders, 5th Edition. Arlington, VA, American Psychiatric Association, 2013

Ammerman S, Tau G: Weeding out the truth: adolescents and cannabis. J Addict Med 10(2):75–82, 2016 26985645

Azofeifa A, Mattson ME, Lyerla R: Supplementary Material. State Level Data: Estimates of Marijuana Use and Related Indicators-National Survey on Drug Use and Health, Colorado, 2002–2014. Rockville, MD, Center for Behavioral Health Statistics and Quality, Substance Abuse and Mental Health Services Administration, 2016a. Available at: https://www.samhsa.gov/sites/default/files/topics/data_outcomes_quality/colorado-2002-2014.pdf. Accessed July23, 2019.

Azofeifa A, Mattson ME, Schauer G, et al: National estimates of marijuana use and related indicators—National Survey on Drug Use and Health, United States, 2002–2014. MMWR Surveill Summ 65(SS-11):1–25, 2016b. Available at: https://www.cdc.gov/mmwr/volumes/65/ss/ss6511a1.htm?s_cid=ss6511a1_w. Accessed July 23, 2019.

Bagot K, Milin R, Kaminer Y: Youth cannabis abuse and the development of early-onset psychotic disorders. Substance Abuse 36:524–533, 2015 25774457

Bonny-Noach H, Sagiv-Alayoff M: Rescuing Israeli travellers: effects of substance abuse, mental health, geographic region of rescue, gender, and age of rescuees. J Travel Med 24(5):1–6, 2017 28931135

Borgelt LM, Franson KL, Nussbaum AM, et al: The pharmacologic and clinical effects of medical cannabis. Pharmacotherapy 33(2):195–209, 2013 23386598

Borges G, Bagge CL, Orozco R: A literature review and meta-analyses of cannabis use and suicidality. J Affect Disord 195:63–74, 2016 26872332

Boyd CJ, Veliz PT, McCabe SE: Adolescents' use of medical marijuana: a secondary analysis of Monitoring the Future data. J Adolesc Health 57(2):241–244, 2015 26206447

Bravo AJ, Anthenien AM, Prince MA, Pearson MR; Marijuana Outcomes Study Team: Marijuana protective behavioral strategies as a moderator of the effects of risk/protective factors on marijuana-related outcomes. Addict Behav 69:14–21, 2017a 28110137

Bravo AJ, Prince MA, Pearson MR; Marijuana Outcomes Study Team: Can I use marijuana safely? An examination of distal antecedents, marijuana protective behavioral strategies and marijuana outcomes. J Stud Alcohol Drugs 78(2):203–212, 2017b 28317500

Brook JS, Lee JY, Brook DW: Trajectories of marijuana use beginning in adolescence predict tobacco dependence in adulthood. Subst Abus 36(4):470–477, 2015 25259421

Burdzovic Andreas J, Pape H, Bretteville-Jensen AL: Who are the adolescents saying "No" to cannabis offers. Drug Alcohol Depend 163:64–70, 2016 27107848

Castellanos-Ryan N, Pingault JB, Parent S, et al: Adolescent cannabis use, change in neurocognitive function, and high-school graduation: a longitudinal study from early adolescence to young adulthood. Dev Psychopathol 29(4):1253–1266, 2017 28031069

Center for Behavioral Health Statistics and Quality: Results From the 2017 National Survey on Drug Use and Health: Detailed Tables. Rockville, MD, Substance Abuse and Mental Health Services Administration, 2017, Available at: https://www.samhsa.gov/data/sites/default/files/cbhsq-reports/NSDUHDetailedTabs2017/NSDUHDetailedTabs2017.htm. Accessed July 23, 2019.

Chen YC, Klig J: Cannabis related emergencies in children and teens. Curr Opin Pediatr March 6, 2019 [Epub ahead of print] 30865027

Conrod PJ: Personality-targeted interventions for substance use and misuse. Curr Addict Rep 3(4):426–436, 2016 27909645

Dai H, Catley D, Richter KP, et al: Electronic cigarettes and future marijuana use: a longitudinal study. Pediatrics 141(5):141, 2018 29686146

Dennis M, Godley SH, Diamond G, et al: The Cannabis Youth Treatment (CYT) study: main findings from two randomized trials. J Subst Abuse Treat 27(3):197–213, 2004 15501373

Dickson B, Mansfield C, Guiahi M, et al: Recommendations from cannabis dispensaries about first-trimester cannabis use. Obstet Gynecol 131(6):1031–1038, 2018 29742676

Di Forti M, Sallis H, Allegri F, et al: Daily use, especially of high-potency cannabis, drives the earlier onset of psychosis in cannabis users. Schizophr Bull 40(6):1509–1517, 2014 24345517

District of Columbia, Department of Health: Medical cannabis: adverse effects & drug interactions. December 22, 2015. Available at: https://dchealth.dc.gov/publication/medical-cannabis-adverse-effects-and-drug-interactions. Accessed May 3, 2019.

D'Souza DC, Perry E, MacDougall L, et al: The psychotomimetic effects of intravenous delta-9-tetrahydrocannabinol in healthy individuals: implications for psychosis. Neuropsychopharmacology 29(8):1558–1572, 2004 15173844

Fergusson DM, Horwood LJ, Swain-Campbell NR: Cannabis dependence and psychotic symptoms in young people. Psychol Med 33(1):15–21, 2003 12537032

Forman-Hoffman VL, Glasheen C, Batts KR: Marijuana use, recent marijuana initiation, and progression to marijuana use disorder among young male and female adolescents aged 12–14 living in US households. Subst Abuse 11:1178221817711159, 2017 28615948

Gates PJ, Sabioni P, Copeland J, et al: Psychosocial interventions for cannabis use disorder. Cochrane Database Syst Rev 5(5):CD005336, 2016 27149547

Gobbi G, Atkin T, Zytynski T, et al: Association of cannabis use in adolescence and risk of depression, anxiety, and suicidality in young adulthood: a systematic review and meta-analysis. JAMA Psychiatry February 13, 2019 [Epub ahead of print] 30758486

Gorelick DA: Pharmacological treatment of cannabis-related disorders. Curr Pharm Des 22(42):6409–6419, 2016 27549375

Gray KM, Carpenter MJ, Baker NL, et al: A double-blind randomized controlled trial of N-acetylcysteine in cannabis-dependent adolescents. Am J Psychiatry 169(8):805–812, 2012 22706327

Hall W: What has research over the past two decades revealed about the adverse health effects of recreational cannabis use? Addiction 110(1):19–35, 2015 25287883

Hall W, Degenhardt L: Adverse health effects of non-medical cannabis use. Lancet 374(9698):1383–1391, 2009 19837255

Hawkins EH: A tale of two systems: co-occurring mental health and substance abuse disorders treatment for adolescents. Annu Rev Psychol 60:197–227, 2009 19035824

Johnston LD, Miech RA, O'Malley PM, et al: Monitoring the Future: National Survey Results on Drug Use: 1975–2017: Overview, Key Findings on Adolescent Drug Use. Ann Arbor, MI, Institute for Social Research, The University of Michigan, 2018

Knapp AA, Lee DC, Borodovsky JT, et al: Emerging trends in cannabis administration among adolescent cannabis users. J Adol Health 64(4):487–493, 2019 30205931

Levine A, Clemenza K, Rynn M, et al: Evidence for the risks and consequences of adolescent cannabis exposure. J Am Acad Child Adolesc Psychiatry 56(3):214–225, 2017 28219487

Manrique-Garcia E, Zammit S, Dalman C, et al: Prognosis of schizophrenia in persons with and without a history of cannabis use. Psychol Med 44(12):2513–2521, 2014 25055170

Martz ME, Schulenberg JE, Patrick ME: Passing on pot: high school seniors' reasons for not using marijuana as predictors of future use. J Stud Alcohol Drugs 79(5):761–769, 2018 30422790

Miech RA, Johnston L, O'Malley PM, et al: Trends in use of marijuana and attitudes toward marijuana among youth before and after decriminalization: the case of California 2007–2013. Int J Drug Policy 26(4):336–344, 2015 25662893

Miech RA, Johnston LD, O'Malley PM, et al: Monitoring the Future: National Survey Results on Drug Use, 1975–2017: Volume 1, Secondary School Students. Ann Arbor, MI, Institute for Social Research, The University of Michigan, 2018. Available at: http://www.monitoringthefuture.org/pubs/monographs/mtf-vol1_2017.pdf. Accessed May 3, 2019.

Meier MH, Caspi A, Ambler A, et al: Persistent cannabis users show neuropsychological decline from childhood to midlife. Proc Natl Acad Sci USA 109(40):E2657–E2664, 2012 22927402

Monte AA, Shelton SK, Mill JE, et al: Acute illness associated with cannabis use, by route of exposure: an observational study. Ann Intern Med March 26, 2019 [Epub ahead of print] 30909297

Morean ME, Kong G, Camenga DR, et al: High school students' use of electronic cigarettes to vaporize cannabis. Pediatrics 136(4):611–616, 2015 26347431

Palamar JJ, Ompad DC, Petkova E: Correlates of intentions to use cannabis among US high school seniors in the case of cannabis legalization. Int J Drug Policy 25(3):424–435, 2014 24589410

Pierre JM: Risks of increasingly potent cannabis: the joint effects of potency and frequency. Current Psychiatry 16(2):15–19, 2017

Reece A: Cannabis problematics include but are not limited to pain management (commentary). JAMA Network, February 2, 2019. Available at: https://jamanetwork.com/journals/jama/article-abstract/2723649. Accessed May 3, 2019.

Rigucci S, Marques TR, Di Forti M, et al: Effects of high-potency cannabis on corpus callosum microstructure. Psychol Med 46(4):841–854, 2015 26610039

Robinson JA, Somasegar S, Shivapour JK, et al: ECG findings in pediatric patients under the influence of marijuana. Cannabis 1(1):28–34, 2018

Rocky Mountain High Intensity Drug Trafficking Area: The Legalization of Marijuana in Colorado: The Impact, Vol 5. Update. 2018. Available at: https://rmhidta.org/files/D2DF/FINAL-%20Volume%205%20UPDATE%202018.pdf. Accessed May 3, 2019.

Salas-Wright CP, Vaughn MG, Ugalde J, Todic J: Substance use and teen pregnancy in the United States: evidence from the NSDUH 2002–2012. Addict Behav 45:218–225, 2015 25706068

Salomonsen-Sautel S, Sakai JT, Thurstone C, et al: Medical marijuana use among adolescents in substance abuse treatment. J Am Acad Child Adolesc Psychiatry 51(7):694–702, 2012 22721592

Salomonsen-Sautel S, Min SJ, Sakai JT, et al: Trends in fatal motor vehicle crashes before and after marijuana commercialization in Colorado. Drug Alcohol Depend 140:137–144, 2014 24831752

Scott JC, Slomiak ST, Jones JD, et al: Association of cannabis with cognitive functioning in adolescent and young adults: a systemic review and meta-analysis. JAMA Psychiatry 75(6):585–595, 2018 29710074

Silins E, Fergusson DM, Patton GC, et al; Cannabis Cohorts Research Consortium: Adolescent substance use and educational attainment: an integrative data analysis comparing cannabis and alcohol from three Australasian cohorts. Drug Alcohol Depend 156:90–96, 2015 26409754

Singh A, Saluja S, Kumar A, et al: Cardiovascular complications of marijuana and related substances: a review. Cardiol Ther 7(1):45–59, 2018 29218644

Stanger C, Ryan SR, Scherer EA, et al: Clinic- and home-based contingency management plus parent training for adolescent cannabis use disorders. J Am Acad Child Adolesc Psychiatry 54(6):445–53.e2, 2015 26004659

Students Against Destructive Decisions: SADD.org survey, 2012

Substance Abuse and Mental Health Services Administration: National Survey on Drug Use and Health: Comparison of 2014-2015 and 2015-2016 Population Percentages (50 States and the District of Columbia). Available at: https://

www.samhsa.gov/data/sites/default/files/NSDUHsaeShortTermCHG2016/ NSDUHsaeShortTermCHG2016.htm. Accessed July 23, 2019.

Swift W, Coffey C, Carlin JB, et al: Adolescent cannabis users at 24 years: trajectories to regular weekly use and dependence in young adulthood. Addiction 103(8):1361–1370, 2008 18855826

Szutorisz H, Hurd YL: Epigenetic effects of cannabis exposure. Biol Psychiatry 79(7):586–594, 2016 26546076

Thurstone C, Riggs PD, Salomonsen-Sautel S, et al: Randomized, controlled trial of atomoxetine for attention-deficit/hyperactivity disorder in adolescents with substance use disorder. J Am Acad Child Adolesc Psychiatry 49(6):573–582, 2010 20494267

Thurstone C, Salomonsen-Sautel S, Mikulich-Gilbertson SK, et al: Prevalence and predictors of injection drug use and risky sexual behaviors among adolescents in substance treatment. Am J Addict 22(6):558–565, 2013 24131163

Thurstone C, Hull M, Timmerman J, Emrick C: Development of a motivational interviewing/acceptance and commitment therapy model for adolescent substance use treatment. J Contextual Behav Sci 6:375–379, 2017

Tocs MS, Farias M, Powell AJ, et al: Myocardial infarct after marijuana inhalation in a 16-year-old adolescent boy. Pediatr Dev Pathol 22(1):80–86, 2019 29958511

Tomko RL, Gilmore AK, Gray KM: The role of depressive symptoms in treatment of adolescent cannabis use disorder with N-acetylcysteine. Addict Behav 85:26–30, 2018 29803870

Tortoriello G, Morris CV, Alpar A, et al: Miswiring the brain: Δ9-tetrahydrocannabinol disrupts cortical development by inducing an SCG10/stathmin-2 degradation pathway. EMBO J 33(7):668–685, 2014 24469251

Vandrey R, Budney AJ, Kamon JL, et al: Cannabis withdrawal in adolescent treatment seekers. Drug Alcohol Depend 78(2):205–210, 2005 15845324

Vo KT, Horng H, Li K, et al: Cannabis intoxication case series: the dangers of edibles containing tetrahydrocannabinol. Ann Emerg Med 71(3):306–313, 2018 29103798

Wang GS, Roosevelt G, Heard K: Pediatric marijuana exposures in a medical marijuana state. JAMA Pediatr 167(7):630–633, 2013 23712626

Williams J, Bretteville-Jensen AL: Does liberalizing cannabis laws increase cannabis use? J Health Econ 36:20–32, 2014 24727348

Wolff V, Jouanjus E: Strokes are possible complications of cannabinoids use. Epilepsy Behav 70(Pt B):355–363, 2017 28237318

Wong SS, Wilens TE: Medical cannabinoids in children and adolescents: a systematic review. Pediatrics 140(5):e20171818, 2017 29061872

10

Youth Opioid Use

Christopher J. Hammond, M.D., Ph.D.

Brian Hendrickson, M.D.

Marc Fishman, M.D.

The current opioid epidemic has devastated families and communities throughout the United States. More than 42,000 opioid overdose deaths occurred in 2016, which equates to approximately 130 Americans dying from an opioid overdose each day (Centers for Disease Control and Prevention 2017; Seth et al. 2018). This epidemic has not bypassed youth—5,455 youth ages 15–24 years died from a drug-related overdose in 2017, with the majority of these deaths attributed to opioids (National Institutes of Health 2019).

Dr. Hammond receives funding from a National Institute on Drug Abuse/American Academy of Child and Adolescent Psychiatrists Physician Scientist Program in Substance Abuse (2K12DA000357).

Amid the growing public health concerns over rising opioid overdose deaths, the U.S. Secretary of Health and Human Services has declared the opiate crisis a national public health emergency (President's Commission on Combating Drug Addiction and the Opioid Crisis 2017).

Opioid misuse is defined as taking an opioid medication in a manner or dose other than as prescribed, such as taking someone else's opioid pain medication or taking an opioid medication to get high. An opioid use disorder (OUD) is a problematic pattern of opioid use that results in serious impairment, distress, or inability to function. Although opioid misuse and OUD affect individuals of all ages, growing evidence points to them being disorders of pediatric origin. OUD has clear neurodevelopmental origins, emerging well before adulthood, and opioid misuse starts in young adulthood for the majority of individuals who go on to develop OUD. Although opioid misuse rates are low during adolescent years, these are the *risk* development years during which vulnerability factors associated with future opioid misuse emerge. In most cases, OUD evolves on a substrate of other substance use disorders (SUDs) such as cannabis use disorder with earlier onset, usually during adolescence (Kaminer 2017; Olfson et al. 2018). Further, young adulthood is the age window during which new-onset opioid misuse and OUD peak. Adolescents and young adults who misuse opioids present with developmentally specific problems as well as opportunities for intervention. Targeting individuals early in their opioid misuse may improve developmental trajectories and reduce morbidity and mortality related to OUD. In this chapter, we present a clinical review of the epidemiology, risk factors, and general prevention and treatment recommendations for youth, including adolescents (ages 13–17 years) and young adults (ages 18–25 years), with opioid misuse and OUD. (A special section on prescription opioids is included in Chapter 11.)

Opioid Pharmacology and Neurobiology

Opioids are a class of drugs, including both naturally derived alkaloids from the opium poppy and synthetic derivatives that exert their pharmacological effect through agonist action at the μ opioid receptor. These drugs can be further categorized as prescription pain medications (e.g., oxycodone, codeine) or illicit drugs (e.g., heroin, street fentanyl analogs). μ Opioid receptors are expressed widely through the brain, with high receptor densities in regions involved in emotion reactivity and regulation, rewards, and pain (Kosten and George 2002). Activation of the body's endogenous opioid system at these brain regions and circuits is thought to explain some of the subjective rewarding, analgesic, and mood-altering effects of these drugs. The expression of μ opioid receptors in regions of the brain stem that regulate breathing is a main factor in the lethality of opioids, because action of opioids on these brain stem regulators results in respiratory depression, the main cause of death during an opioid overdose (Imam et al. 2018).

Epidemiology

Over 11 million American adults 18 years and older, representing 4.2% of the total population, misused opioids within the past year (Center for Behavioral Health Statistics and Quality 2018). The most common type of opioids misused is prescription opiate pain medications, with hydrocodone products topping the list of the most commonly misused pain medications. Young adults living in the United States have the highest rates of opioid misuse of any age group. Prevalence rates vary slightly depending on the survey questions asked and the age range queried. Data from the National Survey on Drug Use and Health (NSDUH) collected in 2016 show that an estimated 3.3 million youth ages 12–25 years reported misusing prescription opioids in the past year, including 3.1% of adolescents (ages 12–17) and 7.5% of young adults (ages 18–25) (Substance Abuse and Mental Health Services Administration 2018). Regarding incident cases of opioid misuse, NSDUH data showed that nearly a half million young adults initiated opioid use in 2016. Data from the Monitoring the Future survey, a large nationally representative cross-sectional survey of U.S. 8th, 10th, and 12th graders, showed that in 2018, 3.4% of U.S. 12th graders had misused opioids in the past year (Johnston et al. 2018). Among adolescents, past-year prescription opioid misuse reached a peak at 9.5% in 2004 before decreasing to its current level of 3.4%.

Compared with prevalence rates of nonmedical prescription opioid misuse, rates of adolescent and young adult heroin use are significantly lower. National survey data show that approximately 0.1% of adolescents' ages 12–17 years and 0.6% of young adults ages 18–25 years reported past-year heroin use (Substance Abuse and Mental Health Services Administration 2018). These lower rates may be driven by high rates of perceived risk and disapproval for heroin use as well as decreased availability. Peak rates of heroin use among 8th, 10th, and 12th graders occurred in the late 1990s and early 2000s, with the lowest estimates of use occurring in 2016, similar to use in 2017. In contrast to the large fluctuations observed in the incidence of nonmedical prescription opioid misuse, the numbers of adolescents and young adults initiating heroin use each year have remained fairly steady since the mid-2000s.

Negative Sequelae of Opioid Misuse and Opioid Use Disorder in Youth

Opioid misuse and OUD are associated with a number of negative sequelae, including criminal justice involvement, educational and vocational failure, elevated rates of sexually transmitted infections, higher rates of concurrent psychiatric and medical disorders, and increased risk of opioid and nonopioid addiction as well as of psychiatric disorders later in life (Subramaniam et al. 2009). The most deadly consequence of opioid misuse is overdose. Overdoses occur when individuals take too much of a drug, resulting in a toxic state that may include altered mental status, medical complications, and death. Overdoses are commonly classified as intentional (purposefully self-inflicted) or unintentional (accidental) and, based on the end outcome, as lethal or nonlethal. During the current opioid epidemic, opioid-related overdoses, both intentional and unintentional, and lethal and nonlethal, have increased dramatically among adolescents and young adults. For example, opioid overdose deaths tripled in adolescents ages 15–19 years from 1999 (0.8 per 100,000) to 2015 (2.4) (Curtin et al. 2017). Adolescent opioid overdose deaths are highest among males and most commonly involve heroin. Compared with adolescent males, adolescent females are at higher risk for intentional opioid overdose deaths.

Risk Factors for Development of Opioid Misuse and Opioid Use Disorder in Youth

A number of demographic and psychosocial risk factors increase the risk for opioid initiation, misuse, and the development of OUD during adolescence and young adulthood (Substance Abuse and Mental Health Services Administration 2016). While many of these risk factors represent shared or common liability factors for all SUDs, some risk factors are specific to opioids. These risk factors can be broadly stratified into individual, family, school, and community-based factors (Table 10–1). Demographically, non-Hispanic white race/ethnicity, older age of adolescence (15–17 years), and female sex are associated with higher levels of nonmedical prescription opioid misuse (Vaughn et al. 2016).

From a developmental perspective, individuals ages 13–25 years (youth) are at higher risk for opioid initiation and developing OUD compared with children younger than 13 years and older adults. Thus, youth is a developmental stage that is, in and of itself, a risk period. Older adolescence to young adulthood represents an age range of increased vulnerability for developing an SUD, including to opioids (Vaughn et al. 2016). This general age-related addiction vulnerability is thought to be due, in part, to the staggered maturation of brain regions involved in motivation and self-regulation from ages 13 to 26 years (Hammond et al. 2014). Longitudinal brain imaging studies of children, adolescents, and young adults show a temporal pattern of early maturation of subcortical reward circuits and delayed maturation of the prefrontal cortex and other subcomponents of the executive control circuit, leading to an imbalance in circuit strength between these brain systems (Casey and Jones 2010). This imbalance is thought to result in greater reward-driven behaviors, increased risk taking, and substance engagement during youth.

Other individual factors, including the presence of psychiatric disorders and nonopioid substance use, can further increase risk. Psychiatric, medical, and psychological factors that increase the risk for opioid initiation include having a past-year history of a psychiatric disorder and having physical health problems (including headache, fatigue, acute and chronic pain) (Substance Abuse and Mental Health Services Administration 2016). The use and misuse of nonopiate substances, including cannabis, alcohol, and cigarettes, during adolescence also increase the odds of later opioid misuse. There is a growing body of data suggesting that cannabis use during adolescence may convey greater risk for progression to opioids than alcohol or tobacco use (Center for Behavioral Health Statistics and Quality 2018) (see section "Complex Relationship Between Youth Cannabis Use and Opioid Use Disorder" later in this chapter for more information). Early age at onset of regular drug use is a robust risk fac-

Table 10–1. Individual, parental, familial, and environmental risk factors for opiate misuse and opioid use disorder (OUD) in youth

Individual factors

Genetic predisposition

- Family history of opioid or other substance use disorder in first-degree relative; common liability factor with shared risk genes across substance use disorders; candidate genes including the *ORM1* gene encoding for the μ-opioid receptor

Sex

- Females at higher risk for nonmedication prescription opioid misuse than males; males at higher risk for developing OUD and for opioid-related overdoses and deaths than females; females at higher risk for intentional opioid overdoses

Ethnicity

- Non-Hispanic white youth at elevated risk for nonmedication prescription opioid misuse and OUD

Temperament

- Difficult temperament, behavioral disinhibition, early-onset aggression, or emotional distress

Personality

- High novelty seeking, aggression, impulsivity, difficulty inhibiting responses

Comorbid psychiatric disorders

- Major depressive disorder, anxiety disorders, posttraumatic stress disorder, conduct disorder

Substance use–related factors

- Early substance use (especially prior to age 13 years)

- Use and misuse of other substances (e.g., tobacco, cannabis, alcohol); nonmedical prescription drug misuse

- Perception that there is little risk in substance use; motivation for use, including pain relief or "getting high"

Medical conditions

- Physical health problems (e.g., headache, fatigue, acute or chronic pain)

- Being prescribed an opioid medication to treat pain

Table 10–1. Individual, parental, familial, and environmental risk factors for opiate misuse and opioid use disorder (OUD) in youth *(continued)*

Parental and family factors

Parental/Parenting

• Parental substance misuse, substance use disorders (including OUD), parental psychiatric disorders, favorable parental attitude toward substance use, low parental monitoring/supervision

Family

• Family conflict, dysfunction, and discord; high interpersonal conflict among family members; parental divorce; negative parent-child relationship

Environmental factors

Peer group

• Peer group with drug use, including prescription drug misuse; peer group delinquent behaviors

School

• School failure and dropout associated with greater risk for OUD

Childhood adversity

• Physical, emotional, and sexual abuse; physical and emotional neglect; adverse childhood experiences, including witnessing a family member overdose

Community

• Lower socioeconomic status; communities with greater availability of drugs and alcohol; communities with views or approval of substance use; lower cost of drugs

tor for developing an SUD in general, and the same pattern is seen related to opioids. Early age at initiation of nonmedical prescription drug misuse (i.e., prior to the age of 13) increases the risk for initiating heroin and for developing OUD by young adulthood (Cerdá et al. 2015). Drug use motivational factors also influence the risk for opioid misuse.

There appear to be two motivational pathways for development of OUD in youth, with one related to use for reward motives (i.e., using opioids to get high) and the other related to use for pain reduction motives (i.e., using opioids to relieve under-controlled pain). Although the reward motive pathway is slightly more common, in both of these groups, nearly half of youth will go on to develop OUD (McCabe and Cranford 2012).

Environmental factors that increase opioid misuse risk include being prescribed an opioid medication, parental divorce, greater number of childhood adverse events, favorable parental attitudes toward substance use, witnessing a family member overdose, greater peer prescription drug misuse and substance use, and weaker social bonds (Substance Abuse and Mental Health Services Administration 2016).

Youth with OUD differ from those with nonopioid SUDs like cannabis or alcohol use disorder in some ways but share a similar background with youth with early-onset SUD (Subramaniam et al. 2009). Among treatment-seeking adolescents, the average age at onset of first use of opioids is 15.1 years, with onset of OUD between ages 15 and 16 years. Very striking is the finding that in both opioid- and non-opioid-using groups, the age at onset of regular cannabis was 13 years, and the age at onset of regular alcohol use was 13.5 years, with SUD onset at 14 years (Subramaniam et al. 2009). Compared with treatment-seeking cannabis and alcohol users, adolescents seeking treatment for OUD are more likely to be non-Hispanic white, to live in a suburban area, and to have dropped out of school. In addition, these adolescents are significantly more likely to be polysubstance users, to have higher substance use severity and delinquent behaviors, and to engage in intravenous drug use.

Prevention Targeting Known Risk Factors

Current strategies to prevent initiation of opioids and progression to the development of OUD include universal and targeted preventions designed to address modifiable risk factors and provide for targeted early interventions. Knowledge of modifiable risk factors for opioid misuse can be used by clinicians as a roadmap to guide risk assessment and stratification along with targeted prevention and early intervention in youth. From a public health perspective, states and institutions would benefit from developing a cascade of care for responding to the opioid epidemic that includes resources to support prevention, early intervention, and specialty treatment efforts (Williams et al. 2019).

Since substance misuse may present with varied and subtle symptoms, the American Academy of Pediatrics (AAP) and the Substance Abuse and Mental Health Services Administration (SAMHSA) recommend using a Screening, Brief Intervention, and Referral to Treatment (SBIRT) framework to address youth substance use as part of routine pediatric health care (Levy et al. 2016). Evidenced-based screening tools may be used to aid the diagnosis of an SUD. Commonsense strategies to prevent opioid misuse include limiting the prescription of opioids for pain, reducing inappropriate prescribing, and educating families on proper disposal of opioid medications and on the signs and symptoms of adolescent substance misuse and SUDs, including opioids (Chadi et al. 2018). Since psychiatric illness and family dysfunction also increase the risk for opioid misuse, screening for, diagnosing, and aggressively treating mental health problems may mitigate risk. Given that a history of substance use (e.g., alcohol, cannabis, nicotine) increases the risk of later opioid misuse and OUD, positive screens or high clinical suspicion of substance use in youth or family should be further assessed and promptly treated.

Clinical Management and Evidence-Based Interventions for Youth Opioid Use Disorder

The first step of clinical management of opioid misuse or OUD is to perform a comprehensive assessment and obtain a proper diagnosis. Any assessment for suspected opioid misuse should include a full medical and psychosocial assessment along with urine drug screening. Because many youth with OUD have multifactorial problems, it is important to characterize family, school/educational, vocational, and mental health histories; living arrangements, custody, and legal and social service involvement; and the role their peers, family, and support system play in the development and maintenance of their drug use behaviors (Bukstein et al. 2005). Perpetuating factors identified during the assessment phase can later be targeted during treatment to reduce the risk for relapse. To obtain an OUD diagnosis using DSM-5 (American Psychiatric Association 2013) criteria, an individual needs to engage in functionally impairing opioid use and to have met 2 or more of the following 11 criteria within the past 12 months:

1. Opioids consumed in larger amounts over a longer period of time than was intended
2. A persistent desire or unsuccessful effort to cut down on opioid use
3. A great deal of time spent in activities related to obtaining and using opioids
4. Craving
5. Failure to fulfill major role obligations at work, school, or home
6. Persistent or recurrent social or interpersonal problems caused or exacerbated by opioid use
7. Important social, occupational, or recreational activities given up as a result of the opioid use
8. Recurrent use of opioids in physically hazardous situations
9. Continued use despite knowledge of persistent psychosocial or psychological problems related to opioid engagement
10. Tolerance
11. Withdrawal

OUD diagnoses, similar to diagnoses of other SUDs, fall along a continuum of severity based on number of DSM-5 symptoms reported: mild (2–3 symptoms), moderate (4–5 symptoms), or severe (6 or more symptoms).

The intensity of clinical management should be based on the severity of OUD and the presence or absence of prognostic factors (i.e., the presence of co-occurring medical or psychiatric conditions, treatment motivation, living situation, and family engagement) (Fishman 2008). The American Society of Addiction Medicine (ASAM) has developed criteria (the ASAM Criteria; Mee-Lee et al. 2013) for patient placement that can aid in guiding level-of-care decisions about whether a youth with an OUD diagnosis should receive treatment in an inpatient, residential, or outpatient setting. Generally, treatment of youth with mild-to-moderate severity OUD and few negative prognostic factors will typically involve provision of evidence-based psychosocial interventions and may include medically assisted detoxification if the youth are experiencing physical withdrawal symptoms. Adolescents with severe OUD or multiple negative prognostic factors usually require higher intensity treatment and are more likely to benefit from maintenance medication for OUD.

The use of medications to treat OUD should always be provided in conjunction with psychosocial interventions.

Addressing sexual and HIV risk behaviors and co-occurring psychiatric conditions is an important component of the clinical management of youth OUD. Many adolescents and young adults with OUD engage in high-risk sexual behaviors, and some administer opioids intravenously. These behaviors increase their risk for a number of medical complications, including sexually transmitted infections, hepatitis C, and HIV/AIDs, as well as pregnancy (Subramaniam et al. 2009). Screening for and treating sexually transmitted infections and providing education to youth about sexual and HIV risk behaviors can help mitigate risk in high-risk youth. Youth with OUD also have high rates of adverse childhood experiences and commonly present with co-occurring psychiatric conditions, including depression, anxiety, and conduct disorders (Volkow et al. 2019). Treating psychiatric comorbidity and addressing traumatic stress are vital and are likely to improve outcomes (Subramaniam et al. 2011). Concurrent treatment of both OUD and the co-occurring psychiatric condition by the same treatment team using integrated treatment approaches is associated with improved functional outcomes compared with parallel or sequential treatment (Bukstein and Horner 2010).

Role for Medication-Assisted Treatment in Youth Opioid Use Disorder

The U.S. Food and Drug Administration (FDA) has approved three medication classes for the maintenance treatment of OUD: 1) buprenorphine (16 years and older), 2) methadone (16 years and older), and 3) naltrexone (18 years and older). The FDA has approved a number of different formulations and administration methods for these classes of medications (e.g., daily oral and monthly intramuscular injection for naltrexone; sublingual film, tablet, monthly intramuscular injection, and 6-month implant for buprenorphine).

Medication-assisted treatment (MAT) is an evidence-base treatment approach that involves prescribing an FDA-approved medication for maintenance treatment of OUD in conjunction with behavioral therapy. MAT with buprenorphine, methadone, or extended-release naltrexone has been shown to reduce morbidity and mortality in adults with OUD (Larochelle et al. 2018;

Volkow et al. 2014). Despite being a first-line treatment for OUD in adults, the use of agonist medications and MAT for OUD in youth has been controversial because of stigma and concerns about the effects of chronic opioid agonist treatment on the developing brain and endocrine systems in youth (Hammond 2016). As such, MAT for OUD is greatly underutilized in adolescent and young adult populations. A recent retrospective cohort study examining data from health insurance claims pertaining to 2.4 million youth ages 13–22 years found that only three out of four youth accessed any treatment within 3 months of receiving an OUD diagnosis, and it was also noted that the rates of receiving such a diagnosis were well below the known population prevalence (Hadland et al. 2018). The majority of youth (52%) received behavioral interventions only, with less than one in four youth receiving MAT (26% of 18- to 22-year-olds and less than 5% of 13- to 17-year-olds). The study further found that timely receipt of buprenorphine, naltrexone, or methadone was associated with increased treatment retention compared with receipt of behavioral interventions alone.

Emerging evidence from clinical studies of youth ages 15–21 years with OUD suggests a role for medications in treating opioid withdrawal during detoxification and a role for medication and MAT approaches in subgroups of youth with OUD who have negative prognostic factors (Borodovsky et al. 2018; Hammond and Gray 2016). Table 10–2 presents medications and their dosing and indications in youth with OUD. There is *no* evidence to support the notion that youth should receive and fail a trial of treatment without medications before treatment with MAT. These findings have led to a shift in guidelines, with the AAP now recommending that adolescents with severe OUD routinely receive MAT.

Medications for Maintenance Treatment in Youth With Opioid Use Disorder

Medications for OUD maintenance pharmacotherapy can broadly be categorized into opioid agonist (buprenorphine and methadone) and opioid antagonist (naltrexone) treatments based on their pharmacological mechanism of action. A Cochrane systematic review of maintenance treatments for opioid-dependent adolescents, completed in 2014, analyzed data from two randomized

Table 10–2. Medications for the treatment of opioid use disorder (OUDs) in youth

Medication	Mechanism of action	Approved age of use	Typical induction dose	Target dosing
Buprenorphine (sublingual)	Partial opioid agonist	16+ years	2–4 mg/day	16–24 mg/day[a]
Buprenorphine/naloxone (sublingual)	Partial opioid agonist/ opioid antagonist	16+ years	2–8 mg/0.5–2 mg/day	16–24 mg/4–6 mg/day
Methadone (oral)	Full opioid agonist	18+ years in licensed methadone maintenance programs	≥10–30 mg/day	≥60–100 mg/day
Naltrexone (oral or intramuscular)	Opioid antagonist	Not yet approved specifically in youth	Start 7–10 days after last use 25–50 mg daily (oral) or 380 mg monthly (intramuscular)	50 mg/day (oral) 380 mg/month (intramuscular)

[a]Combination product generally preferred to avoid diversion for injection use.

controlled trials that included a total of 189 participants (Minozzi et al. 2014). Preliminary evidence from the observational and controlled studies suggested that agonist therapies, including methadone and buprenorphine, may be effective during active treatment. A recent review (Borodovsky et al. 2018) summarizes the evidence for the benefits of MAT in youth.

Methadone

Methadone is a μ opioid receptor agonist used in restricted clinical settings to treat individuals with OUD. A series of observational and naturalistic studies published in the 1970s showed that methadone is safe and associated with better treatment engagement than behavioral therapy alone for youth addicted to heroin (Hopfer et al. 2003). Today, methadone can be prescribed as a maintenance treatment for adolescents 16 years and older with severe OUD at licensed and regulated methadone maintenance treatment (MMT) programs (also referred to as opioid treatment programs). Service regulations require documentation that a youth has failed two treatment episodes of drug-free detoxification followed by behavioral therapy. In practice, few MMT programs offer methadone for youth under age 18. In general, most methadone programs would not be expected to have developmentally specific treatment components targeting adolescents or young adults.

Buprenorphine

Buprenorphine is a μ opioid receptor partial agonist that has received FDA approval for OUD maintenance treatment in individuals age 16 years and older. It requires additional training and licensure by physicians and is used in both outpatient and inpatient settings.

A multisite randomized clinical trial run through the National Institute on Drug Abuse Clinical Trials Network examined treatment outcomes in adolescents and young adults ($N=152$) randomly assigned to receive either 2-week short-term buprenorphine-naloxone detoxification (detox group) or 8-week extended MAT with buprenorphine-naloxone (Bup-Nal group), with both groups receiving behavioral therapy (Woody et al. 2008). The results of the study showed that compared with the detox group, the Bup-Nal group had higher treatment retention and more opioid-negative urine samples during active treatment, but that after discontinuing the buprenorphine-naloxone, youth in the Bup-Nal group generally relapsed (reverting to the trajectory of the comparison condition). The findings of this study parallel those from naturalistic observational studies in young adults (Borodovsky et al. 2018) and those reported in the adult literature and suggest that continued maintenance treatment with buprenorphine-naloxone may be crucial for sustaining opioid abstinence in youth.

Naltrexone

Naltrexone is a μ opioid receptor antagonist that blocks the rewarding effects of opioids. It is available in daily oral (oral naltrexone) and monthly injectable (extended-release naltrexone [XR-naltrexone]) formulations. A single open-label prospective case series in adolescents and young adults enrolled in community-based substance use treatment has shown early promise for XR-naltrexone (Fishman et al. 2010). A small, naturalistic cohort study in young adults showed similar results for buprenorphine and XR-naltrexone (Vo et al. 2016), and a small case series described promising results for an innovative model of home delivery of XR-naltrexone (Vo et al. 2016, 2018).

Medications for Opioid Withdrawal in Youth

Opioid withdrawal manifests 48–72 hours after abrupt discontinuation of opioids in chronic users and includes symptoms of anxiety, restlessness, bone or joint aches, lacrimation (tearing), rhinorrhea (runny nose), mydriasis (dilated pupils), yawning, tremor, abdominal cramping, diarrhea, tachycardia (elevated heart rate), and diaphoresis (sweating). Onset and duration of opioid withdrawal depend on the half-life of the opioid most frequently used. In adolescents and young adults, buprenorphine-naloxone and clonidine, an α_2-agonist and nonopioid withdrawal management (also known as *detoxification*) medication, have both been shown to effectively reduce opioid withdrawal symptoms (Marsch et al. 2005). Clinical studies in older adolescents and in adults comparing the efficacy of buprenorphine and clonidine as part of an outpatient opioid withdrawal management program have shown that both medications effectively reduce opioid withdrawal symptoms, but that compared with those receiving clonidine, individuals receiving buprenorphine have fewer opioid-positive urine drug tests and are more likely to remain in treatment (Ling et al. 2005; Marsch et al. 2005). Given these findings, bupre-norphine should be the withdrawal treatment agent of choice in youth with moderate to severe OUD. For youth who have less severe OUD or those who are interested in nonopioid detoxification medications, clonidine and other agents for symptomatic relief are a reasonable choice to target withdrawal symptoms. Nonopioid withdrawal medications may sometimes have a pref-erential role in acceleration of the transition to XR-naltrexone when that treat-ment is chosen.

Opioid Overdose Prevention

With the rising rates of opioid overdose deaths in youth, clinicians should, whenever possible, work with the presenting patient and their family members and establish an opioid overdose response plan. To help clinicians, SAMHSA has developed an opioid overdose prevention toolkit that can be used to guide pre-vention planning sessions with families (Substance Abuse and Mental Health Services Administration 2014). Components of an opioid overdose preven-tion plan include teaching patients and families how to recognize and respond to a suspected opioid overdose. Many states have passed "Good Samaritan" laws to protect individuals who help someone experiencing a suspected over-dose or drug-related medical emergency from being charged or prosecuted for drug-related crimes and from liability if administering naloxone. Clinicians should become knowledgeable about local and state laws and educate patients and families about these laws.

Naloxone

Naloxone is an opioid antagonist rescue agent that is prescribed as an opioid overdose antidote. According to the World Health Organization, people likely to witness an opioid overdose, such as family and friends of opioid users, should have access to naloxone and be trained in how to administer it for emer-gency management of respiratory depression during a suspected opioid over-dose. The FDA has approved an intranasal formulation of naloxone for opioid overdose, which has been increasingly widely disseminated for use by non-medical personnel. Clinicians who work with youth opioid misusers should strongly consider prescribing intranasal naloxone and provide education and training about how to use it in the event of a suspected overdose (Hammond 2016; Wilson et al. 2018). Parents and other family members of youth with OUD may be particularly good targets for deployment of naloxone.

Alternative Medicines for Opioid Use Disorder and the Case of Kratom

Clinicians should be aware of different complementary and alternative medical treatments that individuals with OUD sometimes use to self-treat their symptoms. Kratom, or *Mitragyna speciosa*, is a psychoactive plant indigenous to Southeast Asia that has received national attention for its use to relieve opioid withdrawal, pain, and mood symptoms, as well as for issues related to toxicity associated with its use (Swogger and Walsh 2018). Kratom acts as a partial agonist and antagonist at μ and κ opioid receptors and does not appear to produce respiratory depression to the same degree as full opioid agonists. Kratom users report using kratom for the purpose of self-treating pain, emotional distress, and opioid withdrawal and describe long-term kratom use as an opioid substitute (Grundmann 2017; Swogger and Walsh 2018).

The use of kratom in the United States has risen significantly since 2010. This increase in kratom use has also coincided with a significant increase in the number of emergency department visits and exposures related to kratom use that have been reported to U.S. poison control centers (Post et al. 2019). For example, U.S. poison control center calls related to kratom increased 10-fold between 2010 and 2015 (Post et al. 2019). Some users of kratom have experienced serious adverse medical outcomes related to their use of this supplement, including agitation/irritability, arrhythmias, and even death (Post et al. 2019). These adverse outcomes are more likely in individuals who combine use of kratom with other drugs.

Additional research is needed to clarify the safety profile, risks, and benefits of kratom use, and whether there may be a role for kratom in OUD pharmacopeia. At present, few data exist on the prevalence and effects of kratom use in youth samples. Given the limited data on kratom and amid safety concerns, clinicians should caution their patients about the potential adverse medical outcomes that have been reported with kratom use.

Opioids and Pediatric Pain Management

Receipt of an opioid prescription for a pain condition by a youth represents a risk factor for opioid misuse and OUD. As such, proper clinical management of pediatric acute and chronic pain is important to reduce this risk. Pediatric pain may be secondary to a medical condition (e.g., inflammatory bowel disease, sickle cell disease, rheumatoid arthritis, cancer) or be a primary pain disorder (e.g., headache, centrally mediated abdominal pain syndromes, complex regional pain syndrome, back pain, musculoskeletal pain) (Liossi and Howard 2016). For acute and postoperative pain, or pain secondary to a primary medical procedure or dental work, general recommendations include the use of multimodal analgesia, nonpharmacological measures such as ice and elevation, nonopioid pain relievers (e.g., acetaminophen and nonsteroidal anti-inflammatories), and limiting of the dosage and quantity of opioid pain prescriptions (Landry et al. 2015). Chronic pediatric pain is often multifactorial and multidimensional and may stem from a combination of neurosensory (nociceptive), affective, sociocultural, behavioral, and cognitive factors. Whenever opioids are recommended or indicated for chronic pediatric pain, a multidisciplinary approach with close monitoring is also recommended.

Complex Relationship Between Youth Cannabis Use and Opioid Use Disorder

In the context of the opioid epidemic and continued rising rates of opioid overdose deaths, there has been growing public interest in the possibility that medical marijuana might curb or prevent opioid misuse and reduce associated negative sequelae (Powell et al. 2018). Several states are considering making OUD an indicated condition for treatment with medical marijuana. The evidence to support this expansion of medical marijuana to address the opioid crisis is limited and highly variable, with some studies showing harm and other studies showing possible benefit. Neurobiologically, there is significant overlap in endogenous opioid and cannabinoid brain systems, and the preclinical literature paints two pictures related to the effects of cannabinoids on opioid administration (Robledo et al. 2008). Animal models using adult rodents have shown an opioid-sparing effect of cannabinoids, suggesting that cannabis may reduce use of opioids related to pain (Nielsen et al. 2017). Conversely, animal models testing youth addiction vulnerability suggest the opposite relationship, showing that exposure to cannabinoids during adolescence produces long-lasting alterations in prefrontal and reward circuits and *increased* heroin self-administration in adulthood (Ellgren et al. 2007). As of this writing, few studies have been published examining the association between cannabis and opioid use in humans. An ecological opioid overdose mortality analysis of state-level data comparing death rates in states that permit and do not permit medical marijuana was recently published showing that opioid overdose deaths were approximately 25% lower in states permitting medical marijuana (Bachhuber et al. 2014). This finding should be interpreted cautiously given the difficulty in controlling for confounding variables in ecological state-level data. Results from an online survey of medical marijuana patients with chronic pain indicated that these patients self-report a decrease in opioid use and improved quality of life since starting medical marijuana (Boehnke et al. 2016). Data from the National Epidemiologic Survey on Alcohol and Related Conditions (NESARC), a longitudinal study using a large sample of nationally representative U.S. adults, showed that cannabis use at Wave 1 was associated with a greater odds of opioid misuse and of developing OUD 3 years later at Wave 2 (Olfson et al. 2018). This association remained significant after the authors controlled for a number of confounding variables. The study also found a dose-response relationship between cannabis use frequency and the risk for developing OUD, with 2.9%, 4.3%, and 4.4% of occasional, frequent, and very frequent cannabis users at Wave 1 going on to develop OUD by Wave 2, compared with 0.5% of non-users of cannabis. Another study examining data from 6,000 high school students in Connecticut over a period of 12 years found that youth who used marijuana had a 14-fold increase in nonmedical prescription opioid misuse and a 4-fold increase in heroin use compared with non–marijuana users (Kaminer 2017). A small number of human trials have examined the impact of cannabinoids on opioid withdrawal and have not shown any robust effects (Bisaga et al. 2015; Lofwall et al. 2016).

In summary, complex relationships exist between cannabis and opioid use. Clinically, there are very few data to support that cannabinoids represent a treatment or substitute for opioids or OUD, despite some preliminary findings suggesting that cannabis could provide benefit for a subgroup of adults with chronic pain and more severe opioid use. Cannabis use by youth appears to increase the risk for opioid initiation and for the development of OUD. Given these findings, youth who use cannabis may be considered an at-risk group for OUD and should be treated accordingly with early interventions for cannabis use and secondary prevention around opioid initiation. More research is critically needed in this area to improve our understanding of cannabis-opioid interactions and to characterize possible harms and benefits of cannabis use on opioid misuse and related health outcomes in different age groups.

Conclusion

Opioid misuse and OUD in youth are associated with multiple negative sequelae and elevated morbidity and mortality. These disorders have clear child and adolescent antecedents and young-adult onset. Overlapping risk, protective, and prognostic factors provide a roadmap for targeted prevention and early intervention strategies in youth. A developmentally informed cascade of care, including provision of universal and targeted prevention for high-risk children and adolescents, early interventions for youth identified as misusing opioids, and specialty treatment for youth who have developed OUD, may improve outcomes. MAT, along with comprehensive psychosocial interventions, should be considered a central treatment component for youth with OUD.

Key Points

- Opioid use, misuse, and opioid use disorder (OUD) are common in older adolescents and young adults (ages 17–25 years), and are associated with multiple negative sequelae including overdose and death.

- A developmentally informed cascade of care, including provision of universal and targeted prevention for high-risk children and adolescents, early interventions for youth identified as misusing opioids, and specialty treatment for youth who have developed OUD may improve outcomes.

- There is a growing consensus that clinical management of youth with OUD should incorporate evidence-based psychosocial interventions along with medication-assisted treatment (MAT), especially in youth with higher-severity OUD and negative prognostic factors.

- Few youth who are in need of treatment ever receive it, and of those who do receive treatment, only a small number receive MAT with buprenorphine, methadone, or extended-release naltrexone, the standard of care for OUD in adults.

- Youth who are at elevated risk for fatal opioid overdose, as well as their families, should receive training on how to identify and respond to a suspected overdose, including the administration of naloxone.

References

American Psychiatric Association: Diagnostic and Statistical Manual of Mental Disorders, 5th Edition. Arlington, VA, American Psychiatric Association, 2013

Bachhuber MA, Saloner B, Cunningham CO, et al: Medical cannabis laws and opioid analgesic overdose mortality in the United States, 1999–2010. JAMA Intern Med 174(10):1668–1673, 2014 25154332

Bisaga A, Sullivan MA, Glass A, et al: The effects of dronabinol during detoxification and the initiation of treatment with extended release naltrexone. Drug Alcohol Depend 154:38–45, 2015 26187456

Boehnke KF, Litinas E, Clauw DJ: Medical cannabis use is associated with decreased opiate medication use in a retrospective cross-sectional survey of patients with chronic pain. J Pain 17(6):739–744, 2016 27001005

Borodovsky JT, Levy S, Fishman M, et al: Buprenorphine treatment for adolescents and young adults with opioid use disorders: a narrative review. J Addict Med 12(3):170–183, 2018 29432333

Bukstein OG, Horner MS: Management of the adolescent with substance use disorders and comorbid psychopathology. Child Adolesc Psychiatr Clin N Am 19(3):609–623, 2010 20682224

Bukstein OG, Bernet W, Arnold V, et al; Work Group on Quality Issues: Practice parameter for the assessment and treatment of children and adolescents with substance use disorders. J Am Acad Child Adolesc Psychiatry 44(6):609–621, 2005 15908844

Casey BJ, Jones RM: Neurobiology of the adolescent brain and behavior: implications for substance use disorders. J Am Acad Child Adolesc Psychiatry 49(12):1189–1201, quiz 1285, 2010 21093769

Center for Behavioral Health Statistics and Quality: 2017 National Survey on Drug Use and Health: Detailed Tables. Rockville, MD, Substance Abuse and Mental Health Services Administration, 2018

Centers for Disease Control and Prevention: Wide-ranging online data for epidemiologic research (WONDER). Atlanta, GA, National Center for Health Statistics, 2017

Cerdá M, Santaella J, Marshall BD, et al: Nonmedical prescription opioid use in childhood and early adolescence predicts transitions to heroin use in young adulthood: a national study. J Pediatr 167(3):605.e1-2–612.e1-2, 2015 26054942

Chadi N, Bagley SM, Hadland SE: Addressing adolescents' and young adults' substance use disorders. Med Clin North Am 102(4):603–620, 2018 29933818

Curtin SC, Tejada-Vera B, Warmer M: Drug overdose deaths among adolescents aged 15–19 in the United States: 1999–2015. NCHS Data Brief 282(282):1–8, 2017 29155681

Ellgren M, Spano SM, Hurd YL: Adolescent cannabis exposure alters opiate intake and opioid limbic neuronal populations in adult rats. Neuropsychopharmacology 32(3):607–615, 2007 16823391

Fishman M: Treatment planning, matching, and placement for adolescents with substance use disorders, in Adolescent Substance Abuse: Psychiatric Comorbidity and High-Risk Behaviors. Edited by Kaminer Y, Winters K. New York, Routledge/Taylor & Francis, 2008, pp 88–110

Fishman MJ, Winstanley EL, Curran E, et al: Treatment of opioid dependence in adolescents and young adults with extended release naltrexone: preliminary case-series and feasibility. Addiction 105(9):1669–1676, 2010 20626723

Grundmann O: Patterns of kratom use and health impact in the US—results from an online survey. Drug Alcohol Depend 176:63–70, 2017 28521200

Hadland SE, Bagley SM, Rodean J, et al: Receipt of timely addiction treatment and association of early medication treatment with retention in care among youths with opioid use disorder. JAMA Pediatr 172(11):1029–1037, 2018 30208470

Hammond CJ: The role of pharmacotherapy in the treatment of adolescent substance use disorders. Child Adolesc Psychiatr Clin North Am25(4):685–711, 2016 27613346

Hammond CJ, Gray KM: Pharmacotherapy for adolescent substance use disorders. J Child Adolesc Subst Abuse 25(4):292–316, 2016 28082828

Hammond CJ, Mayes LC, Potenza MN: Neurobiology of adolescent substance use and addictive behaviors: treatment implications. Adolesc Med State Art Rev 25(1):15–32, 2014 25022184

Hopfer CJ, Khuri E, Crowley TJ: Treating adolescent heroin use. J Am Acad Child Adolesc Psychiatry 42(5):609–611, 2003 12707565

Imam MZ, Kuo A, Ghassabian S, et al: Progress in understanding mechanisms of opioid-induced gastrointestinal adverse effects and respiratory depression. Neuropharmacology 131:238–255, 2018 29273520

Johnston LD, Miech RA, O'Malley PM, et al: Monitoring the Future: National Survey Results on Drug Use: 1975–2017: Overview, Key Findings on Adolescent Drug Use. Ann Arbor, MI, Institute for Social Research, The University of Michigan, 2018

Kaminer Y: The denial of the association between youth cannabis and opiate use: a "Split Brain Syndrome"? Subst Abus 38(4):367–368, 2017 28910591

Kosten TR, George TP: The neurobiology of opioid dependence: implications for treatment. Sci Pract Perspect 1(1):13–20, 2002 18567959

Landry BW, Fischer PR, Driscoll SW, et al: Managing chronic pain in children and adolescents: a clinical review. PM R 7(11)(suppl):S295–S315, 2015 26568508

Larochelle MR, Bernson D, Land T, et al: Medication for opioid use disorder after nonfatal opioid overdose and association with mortality: a cohort study. Ann Intern Med 169(3):137–145, 2018 29913516

Levy SJ, Williams JF; Committee on Substance Use and Prevention: Substance use screening, brief intervention, and referral to treatment. Pediatrics 138(1):e20161211, 2016 27325634

Ling W, Amass L, Shoptaw S, et al; Buprenorphine Study Protocol Group: A multicenter randomized trial of buprenorphine-naloxone versus clonidine for opioid detoxification: findings from the National Institute on Drug Abuse Clinical Trials Network. Addiction 100(8):1090–1100, 2005 16042639

Liossi C, Howard RF: Pediatric chronic pain: Biopsychosocial assessment and formulation. Pediatrics 138(5):e20160331, 2016 27940762

Lofwall MR, Babalonis S, Nuzzo PA, et al: Opioid withdrawal suppression efficacy of oral dronabinol in opioid dependent humans. Drug Alcohol Depend 164:143–150, 2016 27234658

Marsch LA, Bickel WK, Badger GJ, et al: Comparison of pharmacological treatments for opioid-dependent adolescents: a randomized controlled trial. Arch Gen Psychiatry 62(10):1157–1164, 2005 16203961

McCabe SE, Cranford JA: Motivational subtypes of nonmedical use of prescription medications: results from a national study. J Adolesc Health 51(5):445–452, 2012 23084165

Mee-Lee D, Shulman GD, Fishman M, et al: The ASAM Criteria: Treatment Criteria for Addictive, Substance-Related, and Co-Occurring Conditions, 3rd Edition. Chevy Chase, MD, American Society of Addiction Medicine, 2013

Minozzi S, Amato L, Bellisario C, et al: Maintenance treatments for opiate -dependent adolescents. Cochrane Database Syst Rev 24(6):CD007210, 2014 24957634

National Institutes of Health: Drug overdoses in youth. April 9, 2019. Available at: https://teens.drugabuse.gov/drug-facts/drug-overdoses-youth. Accessed May 6, 2019.

Nielsen S, Sabioni P, Trigo JM, et al: Opioid-sparing effects of cannabinoids: a systematic review and meta-analysis. Neuropsychopharmacology 42(9):1752–1765, 2017 28327548

Olfson M, Wall MM, Liu SM, et al: Cannabis use and risk of prescription opioid use disorder in the United States. Am J Psychiatry 175(1):47–53, 2018 28946762

Post S, Spiller HA, Chounthirath T, Smith GA: Kratom exposures reported to United States poison control centers: 2011–2017. Clin Toxicol (Phila) 57(10):857–854, 2019 30786220

Powell D, Pacula RL, Jacobson M: Do medical marijuana laws reduce addiction and deaths related to painkillers? J Health Econ 58:29–42, 2018 29408153

President's Commission on Combating Drug Addiction and the Opioid Crisis: Report. November 1, 2017. Available at: https://www.whitehouse.gov/sites/whitehouse.gov/files/images/Final_Report_Draft_11-1-2017.pdf. Accessed May 6, 2019.

Robledo P, Berrendero F, Ozaita A, et al: Advances in the field of cannabinoid—opioid cross-talk. Addict Biol 13(2):213–224, 2008 18482431

Seth P, Scholl L, Rudd RA, et al: Overdose deaths involving opioids, cocaine, and psychostimulants – United States, 2015–2016. MMWR Morb Mortal Wkly Rep 67(12):349–358, 2018 29596405

Subramaniam GA, Stitzer ML, Woody G, et al: Clinical characteristics of treatment-seeking adolescents with opioid versus cannabis/alcohol use disorders. Drug Alcohol Depend 99(1–3):141–149, 2009 18818027

Subramaniam GA, Warden D, Minhajuddin A, et al: Predictors of abstinence: National Institute of Drug Abuse multisite buprenorphine/naloxone treatment trial in opioid-dependent youth. J Am Acad Child Adolesc Psychiatry 50(11):1120–1128, 2011 22024000

Substance Abuse and Mental Health Services Administration: SAMHSA Opioid Overdose Prevention Toolkit (HHS Publ No SMA 14-4742). Rockville, MD, Substance Abuse and Mental Health Services Administration, 2014

Substance Use and Mental Health Services Administration: Preventing Prescription Drug Misuse: Overview of Factors and Strategies. Rockville, MD, Center for the Application of Prevention Technologies, 2016

Substance Abuse and Mental Health Services Administration: Key Substance Use and Mental Health Indicators in the United States: Results From the 2017 National Survey on Drug Use and Health (HHS Publ No SMA 18-5068, NSDUH Series

H-53). Rockville, MD, Center for Behavioral Health Statistics and Quality, Substance Abuse and Mental Health Services Administration, 2018

Swogger MT, Walsh Z: Kratom use and mental health: a systematic review. Drug Alcohol Depend 183:134–140, 2018 29248691

Vaughn MG, Nelson EJ, Salas-Wright CP, et al: Racial and ethnic trends and correlates of non-medical use of prescription opioids among adolescents in the United States 2004–2013. J Psychiatr Res 73:17–24, 2016 26679761

Vo HT, Robbins E, Westwood M, et al: Relapse prevention medications in community treatment for young adults with opioid addiction. Subst Abus 37(3):392–397, 2016 26820059

Vo HT, Burgower R, Rozenberg I, et al: Home-based delivery of XR-NTX in youth with opioid addiction. J Subst Abuse Treat 85:84–89, 2018 28867062

Volkow ND, Frieden TR, Hyde PS, et al: Medication-assisted therapies—tackling the opioid-overdose epidemic. N Engl J Med 370(22):2063–2066, 2014 24758595

Volkow ND, Jones EB, Einstein EB, et al: Prevention and treatment of opioid misuse and addiction. JAMA Psychiatry 76(2):208–216, 2019 30516809

Williams AR, Nunes EV, Bisaga A, et al: Development of a cascade of care for responding to the opioid epidemic. Am J Drug Alcohol Abuse 45(1):1–10, 2019 30675818

Wilson JD, Berk J, Adger H, et al: Identifying missed clinical opportunities in delivery of overdose prevention and naloxone prescription to adolescents using opioids. J Adolesc Health 63(2):245–248, 2018 30149925

Woody GE, Poole SA, Subramaniam G, et al: Extended vs short-term buprenorphine-naloxone for treatment of opioid-addicted youth: a randomized trial. JAMA 300(17):2003–2011, 2008 18984887

Youth Club, Prescription, and Over-the-Counter Drug Use

Charles Albert Whitmore, M.D., M.P.H.

Christian Hopfer, M.D.

Abuse of hallucinogens and dissociative drugs, prescription opioids and anxiolytics, and over-the-counter (OTC) medications is a significant problem among adolescents and young adults. The use of hallucinogenic and dissociative substances, commonly referred to as "club drugs," became popular during the 1990s. Despite the overall declining trend in adolescents' use of club drugs since the early 2000s (Johnston et al. 2018), the use of these substances is associated with potential health effects such as dangerous or irrational behavior, confusion, respiratory depression, arrhythmia, and prolonged episodes of symptoms similar to psychosis (National Institute on Drug Abuse 2015). Additionally, adolescents continue to misuse prescription and OTC cough and cold medicine, a practice called "pharming" that became more common during the early 2000s (Levine 2007; Johnston et al. 2008). Pharming is associated with various potential health effects, including increasing risk of using multiple substances, developing a formal substance use disorder, and experiencing harm from ingredients commonly found in these medications, such as acetaminophen-related liver damage or ibuprofen-related kidney damage (Cooper 2013).

In this chapter we address the abuse of club drugs, prescription medications, and OTC cough and cold medication. The following drugs, along with associated treatment-related issues, are reviewed: MDMA (3,4-methylenedioxymethamphetamine; "ecstasy"); GHB (γ-hydroxybutyrate); methamphetamine; ketamine; LSD (lysergic acid diethylamide); prescription opioids such as hydrocodone; prescription benzodiazepines; and dextromethorphan ([+]-3-methoxy-*N*-methylmorphinan), which is an active ingredient in cough suppressants and cold medicines.

Club Drugs

Overview

During the 1990s, epidemiological surveys detected the increased use of a group of drugs that were commonly associated with all-night dance parties called "raves," which were frequented by older adolescents and young adults. The moniker "club drugs" was coined as an umbrella term referring to substances commonly consumed at raves or at other dance clubs. This category of drugs is quite broad and includes MDMA, LSD, GHB, ketamine, and methamphetamine (National Institute on Drug Abuse 2019). These substances, with the exception of GHB, have hallucinogenic properties that "enhance" the experience of dancing to electronic music and/or facilitate the ability to participate in all-night dances by increasing energy or depressing the need for food or sleep. Although initially associated with all-night dance parties and dance clubs, these substances are now consumed by adolescents and young adults outside of this particular milieu (Hopfer et al. 2006).

MDMA

Brief History

MDMA was initially synthesized in 1891 as an appetite suppressant (Haber 1891); however, it was not widely used until the 1970s. Some psychotherapists reported that its use facilitated introspective states and closeness with the therapist. It gradually became more popular as an illicit substance and became most commonly known as "ecstasy" in its street form. MDMA use was first reported to be part of a youth subculture in the early 1980s, with reports initially surfacing in Europe and later appearing in North America in the early 1990s. It has a significant potential for abuse and neurotoxicity (Cottler et al. 2001; Freese et al. 2002; Scheier et al. 2008).

Chemical Name and Mechanisms of Action

MDMA is a semisynthetic substance that can produce both stimulant and psychedelic effects. As indicated by its chemical name, 3,4-methylenedioxymethamphetamine, MDMA is a member of the amphetamine class. However, it also shares chemical similarities to the hallucinogen mescaline (Koesters et al. 2002). It functions as an indirect sympathomimetic, acting at dopaminergic and adrenergic receptors, but also inhibiting the reuptake of serotonin, which is thought to be related to its hallucinogenic properties.

Street Names and Typical Doses

MDMA is most commonly known as "ecstasy," "Molly," or "X." Other names include "E," "the love drug," "the hug drug," "Adam," and "Stacey." Studies of actual street MDMA tablets report that doses typically range from 75 to 150 mg.

Route of Administration

MDMA is taken orally in a tablet or a capsule form.

Physical and Psychological Effects

MDMA typically has an onset of action of 20–40 minutes, with a peak effect at 60–90 minutes, and the effects last about 3–6 hours. The reported desired effects of MDMA include elevated mood; a sense of intimacy, sensuality, and a desire to be touched (ergo the names "the love drug" and "the hug drug"); altered visual, sensual, or emotional feelings; and increased energy and self-confidence. Adverse effects may include increases in both heart rate and blood pressure. Because it is often used in raves with extended dancing, MDMA may cause dangerous increases in body temperature and dehydration, which might lead to medical complications and death (Grob 1998). Other possible adverse effects include derealization and depersonalization, jaw clenching, gait disturbances, and hyponatremia (Koesters et al. 2002).

Epidemiology

In the 2017 Monitoring the Future survey, 4.9% of 12th graders, 2.8% of 10th graders, and 1.5% of 8th graders reported having ever using MDMA. Annual prevalence of use was 2.6%, 1.7%, and 0.9%, respectively. Past 30-day prevalence was 0.9%, 0.5%, and 0.4%, respectively (Miech et al. 2018).

Patterns of Use and Risk of Abuse and Dependence

Studies of MDMA users have observed withdrawal symptoms associated with regular use and physiological dependence distinct from the acute "crash" or "come-down" sequelae of using this drug (McKetin et al. 2014). Symptoms may include generalized fatigue, agitation, trouble concentrating, anxiety, depression, hyperphagia, and insomnia and may last 1–3 days (Curran and Travill 1997). Of MDMA users, 20% report a "severe-dependent" cluster of behavioral and psychological symptoms, underscoring the risk of developing severe dependence on MDMA (Scheier et al. 2008). Furthermore, MDMA use typically co-occurs with use of other drugs (Wu et al. 2006), and MDMA users have a significantly higher risk of developing dependence than do LSD users (Leung and Cottler 2008).

Specific Treatment Issues

The typical length of time that MDMA is detectable through urine toxicology is 1–2 days; thus, a frequent program of random urine monitoring is necessary to detect MDMA use. MDMA is not always detected in standard urinalyses, although it may cross-react with and be detected as amphetamines. Thus, it is important to clarify that the laboratory one is using detects MDMA.

Two particular clinical issues deserve additional attention: concerns about neurotoxicity stemming from chronic MDMA abuse, and the medical management of MDMA overdoses. One of the major concerns about MDMA use is whether, in addition to developing abuse or dependence, users may experience chronic neurotoxic effects. Animal studies demonstrate that MDMA use results in substantial loss of serotonergic neurons. Human studies are all complicated by the fact that MDMA users tend to use other substances, so it is difficult to isolate the effects of MDMA. However, substantial evidence exists for one to suspect that chronic MDMA use is associated with a range of psychiatric problems, including sleep disturbances, neuropsychological impairment, and mood and anxiety disorders (Montoya et al. 2002). Acute MDMA toxicity may include hyperthermia, seizures, cardiac arrhythmias, and hyponatremia.

GHB

Brief History

GHB's history dates back to its development in the 1960s as a possible analog for γ-aminobutyric acid (GABA) and as an anesthetic. It later was found to be an endogenous product of the human brain, with GHB-specific receptors being identified (Okun et al. 2001). GHB was legally available in the early 1990s and was marketed for its effects as an anabolic agent and also sold in health food stores as a possible treatment for narcolepsy and alcohol dependence and withdrawal. Because of numerous reports of adverse effects, including comas and seizures, the Drug Enforcement Administration placed it in Schedule I of the Controlled Substances Act in 2000. GHB has been used as a treatment for alcoholism and is approved as a treatment for narcolepsy in Europe.

Chemical Name and Mechanisms of Action

GHB, which stands for γ-hydroxybutyrate, is chemically similar to the inhibitory neurotransmitter GABA and has some limited activity at the GABA receptor. The brain has specific GHB receptors, and GHB's mechanism of action is thought to be mediated through these specific GHB receptors as well as through GABA receptors and the inhibitory actions on dopaminergic receptors (Okun et al. 2001).

Street Names and Typical Doses

The most common street names of GHB are "G" and "liquid ecstasy." Other names for GHB include "easy lay," "soap," "Georgia homeboy," "liquid X," "goop," "scoop," "salty water," and "grievous bodily harm." It is typically sold as a clear, salty liquid and is taken in teaspoons or capsules. The concentrations can vary markedly, ranging from 500 mg to 5 g per dose, which may account for cases of overdose.

Route of Administration

GHB is available in a liquid, a capsule, or a powder form and is orally administered.

Physical and Psychological Effects

GHB is rapidly absorbed and has a rapid onset of action, often within 15 minutes. It reaches peak concentrations in 20–60 minutes and is metabolized rapidly, with a half-life of 30 minutes. The duration of effect is usually 2–6 hours. Substantial individual variation occurs in response to GHB, and effects can include sedation or coma. The desired effects are described as similar to alcohol intoxication; however, the effects are typically more unpredictable. Users report enhanced social activity or improved sleep. Side effects can include drowsiness, vomiting, nystagmus, and ataxia, with possible death resulting from high doses (Freese et al. 2002). GHB is also considered a "date rape" drug because it can easily be added to drinks and render the victim disinhibited or unconscious, and thus vulnerable to rape.

Epidemiology

GHB use is fairly uncommon among adolescents. In the 2017 Monitoring the Future study, the annual reported use was 0.4% among 12th graders (Miech et al. 2018).

Patterns of Use and Risk of Abuse and Dependence

Knowledge about typical patterns of GHB use is very scarce. Most use occurs in the context of polysubstance use, and daily users may develop withdrawal syndromes (Degenhardt et al. 2002; Miotto et al. 2001). Case reports indicate that users can develop severe dependence, which may be characterized by very heavy use. There are reports of "round-the-clock" users who take GHB every 2–4 hours (Freese et al. 2002). If patients take GHB to be able to sleep, the rapid elimination of GHB often results in rebound insomnia after 2–3 hours, and users might take additional doses to return to sleep. Because physical tolerance can develop to GHB and dependent users might escalate their intake, dependent users might take 25–100 g of GHB per day (Freese et al. 2002).

Withdrawal also can occur in dependent users and can be severe because the withdrawal syndrome is similar to benzodiazepine or alcohol withdrawal. Onset may begin 1–6 hours after last use, and early symptoms include anxiety, insomnia, tremors, nausea, and vomiting. Autonomic instability can develop, and diaphoresis, hypertension, tremor, and tachycardia may be present. Severe cases of withdrawal may present as similar to delirium tremens (van Noorden et al. 2009). Longer term, a protracted withdrawal state may last for 3–6 months, characterized by dysphoria, memory problems, anxiety, and insomnia.

Specific Treatment Issues

Because of the rapid elimination of GHB, urine detection is possible only within an 8-hour time frame; therefore, frequent random urinalysis is required to detect GHB abuse. Treatment of GHB-induced coma is generally conservative, focusing on taking aspiration precautions and observing pulse oximetry. Gastric lavage is not indicated for GHB overdose because of the rapid absorption of this drug. Neither naloxone nor flumazenil has been shown to reverse GHB-induced coma. Recovery usually occurs rapidly, typically within 4–6 hours. Physostigmine, 2 mg intravenously, may be used to reverse the effects of GHB if necessary, but its routine use is not recommended (Okun et al. 2001).

Methamphetamine

Brief History

Methamphetamine was initially synthesized from ephedrine in 1887 but was not widely used until World War II, when it was taken by soldiers to maintain alertness. Its use as an illicit substance became more widespread in the 1970s and continues to be a growing problem. Methamphetamine can be fairly easily synthesized by a reduction reaction from precursor compounds ephedrine or pseudoephedrine, a fact that has led to laws regulating the distribution of these agents.

Chemical Name and Mechanisms of Action

Methamphetamine ([2S]-N-methyl-1-phenylpropan-2-amine) has two isomers: a levorotatory (R-form) isomer, which is used as a nasal decongestant, and a dextrorotatory (S-form) isomer, which is the active ingredient in the illicit substance of abuse. Methamphetamine is structurally similar to amphetamine, but the methyl group both increases methamphetamine's ability to cross the blood-brain barrier and makes it more resistant to degradation by monoamine oxygenase. Methamphetamine is a stimulant and acts by stimulating the release of dopamine, norepinephrine, and serotonin. At higher doses, it also inhibits the reuptake of these neurotransmitters (Cook et al. 1992, 1993).

Street Names and Typical Doses

Methamphetamine is known by a variety of street names, including "speed," "ice," "crystal," "glass," and "crank." Typical street doses vary but range from 100 to 250 mg.

Route of Administration

Methamphetamine can be smoked or can be administered intranasally, intravenously, or subcutaneously.

Physical and Psychological Effects

Methamphetamine has a rapid onset of action and a half-life of 9–15 hours; effects can last up to 30 hours. Desired effects of methamphetamine include increased energy, sense of well-being, libido, alertness, and activity; excitement; and decreased appetite. Physical effects include elevated blood pressure, body temperature, and respiration. Adverse effects include medical problems associated with excess doses and may include seizures or strokes, as well as hypertensive crises. Psychological effects may include the development of paranoia and hallucinations, psychosis, and suicidal or homicidal ideation, as well as cognitive impairments. Insomnia is a common effect of methamphetamine use, resulting in patterns of staying awake for days and then "crashing." Withdrawal depression is common. Methamphetamine use has also been linked with engaging in high-risk sexual behaviors.

Epidemiology

In the 2017 Monitoring the Future survey, 1.1% of 12th graders, 0.9% of 10th graders, and 0.7% of 8th graders reported having ever using methamphetamines. Annual prevalence of use was 0.6%, 0.4%, and 0.5%, respectively, and past 30-day prevalence was 0.3%, 0.1%, 0.2%, respectively (Miech et al. 2018).

Patterns of Use and Risk of Abuse and Dependence

Methamphetamine is a highly addictive substance, and there is a strong likelihood of users becoming dependent (National Institute on Drug Abuse 2013). A review of studies of adolescent methamphetamine users concluded that use of methamphetamine was associated with other drug use and engaging in risky behaviors (Russell et al. 2008). Others reported that compared with a sample of marijuana-abusing youth, methamphetamine-abusing youth were older, were more likely to be white and female, were more likely to have had prior treatment episodes, and had poorer treatment retention (Gonzales et al. 2008). Of particular clinical note is that girls who use methamphetamine may do so for reasons such as weight control, and particular attention should be given to this concern during treatment.

Specific Treatment Issues

Methamphetamine is detectable for 2–3 days by urinalysis; thus, a program of one or two weekly random urine drug screens should detect most dependent users. Typical approaches to treatment include contingency management approaches, 12-step group facilitation, and cognitive-behavioral approaches. A practical clinical issue is what to do if users complain about problems with attention after desisting from use (Kalechstein et al. 2003). There are numerous reports of methamphetamine use being associated with subsequent neuropsychological impairment, and many users may have preexisting problems with attention-deficit/hyperactivity disorder (ADHD). Laboratories can discriminate between amphetamines prescribed for ADHD and methamphetamines; however, a discussion should be held with the laboratory to confirm their procedures for making this differentiation. Essentially, because methamphetamines are metabolized to amphetamines, if amphetamines are prescribed, urinalysis should reveal only amphetamines, not methamphetamine. Clinically, it is important to be clear with patients in advance how testing will be conducted and what consequences may occur if methamphetamines are detected in the urine, which would be considered a relapse.

In general, treatment for ADHD in patients with a history of methamphetamine use should focus on treatment with medications without abuse potential such as atomoxetine or α-agonists. If a determination is made that stimulants would be the best treatment option, the clinician should clarify whether the lab can with confidence detect the difference between methamphetamine use and use of prescription stimulants.

Ketamine

Brief History

Ketamine was initially developed in 1962 and used as an anesthetic agent in adult surgical patients; however, after reports emerged of severe adverse reactions, its use rapidly diminished (Wolff and Winstock 2006). Because of its hallucinogenic properties, ketamine came into use as a street drug. It first gained popularity in the 1980s, when large doses were found to cause dreamlike states similar to those associated with phencyclidine (PCP) use. Recently, ketamine has been studied for its potential mood properties (Sanacora et al. 2017), though when used to treat depression, it is delivered at substantially lower doses than those used recreationally.

Chemical Name and Mechanisms of Action

Ketamine (2-[2-chlorophenyl]-2-[methylamino]cyclohexanone) is a derivative of PCP (l-[l-phenylcyclohexyl]piperidine). Ketamine is classified as an antagonist of the *N*-methyl-D-aspartate (NMDA) receptor; however, it also has activity at the opiate, serotonin, and acetylcholine receptors (Wolff and Winstock 2006).

Street Names and Typical Doses

Ketamine, known as "K," "special K," "kat food," and "vitamin K," is an anesthetic approved for both human and animal use, although about 90% of the ketamine sold today is intended for veterinary use only. Street preparations typically include powder forms for intranasal use of approximately 100–400 mg, and liquid, capsule, and powder forms for ingestion in doses of about 300–500 mg.

Route of Administration

Ketamine can be administered orally, intravenously, intranasally, and subcutaneously.

Physical and Psychological Effects

Ketamine has a short half-life, and effects typically last 1–3 hours. Onset of action is typically rapid, within 30 minutes. Desired effects of ketamine include mood elevation and some perceptual changes, including visual hallucinations and experiences of derealization or depersonalization. Low doses also may result in impaired attention, learning ability, and memory. At high doses, ketamine can cause delirium, amnesia, impaired motor function, high blood pressure, depression, vomiting, slurred speech, and potentially fatal respiratory problems. High-dose users report intense dissociative experiences, including out-of-body and near-death experiences. Visual disturbances can occur weeks after use (Wolff and Winstock 2006).

Epidemiology

Ketamine use is relatively rare among adolescents. In the 2017 Monitoring the Future study, the annual reported use was 1.2% among 12th graders (Miech et al. 2018).

Patterns of Use and Risk of Abuse and Dependence

Studies of ketamine users are limited. Many users also appear to be users of other club drugs (Dillon et al. 2003). In case studies, dependent users have reported loss of control over use, as well as other cognitive and behavioral changes associated with a dependence syndrome (Hurt and Ritchie 1994).

Specific Treatment Issues

Users of ketamine may report persistent perceptual problems similar to those that occur with use of LSD. Management of acute toxicity is typically supportive. Haloperidol has limited effects on the psychosis associated with ketamine (Wolff and Winstock 2006), and benzodiazepines may be useful to combat agitation. Long-term users may experience persistent cognitive difficulties. Pharmacological management may include medications that improve attention and focus.

LSD

Brief History

Although LSD was first synthesized in 1938, its psychedelic properties were not recognized until 5 years later. Initial tests by researchers at the Swiss company Sandoz resulted in reports that even very small doses measured in micrograms produced hallucinogenic effects (National Institute on Drug Abuse 2015). It has been manufactured and sold illegally since the 1960s in the United States. LSD use has waxed and waned in popularity, with its use rising in the 1960s, declining in the 1970s and 1980s, and experiencing a resurgence in the 1990s (Johnston et al. 2008). In the 2000s, rates of use have trended down from their high rates in the 1990s and remain considerably lower than their prior peak use (Johnston et al. 2018).

Chemical Name and Mechanisms of Action

LSD (lysergic acid diethylamide) is synthesized from lysergic acid, an ergot. It affects a large number of G protein–coupled receptors, including dopamine and serotonergic receptors. Its mechanism of action is complex and not completely understood, but its psychotropic effects appear to be due in part to agonism of the serotonin 5-HT$_{2A}$ receptors (Freese et al. 2002).

Street Names and Typical Doses

The most common street name for LSD is "acid," although other names include "yellow sunshines" and "boomers." LSD doses are much smaller than those for most other pharmacologically active substances, having effects at the microgram level. Minimal doses that have some psychotropic effects are between 20 and 25 µg, with typical doses being between 100 and 500 µg.

Route of Administration

LSD typically is sold as a liquid (often packaged in small bottles designed to hold breath freshener drops) or applied to blotter paper, sugar cubes, gelatin squares, or tablets. It is orally ingested.

Physical and Psychological Effects

As a hallucinogen, LSD produces abnormalities in sensory perception. Its effects are unpredictable depending on dose, surroundings, and the user's mood and personality. Typically taking the drug by mouth in tablet or blotter paper form, an LSD user begins to feel effects within 30–90 minutes. These effects include dilated pupils, increased body temperature, increased heart rate and blood pressure, sweating, dry mouth, and tremors. Long-term problems associated with LSD include persistent psychosis and hallucinogen persisting perception disorder (i.e., flashbacks) (Abraham et al. 1996; Halpern and Pope 2003). A rare yet serious effect reported in adults and youth is LSD-induced chronic visual disturbance (Kaminer and Hrecznyj 1991).

Epidemiology

In the 2017 Monitoring the Future survey, 5.0% of 12th graders, 3.0% of 10th graders, and 1.3% of 8th graders reported having ever using LSD. Annual prevalence of use was 3.3%, 2.1%, and 0.9%, respectively, and past 30-day prevalence was 1.2%, 0.8%, and 0.3%, respectively (Miech et al. 2018).

Patterns of Use and Risk of Abuse and Dependence

LSD use is typically not characterized by the development of a dependence syndrome, although heavy users might ingest LSD daily (Abraham et al. 1996).

Specific Treatment Issues

Detection of LSD use requires special laboratory procedures, and clinicians must specifically request testing because the drug is not normally detected by standard urine toxicology tests. Because of its low concentrations, LSD typically is not tested for using standard procedures, and detection is difficult. LSD is detectable for up to 7–10 days with special procedures. Management of LSD-related persistent perceptual disorders may include selective serotonin reuptake inhibitors (SSRIs), antipsychotic agents, or benzodiazepines (Halpern and Pope 2003).

Prescription and Over-the-Counter Medications

Overview

Abuse of prescription and OTC medications is common among youth for several reasons: these medications are readily available at home and in the pharmacy, are inexpensive, may be easily purchased on the Internet, are legal, and are erroneously perceived as harmless (Levine 2007). Abuse of medications prescribed for medical or psychiatric conditions remains a major area of concern, particularly among adolescents and young adults who experiment with opiates/opioids more frequently than with illicit drugs, except marijuana (Compton and Volkow 2006; National Institute on Drug Abuse 2018). On the basis of a survey of 103, 920 adolescents (ages 12–17 years), the most common prescription drug misuse source was friends or family for free (29%–33%), followed by physician sources for opioids (24%) and purchases for stimulants and tranquilizer/sedatives 23% each; 70% used multiple sources (Schepis et al. 2018). At least 70% of prescription drug misusers who reported multiple sources had at least 1 past year of substance use disorder (McCabe et al. 2018).

There has been a substantial increase in deaths attributable to prescription drugs, primarily opioids, over the past decade (Jones et al. 2018). Additionally, abuse of OTC medications, primarily dextromethorphan, which is an active ingredient in cough suppressants, has received increased attention (Bryner et al. 2006). In the following subsections we focus on prescription opioid and benzodiazepine dependence, as well as abuse of dextromethorphan.

Prescription Medications: Opioids

Brief History

Opioids have long been used by humans to induce euphoria and manage pain. Illicit opioid use in the United States involves primarily heroin and fentanyl, a synthetic analog, and is rare among adolescents. However, a growing concern is the nonmedical use of prescription opioids by adolescents, with morbid and lethal consequences. The United States has been experiencing an opiate epidemic (Woody et al. 2008), and adolescents have not been immune from this rise in opiate-related fatalities. In the following subsections, the focus is on the most common prescription opioids abused by adolescents. These include oxycodone, most commonly marketed as OxyContin, and hydrocodone, most commonly in the form of Vicodin.

Chemical Name and Mechanisms of Action

OxyContin (oxycodone) is a strong opioid analgesic typically used to treat moderate to severe chronic pain. Vicodin (hydrocodone bitartrate–acetaminophen) is a combination drug consisting of acetaminophen and hydrocodone, a synthetic opioid analgesic also typically used for pain control.

Street Names and Typical Doses

OxyContin is most frequently known on the street as "OC," "OX," "oxy," "oxycotton," "Hillbilly heroin," and "kicker." Typical OxyContin doses are between 10 and 80 mg.

Vicodin is known as "vike" and "Watson-387" (this refers to the imprint on the pill). Vicodin tablets typically contain 5 mg of hydrocodone and 500 mg of acetaminophen.

Route of Administration

Typically, both OxyContin and Vicodin are administered orally, although they can be injected.

Physical and Psychological Effects

The use of opioids results in the relief of pain and the induction of euphoria. Opiates typically cause respiratory depression and reduced gastrointestinal motility, along with drowsiness. Constricted pupils are a hallmark of opiate use. Regular use induces substantial tolerance, and withdrawal states may occur upon discontinuation. Withdrawal may be characterized by diarrhea, muscle pain, nausea, piloerection, and dilated pupils. Withdrawal may last 3–7 days (Jasinski 1981).

Epidemiology

In the 2017 Monitoring the Future survey, 6.8% of 12th graders reported lifetime nonmedical use of opioids other than heroin, 4.2% of 12th graders reported annual use, 1.6% of 12th graders reported past-30-day use, and 0.1% reported daily use. Annual prevalence of OxyContin use was 2.7% of 12th graders, 2.2% of 10th graders, and 0.8% of 8th graders. Annual prevalence of Vicodin use was 2.0% of 12th graders, 1.5% of 10th graders, and 0.7% of 8th graders (Miech et al. 2018).

Patterns of Use and Risk of Abuse and Dependence

A population-based study of adolescents found that of those who misused prescription medications (primarily opioids), approximately 17% reported symptoms of either substance abuse or dependence (Schepis and Krishnan-Sarin 2008).

Specific Treatment Issues

A comparison was made between treatment-seeking prescription opioid abusers and heroin-using adolescents with opioid use disorder (Subramaniam and Stitzer 2009). Both groups were older (mean = 17 years), predominantly suburban white youth with high rates of psychiatric comorbidity (83%). Youth in the heroin-using group were more likely to drop out of school, be dependent on opioids, and inject drugs. The prescription opioid–using youth were more likely to have symptoms that met criteria for multiple substance use disorders (including prescription sedatives and psychostimulants) and current ADHD, as well as to report selling drugs. These differences may have implications for the design of treatment programs, specifically indicating the need for more psychiatric services in these populations to address comorbidity.

For opioid use disorder, pharmacotherapy is the first line of treatment. Patients should be treated with either agonist medications, such as buprenorphine-naloxone, or antagonist medications, such as naltrexone (Fishman et al. 2010; Sigmon et al. 2012; Woody et al. 2008). Although clinicians may be unfamiliar with this treatment or consider it inappropriate for adolescents, careful consideration must be given to the risk of death from continued opiate use and the risk of progressing from prescription opiate misuse to either prescription or other opioid use disorder, which is associated with substantial morbidity and mortality (Borodovsky et al. 2018). Agonist therapy may help stabilize the patient and allow him or her to engage in psychosocial treatments.

If detoxification from opioids is attempted, usually by utilizing other agonist therapies such as buprenorphine or methadone, it should be followed by antagonist therapy. Methadone treatment can be administered only by a clinic licensed to treat opioid dependence (Hopfer et al. 2003), however, treatment with buprenorphine is more common currently. It is noteworthy that patients need to be educated that if they detoxify from opioids, then they will not be as tolerant to opiates as they were when they were using. Additionally, they should understand that if they relapse, they are at significant risk for overdosing, and thus antagonist therapy such as injectable naltrexone is strongly recommended (Fishman et al. 2010). Another clinical issue of substantial importance is distinguishing legitimate use of prescription medications from misuse, abuse, or dependence. Symptoms of misuse and a formal use disorder include diversion of medications, nonadherence behaviors, losing prescriptions, and demonstrating signs of declining functioning (Hertz and Knight 2006). Any pharmacological treatment should be integrated with other evidence-based psychosocial treatment approaches to managing substance use disorders (see Chapter 10 in this manual for more information about opioids and Chapters 13–15 for a discussion of psychosocial approaches).

Prescription Medications: Benzodiazepines

Brief History

Benzodiazepines were developed in the 1950s and became more widespread as therapeutic agents in the 1960s. The growing recognition that this class of medications has abuse and dependence potential led to their being declared controlled substances.

Misuse of prescription benzodiazepines is the second most common form of misuse of prescription medications, after misuse of prescription opioids. Additionally, the benzodiazepine flunitrazepam (Rohypnol), which is not available as a prescription benzodiazepine in the United States, is considered a club drug (Wu et al. 2006).

Chemical Name and Mechanisms of Action

A large number of benzodiazepines have been developed, all with different half-lives and different degrees of sedative or hypnotic properties. All act by modulation of the GABA receptors. Duration of effect varies depending on half-life.

Street Names and Typical Doses

Most street names of benzodiazepines are similar to the brand name of the benzodiazepine. Doses are similar to those used therapeutically.

Route of Administration

The typical route of administration of benzodiazepines is oral; however, these medications can also be injected.

Physical and Psychological Effects

Benzodiazepines reduce anxiety and can cause sedation at higher doses. In combination with other central nervous system depressants, there is a risk of respiratory depression. Tolerance will develop if benzodiazepines are used regularly, and withdrawal can result in seizures.

Epidemiology

Abuse or misuse of prescription benzodiazepines has remained fairly steady among adolescents since 2000. In the 2017 Monitoring the Future study, the lifetime reported use of nonmedical "tranquilizers" was 7.5% of 12th graders, 6.0% of 10th graders, and 3.4% of 8th graders (Miech et al. 2018). Annual prevalence of use was 4.7%, 4.1%, and 2.0%, respectively, and past-30-day prevalence was 2.0%, 1.5%, and 0.7%%, respectively. This same study found that the lifetime reported use of flunitrazepam was 0.7% of 10th graders and 0.6% of 8th graders. Annual prevalence of use was 0.8%, 0.3%, and 0.4% respectively, and past-30-day prevalence was less than 0.05% of 10th graders and 0.1% of 8th graders.

Patterns of Use and Risk of Abuse and Dependence

The rate at which adolescents progress from misuse of benzodiazepines to a formal use disorder is not known. Clinically, physiological dependence on benzodiazepines is characterized by the DSM-5 constellation of symptoms that constitute dependence (American Psychiatric Association 2013).

Specific Treatment Issues

A practical concern for clinicians treating adolescents is how to recognize whether an adolescent being treated for an anxiety disorder is developing abuse of or dependence on benzodiazepines. Requests for more medications do not by themselves indicate dependence. Signs to look for are evidence of engaging in antisocial or manipulative behaviors around benzodiazepine use, as well as evidence of intoxication on benzodiazepines or problems fulfilling role obligations. If patients are determined to be dependent on benzodiazepines, generally it is advisable to taper them off benzodiazepines and engage them in substance abuse treatment. A difficult issue is the management of complaints of anxiety, which may worsen when a patient is tapering off benzodiazepine use. SSRIs and buspirone may be helpful, as may cognitive-behavioral therapies that focus on managing anxiety (Martin and Volkmar 2007).

Over-the-Counter Medications: Dextromethorphan

Brief History

Although a number of OTC medications have abuse potential, abuse of dextromethorphan is clinically most concerning. Dextromethorphan has been used for many years as a cough suppressant in many OTC cold and cough preparations, such as Coricidin.

Chemical Name and Mechanisms of Action

Dextromethorphan ([+]-3-methoxy-*N*-methylmorphinan) is a morphine derivative and acts on the σ opioid receptor, and therefore is thought to not have abuse potential. However, it is a prodrug of dextrorphan, which acts on the NMDA receptor. These effects become clinically relevant when very high doses are taken, and the result is similar to that of PCP and ketamine. Typically, dextromethorphan takes about 30–60 minutes to have effects, and effects usually last about 6 hours.

Street Names and Typical Doses

Street names include most commonly "DXM," and also "CCC," "Triple C," "Dex," "poor man's PCP," "Robo," and "Skittles."

Route of Administration

Dextromethorphan is taken orally as a capsule or syrup.

Physical and Psychological Effects

Dextromethorphan is primarily an antitussive agent. In high doses, such as those greater than 180 mg, however, it has dissociative hallucinogenic properties.

Epidemiology

In the 2017 Monitoring the Future study, the annual prevalence of misusing OTC cough and cold medications was 3.2% of 12th graders, 3.6% of 10th graders, and 2.1% of 8th graders (Miech et al. 2018).

Patterns of Use and Risk of Developing a Use Disorder

Most users of dextromethorphan do not abuse it, and the risk of developing abuse or dependence is unknown. Cases of abuse have been reported since the 1960s (Williams and Kokotailo 2006).

Specific Treatment Issues

Treatment of dextromethorphan abuse or dependence involves the usual strategies to address substance abuse disorders. High doses, particularly when combined with alcohol, may result in death. Typically, management of dextromethorphan overdoses is supportive. Case reports have indicated that naltrexone assists with reducing cravings for dextromethorphan (Williams and Kokotailo 2006).

Conclusion

In this chapter, we have reviewed a broad range of substances with varying pharmacological and addictive properties. However, a few practical issues bear noting. The first is that opioid use disorder, whether in adolescents or in adults, is one of the few substance use disorders for which pharmacotherapy, typically with agonists such as methadone or buprenorphine, is a first line of therapy. Although clinicians may be unfamiliar with this treatment or consider it inappropriate for adolescents, careful consideration must be given to the risk of death from continued opioid use and the risk of progressing from prescription opioid dependence to heroin dependence, which is associated with substantial morbidity and mortality. Agonist therapy may help stabilize the patient and allow him or her to engage in psychosocial treatments. If this is not an option, antagonist therapy should be utilized.

Another practical issue is how to manage comorbid psychiatric or medical problems, such as anxiety, in the presence of benzodiazepine dependence, pain in the management of opiate dependence, or ADHD when patients are abusing stimulants or other drugs and/or have a history of MDMA or methamphetamine dependence. Clinically, it is highly advisable to avoid controlled substances when treating these comorbid conditions, and if they are used, to consider how abuse or dependence could be detected and be differentiated from appropriate use. This may require consultation with a laboratory that conducts urinalysis to confirm that the specific medications being prescribed are detectable, as well as substances that are likely to be abused, and clarify which metabolites may be detected (e.g., whether methamphetamine can be distinguished from prescription stimulants).

Key Points

- Physicians need to be aware of the risk of diversion and abuse of prescription medications, such as painkillers and stimulants. This is particularly important in families in which substance abuse has been diagnosed.

- Clinicians should provide education to parents and adolescents regarding the peril of abusing prescription and over-the-counter medications.

- Prescription medications should be stored in a place that cannot be accessed by adolescents. Pills should be frequently counted, and any discrepancy should be reported immediately to the prescribing physician.

- Opioid use disorder should be treated with pharmacotherapy in almost all circumstances. This could include either agonist therapy or antagonist therapy.

References

Abraham HD, Aldridge AM, Gogia P: The psychopharmacology of hallucinogens. Neuropsychopharmacology 14(4):285–298, 1996 8924196

American Psychiatric Association: Diagnostic and Statistical Manual of Mental Disorders, 5th Edition. Arlington, VA, American Psychiatric Association, 2013

Borodovsky JT, Levy S, Fishman M, et al: Buprenorphine treatment for adolescents and young adults with opioid use disorders: a narrative review. J Addict Med 12(3):170–183, 2018 29432333

Bryner JK, Wang UK, Hui JW, et al: Dextromethorphan abuse in adolescence: an increasing trend: 1999–2004. Arch Pediatr Adolesc Med 160(12):1217–1222, 2006 17146018

Compton WM, Volkow ND: Abuse of prescription drugs and the risk of addiction. Drug Alcohol Depend 83 (suppl 1):S4–S7, 2006 16563663

Cook CE, Jeffcoat AR, Sadler BM, et al: Pharmacokinetics of oral methamphetamine and effects of repeated daily dosing in humans. Drug Metab Dispos 20(6):856–862, 1992 1362938

Cook CE, Jeffcoat AR, Hill JM, et al: Pharmacokinetics of methamphetamine self-administered to human subjects by smoking S-(+)-methamphetamine hydrochloride. Drug Metab Dispos 21(4):717–723, 1993 8104133

Cooper RJ: Over-the-counter medicine abuse—a review of the literature. J Subst Use 18(2):82–107, 2013 23525509

Cottler LB, Womack SB, Compton WM, et al: Ecstasy abuse and dependence among adolescents and young adults: applicability and reliability of DSM-IV criteria. Hum Psychopharmacol 16(8):599–606, 2001 12404539

Curran HV, Travill RA: Mood and cognitive effects of +/-3,4-methylenedioxymethamphetamine (MDMA, "ecstasy"): week-end "high" followed by mid-week low. Addiction 92(7):821–831, 1997 9293041

Degenhardt L, Darke S, Dillon P: GHB use among Australians: characteristics, use patterns and associated harm. Drug Alcohol Depend 67(1):89–94, 2002 12062782

Dillon P, Copeland J, Jansen K: Patterns of use and harms associated with non-medical ketamine use. Drug Alcohol Depend 69(1):23–28, 2003 12536063

Fishman MJ, Winstanley EL, Curran E, et al: Treatment of opioid dependence in adolescents and young adults with extended release naltrexone: preliminary case-series and feasibility. Addiction 105(9):1669–1676, 2010 20626723

Freese TE, Miotto K, Reback CJ: The effects and consequences of selected club drugs. J Subst Abuse Treat 23(2):151–156, 2002 12220613

Gonzales R, Ang A, McCann MJ, et al: An emerging problem: methamphetamine abuse among treatment seeking youth. Subst Abus 29(2):71–80, 2008 19042326

Grob C: MDMA research: preliminary investigations with human subjects. International Journal of Drug Policy 9(2):119–124, 1998

Haber F: Uber einige derivate des piperonals. Berichte der Deutschen Chemischen Gesellschaft 24(1):617–626, 1891

Halpern JH, Pope HG Jr: Hallucinogen persisting perception disorder: what do we know after 50 years? Drug Alcohol Depend 69(2):109–119, 2003 12609692

Hertz JA, Knight JR: Prescription drug misuse: a growing national problem. Adolesc Med Clin 17(2):751–769; abstract xiii, 2006 17030290

Hopfer CJ, Khuri E, Crowley TJ: Treating adolescent heroin use. J Am Acad Child Adolesc Psychiatry 42(5):609–611, 2003 12707565

Hopfer CJ, Mendelson B, Van Leeuwen JM, et al: Club drug use among youths in treatment for substance abuse. Am J Addict 15(1):94–99, 2006 16449098

Hurt PH, Ritchie EC: A case of ketamine dependence (letter). Am J Psychiatry 151(5):779, 1994 8166324

Jasinski DR: Opiate withdrawal syndrome: acute and protracted aspects. Ann N Y Acad Sci 362:183–186, 1981 6942707

Johnston LD, O'Malley PM, Bachman JG, et al: Monitoring the Future National Survey Results on Drug Use, 1975–2007, Volume I: Secondary School Students (NIH Publ No 08-6418A). Bethesda, MD, National Institute on Drug Abuse, 2008

Johnston LD, Miech RA, O'Malley PM, et al: Monitoring the Future: National Survey Results on Drug Use: 1975–2017: Overview, Key Findings on Adolescent Drug Use. Ann Arbor, MI, Institute for Social Research, The University of Michigan, 2018

Jones CM, Einstein EB, Compton WM: Changes in synthetic opioid involvement in drug overdose deaths in the United States, 2010–2016. JAMA 319(17):1819–1821, 2018 29715347

Kalechstein AD, Newton TF, Green M: Methamphetamine dependence is associated with neurocognitive impairment in the initial phases of abstinence. J Neuropsychiatry Clin Neurosci 15(2):215–220, 2003 12724464

Kaminer Y, Hrecznyj B: LSD induced chronic visual disturbances in an adolescent. J Nerv Ment Dis 179:173–174, 1991 1997667

Koesters SC, Rogers PD, Rajasingham CR: MDMA ("ecstasy") and other "club drugs." The new epidemic. Pediatr Clin North Am 49(2):415–433, 2002 11993291

Leung KS, Cottler LB: Ecstasy and other club drugs: a review of recent epidemiologic studies. Curr Opin Psychiatry 21(3):234–241, 2008 18382220

Levine DA: "Pharming": the abuse of prescription and over-the-counter drugs in teens. Curr Opin Pediatr 19(3):270–274, 2007 17505185

Martin A, Volkmar FR: Lewis's Child and Adolescent Psychiatry: A Comprehensive Textbook, 4th Edition. Baltimore, MD, Lippincott Williams & Wilkins, 2007

McCabe SE, Teter CJ, Boyd CJ, et al: Sources of prescription medication misuse among young adults in the U.S.: the role of educational status. J Clin Psychiatry 79(2):17m11958, 2018 29570970

McKetin R, Copeland J, Norberg MM, et al: The effect of the ecstasy 'come-down' on the diagnosis of ecstasy dependence. Drug Alcohol Depend 139:26–32, 2014 24703083

Miech RA, Johnston LD, O'Malley PM, et al: Monitoring the Future: National Survey Results on Drug Use, 1975–2017: Volume I, Secondary School Students. Ann Arbor, MI, Institute for Social Research, The University of Michigan, 2018

Miotto K, Darakjian J, Basch J, et al: Gamma-hydroxybutyric acid: patterns of use, effects and withdrawal. Am J Addict 10(3):232–241, 2001 11579621

Montoya AG, Sorrentino R, Lukas SE, Price BH: Long-term neuropsychiatric consequences of "ecstasy" (MDMA): a review. Harv Rev Psychiatry 10(4):212–220, 2002 12119307

National Institute on Drug Abuse: Research Report Series: Methamphetamine: abuse and addiction (NIH Publ No 06-4210). September 2006, revised September 2013. Available at: https://www.drugabuse.gov/publications/research-reports/methamphetamine/letter-director. Accessed May 6, 2019.

National Institute on Drug Abuse: Research Report Series: Hallucinogens and dissociative drugs, including LSD, PCP, ketamine, and dextromethorphan (NIH Publ No 01-4209). March 2001, revised February 2015. Available at: https://www.drugabuse.gov/publications/research-reports/hallucinogens-dissociative-drugs/director. Accessed May 6, 2019.

National Institute on Drug Abuse: Research Report Series: Prescription drugs: abuse and addiction (NIH Publ No 05-4881). August 2005, revised January 2018. Available at: https://www.drugabuse.gov/publications/research-reports/misuse-prescription-drugs/summary. Accessed May 6, 2019.

National Institute on Drug Abuse: Club drugs. 2019. Available at: https://www.drugabuse.gov/drugs-abuse/club-drugs. Accessed January 23, 2019.

Okun MS, Boothby LA, Bartfield RB, et al: GHB: an important pharmacologic and clinical update. J Pharm Pharm Sci 4(2):167–175, 2001 11466174

Russell K, Dryden DM, Liang Y, et al: Risk factors for methamphetamine use in youth: a systematic review. BMC Pediatr 8:48, 2008 18957076

Sanacora G, Frye MA, McDonald W, et al; American Psychiatric Association (APA) Council of Research Task Force on Novel Biomarkers and Treatments: A consensus statement on the use of ketamine in the treatment of mood disorders. JAMA Psychiatry 74(4):399–405, 2017 28249076

Scheier LM, Ben Abdallah A, Inciardi JA, et al: Tri-city study of Ecstasy use problems: a latent class analysis. Drug Alcohol Depend 98(3):249–263, 2008 18674872

Schepis TS, Krishnan-Sarin S: Characterizing adolescent prescription misusers: a population-based study. J Am Acad Child Adolesc Psychiatry 47(7):745–754, 2008 18520963

Schepis TS, Wilens TE, McCabe SE: Prescription drugs misuse: sources of controlled medications in adolescents. J Am Acad Child Adolesc Psychiatry October 30, 2018 [Epub ahead of print] 30768405

Sigmon SC, Bisaga A, Nunes EV, et al: Opioid detoxification and naltrexone induction strategies: recommendations for clinical practice. Am J Drug Alcohol Abuse 38(3):187–199, 2012 22404717

Subramaniam GA, Stitzer MA: Clinical characteristics of treatment-seeking prescription opioid vs. heroin-using adolescents with opioid use disorder. Drug Alcohol Depend 101(1–2):13–19, 2009 19081205

van Noorden MS, van Dongen LC, Zitman FG, et al: Gamma-hydroxybutyrate withdrawal syndrome: dangerous but not well-known. Gen Hosp Psychiatry 31(4):394–396, 2009 19555805

Williams JF, Kokotailo PK: Abuse of proprietary (over-the-counter) drugs. Adolesc Med Clin 17(3):733–750; abstract xiii, 2006 17030289

Wolff K, Winstock AR: Ketamine: from medicine to misuse. CNS Drugs 20(3):199–218, 2006 16529526

Woody GE, Poole SA, Subramaniam G, et al: Extended vs short-term buprenorphine-naloxone for treatment of opioid-addicted youth: a randomized trial. JAMA 300(17):2003–2011, 2008 18984887

Wu LT, Schlenger WE, Galvin DM: Concurrent use of methamphetamine, MDMA, LSD, ketamine, GHB, and flunitrazepam among American youths. Drug Alcohol Depend 84(1):102–113, 2006 16483730

PART III

Specific Interventions for Youth
With Substance Use Disorders

12

Continuity of Care for Abstinence and Harm Reduction

Yifrah Kaminer, M.D., M.B.A.

Mark D. Godley, Ph.D.

Ken C. Winters, Ph.D.

Kara S. Bagot, M.D.

Adolescence is a critical period for the potential initiation of substance use, substance use disorders (SUDs), and associated negative consequences that present significant public health concerns. It is estimated that only a small segment of the adolescent subpopulation with SUDs end up in treatment.

This chapter has three objectives: First, to present potential therapeutic variables that affect treatment processes and outcomes, which will include addressing mechanisms of behaviorial change (MOBCs) in treatment. Second, to discuss aftercare/continuing care and the emerging adaptive treatment approach in order to provide continuity of care that will maintain treatment gains, enhance treatment outcomes for poor responders, and prevent relapse in youth who achieved abstinence. Third, to address future directions of research, including non-abstinence-oriented treatment outcomes such as harm reduction (HR) for youth.

Progress in Youth Treatment Research

Great advances have been made since the 1990s in the development and evaluation of treatments for adolescent SUDs (Dennis and Kaminer 2006; Hogue et al. 2018). These advances are reflected in the use of assessment tools developed and validated on adolescents; treatment manuals with specific protocols that permit treatment replication; and an increased rigor in evaluating the effectiveness of these protocols.

This body of treatment evaluation research focuses on varying interventions using different theory-driven approaches. There is solid evidence that family systems–based treatments; motivational enhancement, 12-step, therapeutic community, community reinforcement, and cognitive-behavioral approaches; and pharmacological approaches either have met standards of evidence-based treatments or have demonstrated modest empirical support (Dennis et al. 2004; Hogue et al. 2018; Winters et al. 2018). Despite prominent differences in design and methodology, the most recent studies employing various treatment modalities in youth with SUDs in general have reported remarkably similar outcomes (Hogue et al. 2018; Waldron and Turner 2008). Brief interventions, including expanded use of Screening, Brief Intervention, and Referral to Treatment (SBIRT; see Chapter 4), are receiving more attention for use in diverse settings, such as in emergency departments, school-based clinics, and juvenile justice settings (Winters 2016). The use of technology-assisted interventions including via the telephone (telepsychiatry), computer, and Internet, has been growing (Kaminer and Napolitano 2010; Marsch and Borodovsky 2016).

The Therapeutic Process, Mechanisms of Behavioral Change, and Outcomes

When Does Treatment for Adolescents Begin and When Does It End?

Most interventions are abstinence oriented. However, only about 30%–40% of adolescents will achieve abstinence on completion of a single episode of treatment. The majority of teens treated in outpatient settings will be partial or poor responders who have not achieved abstinence (Black and Chung 2014; Passetti et al. 2016), and many who achieve abstinence will relapse 3–6 months later (Waldron and Turner 2008). Thus, the long-term view of recovery for adolescents includes a range of trajectory patterns involving a mix of abstinence, remissions, and relapse (see Chapter 1 in this manual).

Despite the fact that evidence-based treatments are theory-driven, tests of the MOBC suggested by the theories on which the interventions are based often do not yield positive results (Apodaca and Longabaugh 2009; Morgenstern and McKay 2007). Some theorists have argued that treatment effects are due primarily to "general" therapeutic factors or nonspecific effects, such as an empathic and caring therapist, and the structure and support provided by regularly scheduled treatment sessions over a prolonged period of time. Increased motivation to change has been cited often as a predictor for positive outcome in both the adult and the youth literature. For example, the seminal controlled studies of giving advice to quit smoking or drinking because it might be harmful to health indicated that more adult participants quit smoking in the month immediately preceding the research interview than quit in the month following a brief intervention (Edwards et al. 1977; Russell et al. 1979). A year later, there were no significant differences in outcome between the two groups.

What differentiates youth from adults in preparation for treatment? Treated adolescents differ from their adult counterparts in length and severity of substance use, typical patterns and context of use, type of substance-related problems most often experienced, and source of referral to treatment (see Chapter 1 for further discussion). Adolescents with SUDs should be evaluated in a developmental perspective. There are subgroups of adolescents who have not yet started using drugs, or who have not yet reached the peak of the trajectory characterizing their drinking or drug use pattern. Therefore, any effort to reduce or eliminate use amounts to "swimming upstream" (see Chapter 2 for more details on prevention). Furthermore, adolescents are also less motivated to change substance use, and often enter treatment because of external pressures by a concerned parent, mental health clinician, school staff, or the legal system (Bagot and Kaminer 2018). Consequently, it appears unlikely that youth will respond to advice only.

In the search to identify the effective ingredients of successful psychotherapy, one therapist characteristic in particular, "accurate empathy," as defined by Carl Rogers (1957), has been shown to be a predictor of therapeutic success. Within the addiction field, the search for critical conditions that are necessary and sufficient to induce change has led to the identification of six critical elements developed by Miller and Sanchez (1994): 1) **Feedback** regarding personal risk or impairment; 2) emphasis on personal **Responsibility** for change; 3) clear **Advice** to change; 4) a **Menu** of alternative change options; 5) therapist **Empathy**; and 6) facilitation of participant optimism about the potential to change and **Self-efficacy**. These six active ingredients of effective brief interventions are represented best by the acronym **FRAMES**. Therapeutic interventions containing some or all of these elements have been effective in initiating change and reducing alcohol use (Arkowitz et al. 2016).

Assessment Reactivity

Participants in some clinics in general and in treatment outcome studies in particular undergo extensive assessment protocols to assess eligibility and to provide information before beginning therapy sessions. Participants might be exposed, therefore, to a professional who does not necessarily function as a therapist, such as a research assistant in a clinical trial or a nurse in an outpatient clinic setting. Such interactions containing some or all of the components or active ingredients of FRAMES might be effective in initiating change and reducing substance use, although, a priori, they were not intended to be therapeutic. This change is defined as *assessment reactivity* (AR) (Clifford et al. 2007). In this case, AR refers to a change of substance use status from positive to negative from baseline to the time of initiation of the first therapy session.

AR has been reported in association with posttreatment follow-up assessments in adults (Clifford et al. 2007), as well as with adolescents in an assessment-only condition (McCambridge and Strang 2005).

Kaminer et al. (2008) conducted a study, first, to examine if a change from positive to negative alcohol use from baseline assessment to the onset of the first session (i.e., pretreatment phase) occurs in adolescents (i.e., baseline assessment reactivity [BAR]); and, second, to compare what mediators differentiate BAR-positive and BAR-negative youth. Participants were 177 adolescents with alcohol use disorder (AUD) in 9 weekly group sessions of cognitive-behavioral therapy. Self-report for alcohol and urinalysis for drug use in the past 30 days before baseline assessment and immediately before the first session of treatment was obtained to determine BAR. For alcohol use, 51% reported abstinence at the first session, while 29% of those who tested positive for other drugs at baseline assessment tested negative for drugs. The finding was highly significant. It was also reported that variables such as age, gender, criminal justice involvement, and duration of wait from baseline assessment to first session were not associated with BAR. The likelihood of manifesting BAR was significantly correlated with the level of readiness to change and with several subscales measuring self-efficacy. In this study, alcohol and other substance use at first session predicted use at last session and participants continued to improve from first to last session. That is, treatment outcome was not solely attributed to BAR. These findings support the validity of BAR as a construct relevant to youth waiting for the initiation of SUD treatment.

Heterogeneity of Response to Adolescent SUD Treatment

Despite prominent differences in design and methodology, the most recent studies employing various treatment modalities in youth with SUDs have reported remarkably similar outcomes. These outcomes suggest that similar MOBCs may be the active ingredients of various treatment modalities that appear different in the way they are administered. Nevertheless, there are no data to support or negate the possibility that, similarly to psychopharmacological treatment, these modalities might share active ingredients of MOBCs. There is an increasing effort invested in studying MOBCs in adolescent substance abuse treatment. Examples of potential mediator variables are readiness to change (Tevyaw and Monti 2004), coping skills (Waldron and Kaminer 2004), and self-efficacy (Burleson and Kaminer 2005).

The traditional experimental designs for youth SUDs have emphasized the comparison of standardized, fixed interventions as the primary method for evaluating treatment efficacy. Despite considerable variation in patient response, most treatments in the addictions strive to deliver essentially the same intervention to all patients, regardless of how the patient is responding. Indeed, treatment planning based on this approach has overlooked the most urgent challenges facing the field: the heterogeneity of adolescent response to treatment, the problem of poor response to treatment, and the difficulty in preventing relapse (Waldron and Turner 2008).

Data from numerous treatment studies indicate that there are large individual differences in patient's responsivity, even to effective treatments that have been standardized and with therapists who show high adherence to treatment manuals (Dennis et al. 2004; Tanner-Smith et al. 2013; Winters et al. 2018). Cluster analysis empirically identified different patterns of treatment response over time while considering severity of use at baseline versus response to treatment (Babbin et al. 2016). The authors recommend investigating homogeneous subgroups, such as low-use responders, high-use responders, relapsers, and nonresponders to initial treatment.

There are usually two types of poor responders to substance abuse treatment: those who are noncompleters of treatment (i.e., dropout and administrative discharge) and those who are retained in treatment and continue to use drugs as evidenced by positive drug urinalysis (i.e., nonresponders to initial treatment). The literature provides little guidance to the question of what to do with poor responders to treatment. A review by Godley and Godley (2009) indicates that only a few programs clearly specify what types of efforts (if any) will be made for linking those who complete the program, and even fewer for linking treatment noncompleters, to continuing care.

Several studies imply that in order to get services for the maintenance of treatment gains, an adolescent has to graduate or complete the treatment program (Stevens and Morral 2003). This popular approach is raising a public health concern because several episodes of treatment, and therefore multiple entries, are the rule rather than the expectation for youth with SUDs. Noncompleters are at higher risk for continued or exacerbated substance use, as well as substance use–related consequences (Kaminer et al. 2008). Godley et al. (2007) posit that noncompleter status does not necessarily indicate that the adolescent may fail to benefit from continuing care. In fact, research demonstrates that noncompleters engaged in assertive continuing care (ACC) had increased abstinence days relative to noncompleters in the control group who failed to attend continuing care. It may be harder to get the first session of the assigned adaptive treatment condition arranged because of the abrupt or unexpected departure of the adolescent from the initial treatment program. However, engaging dropouts has not been as difficult as might be perceived when an effective tracking system is in place (Dennis and Scott 2012; Godley et al. 2014).

Aftercare/Continuing Care for Youth With SUDs

There is a growing consensus that SUD is a chronic disorder with a relapsing-remitting course (McLellan et al. 2000). Very little has been done among community-based programs, however, to link and engage patients with aftercare programs and services (McKay 2009). Often, there is no coordinated effort to provide a system of continuing care. The lack of posttreatment support and monitoring of clients leaves them vulnerable to resuming pretreatment levels of use or frequent relapse. Also, there is substantial variability within and between programs in terms of the success in achieving goals for continuing care. The most common approach to reducing recurrence of psychiatric disorders has been continuing care by the addition of "booster" sessions, typically at a reduced frequency, after the end of more intensive acute treatments. A common growing view of addiction treatment is that it is a process that requires a continuum of care, including management and monitoring methods similar to those used in chronic disease management (McKay 2009; Scott et al. 2005).

The majority of the research on continuing care has been conducted with adults; however, a growing number of youth continuing care studies have been published (Godley et al. 2007; Kaminer et al. 2008, 2017). Research on ACC (Godley et al. 2007) has been guided by the principle that rapid linkage into continuing care without regard for treatment completion status will improve continuing care initiation, retention, and clinical outcomes relative to usual continuing care (UCC), The continuing care program should include an evidence-based intervention (in this case the Adolescent Community Reinforcement Approach; see Chapter 14 in this manual) and case management, with all program services delivered to youth in home, at school, or in other convenient locations. In the first trial (Godley et al. 2007),183 youth ages 12–17 years discharged from residential treatment were randomly assigned to participate in either ACC or UCC. The ACC group received 3 months of ACC assistance and were compared with the UCC group, which had ad lib availability of services throughout the study. Results over 3-, 6-, and 9-month follow-up intervals demonstrated the superiority of ACC on continuing care initiation, engagement, retention, and substance use outcomes. Although encouraging, the overall treatment effects were in the small to medium range, suggesting the opportunity to further improve ACC.

Godley and colleagues (2014) next tested ACC with the addition of contingency management (CM) to provide escalating opportunities to earn/win client-selected prizes for increasing verifiable prosocial activities and abstinence from all drugs. In this study, 337 youth ages 12–18 years were randomly allocated to either UCC, ACC, CM, or ACC+CM. All experimental interventions occurred in the first 3 months postresidential discharge with 9 additional months of follow-up. The results essentially replicated those of the first study for the ACC condition and the CM condition relative to UCC. However, the combination of ACC+CM was not statistically different from UCC. While it is clear that motivational approaches like CM and assertive outreach approaches like ACC are likely to perform better in practice than UCC, treatment providers have expressed difficulty in obtaining reimbursement for such services.

Dennis and Scott (2012) suggested that longer-term recovery monitoring and support was necessary to produce stable remission. Difficulties with ACC implementation and the need for extended monitoring and support led Godley et al. (2019) to revise the approach. They developed a less intensive form of ACC that would retain some of its features (rapid initiation following discharge, without regard for treatment completion status) but extend a recovery monitoring and support intervention via telephone and text messaging for a much longer period than the prior ACC work. In a randomized trial, 403 youth were assigned either to the recovery monitoring and support condition or to services as usual. Under the supervision of a study leader, trained volunteers made recovery monitoring and support contacts for 9 months. Volunteers were undergraduate or graduate students in training for nursing, psychology, or social work. The results were encouraging, and the remission rate increased proportionately to support session completion rate. Moreover, the hypothesis that the new recovery monitoring and support intervention would increase pro-recovery peers and activities (proximal) outcomes and subsequently improve substance use and remission (distal) outcomes was supported (Godley et al. 2019).

Another possible mechanism that accounts for the relationship between aftercare and improved outcomes is the maintenance of during-treatment proximal outcome gains afforded by continuing care (e.g., increased self-efficacy, improved readiness to change). One of the crucial goals of continuing care should be to prepare for coping effectively with high-risk situations for relapse. Indeed, McKay (2009) suggested that an individualized relapse prevention program might be helpful in facilitating maintenance of abstinence or in initiating abstinence for those who failed to achieve it during treatment.

Kaminer et al. (2008) studied aftercare for youth in an outpatient program for the following reasons: 1) the rates of continued use and of relapse for adolescents posttreatment are high; 2) the literature provides little guidance for the implementation of continuing care programs for youth after a treatment episode in an outpatient clinic; and 3) very little research has been done to investigate the relationship between self-efficacy, readiness to change, and social support and engagement as it pertains to outcomes of continuing care for adolescents with SUD. The study was developed to test the relative efficacy of three randomized aftercare conditions for treatment completers only during the 3-month period following treatment. They included a) individualized 50-minute in-person sessions involving integrated motivational enhancement and cognitive-behavioral therapies; b) brief therapeutic phone contacts, limited to 15 minutes only, involving individualized integrated motivational enhancement and cognitive-behavioral therapies; and c) a no-active aftercare (NA) condition as control. Among treatment completers, 90% finished the assigned aftercare conditions. The phone intervention was found to be feasible and acceptable to both adolescents and therapists (Burleson and Kaminer 2005). There was a significant reduction in number of drinking occasions, heavy drinking occasions, and drinks per occasion, and in highest number of drinks per occasion, as a function of combined active aftercare conditions versus the no-active aftercare condition.

More than 80% of the cohort had use that met criteria for cannabis use disorder (CUD). There was also a significant change in readiness to change in marijuana use, such that youth in the two active aftercare conditions collectively showed significantly more readiness to change than youth in the NA group. Similar to the findings regarding AUD, there was a significant reduction in cannabis positive urinalysis as a function of combined active aftercare conditions versus the NA condition. There was no significant difference between the two active interventions regarding AUD or CUD (Kaminer et al. 2008). These results were maintained 12-month post aftercare completion (Burleson et al. 2012).

In a pilot study, Gonzales et al. (2016) studied the effects of a 12-week mobile texting aftercare program, using a randomized controlled design. The program was based on disease management components, including monitoring, feedback, helpful recovery reminders, and education and support. Participants also responded to prompts to provide information back to the web platform that allowed for tailored feedback to be provided. Youth receiving the short-term texting intervention achieved and maintained significantly higher 12-step meeting attendance as well as reductions in their primary drug of use out to a 9-month follow-up compared with the aftercare-as-usual group. This technology-based intervention shows promise for further study, especially its possible expansion to all drugs used by youth in treatment, not just their primary drug of choice, as well as its provision over an extended basis to promote long-term remission and recovery. See Chapter 16 in this manual for more information on technology-supported interventions.

Adaptive Treatment for Youth

Adaptive treatment research for adult substance abusers has been developing during the last decade to address the heterogeneity in both clinical severity and treatment response (Collins et al. 2004; Murphy et al. 2007). This is a promising performance-based procedure in which individuals who respond poorly to an initial level of evidence-based efficacious treatment are then provided a different or more enhanced version of the same treatment (McKay 2009). The definitions of nonresponse or poor response and the timing of change are pivotal decision rules in an adaptive treatment protocol, which includes an algorithm of intervention options.

Most of the 15 adaptive treatment studies reviewed by McKay (2009) yielded significant results in which adaptive procedures led either to better substance use outcomes or to equivalent outcomes in treatments with other advantages (e.g., lower cost, lower patient burden, greater safety) or produced algorithms that specified which patients would benefit most from what continuing care treatments.

One of the key questions in treatment is what to do with patients who do not respond to an initial treatment. Should their initial treatment be switched to something else? If so, to what treatment? Or, should they receive another treatment to augment what they are already taking (McKay 2009)? Several models for adapting treatment have been proposed, often guided by theory as to how to respond when a client is not responding to the first line of treatment. The stepped-care approach has received a great deal of attention in the literature. With this model, the patient begins by receiving the lowest-intensity appropriate level of care, and is then "stepped up" to more intensive treatment if warranted by poor initial response. This approach has the potential to increase rates of participation, as it may be more palatable to patients because it places a lower burden on them at the beginning of treatment. Stepped care may also increase cost-effectiveness, because lower-intensity treatments are also often less costly (McKay 2009).

Adaptive or stepped-care treatment algorithms have been developed and evaluated for a number of disorders, including depression and anxiety (Fava et al. 2006; Otto et al. 2000; Scogin et al. 2003). Although practicing child and adolescent psychiatrists have developed their own algorithms to address the issue of nonresponse (most notably, e.g., the Texas Children's Medication Algorithm Project, Hughes et al. 2007), the field of adolescent substance abuse treatment, which relies mostly on psychosocial interventions, has not generated an empirically supported set of tailoring variables and decision rules specifying the intervention that is most likely to be effective in the face of initial nonresponse.

Brown et al. (2013) reported that initiation of abstinence in adolescents treated for CUD occurred by the sixth week of treatment for 94% of teens, suggesting that alternative, clinical approaches should be considered for those not responding by week 6. Kaminer et al. (2017) tested the hypothesis that adaptive treatment improves outcomes for poor responders to evidence-based practice interventions. A total of 161 adolescents, 13–18 years of age, diagnosed with DSM-IV CUD were enrolled in this randomized outpatient study. Following a 7-session weekly motivational enhancement and cognitive-behavioral therapy intervention, only poor responders (defined as those failing to achieve abstinence at week 7 for any reason) were randomly assigned to a 10-week adaptive treatment phase of either an individualized enhanced cognitive-behavioral therapy or an Adolescent Community Reinforcement Approach intervention. Good responders enrolled only in follow-up assessments starting at the completion of the adaptive treatment phase (week 17). Eighty adolescents (50%) met the criterion for poor response to treatment; of these poor responders, 37% completed the adaptive treatment phase, and 27% of them achieved abstinence. There was no significant difference in retention and abstinence rates between the adaptive treatment conditions. Although the majority of good responders had relapsed by week 17, they significantly differed from poor responders both on drug use (71% vs. 91%, respectively; $P<0.05$) and on reporting to scheduled assessment on that week (78% vs. 54%, respectively; $P<0.01$). Continuing care to achieve abstinence among poor responders remains a therapeutic necessity and a research challenge. Examining innovative adaptive treatment–designed interventions including potential integrative approaches should be further studied in order to improve treatment outcomes. Another possibility is the study of HR for youth (see next section).

The most sophisticated yet challenging designs of adaptive treatments are the multiphase optimization strategy (MOST) and the sequential multiple assignment randomized trial (SMART). However, in order to secure acceptable power for analyses, these designs require a very large number of subjects who can be recruited only in multicenter trials (Collins et al. 2007). No studies involving youth with SUD have been reported yet. A pilot test of SMART design reported that feasibility and acceptability to prevent adolescent conduct problems were promising (August et al. 2016).

Harm Reduction (Versus Abstinence) in Youth With Substance Use Disorders

Abstinence has traditionally been the ultimate goal of SUD treatment. However, it has been a challenge to develop effective evidence-based treatments that result in achieving and maintaining durable abstinence for youth with SUDs. Most evidence-based therapies, regardless of modality provided in outpatient settings, have resulted in similar outcomes, including low rates of abstinence (30%–50% of participants) and high rates of relapse (60% of participants) at

3 months after treatment completion (Hogue et al. 2018). Research-based treatments have not adequately considered the impact of the heterogeneity of personal characteristics on response to treatment. These characteristics include co-occurring psychiatric disorders, baseline clinical severity, motivation to change, self-efficacy, coping skills, goal setting, goal commitment, and/or impact of treatment referral sources (Passetti et al. 2016).

Since achieving abstinence remains an elusive goal for many youth with SUD, we examine HR for youth with SUDs; discuss the rational, potential implementation of these interventions; and address considerations for revising its definition to meet relevant developmental stage needs.

Unlike adults, a considerable number of adolescents evaluated for treatment do not believe abstinence is necessary. Many prefer to reduce the frequency and dosage of their drug of choice to a level they believe is controllable to stay out of "harm's way," such as suspension from school or other legal penalties. Therefore, it is important to examine harm minimization or harm reduction and evaluate whether this approach might accommodate a segment of youth referred to treatment.

Traditionally, HR focuses on reduction of negative consequences related to substance use behaviors, such as medical problems and school dropout, and not primarily on abstinence per se as an outcome (Marlatt and Witkiewitz 2010). Common examples of HR include needle exchange programs, educational/vocational training, and approaches for addressing homelessness and domestic violence.

As a way to address HR for adolescent SUD, reduction of negative consequences related to substance use behaviors (e.g., driving or being driven under the influence of substances, drug use on school grounds) merits consideration. However, we further posit that the definition of HR for youth (HR-Y) should include reduction of substance consumption (i.e., frequency, quantity, or duration) and of more harmful delivery methods of use (e.g., injection, inhaling drugs) as proximal outcomes for adolescents in treatment even when the explicit treatment goal is abstinence/remission.

Increasing Motivation for Change

It is imperative to understand the process leading to behavior change, including increasing motivation, goal setting, and goal commitment while enhancing youth input in the process and the target outcome (i.e., personal needs and wants). This procedure is known as *functional analysis* (Black and Chung 2014). Within the addiction field, the motivational interviewing approach, and its manualized format, motivational enhancement therapy, were initially grounded in research on processes of change. Motivational interviewing and motivational enhancement therapy begin at the stage of change at which the patient is at the time of treatment and assist in moving him or her through the stages toward action and maintenance of treatment gains. Motivational interviewing decreases the likelihood of being drawn into a power struggle with an ambivalent client about the need for, and degree of, change by developing a therapeutic alliance around the adolescent's perspective of the problem behavior(s) and facilitating identification of the impact of behaviors on ability to achieve client-stated goals. The motivational interviewing approach is supported by research reporting that low readiness to change contributes to attrition and that external coercion from juvenile justice, family members, and/or school is negatively associated with motivation and treatment retention (Bagot and Kaminer 2018). Chapter 13 in this manual includes a more detailed review of motivational interviewing.

Goal Setting

According to the goal-setting theory, specific goal setting is associated with higher performance because of reduced ambiguity in process and outcome. A study on youth SUD outcomes and goal setting found that goal setting and motivation that precedes goal setting predict lower cannabis use in treated adolescents (Spinola et al. 2017). Further, adolescents with lower frequency of cannabis use appear to be more likely to set abstinence-related goals. Kaminer and colleagues (2016) studied "goal commitment to change" as a potential mediator and a MOBC for adolescents in treatment for SUD using the Adolescent Substance Abuse Goal Commitment questionnaire. The authors reported that greater commitment to abstinence is associated with reduced use of alcohol as well as cannabis use, whereas commitment to HR did not predict any of the drinking outcomes (Kaminer et al. 2018).

What's a Therapist to Do?

There is a clear consensus that adolescent biopsychosocial development and ecological influences have an impact on treatment process and outcome. Furthermore, they contribute to engagement in treatment and provide personal meaning to the individual's potential set of treatment goals. Adolescents' ability to achieve abstinence already by 6 weeks of treatment (earlier than the fixed 12-week treatment programs generally afford) supports the development of short-term, flexible, proximal goals for those who are unable to achieve abstinence by then. We propose adding HR-Y to our treatment armamentarium as a proximal outcome for those who are unable to achieve abstinence by week 6 of abstinence-oriented treatment (Figure 12–1). Continuing care monitoring and support should follow all clients.

Conclusion and Future Directions

For many adolescents in abstinence-oriented treatment, outcome at 12 weeks from treatment initiation can be predicted by week 6 of treatment. For those who are unable to achieve abstinence, HR-Y may be a viable option for reduction in use as a proximal outcome on a path to abstinence. HR-Y also allows adolescents to identify and enact internally motivated goals, reinforcing healthy developmental processes, and potentially improving self-efficacy for future abstinence. Promising research designs should examine the effectiveness of HR-Y prospectively compared with treatment as usual or other controlled conditions. Further, the role of co-occurring disorders, and referral sources such as families and other systems (e.g., schools, juvenile justice), within the HR-Y framework requires further exploration, as system goals may not align with a nonabstinence proximal outcome.

Perhaps the most important future research priority in this field is to address the question of how to best address poor response to treatment. Little research attention has been directed toward enhancing treatment engagement strategies, and only a few programs clearly specify what types of efforts (if any) will be made for linking adolescent clients to continuing care (Godley and Godley 2009). Because research has started to identify some factors that influence recovery—aftercare involvement, coexisting disorders, coping skills, peer drug use, parental support, and motivational factors—a high priority for research is to identify ways to tailor treatment approaches in order to promote engagement that leads to improved treatment response.

Future research of enhanced engagement and promotion of outcomes should continue to explore outreach to adolescents via daily monitoring of harmful activity and on-demand support or interventions by improved technological approaches (e.g., smartphones, text messaging).

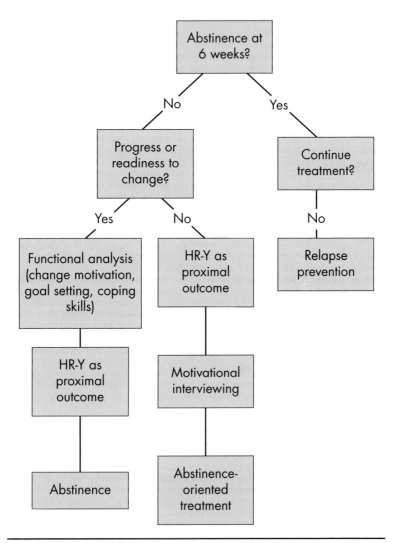

Figure 12–1.   Initial treatment phase decision tree.

HR-Y = harm reduction for youth.

Key Points

- Baseline assessment reactivity should be considered when evaluating treatment outcomes.

- Regardless of varying treatment modalities, treatment outcomes across conditions have been similar in part because of common mechanisms of behavior change, as well as the lack of treatment options tailored to the initial response to treatment.

- Standardized treatment manuals and specific protocols that permit treatment replication are available for a variety of interventions.

- There is a need for aftercare/continuing care in order to maintain treatment gains and prevent relapse.

References

Apodaca TR, Longabaugh R: Mechanisms of change in motivational interviewing: a review and preliminary evaluation of the evidence. Addiction 104(5):705–715, 2009 19413785

Arkowitz H, Miller WR, Rollnick S (eds): Motivational Interviewing in the Treatment of Psychological Problems. New York, Guilford, 2016

August GJ, Piehler TF, Bloomquist ML: Being "SMART" about adolescent conduct problems prevention: executing a SMART pilot study in a juvenile diversion agency. J Clin Child Adolesc Psychol 45(4):495–509, 2016 25256135

Babbin SF, Stanger C, Scherer EA, et al: Identifying treatment response subgroups for adolescent cannabis use. Addict Behav 59:72–79, 2016 27082747

Bagot KS, Kaminer Y: Harm reduction for youth in treatment for substance use disorders: one size does not fit all. Current Addiction Reports 5(3):379–385, 2018

Black JJ, Chung T: Mechanisms of change in adolescent substance use treatment: how does treatment work? Subst Abus 35(4):344–351, 2014 24901750

Brown PC, Budney AJ, Thostenson JD, et al: Initiation of abstinence in adolescents treated for marijuana use disorders. J Subst Abuse Treat 44(4):384–390, 2013 23085041

Burleson J, Kaminer Y: Self-efficacy as a predictor of relapse in adolescent substance use disorders. Addict Behav 20:751–764, 2005 16095844

Burleson JA, Kaminer Y, Burke RH: Twelve-month follow-up of aftercare for adolescents with alcohol use disorders. J Subst Abuse Treat 42(1):78–86, 2012 21868186

Clifford PR, Maisto SA, Davis CM: Alcohol treatment research assessment exposure subject reactivity effects: part I. Alcohol use and related consequences. J Stud Alcohol Drugs 68(4):519–528, 2007 17568955

Collins LM, Murphy SA, Bierman KL: A conceptual framework for adaptive preventive interventions. Prev Sci 5(3):185–196, 2004 15470938

Collins LM, Murphy SA, Strecher V: The multiphase optimization strategy (MOST) and the sequential multiple assignment randomized trial (SMART): new methods for more potent eHealth interventions. Am J Prev Med 32 (5, suppl):S112–S118, 2007 17466815

Dennis ML, Kaminer Y: Introduction to special issue on advances in the assessment and treatment of adolescent substance use disorders. Am J Addict 15 (suppl 1):1–3, 2006 17182414

Dennis ML, Godley SH, Diamond G, et al: The Cannabis Youth Treatment (CYT) Study: main findings from two randomized trials. J Subst Abuse Treat 27(3):197–213, 2004 15501373

Dennis ML, Scott CK: Four-year outcomes from the Early Re-Intervention Experiment (ERI) with Recovery Management Checkups (RMCs). Drug Alcohol Depend 121(1–2):10–17, 2012 21903347

Edwards G, Orford J, Egert S, et al: Alcoholism: a controlled trial of "treatment" and "advice." J Stud Alcohol 38(5):1004–1031, 1977 881837

Fava M, Rush AJ, Wisniewski SR, et al: A comparison of mirtazapine and nortriptyline following two consecutive failed medication treatments for depressed outpatients: a STAR*D report. Am J Psychiatry 163(7):1161–1172, 2006 16816220

Godley MD, Godley SH: Continuing care following residential treatment: history, current practice, critical issues, and emerging approaches, in Understanding and Treating Adolescent Substance Use Disorders. Edited by Jainchill N. Kingston, NJ, Civic Research Institute, 2009

Godley MD, Godley SH, Dennis ML, et al: The effect of assertive continuing care on continuing care linkage, adherence and abstinence following residential treatment for adolescents with substance use disorders. Addiction 102(1):81–93, 2007 17207126

Godley MD, Godley SH, Dennis ML, et al: A randomized trial of assertive continuing care and contingency management for adolescents with substance use disorders. J Consult Clin Psychol 82(1):40–51, 2014 24294838

Godley MD, Passetti LL, Hunter BD, et al: A randomized trial of Volunteer Recovery Support for Adolescents (VRSA) following residential treatment discharge. J Subst Abuse Treat 98:15–25, 2019 30665599

Gonzales R, Hernandez M, Murphy DA, et al: Youth recovery outcomes at 6 and 9 months following participation in a mobile texting recovery support aftercare pilot study. Am J Addict 25(1):62–68, 2016 26689171

Hogue A, Henderson CE, Becker SJ, et al: Evidence base on outpatient behavioral treatments for adolescent substance use, 2014–2017: outcomes, treatment delivery, and promising horizons. J Clin Child Adolesc Psychol 47(4):499–526, 2018 29893607

Hughes CW, Emslie GJ, Crismon ML, et al; Texas Consensus Conference Panel on Medication Treatment of Childhood Major Depressive Disorder: Texas Children's Medication Algorithm Project: update from Texas Consensus Conference Panel on Medication Treatment of Childhood Major Depressive Disorder. J Am Acad Child Adolesc Psychiatry 46(6):667–686, 2007 17513980

Kaminer Y, Napolitano C: Dial for Therapy: Manual for the Aftercare of Adolescents With Alcohol and Other Substance Use Disorders. Minneapolis, MN, Hazelden, 2010

Kaminer Y, Burleson JA, Burke RH: Efficacy of outpatient aftercare for adolescents with alcohol use disorders: a randomized controlled study. J Am Acad Child Adolesc Psychiatry 47(12):1405–1412, 2008 18978635

Kaminer Y, Ohannessian CM, McKay JR, et al: The Adolescent Substance Abuse Goal Commitment (ASAGC) questionnaire: an examination of clinical utility and psychometric properties. J Subst Abuse Treat 61:42–46, 2016 26531893

Kaminer Y, Ohannessian CM, Burke RH: Adolescents with cannabis use disorders: adaptive treatment for poor responders. Addict Behav 70:102–106, 2017 28232290

Kaminer Y, Ohannessian CM, McKay JR, et al: Goal commitment predicts treatment outcome for adolescents with alcohol use disorder. Addict Behav 76:122–128, 2018 28800496

Marlatt GA, Witkiewitz K: Update on harm-reduction policy and intervention research. Annu Rev Clin Psychol 6:591–606, 2010 20192791

Marsch LA, Borodovsky JT: Technology-based interventions for preventing and treating substance use among youth. Child Adolesc Psychiatr Clin N Am 25(4):755–768, 2016 27613350

McCambridge J, Strang J: Deterioration over time in effect of motivational interviewing in reducing drug consumption and related risk among young people. Addiction 100(4):470–478, 2005 15784061

McKay JR: Continuing care research: what we have learned and where we are going. J Subst Abuse Treat 36(2):131–145, 2009 19161894

McLellan AT, Lewis DC, O'Brien CP, et al: Drug dependence, a chronic medical illness: implications for treatment, insurance, and outcomes evaluation. JAMA 284(13):1689–1695, 2000 11015800

Miller WR, Sanchez V: Motivating young adults for treatment and lifestyle change, in Issues in Alcohol Use and Misuse by Young Adults. Edited by Howard G, Nathan P. Notre Dame, IN, University of Notre Dame Press, 1994, pp 51–81

Morgenstern J, McKay JR: Rethinking the paradigms that inform behavioral treatment research for substance use disorders. Addiction 102(9):1377–1389, 2007 17610541

Murphy SA, Lynch KG, Oslin D, et al: Developing adaptive treatment strategies in substance abuse research. Drug Alcohol Depend 88 (suppl 2):S24–S30, 2007 17056207

Otto MW, Pollack MH, Maki KM: Empirically supported treatments for panic disorder: costs, benefits, and stepped care. J Consult Clin Psychol 68(4):556–563, 2000 10965630

Passetti LL, Godley MD, Kaminer Y: Continuing care for adolescents in treatment for substance use disorders. Child Adolesc Psychiatr Clin N Am 25(4):669–684, 2016 27613345

Rogers CR: The necessary and sufficient conditions for therapeutic personality change. J Consult Psychol 21(2):95–103, 1957 13416422

Russell MA, Wilson C, Taylor C, et al: Effect of general practitioner's advice against smoking. Br Med J 2(6184):231–235, 1979 476401

Scogin FR, Hanson A, Welsh D: Self-administered treatment in stepped-care models of depression treatment. J Clin Psychol 59(3):341–349, 2003 12579549

Scott CK, Dennis ML, Foss MA: Utilizing Recovery Management Checkups to shorten the cycle of relapse, treatment reentry, and recovery. Drug Alcohol Depend 78(3):325–338, 2005 15893164

Spinola S, Park A, Maisto SA, et al: Motivation precedes goal setting in prediction of cannabis treatment outcomes in adolescents. J Child Adolesc Subst Abuse 26(2):132–140, 2017 29242699

Stevens SJ, Morral AR (eds): Adolescent Substance Abuse Treatment in the United States: Exemplary Models From a National Evaluation Study. Binghamton, NY, Haworth Press, 2003

Tanner-Smith EE, Wilson SJ, Lipsey MW: The comparative effectiveness of outpatient treatment for adolescent substance abuse: a meta-analysis. J Subst Abuse Treat 44(2):145–158, 2013 22763198

Tevyaw TO, Monti PM: Motivational enhancement and other brief interventions for adolescent substance abuse: foundations, applications and evaluations. Addiction 99 (suppl 2):63–75, 2004 15488106

Waldron HB, Kaminer Y: On the learning curve: the emerging evidence supporting cognitive-behavioral therapies for adolescent substance abuse. Addiction 99 (suppl 2):93–105, 2004 15488108

Waldron HB, Turner C: Evidence-based psychosocial treatments for adolescent substance abuse. J Clin Child Adolesc Psychol 37(1):238–261, 2008 18444060

Winters KC: Brief interventions for adolescents. J Drug Abuse 2(1):14, 2016 27182561

Winters KC, Botzet AM, Fahnhorst T, et al: Adolescent substance abuse treatment: a review of evidence-based research, in Handbook on the Prevention and Treatment of Substance Abuse in Adolescence, 2nd Edition. Edited by Leukefeld C, Gullotta T, Staton Tindall M. New York, Springer, 2018, pp 141–171

13

Brief Motivational Interventions, Cognitive-Behavioral Therapy, and Contingency Management

Anthony Spirito, Ph.D., A.B.P.P.

Yifrah Kaminer, M.D., M.B.A.

Kimberly H. McManama O'Brien, Ph.D., L.I.C.S.W.

Research has shown that early-onset substance use problems can predict continuing substance abuse problems in adulthood (Hill et al. 2000). Individuals who seek help at earlier stages of drug dependence often experience more favorable outcomes, highlighting the importance of working with adolescents who are beginning their involvement with drugs. In 2014, a comprehensive review concluded that ecological family-based treatment, as well as individual and group cognitive-behavioral therapies, were well-established treatments for adolescent substance use (Hogue et al. 2014). An update (Hogue et al. 2018) concluded that behavioral family-based treatment and motivational interviewing (MI) were probably efficacious treatments, and five different types of multicomponent treatments (i.e., treatments combining more than one approach), three of which include contingency management (CM), were well established or probably efficacious In this chapter we review outpatient brief motivational interventions (BMIs), cognitive-behavioral therapy (CBT), and CM reinforcement approaches for youth with alcohol use disorder and/or substance use disorders (SUDs).

Brief Motivational Interventions

The theoretical basis for BMIs is grounded in client-centered therapy (Rogers 1957), social learning theory (Bandura 1977), cognitive-behavioral approaches (Marlatt and Gordon 1985), and the transtheoretical paradigm of change (Prochaska et al. 1992). The gradual shift from viewing motivation as a "trait" to a "state" also played a significant role in the advancement of BMIs.

In the search to identify the effective ingredients of successful psychotherapy, one therapist characteristic in particular, "accurate empathy," as defined by Carl Rogers (1957), has been shown to be a predictor of therapeutic success. Within the addiction field, the search for critical conditions that are necessary to induce change has included empathy as well as additional factors.

MI approaches are further grounded in research on processes of change (Prochaska et al. 1992). The "transtheoretical model" describes five stages of change that people progress through in modifying problem behaviors: precontemplation, contemplation, preparation, action, and maintenance. MI and motivational enhancement therapy (MET; discussed later in this chapter) approaches explore where clients are currently located in the cycle of change and assist them to move through the stages toward action and maintenance. Miller and Rollnick (2012) note that MI pertains to both a style of relating to others and a set of techniques to facilitate that process. To embrace this style, or "MI spirit," the therapist must embody four core qualities: partnership, acceptance, compassion, and evocation (Miller and Rollnick 2012). By embodying these characteristics and focusing responsibility for change on the client, the MI therapist decreases the likelihood of being drawn into a power struggle and arguing with the resistant (i.e., precontemplator) or ambivalent (i.e., contemplator) patient about the need to change.

In addition to embracing the MI spirit, the therapist intentionally uses a four-process method, as well as specific MI techniques, to evoke change in the client (Miller and Rollnick 2012). The four processes are engaging, focusing, evoking, and planning, although not necessarily used in that order or in a linear manner. Clients move through the processes at different rates and go back and forth between processes, depending on their needs and the flow of the session. The specific MI techniques can be remembered with the acronym OARS, which stands for Open questions, Affirming, Reflections, and Summarizing (Miller and Rollnick 2012). Perhaps the most important MI skill is reflection—that is, a listening response wherein the therapist restates a key aspect of a client's previous statement, demonstrating a true understanding of the client's thoughts, feelings, and/or experience. When the therapist provides reflections rather than a series of questions, the session will feel more like a collaborative partnership than a one-way interrogation, which, in turn, may lead to further progress toward change.

During the MI process, it is common for the patient to express ambivalence, which is the simultaneous presence of competing motivations for and against change. When ambivalence is present, it is important for the therapist to develop discrepancies—that is, help clients to see the distance between the current status and one or more of their change goals (e.g., improving school performance). This can be done by engaging the patient in a conversation about the benefits and drawbacks of substance use, as well as short-and long-term goals and how the addictive behavior affects the process of achieving these goals (Miller and Rose 2015). The overall aim of the MI session is for the therapist to evoke change talk in the patient, which is any patient speech that favors movement toward a particular change goal, such as reducing the number of drinks on a weekend. When the therapist hears an adolescent patient use change talk, the change talk is then reflected back to the patient (Miller and Rollnick 2012).

Mechanisms of behavioral change (MOBCs) for different psychotherapies constitute an important area of investigation. Apodaca and Longabaugh (2009) reviewed the literature for the following constructs of therapist behavior in MI: MI spirit, MI-consistent behaviors, MI-inconsistent behaviors, and therapist use of specific techniques. Five constructs of behavior were evaluated: change talk/intention, readiness to change, involvement/engagement, resistance, and the client's experience of discrepancy. The most consistent evidence was found for three constructs: client change talk/intention (Moyers et al. 2007) and client experience of discrepancy (both related to better outcomes) and therapist MI-inconsistent behavior (related to worse outcomes). Regarding use of specific techniques, use of a decisional balance exercise showed the strongest association with better outcomes. Another study noted that overall MI spirit might be more important than particular MI techniques (Gaume et al. 2009). In fact, a recent systemic review found MI spirit and motivation to be the most promising MOBCs in MI interventions (Copeland et al. 2015).

While most studies label their intervention as MI, many of these interventions are more properly called *motivational enhancement therapy.* MET is a variation on MI that is commonly used in both clinical practice and clinical research (Miller et al. 1995), especially with adolescents. Although MI and MET share the same principles and core techniques, they differ in that MET is more structured and typically includes techniques that are specifically used to enhance motivation to change, such as a decisional balance and personalized feedback. Table 13–1 contains a transcript contrasting a directive approach with a MET approach.

Evidence for BMI With Adolescents

There is a growing evidence base for BMIs with adolescents who use alcohol and/or other drugs. In the review that follows, we typically refer to MI as the intervention because the interventions are reported as such by the authors, but many are better described as MET.

A meta-analysis by Tanner-Smith and Lipsey (2015) found that alcohol BMIs with adolescents led to significant reductions in alcohol use and alcohol-related problems, and that the effects were maintained for up to 1 year postintervention. The authors found decisional balance and goal-setting exercises to be particularly helpful components of these brief interventions. Another meta-analysis of 21 studies of MI for adolescent substance use found small but significant effect sizes that retained their effect over time (Jensen et al. 2011). These findings were supported by Hogue et al.'s (2018) review of outpatient behavioral treatment, which categorized MI interventions as probably efficacious. A review by Barnett et al. (2012) found that while there was no difference between telephone or in-person follow-ups, providing feedback face-to-

Table 13–1.   A transcript with "Tim" contrasting a directive approach with a motivational enhancement therapy (MET) approach

Assessment using directive approach	Assessment using MET approach	MET technique
Therapist: Tell me about your drug problem.	What brings you here today?	Active listening Empathy
Tim: I don't have a drug problem.	I'm only here because my Dad made me come.	
Therapist: What do you mean you do not have a drug problem?	Tell me more about that.	Roll with resistance Maintain empathy
Tim: I use drugs, no problem....	My Dad thinks that I have a drug problem.	
Therapist: I have reliable information in this chart about your use.	Care to tell me why he thinks so?	Begin to develop discrepancy between Tim's understanding of his substance use disorder and the concerns of others who care for him
Tim: You sound like my Dad or a probation officer.	I've been using and it kinda got me in trouble a couple of times.	
Therapist: Sounds like you are in denial of your drug use and consequences. We need to work on changing your negative attitude, otherwise you could be in trouble.	Sounds as if you went through some difficulties.	Active listening Empathy Develop discrepancy
Tim: [*Goes silent*] I don't want to work with you.	I got problems in school and with the police. I don't see how coming to a place like this is gonna be helpful with that.	

Table 13–1.   A transcript with "Tim" contrasting a directive
approach with a motivational enhancement therapy
(MET) approach *(continued)*

Assessment using directive approach	Assessment using MET approach	MET technique
Therapist: I have a lot of experience working with teenagers like you and I want to help you. However, you have to listen to me in order to make some changes in order not to ruin your life.	I appreciate your honesty. I am glad that we have an opportunity to talk. If you want we can meet several times and work together to solve these problems. Shall we schedule a meeting to continue?	Roll with resistance Support self-efficacy Continue to identify opportunities to highlight discrepancy
Tim: I don't need this lecture. I'm outta here.	Well, OK.	

face was superior to computerized feedback, and involving parents improved results.

BMIs have demonstrated an effect on reducing cannabis use (McCambridge and Strang 2004), with studies maintaining effects at 6- and 12-month follow-up (Walker et al. 2011). A review of BMI for adolescent smoking cessation found a small but significant increase in quitting use of tobacco (Lindson-Hawley et al. 2015).

BMI for Adolescents in the Emergency Department

Health care settings provide a unique opportunity to reach adolescents and are conducive to providing initial services for substance misuse and referral for additional treatment as needed. One reason to conduct interventions in medical settings such as the emergency department (ED) is to capitalize on a "teachable moment" or a possible "window of opportunity" (Tevyaw and Monti 2004). The salience of an alcohol-related event may increase the adolescent's sense of vulnerability and thereby increase receptivity to an intervention. MI is particularly suitable for use in an ED because of its brevity and its fit with the "teachable moment" perspective. A recent meta-analysis of six BMI trials delivered in ED settings found that drinking frequency and quantity decreased significantly more among adolescents receiving MI versus a control condition (Kohler and Hofmann 2015).

Monti and colleagues (1999) evaluated the use of an MI approach to reduce alcohol-related use and negative consequences among 18- and 19-year-old adolescents treated in an urban hospital ED. Ninety-four adolescents who were being treated in the ED for an alcohol-related event were randomly assigned to receive either a 40-minute MI intervention or a 5-minute "standard care" intervention (i.e., receiving a handout on avoiding drinking and driving and a substance treatment referral list). At the 6-month follow-up assessment, participants who were randomly assigned to the MI condition were more likely to show decreased drinking and driving, traffic violations, and alcohol-related problems than those in the standard care condition. In a related study, the same brief MI intervention was conducted with 152 younger adolescents (ages 13–17 years) treated in the same ED (Spirito et al. 2004). Both the MI and standard care conditions resulted in reduced quantity of drinking during the 12 months of follow-up, while alcohol-related negative consequences were relatively low and stayed low at follow-up in both groups. However, adolescents who screened positive for problematic alcohol use at the baseline assessment in the ED reported significantly more improvement on average number of drinking days per month and frequency of high-volume drinking if they received MI compared with standard care.

In a follow-up study, this research group later tested the effects of a combined parent and adolescent BMI among a sample of families of adolescents (ages 13–17) treated in an urban ED for an alcohol-related event. Participants were randomly assigned to receive either an individual adolescent BMI only or the individual adolescent BMI plus a parent BMI, based on the Family Check-Up (FCU; Dishion and Stormshak 2007; Dishion et al. 2003). Both groups had reduced alcohol and marijuana use over the 12-month follow-up. Notably, the strongest intervention effects were present at 3 and 6 months for both groups, and the combined adolescent and parent BMI was associated with fewer high-volume drinking days at 3 months than the individual BMI (Spirito et al. 2011).

The BMI (Spirito et al. 2011), described in greater detail below, consisted of the following components: establishing rapport, assessing drinking behavior, exploring motivation to change, providing motivational enhancement with personalized feedback, establishing a change plan, anticipating barriers to change, and enhancing coping self-efficacy. These components are common to BMI programs conducted in other settings as well, such as schools and pediatric clinics (see Chapter 4).

Establishing Rapport

The MET session is introduced as an opportunity to talk about thoughts and feelings regarding the event that resulted in the ED visit, to reflect on drinking and its effects, and to spend some time talking about ways to avoid similar events in the future. Clinicians emphasize that they will not tell the adolescent what to do but that it is up to the adolescent to make his or her own choices about drinking. The circumstances that precipitated the ED visit are then reviewed, including how much the adolescent had been drinking, whom he or she was with, and any injuries sustained or negative consequences suffered.

Open-ended questions are used as the primary means to develop rapport and minimize defensiveness in order to encourage the adolescent to discuss recent drinking. The clinician uses an MI style (Miller and Rollnick 2012) to present as empathic and concerned with a nonauthoritarian and nonjudgmental stance. It is important for the clinician to be respectful of the adolescent's ideas, to appear interested in hearing about the adolescent's experiences, and to avoid disapproving statements about any behavior.

Assessing Drinking Behavior

The assessment is used to provide personalized feedback during the MET session. Measures are administered after the basic structure of the MET session has been described to the adolescent. It is important to choose assessments that provide adolescents with a perspective on how they compare on their drinking behaviors (frequency and quantity) to others of the same gender and age. In order to provide such normative information, it is necessary to use measures that have age and gender norms available, such as local and national data provided by the Monitoring the Future survey (www.monitoringthefuture.org) and the Youth Risk Behavior Survey (www.cdc.gov/healthyyouth/data/yrbs/data.htm).

Exploring Motivation to Change

Once the assessment is complete, the adolescent is asked what he or she likes and does not like about drinking. Open-ended questions and reflective listening statements are used to help the adolescent generate as many likes and dislikes (i.e., pros and cons) as possible. The adolescent is always asked first about positive aspects of drinking (e.g., less anxious in social situations). The adolescent is also asked to elaborate on potential negative effects of such risk behaviors, including the worst thing he or she could imagine happening. The adolescent is asked to elaborate on his or her parents' and friends' attitudes toward drinking and engaging in risky behavior while drinking. This discussion is followed by inquiring about how such attitudes might affect the youth's drinking behaviors.

There are several goals of this section of the MET session. First, the clinician tries to gain an understanding of how the adolescent weighs the positive and negative aspects of drinking. By listing pros and cons, the clinician and adolescent can develop a shared understanding of positive reinforcers for drinking as well as the adolescent's perceived negative consequences of drinking. The clinician can then tailor the MET to these personalized pros and cons, while keeping in mind the adolescent's stage of readiness for changing drinking behavior. At the end of this discussion, the clinician should be able to identify peer and parental behavior and attitudes that influence the adolescent's behavior.

Providing Motivational Enhancement With Personalized Feedback

The purpose of this part of MET is to enhance the adolescent's understanding of his or her alcohol use, to provide information about any signs of problem drinking, and to encourage the adolescent in making positive changes to reduce hazardous drinking behavior. This can be done in three ways.

First, the clinician can provide personalized feedback from the assessment battery, including interpretation of the adolescent's drinking compared with age and gender norms. Age- and gender-based normative information can be provided in the form of percentile ranks in graphs and pie charts. Frequency of high-volume drinking, alcohol-related problems, and examples of risk taking related to alcohol use can also be summarized. The clinician decides what portions of the feedback to emphasize. Then, the adolescent is asked what he or she was most surprised by and what was most upsetting. The clinician needs to make sure that the adolescent interprets the meaning of the feedback correctly. For example, teens with relatively benign profiles can be encouraged to consider changes in behavior that might further limit future risk.

Second, the clinician can provide information about alcohol's effects on adolescents in general, such as how it impairs judgment. When relevant, information about blood alcohol concentration (BAC) level and alcohol's effects on driving and other behaviors can be provided. Adolescents who are tested for their BAC upon admission to the ED are typically interested in learning their BAC level. They also are usually receptive to facts about the effects of alcohol at different BAC levels. The fact that even low levels of alcohol can impair driving is often a surprise to adolescents.

Finally, the clinician can enhance motivation by asking the adolescent to imagine the future if his or her drinking were to remain the same, or if it were to change. If there is a discrepancy between an adolescent's current drinking pattern and goals for the future, it is highlighted in order to enhance motivation to change. Some areas to introduce are the possible reactions of family and friends to this behavioral change. Prompts might include, "What would be different [easier, harder] if you were to change your drinking?"

Establishing a Change Plan

The teen's interest in changing by establishing a plan and committing to one should be assessed. We use open-ended questions such as "What, if anything, would you like to change?" If the adolescent is able to generate appropriate ways to reduce drinking, the clinician's task is to help him or her address potential barriers to implementation of these strategies. However, adolescents are often vague about what they will do differently, and the clinician must then help them develop a list of specific strategies. For example, an adolescent might say, "I'll just cut down on my drinking." The clinician's task in this case would be to help the adolescent specify a reduction goal that would lower the adolescent's risk. Open-ended exploration questions such as "Tell me how you might cut down" are preferred. If such an approach is not successful, a more direct response would be, "If you were to have no more than one drink an hour, your blood alcohol level would stay fairly low, although it would still put you at risk. Would that be a reasonable goal?"

Developing a plan with adolescents who are not interested in making changes in their drinking is difficult. Focusing on potentially harmful behaviors, rather than alcohol consumption per se, might be a productive approach in this situation. In other cases, an adolescent may be willing to keep track of drinking, using self-monitoring procedures. This is still a useful goal because it may increase the adolescent's awareness of his or her drinking, especially problematic drinking.

Goal setting is most successful when goals are personalized and simple and include a timeline. A list of goals and target dates should be given to the adolescent at the session. Specific and clear behavior change strategies should be listed (e.g., "After having an alcoholic drink I will have a nonalcoholic drink," "I won't 'chug' or 'shotgun' drinks"). If the adolescent is unable to generate options, examples of things that other adolescents have tried can be supplied. A variety of change strategies should be introduced so that the adolescent will be exposed to strategies he or she might not have envisioned but might be interested in trying.

Anticipating Barriers to Change

In working on a behavior change plan, the clinician should help the adolescent imagine how the change strategies might, or might not, work. For example, the clinician could ask how the adolescent imagines friends will react to the adolescent's decision to limit the number of drinks consumed on weekends. Asking the adolescent to anticipate what might be difficult about carrying out such a plan helps identify ways to handle barriers to implementation, and to develop further strategies to ensure success. This process may help to enhance self-efficacy.

Enhancing Coping Self-Efficacy

Coping self-efficacy has been found to increase the probability that one will resist urges and pressures to relapse. Therefore, the clinician's final task is to enhance the adolescent's sense that he or she can effectively make changes. This can be done by making supportive statements about the adolescent's strengths to successfully carry out the change plan.

* * *

In sum, BMI may be a treatment option because it can be delivered effectively in a relatively brief period and is flexible enough to be applied to individuals who demonstrate a wide range of readiness to change (Tevyaw and Monti 2004). Clinicians and researchers have noted the difficulty in retaining adolescents in treatment. Engaging adolescents in treatment has been challenging. Many adolescents have explicitly or implicitly been coerced into attending treatment, such as by being excluded from the decision-making process about seeking treatment, having treatment imposed on them, and being subject to restraints to retain them in treatment (Bonnie and Monahan 2005). Coercive pressure to seek and continue treatment is not conducive to the behavior change process. Although a BMI may not be sufficient as a standalone treatment, it can be successful when front-loaded onto adolescent treatments, such as CBT, because of its ability to increase readiness and motivation to change.

Cognitive-Behavioral Therapy

CBT approaches integrate strategies derived from classical conditioning, operant, and social learning perspectives. Experimental research within each theoretical perspective has focused on unique aspects of substance use behavior, resulting in the development of distinct intervention techniques that are often combined into a multicomponent cognitive-behavioral intervention. Operant perspectives view substance misuse as a behavior that follows an antecedent (i.e., a trigger) that may lead to negative consequences. A functional analysis is conducted with the patient in order to identify contextual factors, such as settings, situations, or states, that may serve as potential triggers for abuse (Witkiewitz and Marlatt 2004). Intervention strategies based on operant learning often include identifying alternative reinforcers that compete with substance use. The social learning model incorporates the influence of environmental events on the acquisition of behavior, but also recognizes the role of cognitive processes in determining behavior (Bandura 1986). Therapists should take into account the developmental level of the adolescent when using CBT approaches. In addition, adolescents who have a history of heavy substance use may not have had sufficient opportunity to acquire alternative social and coping skills normally developed during adolescence, and skills training may need to be incorporated into CBT protocols.

The most prominent active ingredients of CBT for substance use are coping skills training and approaches that increase the adolescent's self-efficacy to abstain from substances (Black and Chung 2014). CBT sessions characteristically include modeling, behavior rehearsal, feedback, and homework assignments to practice skills taught in session. Studies focused on the hypothesized mechanisms of change underlying CBT have found some core components that promote change in substance use. Coping with situations that might trigger a relapse has been identified as a significant predictor of treatment outcome (Myers et al. 1993). Wishful thinking and social support were found to contribute significantly to prediction of total days using substances and length of initial abstinence, respectively, highlighting the importance of positivity and utilizing social resources (Myers et al. 1993). Self-efficacy to resist alcohol or substance use was found to predict subsequent abstinence among adolescents in treatment (Burleson and Kaminer 2005). A comprehensive review found that CBT and MI share some core mechanisms of change for substance use, including having a supportive therapeutic and/or other relationship, increasing motivation to reduce substance use, improving coping skills, increasing self-efficacy to reduce use, and improving affect regulation (Black and Chung 2014).

Evidence for CBT With Adolescents

Recent adolescent substance use treatment studies have employed more rigorous designs, larger samples, random assignment, direct comparisons of two or more active treatments, improved measures of substance use and other variables, manual-guided interventions, and longer-term outcome assessments, adding significantly to the empirical support for CBT (Waldron and Turner 2008). In a recent update of the evidence base for outpatient behavioral treatments, Hogue et al. (2018) found individual and group CBT to remain well-established stand-alone approaches. Notably, some research indicates that BMIs can be effective when delivered as a precursor to CBT, suggesting that the combination of motivational interventions and CBT may be more effective than MI/MET as a stand-alone approach (Hogue et al. 2014).

A combined MI/MET + CBT protocol was used in the Cannabis Youth Treatment (CYT) study, a randomized field trial involving 600 adolescents that compared five interventions, in various combinations, across four sites (Dennis et al. 2004). The study was designed to address the differential efficacy of the treatments implemented and the effect of treatment dose on outcome. Two group CBT interventions were offered. Both began with 2 individual MET sessions, followed by either 3 CBT sessions (MET/CBT-5; Sampl and Kadden 2001) or 10 CBT sessions (MET/CBT-5 + CBT-7; Webb et al. 2002). A third intervention represented a family-based add-on intervention involving MET/CBT-5 + CBT-7 plus a 6-week family psychoeducational intervention (Hamilton et al. 2001). In addition, a 12-session individual Adolescent Community Reinforcement Approach (Godley et al. 2001) and a 12-week multidimensional family therapy condition (Liddle 2002) were included. All five interventions produced similarly significant reductions in cannabis use and negative consequences of use from pretreatment to the 3-month follow-up, and these reductions were sustained through the 12-month follow-up. Changes in marijuana use were accompanied by short-term reductions in behavioral problems, family problems, school problems, school absences, argumentativeness, violence, and illegal activity. The best predictor of long-term outcomes was initial level of change.

Treatment Modality: Group Versus Individual Intervention

This consistent empirical support of group CBT for adolescent substance use (Burleson et al. 2006) stands in contrast to the iatrogenic "deviant" peer-group effects reported in some studies for group interventions (see, e.g., Dodge et al. 2006). Neither the CYT study group, in its interventions, nor other studies in outpatient settings that included a significant percentage of adolescents with conduct disorders have experienced any severe or unmanageable problems conducting group therapy (e.g., need to eject subjects, discontinuation of a session, physical abuse). In most situations, diverse referral sources allow for a mix of adolescents who are manageable in a group setting by an experienced therapist once a clearly communicated behavioral contract for ground rules is introduced.

Contingency Management Reinforcement Approach

Most adolescent studies have not shown any long-term benefit of one treatment modality over another (Hogue et al. 2018; Waldron and Turner 2008). There are small sustained benefits in substance use outcomes across all interventions. CM reinforcement procedures have traditionally provided rewards for clean (i.e., negative) urinalysis. Drug abstinence can be improved by providing tangible incentives that are contingent on providing objective evidence of abstinence. An abstinence reinforcement system used in combination with an intensive behavioral treatment program has produced impressive outcomes in adult substance abusers (Higgins et al. 1994; Stitzer and Petry 2015). CM treatment is based on the scientific principles and conceptual framework of behavior analysis and behavioral pharmacology. In that framework, the use of abused drugs is considered a special case of operant behavior maintained by the reinforcing effects of the drugs involved. Higgins and colleagues (1994) have stressed the following core strengths of CM: 1) conceptual clarity, 2) empiricism and operationism, 3) compatibility with pharmacotherapies, 4) clinical breadth, and 5) demonstrable efficacy.

The strategy employed in CM is to rearrange the substance user's environment so that drug use and abstinence are readily detected, drug abstinence is positively reinforced, drug use results in an immediate loss of reinforcement, and the density of reinforcement derived from nondrug sources is increased to compete with the reinforcing effects of drugs.

Controlled clinical research has demonstrated the efficacy of CM in laboratory animals and adults with different substances of abuse. In addition to the obvious need to reduce or eliminate drug use, other behaviors to reinforce may also include attendance, compliance with treatment plan, and changes in behaviors or lifestyle that may facilitate abstinence (Stitzer and Petry 2015). A treatment regimen based on CM procedures has shown excellent feasibility. It is highly acceptable to patients; the vast majority of individuals who have been offered the treatment have accepted. Treatment acceptability is very important, in particular among individuals with SUDs, who are often unmotivated for initiation and/or maintenance of treatment. It is noteworthy that marijuana use (the most commonly abused drug in adolescence) is readily modifiable via a direct CM intervention, although such changes appear to dissipate when the contingency is removed (Stanger et al. 2016). CM procedures can use a variety of reinforcers, many of which are commonly used in, or readily adaptable to, standard clinic settings for adolescents. These include cash, vouchers, and on-site retail items.

Although CM research in youth has lagged behind that of adults, data have been accumulating supporting its effectiveness for various objectives, as reviewed by Randall (2017) and Stanger et al. (2016). In addition to abstinence, these objectives include retention in treatment and/or promotion of healthy lifestyle and activities. These CM interventions have shown strong effects when they are used to supplement other evidence-based strategies in youth, such as CBT (Stanger et al. 2015), multisystemic therapy (Henggeler et al.

2012) and Adolescent Community Reinforcement Approach (Godley et al. 2014). Studies show that keeping youth engaged for longer durations increases the likelihood that therapeutic exposure is efficacious. Therefore, the addition of a CM protocol is intended to improve retention rates. Employing low-cost CM has been shown to increase attendance in community adolescent SUD treatment programs (Branson et al. 2012). Furthermore, increased clinical billing by the increased attendance may exceed the costs of implementing low-cost CM program and diminish concerns and objections regarding dissemination (Lott and Jencius 2009). Consequently, bias and concerns about feasibility and costs should not be considered as valid barriers (Stanger et al. 2016). From results of studies employing adaptive treatment for poor responders, it was concluded that the addition of incentives in the form of CM for improved retention and/or abstinence is warranted (see Chapter 12).

Practical Implications

Petry (2000) and Stanger et al. (2016) recommend the following when CM procedures are being designed and implemented:

1. Target the most important behavior to be changed, and choose one that can be quantified objectively and occurs frequently, such us marijuana abstinence or treatment attendance.
2. Choose a reinforcer and specify magnitude. Vouchers, cash, and prizes are desirable reinforcers by clients and agreeable to staff.
3. Utilize behavioral principles and keep them simple so that staff can apply the system consistently and clients can understand it.
4. Draw up a time-limited behavioral contract. Be specific regarding the targeted behavior, monitoring procedures (e.g., drug urinalysis), and reinforcement schedule.
5. Ensure the consistent implementation of the contract by staff and clients.
6. Keep on improving the CM procedures by keeping records, consulting with staff, and receiving feedback from clients regarding problems in the implementation process and what does or does not work.

An example for the development of a new CM-based approach for interventions targeting adolescent SUD is home-based incentives involving parents

(Stanger et al. 2015). Combined clinic- and home-based incentives for cannabis abstinence, when added to MET/CBT-5 + CBT-7, consistently increased rates of abstinence during treatment among teens. Home-based CM involves teaching parents to develop and use a substance monitoring contract (SMC) that specifies positive and negative consequences to be implemented weekly in response to abstinence or substance use. The first two sessions review the structure of the contract and how to select rewards and consequences. The adolescent's input on selecting rewards is solicited during individual sessions with the therapist. At session 3, the contract is implemented; abstinence is determined based on the criteria outlined above. The delay to week 3 in implementing the home-based contract provides additional time for the teen to achieve abstinence before the contract, which includes both incentives and consequences, begins. Subsequent parent sessions focus on adherence to the SMC, evaluation of its impact, and modifications as necessary. More than half (56%) of youth cannabis users who received CM were abstinent at the end of treatment compared with 33% who received MET/CBT-5 + CBT-7 only (Stanger et al. 2015).

Training protocols for CM implementations are available (Litt et al. 2008). Competence of CM implementation can be measured with the Contingency Management Competence Scale (Petry et al. 2010). As an alternative to the traditional low- or high-cost CM using vouchers as incentives for adults, a feasible, low-cost CM procedure known as the "fishbowl-drawing procedure" was developed by Petry and Martin (2002). It was successfully utilized with adolescent substance abusers (Branson et al. 2012; Godley et al. 2014). For example, the drawing bowl may contain 50 slips of paper, all of which will be "winning" slips: 39 will be worth $1; 10 slips will be worth $10, and 1 of the 50 slips will be a "big prize" worth $20 or more. Patients in CM conditions who attend a treatment session or are abstinent (based on the objective of the incentives program) will earn the opportunity to draw from the fishbowl and will continue to earn extra draws for each consecutive week they attend treatment or are abstinent. If a session is missed or the person has been using drugs (as reported by the person or as a result of a positive urinalysis), that person will return to one draw for the next session when the objective was achieved, but may return to the prior level achieved after two consecutive successful sessions. Payments can be made in a variety of ways, including remotely by staff on reloadable credit cards.

Challenges and Limitations

One of the obvious limitations has been that once the CM procedure has been completed, treatment gains and overall differences between treatment conditions are not maintained across follow-ups (Stanger et al. 2016). Other barriers to implementation include lack of sufficient training and lack of incentives to implement CM with fidelity (Randall 2017). Furthermore, negative clinician and administrator attitudes regarding CM efficacy due mainly to ideological differences (e.g., "Why pay a patient to remain abstinent?") can play a role. Public opinion may be opposed to such procedures, even if efficacious, because of concerns regarding the likelihood of patients to purchase drugs. However, these rewards are too little to maintain a "drug habit," and the frequent monitoring of urine for drugs precludes the possibility of continued use without detection. These barriers should be addressed by improved education and dissemination of knowledge about CM implementation protocols and the advantages of this strategy. In addition, cost-effectiveness analysis should be examined comparing low and high costs of CM protocols in order to optimize implementation by utilizing resources adequately.

Key Points

- The theoretical basis of brief motivational interventions is grounded in client-centered therapy.

- The purported mechanisms of action, or mediators, in cognitive-behavioral therapy (CBT) include self-efficacy and behavioral skills.

- The consistent empirical support of group CBT for substance-abusing adolescents and possible iatrogenic "deviant" peer-group effects can be managed by experienced therapists in group interventions.

- Contingency management reinforcement interventions have shown strong effects when used to supplement other evidence-based strategies in youth.

- Little evidence is available to suggest that one therapy is more effective than another therapy. Even less is known about what therapy works for different subpopulations, including ethnic or cultural groups.

References

Apodaca TR, Longabaugh R: Mechanisms of change in motivational interviewing: a review and preliminary evaluation of the evidence. Addiction 104(5):705–715, 2009 19413785

Bandura A: Social Learning Theory. Englewood Cliffs, NJ, Prentice Hall, 1977

Bandura A: Social Foundations of Thought and Action: A Social Cognitive Theory. Englewood Cliffs, NJ, Prentice Hall, 1986

Barnett E, Sussman S, Smith C, et al: Motivational interviewing for adolescent substance use: a review of the literature. Addict Behav 37(12):1325–1334, 2012 22958865

Black JJ, Chung T: Mechanisms of change in adolescent substance use treatment: how does treatment work? Subst Abus 35(4):344–351, 2014 24901750

Bonnie RJ, Monahan J: From coercion to contract: reframing the debate on mandated community treatment for people with mental disorders. Law Hum Behav 29(4):485–503, 2005 16133951

Branson CE, Barbuti AM, Clemmey P, et al: A pilot study of low-cost contingency management to increase attendance in an adolescent substance abuse program. Am J Addict 21(2):126–129, 2012 22332855

Burleson JA, Kaminer Y: Self-efficacy as a predictor of treatment outcome in adolescent substance use disorders. Addict Behav 30(9):1751–1764, 2005 16095844

Burleson JA, Kaminer Y, Dennis ML: Absence of iatrogenic or contagion effects in adolescent group therapy: findings from the Cannabis Youth Treatment (CYT) study. Am J Addict 15 (suppl 1):4–15, 2006 17182415

Copeland L, McNamara R, Kelson M, et al: Mechanisms of change within motivational interviewing in relation to health behaviors outcomes: a systematic review. Patient Educ Couns 98(4):401–411, 2015 25535015

Dennis M, Godley SH, Diamond G, et al: The Cannabis Youth Treatment (CYT) Study: main findings from two randomized trials. J Subst Abuse Treat 27(3):197–213, 2004 15501373

Dishion TJ, Stormshak E: Intervening in Children's Lives: An Ecological, Family-Centered Approach to Mental Health care. Washington, DC, American Psychological Association, 2007

Dishion TJ, Nelson SE, Kavanagh K: The Family Check-Up with high-risk young adolescents: preventing early onset substance use by parent monitoring. Behavior Therapy 34(4):553–571, 2003

Dodge KA, Dishion TJ, Lansford JE: Deviant Peer Influences in Programs for Youth: Problems and Solutions. New York, Guilford, 2006

Gaume J, Gmel G, Faouzi M, et al: Counselor skill influences outcomes of brief motivational interventions. J Subst Abuse Treat 37(2):151–159, 2009 19339147

Godley MD, Godley SH, Dennis ML, et al: A randomized trial of assertive continuing care and contingency management for adolescents with substance use disorders. J Consult Clin Psychol 82(1):40–51, 2014 24294838

Godley SH, Meyers RJ, Smith JE, et al: Adolescent Community Reinforcement Approach (ACRA) for Adolescent Cannabis Users: Cannabis Youth Treatment (CYT) Manual Series, Vol 4. Rockville, MD, Center for Substance Abuse Treatment, Substance Abuse and Mental Health Services Administration, 2001

Hamilton N, Brantly L, Tims F, et al: Family Support Network (FSN) for Adolescent Cannabis Users. Substance Abuse and Mental Health Services Administration; Cannabis Youth Treatment (CYT) Manual Series, Vol 4. Rockville, MD, Center for Substance Abuse, 2002

Henggeler SW, McCartMR, Cunningham PB, Chapman JE: Enhancing the effectiveness of juvenile drug courts by integrating evidence-based practices. J Consult Clin Psychol 80(2):264–275, 2012 22309470

Higgins ST, Budney AJ, Bickel WK: Applying behavioral concepts and principles to the treatment of cocaine dependence. Drug Alcohol Depend 34(2):87–97, 1994 8026305

Hill KG, White HR, Chung IJ, et al: Early adult outcomes of adolescent binge drinking: person- and variable-centered analyses of binge drinking trajectories. Alcohol Clin Exp Res 24(6):892–901, 2000 10888080

Hogue A, Henderson CE, Ozechowski TJ, Robbins MS: Evidence base on outpatient behavioral treatments for adolescent substance use: updates and recommendations 2007–2013. J Clin Child Adolesc Psychol 43(5):695–720, 2014 24926870

Hogue A, Henderson CE, Becker SJ, et al: Evidence base on outpatient behavioral treatments for adolescent substance use, 2014–2017: outcomes, treatment delivery, and promising horizons. J Clin Child Adolesc Psychol 47(4):499–526, 2018 29893607

Jensen CD, Cushing CC, Aylward BS, et al: Effectiveness of motivational interviewing interventions for adolescent substance use behavior change: a meta-analytic review. J Consult Clin Psychol 79(4):433–440, 2011 21728400

Kohler S, Hofmann A: Can motivational interviewing in emergency care reduce alcohol consumption in young people? A systematic review and meta-analysis. Alcohol Alcohol 50(2):107–117, 2015 25563299

Liddle HA: Multidimensional Family Therapy for Adolescent Cannabis Users. Cannabis Youth Treatment (CYT) Manual Series, Vol 5 (DHHS Publ No SMA 02-3660). Rockville, MD, Center for Substance Abuse, 2002

Lindson-Hawley N, Thompson TP, Begh R: Motivational interviewing for smoking cessation. Cochrane Database Syst Rev (3):CD006936, 2015 25726920

Litt MD, Kadden RM, Kabela-Cormier E, Petry NM: Coping skills training and contingency management treatments for marijuana dependence: exploring mechanisms of behavior change. Addiction 103(4):638–648, 2008 18339108

Lott DC, Jencius S: Effectiveness of very low-cost contingency management in a community adolescent treatment program. Drug Alcohol Depend 102(1–3):162–165, 2009 19250774

Marlatt GA, Gordon JR: Relapse Prevention: Maintenance Strategies in the Treatment of Addictive Behaviors. New York, Guilford, 1985

McCambridge J, Strang J: The efficacy of single-session motivational interviewing in reducing drug consumption and perceptions of drug-related risk and harm among young people: results from a multi-site cluster randomized trial. Addiction 99(1):39–52, 2004 14678061

Miller WR, Rollnick S: Motivational Interviewing: Preparing People for Change, 3rd Edition. New York, Guilford, 2012

Miller WR, Rose GS: Motivational interviewing and decisional balance: contrasting responses to client ambivalence. Behav Cogn Psychother 43(2):129–141, 2015 24229732

Miller WR, Zweben A, DiClemente CC, et al: Motivational Enhancement Therapy Manual: A Clinical Research Guide for Therapists Treating Individuals With Alcohol Abuse and Dependence. Rockville, MD, National Institute on Alcohol Abuse and Alcoholism, 1995

Monti PM, Colby SM, Barnett NP, et al: Brief intervention for harm reduction with alcohol-positive older adolescents in a hospital emergency department. J Consult Clin Psychol 67(6):989–994, 1999 10596521

Moyers TB, Martin T, Christopher PJ, et al: Client language as a mediator of motivational interviewing efficacy: where is the evidence? Alcohol Clin Exp Res 31 (10, suppl):40s–47s, 2007 17880345

Myers MG, Brown SA, Mott MA: Coping as a predictor of adolescent substance abuse treatment outcome. J Subst Abuse 5(1):15–29, 1993 8329878

Petry NM: A comprehensive guide to the application of contingency management procedures in clinical settings. Drug Alcohol Depend 58(1–2):9–25, 2000 10669051

Petry NM, Martin B: Low-cost contingency management for treating cocaine- and opioid-abusing methadone patients. J Consult Clin Psychol 70(2):398–405, 2002 11952198

Petry NM, Alessi SM, Ledgerwood DM, et al: Psychometric properties of the Contingency Management Competence Scale. Drug Alcohol Depend 109(1–3):167–174, 2010 20149950

Prochaska JO, DiClemente CC, Norcross JC: In search of how people change. Applications to addictive behaviors. Am Psychol 47(9):1102–1114, 1992 1329589

Randall J: Challenges and possible solutions for implementing contingency management for adolescent substance use disorder in community-based settings. J Child Adolesc Subst Abuse 26(4):332–337, 2017

Rogers CR: The necessary and sufficient conditions of therapeutic personality change. J Consult Psychol 21(2):95–103, 1957 13416422

Sampl S, Kadden R: Motivational Enhancement Therapy and Cognitive Behavioral Therapy for Adolescent Cannabis Users: 5 Sessions. Cannabis Youth Treatment Series, Vol 1 (DHHS Publ No SMA 01-3486). Rockville, MD, Center for Substance Abuse Treatment, Substance Abuse and Mental Health Services Administration, 2001

Spirito A, Monti PM, Barnett NP, et al: A randomized clinical trial of a brief motivational intervention for alcohol-positive adolescents treated in an emergency department. J Pediatr 145(3):396–402, 2004 15343198

Spirito A, Sindelar-Manning H, Colby SM, et al: Individual and family motivational interventions for alcohol-positive adolescents treated in an emergency department: results of a randomized clinical trial. Arch Pediatr Adolesc Med 165(3):269–274, 2011 21383276

Stanger C, Ryan SR, Scherer EA, et al: Clinic- and home-based contingency management plus parent training for adolescent cannabis use disorders. J Am Acad Child Adolesc Psychiatry 54(6):445.e2–453.e2, 2015 26004659

Stanger C, Lansing AH, Budney AJ: Advances in research on contingency management for adolescent substance use. Child Adolesc Psychiatr Clin N Am 25(4):645–659, 2016 27613343

Stitzer M, Petry N: Contingency management, in The American Publishing Textbook of Substance Abuse Treatment, 5th Edition. Edited by Galanter M, Brady KT. Arlington, VA, American Psychiatric Publishing, 2015, pp 423–439

Tanner-Smith EE, Lipsey MW: Brief alcohol interventions for adolescents and young adults: a systematic review and meta-analysis. J Subst Abuse Treat 51:1–18, 2015 25300577

Tevyaw TO, Monti PM: Motivational enhancement and other brief interventions for adolescent substance abuse: foundations, applications and evaluations. Addiction 99 (suppl 2):63–75, 2004 15488106

Waldron HB, Turner CW: Evidence-based psychosocial treatments for adolescent substance abuse. J Clin Child Adolesc Psychol 37(1):238–261, 2008 18444060

Walker DD, Stephens R, Roffman R, et al: Randomized controlled trial of motivational enhancement therapy with nontreatment-seeking adolescent cannabis users: a further test of the teen marijuana check-up. Psychol Addict Behav 25(3):474–484, 2011 21688877

Webb C, Scudder M, Kaminer Y, et al: The Motivational Enhancement Therapy and Cognitive Behavioral Therapy Supplement: 7 Sessions of Cognitive Behavioral Therapy for Adolescent Cannabis Users. Cannabis Youth Treatment Series, Vol 2 (DHHS Publ No SMA 02-659). Rockville, MD, Center for Substance Abuse Treatment, Substance Abuse and Mental Health Services Administration, 2002

Witkiewitz K, Marlatt GA: Relapse prevention for alcohol and drug problems: that was Zen, this is Tao. Am Psychol 59(4):224–235, 2004 15149263

14

Family and Community-Based Therapies

Molly Bobek, L.C.S.W.

Susan H. Godley, Rh.D.

Aaron Hogue, Ph.D.

In this chapter we summarize the evidence base on family therapy and Adolescent Community Reinforcement Approach (A-CRA), a multicomponent treatment for adolescent substance use (ASU). Family therapy and multicomponent treatments both prioritize the value of a fundamentally multidimensional strategy to treating ASU. Family therapy is a multisystem approach that predominantly targets family factors and other key influences in a given adolescent's developmental ecosystem (e.g., peer, school, juvenile justice factors). Multicomponent treatments contain two or more ASU intervention approaches that collectively target several aspects of adolescent functioning, often including family factors and other ecosystem influences. We conclude the chapter with several brief clinical guidelines that are intended to support and encourage therapists in delivering these complex but potent interventions in everyday practice.

Family Therapy

Family therapy is an evidence-based approach to treating ASU that focuses on promoting developmentally calibrated parenting strategies, intervening directly with family members to repair and bolster intrafamilial relationships, and addressing challenges encountered by adolescents and caregivers in key extrafamilial systems. A recent comprehensive review of the evidence base for ASU outpatient treatment determined that the family therapy approach has achieved the highest level of empirical support (Hogue et al. 2018). Family therapy also has the highest level of support for treating adolescent disruptive behaviors that commonly co-occur with ASU, such as oppositional behavior, conduct disorder, and delinquency (McCart and Sheidow 2016). Studies of family therapy for ASU also frequently report significant reductions in internalizing symptoms and gains in prosocial functioning (Hogue and Liddle 2009). Family therapy is particularly effective at promoting treatment attendance and therapeutic alliance, whereas other ASU treatment approaches show mixed success in this light (Hogue et al. 2018).

Within the broader family therapy approach there exists a handful of "brand name," manualized family therapy models specifically designed to treat ASU. Two of these manualized models—functional family therapy (FFT) and multidimensional family therapy (MDFT)—have achieved research benchmarks for being *well established*—that is, efficacy has been demonstrated for the models in at least two independent research settings with rigorous methods design *and* by two independent investigatory teams showing the treatment to be statistically significantly superior either to psychological placebo or to another active treatment. Two other manualized models—brief strategic family therapy (BSFT) and family behavior therapy (FBT)—have met benchmarks for being *probably efficacious*—at least two good experiments with rigorous methods designs have shown the treatment is superior (statistically significantly so) to a wait-list control group *or* one or more good experiments meeting the well-established treatment level (Hogue et al. 2018). Meta-analyses of controlled trials demonstrate that manualized family therapy consistently prevails against other manualized ASU approaches as well as usual care, and produces the largest average effect sizes by a wide margin (Baldwin et al. 2012; Riedinger et al. 2017; Tanner-Smith et al. 2013). Of note, there is currently no evidence of relative superiority among the various manualized family therapy models, although power for such comparisons via meta-analysis is limited (Baldwin et al. 2012) and the various models have not been tested against one another in the same study.

To complement the extensive evidence base on manualized family therapy, recent research has investigated the effectiveness of "naturalistic" family therapy for treating ASU. Hogue and colleagues (2015) conducted a randomized trial of nonmanualized family therapy delivered by community therapists as the routine standard of care for youth behavioral problems in outpatient services, compared with alternative treatment services featuring nonfamily approaches delivered in comparable settings. They found that routine family therapy significantly outperformed alternative treatments in reducing ASU and co-occurring externalizing and internalizing symptoms at 1-year follow-up. Moreover, the routine family therapy condition exceeded a research-defined fidelity benchmark for adherence to family therapy techniques that are signature interventions of manualized models, and equaled an outcomes benchmark for long-term client improvement established by manualized models across numerous controlled trials (Hogue et al. 2017a). These findings indicate that naturalistic family therapy implemented in usual care can achieve performance standards that match those of empirically supported brand-name models—results that present new intervention opportunities for evidence-minded therapists treating ASU in agency settings.

Core Elements

Given that family therapy has the strongest evidence base for treating ASU, as well as promising evidence for naturalistic family therapy in usual care, this approach appears highly suitable for widespread dissemination. As described by Chorpita and Daleiden (2009), the core-elements approach seeks to define a reduced set of intervention techniques that are common ingredients in multiple evidence-based treatments for a given disorder. This is achieved by a) specifying the discrete techniques prescribed by similar manuals and b) distilling these techniques into a smaller number of overlapping elements that are core features (and presumptive active ingredients) of each manual. As a result, the distilled core practice elements are approach specific (i.e., identified with a particular treatment orientation and/or modality) but model free (i.e., not inextricably bound to a single manual or intervention sequence). Given the number of effective manualized family therapy treatments, the core-elements approach would appear to be a natural fit for these models. In Chorpita and Daleiden's (2009) distillation project, however, which included more than 300 controlled trials, family-based treatment could be distilled to one element only, family therapy, underscoring the need for further elucidation of potential core components.

In understanding more meaningfully the evidence base for core components of family therapy for ASU, it is important to understand how the "packages," or the different forms of manualized family therapies, are described and classified. The five major categories of FBT are behavioral, systems, functional, ecological, and educational. These are labeled in large part on the basis of the focus of the intervention for ASU; that is, whether the focus is within and/or outside the system of the family (Becker and Curry 2008). Hogue and colleagues' (2018) review identified ecological family therapy as the approach most supported by evidence. Manualized models of evidence-based ecological family therapy, some of which were discussed earlier, include MDFT, BSFT, and FFT. Although these models differ in the specific nature of their interventions, coordination techniques, and level of expected adherence to the therapeutic techniques within model, all are associated with improved clinical outcomes.

Our process of identifying core components of family therapy began by examining the observational fidelity scales in which discrete techniques are operationalized from MDFT, BSFT, and FFT. The core components derived by this exploration are thematic clinical strategies that are 1) common across all three models, 2) theoretically important and relevant to the family therapy approach, and 3) embodied by multiple items from all three scales. This distillation process has yielded four core components: family engagement, relational reframing, family behavior change, and family restructuring.

Family Engagement

This component incorporates interventions that simultaneously aim to build the relationship between the therapist and all family members and encourage family members' participation in therapy and investment in treatment goals. Engagement is more than attendance, and this component aims to invite involvement of all family members in the goal of systemic change. Therapists trained in family engagement interventions view engagement as a process influenced by the family, the therapist, the interactions between them, and the social context. Engagement difficulties are natural experiences that are systemic and are expected and meant to be explored rather than characterized as "resistance." Family engagement interventions are invariably specified by manualized family therapy models as taking place during the early part of treatment and include building balanced alliances with teens, parents, and siblings. The goal of family engagement in ASU treatment is to support family members in identifying therapy as a benefit to the adolescent, their substance use disorder, their family relationships, and any other challenges identified in the engagement process. In order to establish credibility and value to all family members, it is vital that the therapist convey acceptance, curiosity, and a nonjudgmental attitude. It is essential for all family members to identify with the goals of systemic and ecological therapy throughout treatment, and engagement activities may need to be continually revisited toward this end.

Relational Reframing

This component consists of therapeutic techniques designed to move away from individual and intrapsychic ways of defining problems and generating solutions, and toward a systemic conceptualization focused on relational processes. Relational reframing techniques include keeping a relational focus, educating family members on behaviors that are part of normative adolescent development, and encouraging family members to adopt a more positive view of a behavior or relationship. Family members are often motivated to make systemic changes by understanding their problems differently. Put another way, relational reframing prepares family members to effect change in their relationships. These interventions also aim to remove pathological descriptions and attributions for behaviors, specifically by removing overly pathological ways of describing ASU. For example, a parent's angry outburst might be reframed by a therapist as an expression of worry and fear of loss of control, and a teen's increase in time away from the home might be reframed as a search for autonomy and independence. While a family might initially experience ASU as evidence of a teen's individual frailty or pathology, relational reframing can create an organizing theme for the family through which to understand ASU, and then can link each person's behavior to that theme. Relational reframing interventions may also include targeting the behaviors and cognitions of caregivers. In ASU treatment, understandably the presenting problem is typically the individual behaviors of the adolescent, and so therapists will endeavor to change this problem definition by presenting alternative, systemic definitions to caregivers.

In understanding the third and fourth core components of family therapy for ASU, it is useful to consider the mechanisms of change as defined by early family therapists: the theory of first- and second-order change. As defined by pioneering family therapists, first-order change consists of family cycles of interactions at the behavioral level only, such that therapists endeavor to bring about observable changes in actions. In second-order change, therapists target underlying beliefs, premises, or family rules; it is hoped that changes in these latent processes will then prompt behavior change. Family members may be instructed on using more effective communication strategies to decrease arguments about an adolescent's drug use (first-order); or, they may explore and then repair relationship ruptures that have created interpersonal distance and conflict (and perhaps led to the ASU itself), which would, in turn, decrease their arguing (second-order). The clinical outcome is the same, but the processes for change are meaningfully different. As implied, it is also a recursive process in which one type of change can beget another: therapists hope that changes in beliefs change behavior, and also that changes in behavior will change beliefs about what is possible in relationships and between family members.

Family Behavior Change

This component constitutes first-order change. Therapists employing therapeutic techniques that address family behavior change aim to teach new, concrete skills to all family members and encourage individual behavior change that will allow for improved family relationships. A key feature of this core component, which is in fact true of all the core components, is that all family members can benefit from changing their behavior, and that all family members may need new skills. Therapists actively teach general skills and specific skills, such as assertive communication, and often assign homework to support skill retention and generalizability. These new skills and behaviors are then positively reinforced and coached, for the individual as well as the entire family. Family behavior change can be implemented with the whole family at once, or therapists can encourage change and teach skills working with subsystems or in meetings with individuals. While individuals are often encouraged to make changes, the goal for the change is to make improvements for the entire family. For example, an adolescent may be coached in conflict resolution skills, in the presence of his family, and encouraged to practice these new skills with his or her family, and family members are also taught the same skills and encouraged to practice both inside and outside the family system. The teen learns how to reduce conflict in his or her own life, and the entire family is supported in engaging in less conflict-laden ways. Other examples of behavior change that family therapists can support are positive communication skills, limit setting, and collaborative problem-solving strategies.

Family Restructuring

Family restructuring constitutes second-order change, that is, change in the way the family system is governed. The premise is that therapists must create a context for change and must work to change beliefs and assumptions rather than behaviors, because endeavoring to change behavior alone is insufficient. Family-restructuring interventions aim to prompt shifts in attachment and emotional processes among family members. For ASU, such interventions can include focusing on process, bringing mindfulness to the present moment and nonverbal exchanges, realigning boundaries, and justifying the importance of new skills. In family restructuring, parents and teens are also encouraged to develop insight into predominant cycles of relational interactions, and how these cycles are linked to observable behaviors. If a parent and teen have developed a cycle of interaction in which they engage only when there is a violation of rules followed by a consequence to enforce, and thus there is a premise that connection equates with conflict, a therapist would want to highlight this dynamic with the family, justify the skill of developing new ways to connect with one another, and explore other unexpressed negative emotions outside of the parent-teen interactions. Therapists can also move toward family restructuring by highlighting strengths in the family and exploring the intergenerational contexts of family structures.

Multicomponent Treatment

Multicomponent treatments refer to intervention models or packages that contain multiple intervention components, some of which include family therapy. Multicomponent treatments seek to leverage multiple treatment mechanisms to address the developmental risk and protective factors that influence ASU, maximizing both the intensity and diversity of interventions delivered. Hogue and colleagues (2018) designated two multicomponent treatments as having the highest level of empirical support (well-established): motivational enhancement therapy plus cognitive-behavioral therapy (MET/CBT) and MET/CBT plus family therapy. A third well-established treatment, A-CRA, was categorized as a singular cognitive-behavioral model but can legitimately be classified as a multicomponent treatment, as discussed below. Another three multicomponent treatments were deemed probably efficacious: family therapy plus contingency management (FT+CM), MET/CBT + CM, and MET/CBT+ FT + CM. A major takeaway from Hogue and colleagues' analysis, and from similar empirical reviews (e.g., Brewer et al. 2017), is that multicomponent treatments for ASU continue to accumulate an impressive empirical record for reducing substance use and co-occurring problems among youth.

Multidomain Treatment

An important distinction should be made between multicomponent treatments versus *multidomain* treatments, which contain at least one component that specifically targets a co-occurring disorder or behavioral problem other than ASU. Treatment packages that target multiple domains of adolescent functioning are a vital asset for evidence-based ASU practice, given that the vast majority of youth receiving substance use services also present with co-morbid mental health disorders (Dennis et al. 2004). One kind of multidomain treatment package is *combined treatment*, in which ASU behavioral treatment is coordinated with pharmacological treatment for a given mental health disorder (see, e.g., Hogue et al. 2016, 2017b; Riggs et al. 2011 for attention disorders; Riggs et al. 2007 for mood disorders).

A second kind of multidomain treatment package is *integrated treatment*, in which at least one behavioral component targeting ASU is coordinated with at least one behavioral component targeting a co-occurring problem. Integrated models can proceed with concurrent delivery, implementing the two components simultaneously throughout treatment (see, e.g., Letourneau et al. 2017; Suarez et al. 2012) or with sequential delivery in which treatment focuses first on one disorder and then the other (see, e.g., Adams et al. 2016).

Example of a Multicomponent Model: Adolescent Community Reinforcement Approach

The A-CRA multicomponents include operant techniques, CBT components, family sessions, and a procedure for medication monitoring and adherence (Godley et al. 2016). The adolescent version of Community Reinforcement Approach (CRA) is a modification of a treatment model with a long history that was originally developed for adults with alcohol disorders and experimentally validated in the 1970s and 1980s (Azrin et al. 1982). The model was later adapted for adolescents as part of the Cannabis Youth Treatment study (Dennis et al. 2004).

The use of the word *community* in the title of the model is drawn from its underlying premise, which is to increase adolescents' access to reinforcing prosocial activities and peers in their community through operant conditioning procedures and skills training procedures so that non-using behaviors compete with or replace substance-using behaviors (Godley et al. 2016; Meyers and Smith 1995). A-CRA consists of 19 procedures, which have their roots in operant and social learning theories. Because of this lineage, there is overlap between CRA and CBT approaches.

Examples of operant components are systematic encouragement (based on the behavior-shaping principle) and positive reinforcement. This procedure helps a youth break down a task into achievable steps, practice making a needed contact (e.g., an appointment with a health clinic) with a role-play, complete the first step of the task so it is easier to complete the remaining steps, and review obstacles and possible solutions. The use of positive reinforcement is considered an essential therapeutic skill during every session. The clinician is trained to listen for clues about potential reinforcers or motivators for each youth. Identifying possible reinforcers is also why A-CRA clinicians are trained to treat the whole person and work with what the youth initially prioritizes (e.g., "emotional problems") when completing life-health rating scale items early in treatment.

Functional Analysis and Anger Management are examples of A-CRA's CBT procedures. Functional analyses are used both for decreasing substance-using behaviors and increasing prosocial behaviors. In these applications, triggers are identified for the behaviors, consequences (both positive and negative) are examined, and information is gleaned and discussed to facilitate future behavior change. Examples of behavioral skills training procedures are problem-solving and communication skills. The latter is helpful because many youth will be more successful with school and juvenile justice authorities and with their peer group if they learn and practice positive communication skills in these relationships.

Two other components of A-CRA are the four family sessions and the procedure to help monitor and maintain medication adherence. Most youth live with one or more family members, and thus family is an important part of the youth's community and could help or hinder change. Because CRA had a long history of addressing relationships between significant others, procedures were adapted for use with youth and their parents. These procedures include a) setting positive expectations for treatment outcome; b) identifying parent reinforcers for continued involvement in treatment; c) shaping and reframing discussion of the adolescent in positive terms based on work from family therapists (Alexander et al. 1989); and d) behavioral skills training based on family relationship assessment scales completed by each participant early in the family sessions.

The Medication Monitoring and Adherence procedure is important because of findings that high percentages of youth present to substance use treatment with one or more other mental health problems (Chan et al. 2008; Grella et al. 2004). This procedure can be used when a youth is prescribed a pharmacological treatment for a co-occurring mental health disorder. It includes a) having a discussion about why the medication is important; and b) training a parent or other family member how to monitor medication taking, communicate with the youth regarding objections that may arise, and provide positive reinforcement for taking the medication.

The multiple components of A-CRA illustrate the advantages of training clinicians in a menu of basic treatment elements, including some that have demonstrated efficacy for co-occurring mental health disorder symptoms (Godley et al. 2014b). Training clinicians to apply the components to other mental health symptoms along with substance use problems per se allows them to provide integrated treatment to address multiple problems. One example is the A-CRA procedure for increasing prosocial activities, which has a similar structure and goals to procedures common to substance use–focused family therapy approaches as well as treatments for depression, trauma, conduct disorders, and attention-deficit/hyperactivity disorder. As described in the following subsection, preliminary evidence supports this approach.

Implementation

Gotham (2004) defines implementation of an evidence-based intervention as delivering it in ways that maintain its quality and effectiveness. These are challenging goals because treatment organizations usually have fewer financial and staff resources than were available during the experimental evaluation of the intervention. The widespread adoption of A-CRA by 408 organizations with thousands of youth has provided lessons related to the training of clinicians and supervisors. A large number of the treatment organizations implemented A-CRA with federal grant funding and were required to collect youth intake, implementation, and follow-up outcome data, which could then be analyzed to determine the effectiveness of the intervention for important youth subgroups.

Given the need to develop a training approach that could facilitate the *rapid and simultaneous* implementation of A-CRA across dozens of treatment organizations, research evaluating clinician training in evidence-based interventions was used to develop a set of standardized training and technology-assisted components (Godley et al. 2011a). Training and certification processes were developed for both clinicians and supervisors. Once certified, supervisors can train and certify additional clinicians within their organization, thus creating a pathway to sustainment. Training components include reading the A-CRA clinical guide (Godley et al. 2016), completing online quizzes, and attending a 3-day training session. Following the training, clinicians begin a certification process that is based on recording actual sessions and uploading digital recordings of those sessions to a secure website to be rated by trained raters using a detailed rating manual (Smith et al. 2007). Online courses are available to address specific clinical needs (e.g., using A-CRA procedures for co-occurring disorders). For the clinician to receive certification, the clinician's session recordings have to receive passing scores on all A-CRA procedures. Supervisors are strongly encouraged to first go through clinician certification and are required to demonstrate competency rating sessions and conducting supervision.

Lessons Regarding Training Clinicians

Since requirements for addiction counselors vary widely by state, ASU clinicians across states have different academic and experiential backgrounds. In a cross-site study of A-CRA implementation, only 54% of 115 clinicians had advanced degrees and only 69% were certified addiction counselors (Tobin et al. 2012). Thus, few assumptions can be made about the training and skills that clinicians will have when beginning an evidence-based intervention training process. Despite their differences in training and experience, addiction counselors favor evidence-based interventions they view as flexible because the counselors are encouraged to use their clinical skills to decide what therapy elements or procedures are appropriate to use at a given time (Godley et al. 2001; Tobin et al. 2012).

Evidence demonstrating the relationship of the clinician's implementation of the intervention to outcomes is important to assure clinicians that quality implementation has meaning. In one study, researchers found that adolescents exposed to at least 12 different A-CRA procedures were significantly more likely to be in recovery at 3- and 6-month post-intake follow-up (Garner et al. 2009). In another study, clinician competence, as measured by the A-CRA procedure fidelity ratings, predicted decreases in adolescent substance use at 3-, 6-, and 12-month follow-up (Campos-Melady et al. 2017).

Lessons Regarding Training Supervisors

In practice, not all substance use treatment organizations have dedicated clinical supervisors. Sustainment of best practices requires some amount of clinical supervisory time allotted for training and ongoing supervision, given that clinician turnover is inevitable. A study of the sustainment of A-CRA 12 months after external funding ended revealed that sustainment was significantly more likely among those organizations that had a certified supervisor at the end of funding (Hunter et al. 2017).

Implementation and Outcomes With Subpopulations

The research-based National Institute on Drug Abuse Principles of Adolescent Substance Use Disorder Treatment (National Institute on Drug Abuse

2014) suggest that treatment should be tailored to the unique needs of the youth, treat the whole person (not just focus on substance use), and address other mental health problems the youth may have. A-CRA is flexible and lends itself to the different strengths, experiences, learning styles, and issues that a youth and family bring into treatment. Clinicians are trained to choose procedures on the basis of individual needs during each session. For example, early treatment rating scales allow youth to tell the clinicians what is important to them and to set goals in those areas, an approach that is likely to increase treatment engagement and salience for youth. Clinicians are also encouraged to implement other needed treatments concurrently (e.g., pharmacological treatments, trauma-focused approaches).

Using the large data set generated from the A-CRA implementation effort, researchers were able to examine whether treatment initiation, engagement, retention, or outcomes were different by gender or ethnic group (Godley et al. 2011b). Initiation (receiving a second treatment session within 14 days of the first), engagement (two additional treatment sessions within 30 days of their first session), and retention rates were high and equivalent across gender and ethnic groups. Satisfaction with treatment was high for all groups (over 95%). Both genders had about the same rate of change in increased days of abstinence and recovery rates. All racial groups reported significant increases in days abstinent from substance use and were equivalent with regard to the percentage in recovery at follow-up. Program evaluation findings from A-CRA implementation sites that served predominantly Hispanic populations in different states provide support for the effectiveness of A-CRA with this population (Ruiz et al. 2011; Strunz et al. 2015).

Researchers also compared engagement and outcomes for adolescents with a) substance use disorders only; b) substance use and externalizing mental health problems; c) substance use and internalizing mental health problems; and d) substance use and both externalizing and internalizing problems. Findings revealed that all groups received equal exposure to A-CRA as measured by engagement and retention, and had equivalent treatment satisfaction. At the 12-month follow-up, adolescents with externalizing mental health problems or those with both externalizing and internalizing problems had significantly greater improvement in their days of abstinence and substance problems relative to adolescents with substance use disorders only. Adolescents reporting symptoms of internalizing, externalizing, or both externalizing and internalizing disorders had significantly greater improvements in days of emotional problems relative to adolescents with substance use disorders only (Godley et al. 2014a).

The juvenile justice system is the largest referral source for adolescents entering community-based substance use treatment. Research findings provided support that participation in A-CRA had a significant, direct relation to reduced substance use; a significant, indirect relation to reduced illegal activity through reductions in substance use; and a significant, indirect relation to reduced juvenile justice system involvement through reductions in both substance use and illegal activity (Hunter et al. 2014). Additionally, a randomized controlled study of youth with substance use disorders and juvenile justice involvement found that A-CRA led to superior substance use outcomes compared with usual services provided by a juvenile probation department (Henderson et al. 2016).

Researchers also compared A-CRA treatment and outcome findings for youth with opioid problem use (OPU) with those for youth with marijuana and alcohol problem use (MAPU). Intake comparisons suggested that youth with OPU presented with significantly greater impairment across mental health and risk behaviors. There was no evidence of differences between groups on A-CRA engagement, retention, family sessions, or treatment satisfaction. Clinical outcome data revealed that both groups decreased substance use significantly over time, but the OPU group decreased alcohol and other drug use at a greater rate and reported greater decreases in their emotional problems, although their substance use and emotional problems remained at significantly greater levels than those in the MAPU group. In addition, the OPU group significantly decreased their opioid use. These findings suggest that youth presenting with OPU can be engaged and retained in A-CRA with clinically significant reductions in use; however, youth with OPU may require longer-term treatment and benefit from combining A-CRA with medication such as buprenorphine (Godley et al. 2017).

Key Points

- Because adolescent problems are often systemic and not just individualized, family therapy is an important strategy that can make the adolescent feel less blamed and allow systemic solutions to emerge.

- Family therapy techniques can be implemented with an adolescent alone or with a parent alone.

- Supervision and ongoing quality assurance protocols are vital to effective use of family therapy techniques and may be particularly helpful when clinicians are struggling to engage parents of adolescents or reframe an adolescent's problem relationally.

- Most adolescents with substance use disorders have problems in multiple domains, and many Adolescent Community Reinforcement Approach procedures have been shown to be effective with co-occurring mental health problems.

References

Adams ZW, McCauley JL, Back SE, et al: Clinician perspectives on treating adolescents with co-occurring post-traumatic stress disorder, substance use, and other problems. J Child Adolesc Subst Abuse 25(6):575–583, 2016 27840568

Alexander JF, Waldron HB, Barton C, et al: The minimizing of blaming attributions and behaviors in delinquent families. J Consult Clin Psychol 57(1):19–24, 1989 2925972

Azrin NH, Sisson RW, Meyers R, et al: Alcoholism treatment by disulfiram and community reinforcement therapy. J Behav Ther Exp Psychiatry 13(2):105–112, 1982 7130406

Baldwin SA, Christian S, Berkeljon A, et al: The effects of family therapies for adolescent delinquency and substance abuse: a meta-analysis. J Marital Fam Ther 38(1):281–304, 2012 22283391

Becker SJ, Curry JF: Outpatient interventions for adolescent substance abuse: a quality of evidence review. J Consult Clin Psychol 76(4):531–543, 2008 18665683

Brewer S, Godley MD, Hulvershorn LA: Treating mental health and substance use disorders in adolescents: What is on the menu? Curr Psychiatry Rep 19(1):5, 2017 28120255

Campos-Melady M, Smith JE, Meyers RJ, et al: The effect of therapists' adherence and competence in delivering the adolescent community reinforcement approach on client outcomes. Psychol Addict Behav 31(1):117–129, 2017 27736146

Chan YF, Dennis ML, Funk RR: Prevalence and comorbidity of major internalizing and externalizing problems among adolescents and adults presenting to substance abuse treatment. J Subst Abuse Treat 34(1):14–24, 2008 17574804

Chorpita BF, Daleiden EL: Mapping evidence-based treatments for children and adolescents: application of the distillation and matching model to 615 treatments from 322 randomized trials. J Consult Clin Psychol 77(3):566–579, 2009 19485596

Dennis M, Godley SH, Diamond G, et al: The Cannabis Youth Treatment (CYT) study: main findings from two randomized trials. J Subst Abuse Treat 27(3):197–213, 2004 15501373

Garner BR, Godley SH, Funk RR, et al: Exposure to Adolescent Community Reinforcement Approach treatment procedures as a mediator of the relationship between adolescent substance abuse treatment retention and outcome. J Subst Abuse Treat 36(3):252–264, 2009 18715742

Godley MD, Passetti LL, Subramaniam GA, et al: Adolescent Community Reinforcement Approach implementation and treatment outcomes for youth with opioid problem use. Drug Alcohol Depend 174:9–16, 2017 28282523

Godley SH, White WL, Diamond GS, et al: Therapists' reactions to manual-guided therapies for the treatment of adolescent marijuana users. Clinical Psychology: Science and Practice 8:405–417, 2001

Godley SH, Garner BR, Smith JE, et al: A large-scale dissemination and implementation model for evidence-based treatment and continuing care. Clin Psychol (New York) 18(1):67–83, 2011a 21547241

Godley SH, Hedges K, Hunter B: Gender and racial differences in treatment process and outcome among participants in the Adolescent Community Reinforcement Approach. Psychol Addict Behav 25(1):143–154, 2011b 21443309

Godley SH, Hunter BD, Fernández-Artamendi S, et al: A comparison of treatment outcomes for Adolescent Community Reinforcement Approach participants with and without co-occurring problems. J Subst Abuse Treat 46(4):463–471, 2014a 24462478

Godley SH, Smith JE, Passetti LL, et al: The Adolescent Community Reinforcement Approach (A-CRA) as a model paradigm for the management of adolescents with substance use disorders and co-ocurring psychiatric disorders. Subst Abuse 35(4):352–363, 2014b 25035906

Godley SH, Smith JE, Meyers RJ, et al: The Adolescent Community Reinforcement Approach: A Clinical Guide for Treating Substance Use Disorders. Normal, IL, Chestnut Health Systems, 2016

Gotham HJ: Diffusion of mental health and substance abuse treatments: development, dissemination, and implementation. Clinical Psychology: Science and Practice 11:160–176, 2004

Grella CE, Joshi V, Hser YI: Effects of comorbidity on treatment processes and outcomes among adolescents in drug treatment programs. J Child Adolesc Subst Abuse 13:13–31, 2004

Henderson CE, Wevodau AL, Henderson SE, et al: An independent replication of the Adolescent-Community Reinforcement Approach with justice-involved youth. Am J Addict 25(3):233–240, 2016 26992083

Hogue A, Liddle HA: Family based treatment for adolescent substance abuse: controlled trials and new horizons in services research. J Fam Ther 31(2):126–154, 2009 21113237

Hogue A, Dauber S, Henderson CE, et al: Randomized trial of family therapy versus nonfamily treatment for adolescent behavior problems in usual care. J Clin Child Adolesc Psychol 44(6):954–969, 2015 25496283

Hogue A, Lichvar E, Bobek M: Pilot evaluation of the Medication Integration Protocol for adolescents with ADHD in behavioral care: treatment fidelity, acceptability, and utilization. J Emot Behav Disord 24:223–234, 2016

Hogue A, Dauber S, Henderson CE: Benchmarking family therapy for adolescent behavior problems in usual care: fidelity, outcomes, and therapist performance differences. Adm Policy Ment Health 44(5):626–641, 2017a 27664141

Hogue A, Evans SW, Levin FR: A clinician's guide to co-occurring ADHD among adolescent substance users: comorbidity, neurodevelopmental risk, and evidence-based treatment options. J Child Adolesc Subst Abuse 26(4):277–292, 2017b 30828239

Hogue A, Henderson CE, Becker SJ, et al: Evidence base on outpatient behavioral treatments for adolescent substance use, 2014–2017: outcomes, treatment delivery, and promising horizons. J Clin Child Adolesc Psychol 47(4):499–526, 2018 29893607

Hunter BD, Godley SH, Hesson-McInnis MS, et al: Longitudinal change mechanisms for substance use and illegal activity for adolescents in treatment. Psychol Addict Behav 28(2):507–515, 2014 24128291

Hunter SB, Han B, Slaughter ME, et al: Predicting evidence-based treatment sustainment: results from a longitudinal study of the Adolescent-Community Reinforcement Approach. Implement Sci 12(1):75, 2017 28610574

Letourneau EJ, McCart MR, Sheidow AJ, et al: First evaluation of a contingency management intervention addressing adolescent substance use and sexual risk behaviors: risk reduction therapy for adolescents. J Subst Abuse Treat 72:56–65, 2017 27629581

McCart MR, Sheidow AJ: Evidence-based psychosocial treatments for adolescents with disruptive behavior. J Clin Child Adolesc Psychol 45(5):529–563, 2016 27152911

Meyers RJ, Smith JE: Clinical Guide to Alcohol Treatment: The Community Reinforcement Approach. New York, Guilford, 1995

National Institute on Drug Abuse: Principles of Adolescent Substance Use Disorder Treatment: A Research-Based Guide. NIH Publ No 14-7953. Rockville, MD, NIDA, January 2014. Available at: https://d14rmgtrwzf5a.cloudfront.net/sites/default/files/podata_1_17_14.pdf. Accessed May 16, 2019.

Riedinger V, Pinquart M, Teubert D: Effects of systemic therapy on mental health of children and adolescents: a meta-analysis. J Clin Child Adolesc Psychol 46(6):880–894, 2017 26467300

Riggs PD, Mikulich-Gilbertson SK, Davies RD, et al: A randomized controlled trial of fluoxetine and cognitive behavioral therapy in adolescents with major depression, behavior problems, and substance use disorders. Arch Pediatr Adolesc Med 161(11):1026–1034, 2007 17984403

Riggs PD, Winhusen T, Davies RD, et al: Randomized controlled trial of osmotic-release methylphenidate with cognitive-behavioral therapy in adolescents with attention-deficit/hyperactivity disorder and substance use disorders. J Am Acad Child Adolesc Psychiatry 50(9):903–914, 2011 21871372

Ruiz BS, Korchmaros JD, Greene A, et al: Evidence-based substance abuse treatment for adolescents: engagement and outcomes. Practice: Social Work in Action 23:215–233, 2011

Smith JE, Lundy SL, Gianini L: Community Reinforcement Approach (CRA) and Adolescent Community Reinforcement Approach (A-CRA) Therapist Coding Manual. Normal, IL, Chestnut Health Systems, 2007

Strunz E, Jungerman J, Kinyua J, et al: Evaluation of an assertive continuing care program for Hispanic adolescents. Glob J Health Sci 7(5):106–116, 2015 26156933

Suarez LM, Belcher HM, Briggs EC, et al: Supporting the need for an integrated system of care for youth with co-occurring traumatic stress and substance abuse problems. Am J Community Psychol 49(3–4):430–440, 2012 21837575

Tanner-Smith EE, Wilson SJ, Lipsey MW: The comparative effectiveness of outpatient treatment for adolescent substance abuse: a meta-analysis. J Subst Abuse Treat 44(2):145–158, 2013 22763198

Tobin T, Huntington N, Lang D, et al: Program Evaluation for Assertive Adolescent and Family Treatment (AAFT): Final Report. Sudbury, MA, Advocates for Human Potential, 2012

15

Twelve-Step and Mutual-Help Programs

John F. Kelly, Ph.D.

Alexandra W. Abry, B.A.

Nilofar Fallah-Sohy, B.S.

Substance use disorder (SUD) is the top cause of premature mortality and morbidity among young people in middle- and high-income countries globally (Gore et al. 2011). Thus, providing effective intervention for adolescents with SUD in countries such as the United States has become a public health priority, yet remains a clinical challenge (Tanner-Smith et al. 2013). Professional treatment often produces significant salutary changes in adolescents' substance use (Dennis et al. 2004; Tanner-Smith et al. 2013) but by itself may be inadequate to address the prodigious and chronic burden of disease attributable to SUD (Stanger et al. 2016). Clinical contingency management models hold more promise for increasing youth and adult abstinence (Stanger et al.

2016), but these protocols typically last only a matter of weeks, and sustaining beneficial effects after the removal of such contingencies has proved challenging. From a broad clinical and public health perspective, utilization of indigenous, ubiquitous, freely available social recovery support services that can provide natural contingencies that promote abstinence and remission in the communities in which people live over the long term is appealing, and evidence for such entities is growing (Kelly et al. 2019).

Social networks play an important role in influencing the onset and offset of alcohol and other drug use. The U.S. National Institute on Drug Abuse, for example, states that there are four main reasons why people begin to use drugs: to feel good, to feel better, to do better, and because other people are doing it (National Institute on Drug Abuse 2018). We would argue that, paradoxically, these are the same four reasons why people *stop* using alcohol and other drugs: to feel good, to feel better, to do better, and *because other people are (not) doing it*. In other words, as an individual passes through the phases of an alcohol and other drug use disorder from the initial pleasure, relief, and performance enhancement that a substance can initially provide, through to the subsequent pain, angst, and diminished performance that the same substance later induces, social influences that once attracted, facilitated, modeled, and reinforced drug use can equally and powerfully attract, facilitate, model, and reinforce *non*–drug use and increase the chances of remission and long-term recovery (Kelly et al. 2019). Such social forces have been leveraged therapeutically in peer-led 12-step mutual-help organizations (MHOs), such as Alcoholics Anonymous (AA), Narcotics Anonymous (NA), Marijuana Anonymous (MA), as well as other non-12-step MHOs like SMART Recovery and LifeRing, for many decades to help people attain and sustain remission from SUD over the long term (Kelly and Yeterian 2013).

Currently, millions of individuals utilize these resources to aid SUD recovery annually (Humphreys 2004). Most adult and youth treatment programs in the United States include 12-step MHO philosophy and practices (Humphreys 2004; Kelly 2003; Roman and Blum 1999; Tonigan et al. 1996) and/or refer patients to community 12-step MHOs to help prevent relapse. Although dozens of high-quality research studies have been conducted and show support for clinical linkages to 12-step MHOs among adult samples in enhancing abstinence and remission, until recently comparatively little was known regarding youth participation and benefits from such entities; however, more rigorous research in this area is now emerging.

In this chapter we provide an overview of the rationale for potential benefits from participation in 12-step MHOs for adolescents and emerging adults and review existing evidence on the clinical and public health utility of MHO participation in this age group with SUD. We examine the developmentally related clinical differences between youth and adults that necessitate youth-specific 12-step groups and 12-step facilitation (TSF); provide an overview on the prevalence of youth participation in 12-step groups; and review the scientific evidence addressing the clinical, public health, and economic utility of 12-step MHOs in the treatment of, and recovery from, alcohol and other drug use disorders among youth. In the final section, we discuss the clinician's role in promoting MHO participation and provide evidence-based strategies for increasing 12-step MHO attendance among youth.

Life Contexts and Youth-Specific 12-Step Groups

The developmental periods of late adolescence and emerging adulthood confer the highest risk for the onset of SUDs. In 2017 in the United States, 4.0% of adolescents ages 12–17 (~990,000 adolescents) and 14.8% of emerging adults ages 18–25 (~5.1 million emerging adults) had substance use that met DSM-IV criteria for a SUD, compared with 6.4% of all adults 26 years and older (Substance Abuse and Mental Health Services Administration 2018). Adolescents and emerging adults differ clinically from adults with SUD and often face additional age- and life-context-related barriers to accessing treatment and recovery support services. Young people tend to have less complex and severe substance use histories than adults, as they often report less frequent substance use, have fewer dependence symptoms, and have fewer withdrawal symptoms and medical complications than adults (Brown 1993; Kelly and Yeterian 2011). They are also less likely to be interested in spiritual concepts and ideas than their older adult counterparts, and the explicitly spiritual/religious language in the 12 steps may pose a further barrier to identification and feeling of belonging. Table 15–1 lists AA's 12 steps highlighting this language and offers a youth-focused interpretation.

Table 15–1.   Interpretation and potential therapeutic outcome of the 12-step process

Step	Theme	Youth-focused interpretation	Therapeutic outcome
1. We admitted we were powerless over our addiction—that our lives had become unmanageable.	Honesty	Recognize that you have an alcohol/drug problem.	Liberation
2. Came to believe that a Power greater than ourselves could restore us to sanity.	Open-mindedness	Remember that help is available and change is possible.	Instillation of hope
3. Made a decision to turn our will and our lives over to the care of God as we understood Him.	Willingness	Decide to get help.	Self-efficacy
4. Made a searching and fearless moral inventory of ourselves.	Self-assessment and appraisal	Take a look at what is bothering you and why.	Insight
5. Admitted to God, to ourselves, and to another human being the exact nature of our wrongs.	Self-forgiveness; accurate self-appraisal	Talk about what is bothering you and why with someone you trust, and who can help you.	Insight; reduced shame and guilt
6. Were entirely ready to have God remove all these defects of character.	Readiness to change	Start to make the necessary changes.	Cognitive consonance
7. Humbly asked Him to remove our shortcomings.	Humility/accurate appraisal	Continue to make the necessary changes.	Cognitive consonance

Table 15–1. Interpretation and potential therapeutic outcome of the 12-step process *(continued)*

Step	Theme	Youth-focused interpretation	Therapeutic outcome
8. Made a list of all persons we had harmed and became willing to make amends to them all.	Taking responsibility and forgiveness of self/others	Attempt to rectify sources of guilt/shame; mend relationships.	Peace of mind
9. Made direct amends to such people wherever possible, except when to do so would injure them or others.	Restitution to others	Talk to those concerned and make amends where necessary.	Peace of mind; self-esteem
10. Continued to take personal inventory and when we were wrong promptly admitted it.	Emotional balance	Keep on taking a look at yourself and correct mistakes as you go.	Affect and self-regulation
11. Sought through prayer and meditation to improve our conscious contact with God, as we understood Him, praying only for knowledge of His will for us and the power to carry that out.	Connectedness and emotional balance	Stay connected; stay mindful.	Awareness; psychological well-being
12. Having had a spiritual awakening as the result of these Steps, we tried to carry this message to addicts, and to practice these principles in all our affairs.	Helping others achieve recovery	Continue to access help, work on yourself and try to help others.	Self-esteem and mastery

Source. Adapted from Kelly JF, Yeterian JD: "Alcoholics Anonymous and Young People," in *Young People and Alcohol: Impact, Policy, Prevention, Treatment.* Edited by Saunders JB, Rey JM. New York, John Wiley & Sons, 2011, Table 17–3. Copyright © 2011 John Wiley & Sons.

Most young people also have a drug other than alcohol, such as cannabis (74.7%), as their primary substance (Kelly and Yeterian 2011). However, young people with SUD also differ from their adult counterparts in their motivation to access treatment. Young people tend to be motivated by extrinsic factors—such as family, school, or the legal system—to enter treatment, rather than by intrinsic factors (Kelly and Yeterian 2011; Wu et al. 2007). Thus, even if young people enter treatment, they may be less motivated to engage in continuing care. Moreover, a lack of independent transportation or freedom to travel at will serves as a logistical barrier that may further decrease the likelihood that adolescents and emerging adults access treatment and recovery resources (Kelly and Yeterian 2011).

Perhaps the most salient factor that affects the development and maintenance of, as well as recovery from, SUD among adolescents and young adults is social context. Social contexts play a role in establishing and maintaining patterns of heavy and frequent substance use among young people that can lead to alcohol and other drug use disorders (Kelly and Yeterian 2011). Yet, social contexts also play an integral role in SUD recovery, particularly among young people. Among adolescents and emerging adults, for example, the majority of relapses occur in social contexts where drugs and alcohol are present (Brown 1993; Kelly and Yeterian 2011). Conversely, the precursors to relapse among adults typically involve interpersonal conflicts, such as a disagreement with a family member, or negative affect, such as anger or depression (Brown 1993; Kelly and Yeterian 2011). Therefore, support services that provide recovery-specific social support, such as 12-step MHOs, have the ability to provide elements of stimulus control, helping to eradicate alcohol and other drug use cue exposure, by providing young people with a group of supportive peers with whom to socialize, thereby reducing relapse risk (Kelly and Yeterian 2011; Kelly et al. 2008).

This is one of the main bases for the founding of the alternative peer group (APG) model for youth in Texas in the early 1970s. APG programs that use the APG model work to attract and engage youth in recovery by integrating peer support and prosocial activities into clinical practice, which often includes 12-step programming (Nash and Collier 2016). Positive social influence of pro-recovery peers is a key therapeutic element of the APG model. It is theorized that participating in regular enjoyable prosocial activities serves to engage and retain youth while promoting long-term relationships with recovering peer role models. Over time in the APG, participants begin to accrue recovery capital and start to value recovery more than substance use, enhancing the possibility of remission and long-term recovery (Nash and Collier 2016; Nash et al. 2015). All programs that use the APG model provide peer support, social activities, family involvement, and linkages to treatment and other recovery support services. Some APGs offer almost daily activities and clinical services akin to intensive outpatient treatment programs, while others function solely as continuing care. Although research on APGs is only emerging, one unpublished study reported 2-year sobriety rates of 89%–92% for youth who completed an intensive outpatient program that used the APG model between 2006 and 2008. Such estimates are obviously limited by selection and attrition biases, and further research is needed to determine the extent to which these entities hold clinical and public health utility.

Youth Mutual-Help Organization Participation

The past 80 years have seen the emergence and proliferation of peer-based 12-step MHOs such as AA, which originated in the United States in the 1930s and has since been adapted for various other 12-step MHOs (e.g., NA, MA) (Humphreys 2004; Kelly and Yeterian 2013; Kelly et al. 2018). Twelve-step MHOs have grown rapidly throughout the world, with millions of individuals across more than 150 countries using these recovery resources each year (Humphreys 2004; Kelly and Yeterian 2013; Kelly et al. 2018). Although 12-step MHOs initially served more middle-aged individuals with chronic and severe SUD, cultural changes over the past 50 years have led to greater knowledge of addiction as a disease that affects a broad range of people, including young people (Kelly et al. 2018). Similar to adult treatment programs (Humphreys 2004; Kelly 2003; Roman and Blum 1999; Tonigan et al. 1996), 12-step practices and philosophy are often incorporated into treatment programs for young people, with nearly half of adolescent SUD treatment programs (47%) requiring participation in 12-step MHOs during treatment, and 85% linking adolescents with 12-step groups (e.g., MA, NA, AA) as part of their continuing care (Knudsen et al. 2008).

There are several prospective studies that suggest 12-step MHO attendance is both safe and beneficial for young people, with significant, modest correlations between greater attendance and better outcomes (Chi et al. 2009; Hsieh et al. 1998; Kelly and Myers 2007; Kelly and Urbanoski 2012; Kennedy and Minami 1993; Mundt et al. 2012). However, despite evidence pointing to the benefits of 12-step MHO participation for young people, young people make up only a small percentage of 12-step MHO members, with AA and NA both reporting in their recent membership surveys that only 1% of members are younger than 21 years old, and that 11% (AA) and 12% (NA) of members are between the ages of 21 and 30 (Alcoholics Anonymous World Services 2014; Narcotics Anonymous World Services 2013). Considering that the average AA and NA member is 50 and 43 years old (Alcoholics Anonymous World Services 2014; Narcotics Anonymous World Services 2013), respectively, the age composition of most 12-step meetings may pose a particularly formidable barrier to youth engagement in 12-step MHOs by potentially limiting identification and a sense of belonging with other members (Kelly and Myers 2007; Kelly et al. 2005; Labbe et al. 2014). In fact, research has shown that teens and emerging adults who attend AA and NA meetings consisting of a substantial proportion of similar-age peers had significantly better substance use outcomes in the early phases posttreatment when compared with youth who attend meetings primarily made up of adults (Kelly et al. 2005; Kelly and Yeterian 2011; Labbe et al. 2013).

Research on youth who participate in 12-step MHOs after inpatient or outpatient treatment points to declining attendance over time. For example, two studies of adolescents treated in 12-step-oriented inpatient treatment programs show that although adolescents had high rates of 12-step attendance immediately following treatment, rates of attendance declined quite quickly over time (Kelly and Yeterian 2011; Kelly et al. 2005, 2008). In one sample of adolescent inpatients (N=74), 72% of the participants attended at least one 12-step meeting in the first 3 months after discharge, with approximately half (51.8%) of participants attending at least one meeting per week (Kelly et al. 2005); during the second follow-up period (4–6 months posttreatment), just over a half (54.1%) attended at least one meeting, and just under a third (30.8%) attended at least one meeting per week. Average rates of attendance also dropped from approximately two meetings per week in the first 3 months to approximately one meeting per week in the next 4–6 months. Moreover, in an 8-year follow-up of adolescent inpatients (N=166), Kelly et al. (2008) found that although rates of 12-step meeting attendance were high in the first 6 months after treatment, with 91% of participants attending at least one meeting, 83%

monthly, and 65% weekly, attendance declined steadily across the 8-year follow-up period (Kelly and Yeterian 2011); 6–8 years after treatment, only 31%
of participants attended at least once, 19% at least monthly, and 6% at least
weekly.

Studies of adolescents treated in outpatient programs have also shown a
decline in 12-step group attendance over time, but with rates of attendance
starting lower than rates following inpatient treatment. For example, in one
study of adolescents ($N = 357$) in an intensive outpatient treatment program,
researchers found that at 1-year post-intake, 29% of participants reported having attended 10 or more 12-step meetings in the past 6 months (Chi et al. 2009;
Kelly and Yeterian 2011). However, 2 years later, at 3 years post-intake, only
14% of the participants had attended 10 or more 12-step meetings in the past
6 months, with 19% having attended at least one 12-step meeting in the prior
6 months (Chi et al. 2009; Kelly and Yeterian 2011). In another study of adolescents ($N = 127$) in an outpatient SUD treatment, 28% of participants attended
at least one 12-step meeting during the 3-month post-intake period, with the
proportion decreasing during the 4- to 6-month post-intake period (Kelly et al.
2010).

In summary, following inpatient and outpatient treatment, young people
have been found to participate at high rates in the early posttreatment periods,
but developmentally specific barriers to participation can create challenges with
getting to meetings and with identifying and affiliating with 12-step MHOs.
There is some evidence that these potential barriers to participation and benefits may be partially overcome through finding youth-specific meetings
where a substantial proportion of similar-age peers attend (see, e.g., Kelly et al.
2005; Labbe et al. 2014).

Evidence for Mutual-Help Organizations and 12-Step Facilitation for Youth

Several studies have examined adolescent AA/NA involvement in relation to
substance use outcomes following inpatient treatment. Kennedy and Minami
(1993) found that AA/NA attendees had four times lower odds of relapse following treatment. Hsieh et al. (1998) found that AA/NA attendance was the
most powerful discriminator of abstinence in a sample of 2,317 youth. We
found that 12-step meeting attendance was associated with better outcomes,

even when controlling for professional aftercare involvement 6 months after inpatient care (Kelly et al. 2000). In addition, in a prospective 8-year follow-up study following inpatient treatment as youth transitioned into young adulthood, we found that more frequent attendance at 12-step meetings during the first 6 months posttreatment predicted better substance use outcomes 4 and 6 years later (Kelly et al. 2008). In the same study, attendance at approximately 3 meetings per week was associated with complete abstinence in the first 6 months postdischarge (Kelly et al. 2008; Figure 15–1). Moreover, across the entire 8-year follow-up, we found that, on average, youth gained 2 days of abstinence for each AA or NA meeting attended, over and above all other factors associated with better outcomes (Kelly et al. 2008).

Another 3-year longitudinal outpatient study found that AA/NA participation was strongly associated with higher abstinence rates during follow-up (Chi et al. 2009). There is a strong linear independent association between 12-step meeting attendance and significantly better substance clinical outcomes among outpatient samples as well (Kelly and Urbanoski 2012; Kelly et al. 2010).

Although these studies used covariate adjustments to estimate causal connections between 12-step MHO participation and improved outcomes, this statistical practice is not a substitute for randomized experimental studies. Because of the challenges of conducting experimental studies directly on MHOs, such as NA and AA, 12-step treatment and related MHO effects have been studied using what has become known as clinically delivered "12-step facilitation" interventions (Table 15–2). These interventions systematically educate patients about the nature, purpose, and scope of MHOs like AA and NA, and facilitate and monitor participation over one to several sessions. Adult TSF interventions have been tested in many different formats and intensities, including brief advice (Kahler et al. 2005), pure multisession TSF (Litt et al. 2009; Project MATCH Research Group 1997b), combined cognitive-behavioral therapy (CBT)–TSF hybrids (Walitzer et al. 2009), and group treatments (Kaskutas et al. 2008), and in brief linkage procedures (typically using a current 12-step peer) following another treatment (Timko and DeBenedetti 2007).

Dozens of randomized clinical trials (RCTs) have demonstrated the efficacy, effectiveness, and cost-effectiveness of TSF treatments among adults for primary cocaine, alcohol, and methamphetamine use disorder (see, e.g., Kaskutas et al.

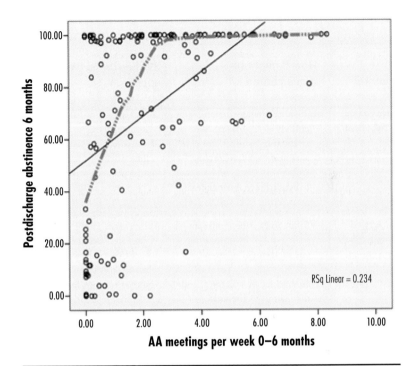

Figure 15–1.   LOWESS graph showing relationship between average number of Alcoholics Anonymous (AA) meetings per week and postdischarge abstinence (PDA).

Exploration of thresholds of AA/Narcotics Anonymous (NA) attendance in relation to concurrent and subsequent PDA using Robust Locally Weighted Scatterplot Smoothing (LOWESS) curves (ordinary least squares regression line also shown).

Source.   Reprinted from Kelly JF, Brown SA, Abrantes A, et al.: "Social Recovery Model: An 8-Year Investigation of Adolescent 12-Step Group Involvement Following Inpatient Treatment." *Alcoholism: Clinical and Experimental Research* 32(8):1468–1478, 2008, Figure 2. Copyright © 2008 John Wiley & Sons. Used with permission.

Table 15–2. Effective ways for clinicians to implement 12-step facilitation (TSF) strategies

Method	How it might be implemented	Studies using the approach
Stand-alone treatment	Individual therapy devoted entirely to facilitating AA attendance by promoting an abstinence goal, increasing willingness to use AA as a tool to help achieve abstinence, and monitoring reactions to AA.	Project MATCH Research Group 1997a Compared TSF as a stand-alone treatment with CBT and MET.
Integrated with other treatment	Within an existing treatment, such as CBT, incorporating encouragement to attend AA, getting patient to agree to attend specific meetings, and discussing AA literature, meetings, and sponsorship.	Walitzer et al. 2009 Compared treatment as usual (5% of time spent discussing AA), motivational AA facilitation (20% AA related), and directive AA facilitation (38% AA related). Kelly et al. 2017 (youth sample) Compared integrated 12-step/MET/CBT treatment with MET/CBT alone, finding better outcomes for the integrated treatment.
Component of a treatment package	Group education and discussion about AA separate from other treatment, with homework assignments to attend meetings, talk to other AA members outside of sessions, and get a sponsor.	Kaskutas et al. 2009 "Making AA Easier," a group intervention to help encourage participation, minimize resistance, and provide education about AA.

Table 15–2. Effective ways for clinicians to implement 12-step facilitation (TSF) strategies *(continued)*

Method	How it might be implemented	Studies using the approach
Modular add-on	Assertive linkage to specific groups, review of 12-step program and common concerns, direct connection to current AA members, and review of client attendance and experiences.	Timko et al. 2006 Compared standard AA referral with intensive treatment.

Note.   AA = Alcoholics Anonymous; CBT = cognitive-behavioral therapy; MET = motivational enhancement therapy.

Source.   Adapted from Kelly JF, Yeterian JD: "Alcoholics Anonymous and Young People," in *Young People and Alcohol: Impact, Policy, Prevention, Treatment.* Edited by Saunders JB, Rey JM. New York, John Wiley & Sons, 2011, Table 17–4. Copyright © 2011 John Wiley & Sons. Used with permission.

2008; Litt et al. 2009; Walitzer et al. 2009). Yet, until recently, no RCTs had examined the utility and efficacy of TSF approaches with adolescents.

While TSF interventions for youth are being developed and tested, it is helpful to focus on the developmentally specific differences between youth and adults noted earlier (see section "Life Contexts and Youth-Specific 12-Step Groups"). For example, TSF interventions for young people may benefit from placing a greater emphasis on NA or MA, rather than AA, because NA and MA may better serve young people, the majority of whom have a primary cannabis use disorder rather than alcohol or other drug use disorder (Kelly and Yeterian 2011). In fact, emerging research points to the benefits of adapting TSF interventions for young people in this way, as researchers have found that young people in a TSF development pilot study (Kelly et al. 2016, 2017) preferred MA and NA treatment "in-services"—in which a young NA member shares his or her story of addiction and recovery and helps facilitate discussion of the benefits of 12-step participation—to AA treatment in-services. This preference was due to the fact that the cannabis-specific experiences of the NA speakers aligned more closely with participants' own experiences when compared with the experience of AA members (Kelly et al. 2016). Although such findings are important for advancing knowledge and efficacy of youth-specific TSF interventions, it is unclear whether matching young people with 12-step fellowship type (e.g., NA, MA) and their primary substance (e.g., cannabis) is necessary for 12-step engagement and the benefits that members derive from long-term engagement. In a prior matching study, we found that despite having a primary "drug of choice" other than alcohol (i.e., cannabis, opioids, stimulants), youth benefited as much from AA attendance as they did from NA attendance in the year following residential SUD treatment, as demonstrated by comparable significant increases in postdischarge abstinence (PDA) in both groups (Kelly et al. 2014). Therefore, it may not be critical for youth to exclusively attend the 12-step group whose fellowship type aligns with their primary substance, but more research is needed to clarify whether young people with primary drug problems would do better in MA or NA when compared with AA, or whether they would do better in another 12-step group.

In the first and only RCT of adolescent-specific TSF, we developed and tested an integrated TSF (iTSF) that included motivational enhancement therapy (MET) and CBT elements in addition to 12-step elements, comparing it with MET/CBT alone. This outpatient protocol was found to double rates of 12-step participation, produce greater effect sizes in terms of enhancing continuous abstinence, and significantly reduce alcohol and other drug use consequences during and in the six months following treatment (Kelly et al. 2017) (see Figure 15–2).

Moderators and Mediators of 12-Step Participation Benefits

As noted previously, some studies have examined moderators and mediators of 12-step MHO benefit. Specifically, in a study with adolescents (Kelly et al. 2005), we found that as the age composition of attended meetings in the first 3 months following discharge from inpatient care became more teen/emerging adult-like, there was a significant increase in PDA. This was also evident between 4 and 6 months postdischarge, but the pattern during that follow-up period showed a potential diminishing return over time. In other words, the apparent benefit of age similarity on PDA declined over time.

This effect was replicated, amplified, and clarified in a subsequent study with emerging adults (18–25 years) (Labbe et al. 2014). This study found that those more ambivalent about 12-step MHO participation, compared with less ambivalent 12-step MHO attendees, had significantly better PDA if they attended 12-step meetings with similar-age peers *early* postresidential treatment discharge, but had *worse* PDA at 12-month follow-up if they were *still* attending purely youth-focused 12-step meetings. These findings suggest that age similarity is good for initial engagement but by itself may be less adept at addressing the ongoing recovery needs of many young people over time, suggesting a need to expand attendance to meetings in which at least some older adults may be present who possess longer recovery time and life experience (Labbe et al. 2014).

Our prior research has shown, too, that beyond these important dynamic age-specific moderator effects of 12-step attendance (i.e., the age composition of the most frequently attended meetings), there may be important differences in the mechanisms of behavior change through which 12-step participation confers recovery benefits for youth compared with older adults. For example, we have found that when compared with older adults, youth 12-step participation similarly enhances and maintains abstinence motivation, self-efficacy, and recovery coping skills, but only abstinence motivation is a full mediator and mechanism of behavior change (Kelly et al. 2000). This finding suggests that unlike adults, for whom all three of these variables have been shown to be significant mechanisms of behavior change (Kelly et al. 2012), adolescents may not exhibit the same degree of impaired control over substance use and may be better able to self-regulate the impulse to use substances once they make a commitment to doing so; 12-step participation appears to help them keep that motivation strong over time, which results in higher abstinence rates.

A further potentially important mediator of outcomes for adolescents is the social network support for substance use. As noted previously, evidence suggests that the precursors to relapse differ developmentally, with the majority of adult relapses being attributed to interpersonal conflict or negative emotional states and most youth relapses being attributed to social situations where alcohol and/or drugs are present (Brown 1993). Thus, youth may benefit from 12-step groups through the replacement of high-risk social situations with low-risk ones (e.g., AA/NA meetings, sober social activities) and a related change in peer network. As support for this notion, in a study of moderated

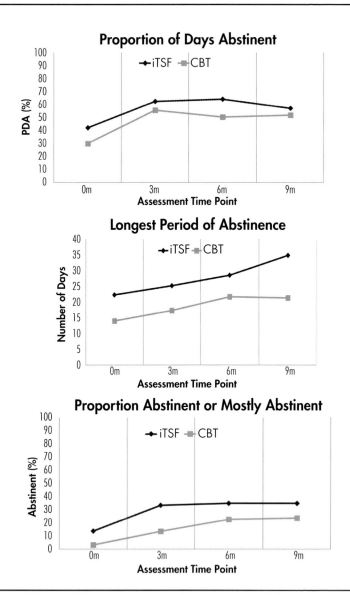

Figure 15–2. Differences in outcomes between integrated 12-step facilitation (iTSF) and cognitive-behavioral therapy (CBT) or motivational enhancement therapy (MET)/CBT in a parallel-group randomized controlled trial.

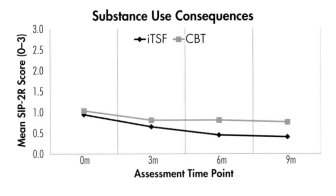

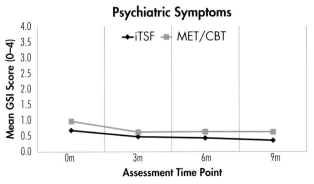

Figure 15–2.   Differences in outcomes between integrated 12-step facilitation (iTSF) and cognitive-behavioral therapy (CBT) or motivational enhancement therapy (MET)/CBT in a parallel-group randomized controlled trial. *(continued)*

GSI = Global Severity Index; PDA = postdischarge abstinence; SIP-2R = Short Inventory of Problems—Recent.

Source.   Adapted from Kelly JF, Kaminer Y, Kahler CW, et al.: "A Pilot Randomized Clinical Trial Testing Integrated 12-Step Facilitation (iTSF) Treatment for Adolescent Substance Use Disorder." *Addiction* 112(12):2155–2166, 2017, Figure 3. Copyright © 2008 John Wiley & Sons. Used with permission.

multiple mediation (Hoeppner et al. 2014; Figure 15–3), we found that compared with older adults, the mechanisms of behavior change via which emerging adults (18–29 years) are helped by 12-step participation is to a much greater extent through its ability to facilitate adaptive changes in their social networks.

Specifically, as shown in Figure 15–3, of the six mediators examined in this rigorous, temporally lagged analysis, by far the largest proportion of the direct effect of AA participation on increasing PDA and decreasing drinks per drinking day (DDD) among emerging adults was through AA's ability to help young people drop alcohol/drug-using social network members from their social networks. This accounted for more than double the mediated effect of that variable among older adults (see Figure 15–3; Hoeppner et al. 2014). Although the age range in this study of emerging adults (18–29 years) was slightly higher than that proposed in the current study (14–21 years), we believe similar mechanisms are likely operating.

Cost-Effectiveness

The economic importance of health care expenditure has continued to grow in recent years alongside rapidly increasing health care costs. Clinical linkages to 12-step MHOs—free, community-based recovery support services—have been shown not only to reduce health care costs but also to enhance clinical outcomes. For example, one study of inpatient SUD treatment programs at the Veterans Health Administration (VHA) found that patients who were treated in professionally led, 12-step-oriented treatment programs attended more AA/NA meetings in the year after treatment when compared with patients treated in CBT programs, who, incidentally, used more professional mental health and addiction services (Humphreys and Moos 2001). The annual health care costs for CBT patients were therefore 65% higher than they were for 12-step patients, which amounted to an additional $4,729 (in 2001 dollars; $6,694 in 2018 dollars) in health care costs per CBT patient ($6,694 in 2018 dollars) (Humphreys and Moos 2001). Moreover, when compared with CBT patients, those patients who received 12-step treatment had significantly higher rates of abstinence at 1-year follow-up (46% in 12-step vs. 36% in CBT) (Humphreys and Moos 2001). Importantly, the CBT and 12-step-oriented groups did not differ by demographic or clinical characteristics at intake. In another study, researchers followed a sample of adolescents for 7 years after they attended intensive outpatient substance use treatment in order to compare health care use and costs among individuals who reported 12-step participation during the follow-up period and those who did not (Mundt et al. 2012). Researchers found that for every 12-step group attended during the follow-up period, there was a $145 per year medical use costs savings (Kelly and Yeterian 2011; Mundt et al. 2012). Researchers attributed these medical cost offsets to a reduced number of alcohol and other drug use treatment costs, inpatient days, and psychiatric visits, and posited that these health care cost offsets could be due, in part, to social network changes as a result of 12-step participation (Mundt et al. 2012). Although the underlying mechanisms that account for the reduction of health care costs among 12-step group participants require further empirical investigation, both studies point to 12-step MHOs as essential recovery resources that not only aid in long-term recovery and remission but also reduce health care use and costs (Humphreys 2004; Kelly and Myers 2007).

In summary, compared with the adult research base on 12-step MHOs, the evidence base for youth is limited in both quantity and quality. Most studies of youth are observational studies following inpatient and outpatient treatment with varying degrees of scientific rigor. As a set of studies, they do show consistency and coherence in showing positive associations between greater attendance and better substance use outcomes up to 8 years following index treatments, with many, but not all, studies controlling for relevant confounds that might account for such positive relationships (e.g., motivation for abstinence, other ongoing treatments). Also, similar to adult studies, one long-term longitudinal youth study found benefits for youth 12-step participation on substance use outcomes and in reduced health care costs (Mundt et al. 2012).

In terms of increased participation and derived recovery benefits, directing youth to meetings where at least some other young people may be in attendance may improve both initial affiliation and clinical outcomes, but over time youth may need to branch out to meetings with a greater age range represented in which members potentially have longer-term sobriety and more life experience. Also, the way in which youth benefit from 12-step MHOs may differ from the way that adults benefit along developmental lines. It appears that a major factor in youth recovery is recovery motivation—the desire to stop or substantially reduce substance use. Compared with adults' treatment samples, youth possess less of this desire intrinsically, on average. Another major aspect of youth recovery appears to be helping them to find social networks that are both conducive to and supportive of recovery. Research so far suggests that 12-step MHOs produce a clinical benefit for young people,

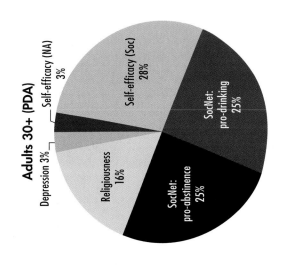

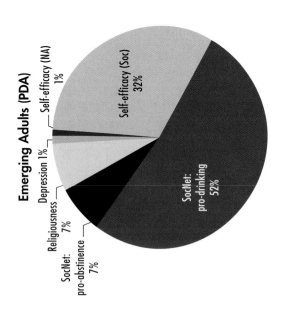

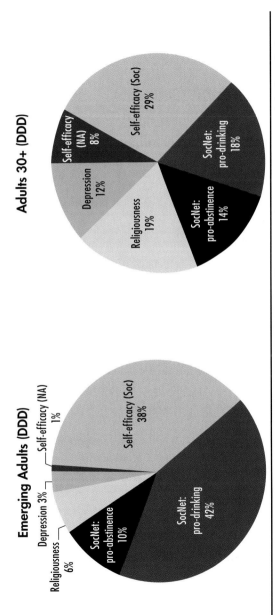

Figure 15–3. Moderated multiple mediation analyses showing differences in the ways emerging adults benefit from Alcoholics Anonymous (AA) compared with older adults.

Differences between emerging adults (18–29 years) and older adults (30+ years) in amount of variance in effect between AA and postdischarge abstinence (PDA) or defined daily dose (DDD), explained by each mechanism of behavior change: decreased depression (Depression); increased religiosity/spirituality (Religiousness); reduced pro-drinkers in one's social network (SocNet: pro-drinking); increased pro-abstainers in one's social network (SocNet: pro-abstinence); self-efficacy to cope with negative affect (Self-efficacy NA); and self-efficacy to cope with risky social situations (Self-efficacy Soc).

Source. Reprinted from Bergman B, Kelly J, Fallah-Sohy N, et al.: "Emerging Adults, Mutual-Help Organizations, and Addiction Recovery," in *Emerging Adults and Substance Use Disorder Treatment: Developmental Considerations and Innovative Approaches.* Edited by Smith DC. New York, Oxford University Press, 2018, Figure 8–2, p. 180. Copyright © 2018 Oxford University Press. Used with permission.

in particular, by enhancing and maintaining recovery motivation over time, and by helping young people drop the negative influence of drug-using peers in favor of prosocial and recovering peers.

Clinical Strategies to Increase 12-Step Participation Among Youth

The consistency and coherence of the systematic research evidence across adult, young adult, and adolescent samples strongly suggest that many youths are likely to derive recovery benefits from 12-step MHO participation. This may have the added advantage of reducing health care costs as these entities are ubiquitous and free of charge apart from voluntary contributions. Given the limited amount of formal research regarding TSF specifically for adolescents (Kelly et al. 2017), in this section we provide clinical guidelines (adapted from Kelly et al. 2018 and based on Kelly et al. 2016) using results derived from the first integrated TSF RCT that developed and tested a manualized outpatient intervention (Kelly et al. 2016, 2017).

Provide Information About 12-Step Meetings

Unlike adults, who often have prior exposure to or knowledge of 12-step meetings, adolescents, particularly those with less severe conditions who are receiving outpatient treatment, often do not have such knowledge or exposure (Kelly et al. 2018). Therefore, providing information about what 12-step organizations are, who they are for, and where to find them, is helpful for young people in treatment. Therapists should inquire about their young patients' knowledge of, or prior experience with, meetings and should provide a brief overview of meetings along with a recommendation to attend them during treatment. It is also advisable for therapists to discuss meeting types, meeting formats, and the culture of 12-step groups to help prepare their patients for their first 12-step meeting. Introducing 12-step concepts can also be helpful for young patients to help them better understand certain language that they might hear at meetings. For example, discussing the Serenity Prayer or slogans such as "One day at a time" or "This too shall pass" can help acquaint young new members with 12-step concepts. After developing a familiarity with meetings over time, therapists can encourage patients to include attending 12-step meetings as a written "step to take" toward their treatment goal so as to elicit a verbal and written commitment to attend during treatment.

Provide a Rationale for Attending 12-Step Meetings During and After Treatment

Asking young patients to provide their own rationale for attending 12-step meetings is also advisable (Kelly et al. 2018). Questions such as "Why do we talk about attending 12-step meetings in treatment?" can help patients generate answers. If answers are not generated by young patients themselves, providers are encouraged to provide the rationale that treatment is short term and that sustained recovery-specific social support is needed to help maintain sobriety over time. Research suggests, however, that young people often generate the correct answers to such questions themselves (Kelly et al. 2016). To further help young patients understand the benefits of 12-step meeting attendance, providers can facilitate discussion of the ways in which attending 12-step meetings can help with treatment-related topics (i.e., social support, coping with urges and cravings, effective communication, and coping with feelings and the challenges of sobriety). When discussing, for example, the importance of avoiding people and places that place the person at risk while in recovery, therapists can facilitate discussion of how attending 12-step meetings can provide access to new sober supports that can help avoid high-risk social situations (e.g., socializing with sober people after meetings).

Facilitate In-House Presentations by Young Members of 12-Step Organizations

Inviting young 12-step members to share their stories of recovery with young people in treatment is strongly advised (Kelly et al. 2018). Exposing young patients to other young people in recovery to whom they can look up to as role models is an effective method of addressing myths and misconceptions of recovery or of 12-step members. Moreover, inviting speakers to address young people in treatment can help increase the chances that patients may be able to identify with 12-step members and receive targeted information relevant to young 12-step members, such as how to find a good young person's meeting. Similarly, inviting speakers who are a good match for the types of drug using experienced by adolescent patients is also advisable. For example, if most patients' primary substance is cannabis, inviting speakers from MA and NA can help facilitate greater identification.

Incorporate Elements of 12-Step Meetings Into Treatment Wherever Possible

Mirroring certain components of 12-step meetings in treatment groups for young people is also advisable (Kelly et al. 2018). Reading aloud a specific group "preamble" and "closing statement" that outline the group's rationale and goals, for example, can help prepare young patients for 12-step meetings. Additionally, providers may choose to distribute "chips" or tokens for group meeting attendance, similar to how chips are awarded at 12-step meetings for sobriety milestones. Members who are new to a treatment group can also be invited to briefly share their personal stories during check-in, which not only mirrors this important aspect of 12-step group meetings but also helps introduce members to one another. Finally, 12-step group rules such as "no crosstalk" can also be adopted into treatment groups in order to further familiarize young people with the 12-step group format.

Have Adolescents Set Weekly Sober Activity Goals and Strongly Encourage 12-Step Attendance

At the end of each group, it is advisable to have youth set a goal to complete at least one sober activity in the following week, such as attending a 12-step meeting or participating in an activity with a sober friend (Kelly et al. 2018). Ideally, young patients will participate in sober activities in addition to 12-step meetings, although giving adolescents the choice to attend 12-step meetings as their sober activity is generally appreciated. Asking young patients to write their goal on a worksheet and read it aloud to the group can help the individual make a public commitment to change, which is associated with an increased likelihood of making the change. During group check-ins each week, it is also advisable to ask young patients to re-read their previous week's goal and report on whether they met it.

Enlist Parental Support for 12-Step Meeting Attendance

Providers should invite parents/guardians of minor patients into at least a portion of individual treatment sessions (e.g., the last 15 minutes) in order to facilitate 12-step meeting attendance during and after treatment (Kelly et al. 2018). It is ideal to have the young patient and their parent/guardian together in a session so that all are privy to providers' recommendations and any other pertinent information, such as research results (ideally graphically presented) showing that adolescents who attend 12-step meetings tend to have better treatment outcomes. During conjoint session time, providers can also help problem-solve barriers to 12-step treatment attendance, such as transportation to 12-step meetings during treatment. The ultimate goal is for the provider to help parents/guardians understand the potential therapeutic value of their child attending 12-step meetings and enlist their support in helping their child get to meetings.

Conclusion

Professional treatment often produces significant salutary changes in adolescents' substance use (Dennis et al. 2004; Tanner-Smith et al. 2013) but by itself may be inadequate to address the prodigious and chronic burden of disease attributable to SUDs. Furthermore, the cost of providing professional care alone for high-volume, high-burden diseases such as SUDs can place a financial burden on many families as well as broader society's economic and human health resources. Given the aim of maximizing the effectiveness of our clinical and public efforts in addressing these endemic public health problems, research suggests that combining proven clinical interventions that link patients with free, ubiquitous, indigenous, community-based recovery support resources that can provide natural prosocial, recovery-related contingencies is likely to enhance remission and long-term recovery rates and simultaneously reduce health care costs. Fortunately, an array of such resources are available in the form of 12-step MHOs and emerging alternative peer groups. Also, newer MHOs that are not 12-step based, such as SMART Recovery and LifeRing, are likely to offer potentially similar utility and benefit but are few in number, and systematic evidence is not available regarding youth participation in such alternatives.

In conclusion, clinical recommendations offered in this chapter are based on sound scientific principles and somewhat limited available evidence, specifically pertaining to young people. Given the devastation that SUDs can cause among young people, including having lifelong ramifications as well as carrying the risk of premature death, much more research is needed to help understand the clinical and public health utility of new and existing MHOs, as well as other recovery support services that might be developed to attract and engage more young people to enhance remission and quality of life.

Key Points

- The consistency and coherence of existing empirical evidence support the clinical and public health utility of facilitating youth participation in 12-step mutual help organizations (MHOs).

- Evidence suggests youth with moderate to severe substance use disorder are likely to become engaged with 12-step MHOs if clinically introduced to 12-step philosophy and practices and encouraged to participate.

- Research indicates that youth who participate in 12-step MHOs are likely to have higher abstinence rates, fewer substance-related consequences, and lower health care costs than youth not participating in these groups.

- Encouraging youth to attend a variety of types of meetings attended by a variety of ages may be better for long-term 12-step MHO retention and substance use outcomes.

- Sophisticated mechanisms of behavior change research suggests that youth may benefit from 12-step MHOs via the ability of such organizations to help these youth shift their social networks from ones dense in substance-using peers to ones that contain more recovering peers.

References

Alcoholics Anonymous World Services: 2014 membership survey. 2014. Available at: http://www.aa.org/assets/en_US/p-48_membershipsurvey.pdf. Accessed May 14, 2019.

Brown SA: Recovery patterns in adolescent substance abuse, in Addictive Behaviors Across the Life Span: Prevention, Treatment, and Policy Issues. Edited by Marlatt GA, Baer JS. Newbury Park, CA, Sage Publications, 1993, pp 161–183

Chi FW, Kaskutas LA, Sterling S, et al: Twelve-step affiliation and 3-year substance use outcomes among adolescents: social support and religious service attendance as potential mediators. Addiction 104(6):927–939, 2009 19344442

Dennis M, Godley SH, Diamond G, et al: The Cannabis Youth Treatment (CYT) Study: main findings from two randomized trials. J Subst Abuse Treat 27(3):197–213, 2004 15501373

Gore FM, Bloem PJ, Patton GC, et al: Global burden of disease in young people aged 10–24 years: a systematic analysis. Lancet 377(9783):2093–2102, 2011 21652063

Hoeppner BB, Hoeppner SS, Kelly JF: Do young people benefit from AA as much, and in the same ways, as adult aged 30+? A moderated multiple mediation analysis. Drug Alcohol Depend 143:181–188, 2014 25150401

Hsieh S, Hoffmann NG, Hollister CD: The relationship between pre-, during-, post-treatment factors, and adolescent substance abuse behaviors. Addict Behav 23(4):477–488, 1998 9698976

Humphreys K: Circles of Recovery: Self-Help Organizations for Addictions. Cambridge, UK, Cambridge University Press, 2004

Humphreys K, Moos R: Can encouraging substance abuse patients to participate in self-help groups reduce demand for health care? A quasi-experimental study. Alcohol Clin Exp Res 25(5):711–716, 2001 11371720

Kahler CW, Strong DR, Read JP: Toward efficient and comprehensive measurement of the alcohol problems continuum in college students: the brief young adult alcohol consequences questionnaire. Alcohol Clin Exp Res 29(7):1180–1189, 2005 16046873

Kaskutas LA, Ye Y, Greenfield TK, et al: Epidemiology of Alcoholics Anonymous participation. Recent Dev Alcohol 18:261–282, 2008 19115774

Kaskutas LA, Subbaraman MS, Witbrodt J, et al: Effectiveness of making Alcoholics Anonymous easier: a group format 12-step facilitation approach. J Subst Abuse Treat 37(3):228–239, 2009 19339148

Kelly JF: Self-help for substance-use disorders: history, effectiveness, knowledge gaps, and research opportunities. Clin Psychol Rev 23(5):639–663, 2003 12971904

Kelly JF, Myers MG: Adolescents' participation in Alcoholics Anonymous and Narcotics Anonymous: review, implications and future directions. J Psychoactive Drugs 39(3):259–269, 2007 18159779

Kelly JF, Urbanoski K: Youth recovery contexts: the incremental effects of 12-step attendance and involvement on adolescent outpatient outcomes. Alcohol Clin Exp Res 36(7):1219–1229, 2012 22509904

Kelly JF, Yeterian JD: Alcoholics Anonymous and young people, in Young People and Alcohol: Impact, Policy, Prevention, Treatment. Edited by Saunders JB, Rey JM. New York, Wiley, 2011, pp 308–326

Kelly JF, Yeterian JD: Mutual-help groups for alcohol and other substance use disorders, in Addictions: A Comprehensive Guidebook. Edited by McCrady BS, Epstein EE. New York, Oxford University Press, 2013, pp 500–525

Kelly JF, Myers MG, Brown SA: A multivariate process model of adolescent 12-step attendance and substance use outcome following inpatient treatment. Psychol Addict Behav 14(4):376–389, 2000 11130156

Kelly JF, Myers MG, Brown SA: The effects of age composition of 12-step groups on adolescent 12-step participation and substance use outcome. J Child Adolesc Subst Abuse 15(1):63–72, 2005 18080000

Kelly JF, Brown SA, Abrantes A, et al: Social recovery model: an 8-year investigation of adolescent 12-step group involvement following inpatient treatment. Alcohol Clin Exp Res 32(8):1468–1478, 2008 18557829

Kelly JF, Dow SJ, Yeterian JD, et al: Can 12-step group participation strengthen and extend the benefits of adolescent addiction treatment? A prospective analysis. Drug Alcohol Depend 110(1–2):117–125, 2010 20338698

Kelly JF, Hoeppner B, Stout RL, et al: Determining the relative importance of the mechanisms of behavior change within Alcoholics Anonymous: a multiple mediator analysis. Addiction 107(2):289–299, 2012 21917054

Kelly JF, Greene MC, Bergman BG: Do drug-dependent patients attending Alcoholics Anonymous rather than Narcotics Anonymous do as well? A prospective, lagged, matching analysis. Alcohol Alcohol 49(6):645–653, 2014 25294352

Kelly JF, Yeterian JD, Cristello JV, et al: Developing and testing twelve-step facilitation for adolescents with substance use disorder: manual development and preliminary outcomes. Subst Abuse 10:55–64, 2016 27429548

Kelly JF, Kaminer Y, Kahler CW, et al: A pilot randomized clinical trial testing integrated 12-step facilitation (iTSF) treatment for adolescent substance use disorder. Addiction 112(12):2155–2166, 2017 28742932

Kelly JF, Cristello JV, Bergman BG: Integrated 12-Step facilitation to promote adolescent mutual-help involvement, in Treating Alcohol and Substance Abuse in Adolescents, 2nd Edition. Edited by Monti PM, Colby SM, O'Leary-Tevyaw TA. New York, Guilford, 2018, pp 405–428

Kelly JF, Abry AW, Fallah-Sohy N, et al: Mutual help and peer support models for opioid use disorder recovery, in Treating Opioid Addiction. Edited by Kelly JF, Wakeman SE. New York, Springer Nature/Humana Press, 2019, pp 139–167

Kennedy BP, Minami M: The Beech Hill Hospital/Outward Bound Adolescent Chemical Dependency Treatment Program. J Subst Abuse Treat 10(4):395–406, 1993 8411298

Knudsen HK, Ducharme LJ, Roman PM, et al: Service delivery and use of evidence-based treatment practices in adolescent substance abuse treatment settings. 2008. Available at: http://ntcs.uga.edu/reports/Adolescent%20Study%20Summary%20Report. Accessed May 14, 2019.

Labbe AK, Greene C, Bergman BG, et al: The importance of age composition of 12-step meetings as a moderating factor in the relation between young adults' 12-step participation and abstinence. Drug Alcohol Depend 133(2):541–547, 2013 23938074

Labbe AK, Slaymaker V, Kelly JF: Toward enhancing 12-step facilitation among young people: a systematic qualitative investigation of young adults' 12-step experiences. Subst Abus 35(4):399–407, 2014 25102256

Litt MD, Kadden RM, Kabela-Cormier E, et al: Changing network support for drinking: network support project 2-year follow-up. J Consult Clin Psychol 77(2):229–242, 2009 19309183

Mundt MP, Parthasarathy S, Chi FW, et al: 12-Step participation reduces medical use costs among adolescents with a history of alcohol and other drug treatment. Drug Alcohol Depend 126(1–2):124–130, 2012 22633367

Narcotics Anonymous World Services: Narcotics Anonymous 2013 membership survey. 2013. Available at: https://www.na.org/admin/include/spaw2/uploads/pdf/PR/NA_Membership_Survey.pdf. Accessed May 14, 2019.

Nash A, Collier C: The alternative peer group: a developmentally appropriate recovery support model for adolescents. J Addict Nurs 27(2):109–119, 2016 27272995

Nash A, Marcus M, Engebretson J, et al: Recovery from adolescent substance use disorder: young people in recovery describe the process and keys to success in an alternative peer group. Journal of Groups in Addiction and Recovery 10(4):290–312, 2015

National Institute on Drug Abuse: Drugs, brain, and behavior: the science of addiction. July 20, 2018. Available at: https://www.drugabuse.gov/publications/drugs-brains-behavior-science-addiction. Accessed May 14, 2019.

Project MATCH Research Group: Matching alcoholism treatments to client heterogeneity: Project MATCH posttreatment drinking outcomes. J Stud Alcohol 58(1):7–29, 1997a 8979210

Project MATCH Research Group: Project MATCH secondary a priori hypotheses. Addiction 92(12):1671–1698, 1997b 9581001

Roman PM, Blum TC: National Treatment Center Study (Summary 3). Athens, GA, University of Georgia, 1999

Substance Abuse and Mental Health Services Administration: Key Substance Use and Mental Health Indicators in the United States: Results From the 2017 National Survey on Drug Use and Health (NSDUH Series H-53, HHS Publ No SMA 18-5068). Rockville, MD, Center for Behavioral Health Statistics and Quality, Substance Abuse and Mental Health Services Administration, 2018

Stanger C, Lansing AH, Budney AJ: Advances in research on contingency management for adolescent substance use. Child Adolesc Psychiatr Clin N Am 25(4):645–659, 2016 27613343

Tanner-Smith EE, Wilson SJ, Lipsey MW: The comparative effectiveness of outpatient treatment for adolescent substance abuse: a meta-analysis. J Subst Abuse Treat 44(2):145–158, 2013 22763198

Timko C, DeBenedetti A: A randomized controlled trial of intensive referral to 12-step self-help groups: one-year outcomes. Drug Alcohol Depend 90(2–3):270–279, 2007 17524574

Timko C, Debenedetti A, Billow R: Intensive referral to 12-step self-help groups and 6-month substance use disorder outcomes. Addiction 101(5):678–688, 2006 16669901

Tonigan JS, Toscova R, Miller WR: Meta-analysis of the literature on Alcoholics Anonymous: sample and study characteristics moderate findings. J Stud Alcohol 57(1):65–72, 1996 8747503

Walitzer KS, Dermen KH, Barrick C: Facilitating involvement in Alcoholics Anonymous during out-patient treatment: a randomized clinical trial. Addiction 104(3):391–401, 2009 19207347

Wu LT, Pilowsky DJ, Schlenger WE, et al: Alcohol use disorders and the use of treatment services among college-age young adults. Psychiatr Serv 58(2):192–200, 2007 17287375

16

Electronic Tools and Resources for Assessing and Treating Youth Substance Use Disorders

Rachel Gonzales-Castaneda, Ph.D., M.P.H.

Kyle C. McCarthy, M.S.

Briana Thrasher, B.A.

T he topic of teens and substance use is of great importance among health professionals, policy makers, and the lay public. A common question frequently raised among these diverse groups is "Why are adolescents more prone to substance use risk taking and addiction (or substance use disorders [SUDs])?" In pursuit of answers to this question, growing attention has focused on the adolescent brain. The research looking at when individuals with SUDs start using alcohol and drugs has established that the risk is higher for those who start early (DeWit

This work was supported in part by grants K01 DA027754 from the National Institute on Drug Abuse and Los Angeles County Contract 2000-S-TG661 from the Department of Public Health.

349

et al. 2000), during their teenage years, given that the maturing brains of adolescents are more likely to make the myriad of changes and adaptations in core systems (learning, reward, and executive control functions) that are associated with the onset, progression, and maintenance of SUDs. Specifically, studies have identified that the heightened activity in the reward center, coupled with the lack of executive constraint in the developing adolescent brain, is a recipe for risk taking and progression toward "pathological compulsive behaviors" (Eaton et al. 2006). We see this reflected in epidemiological studies that report on steady prevalence rates of use of tobacco, alcohol, cannabis, and other illicit drugs each year, as well as growing rates of treatment admissions, which soared to 20.7 million Americans (7.6%) over the age of 12 seeking substance use treatment in 2016 (Substance Abuse and Mental Health Services Administration 2017). These epidemiological and treatment trends are concerning and raise another common question asked among diverse circles: "What are effective ways to address (prevent and treat) adolescent substance use risk issues?"

Increasingly attention has been given to the use of technology applications for the prevention and treatment of substance use among adolescents given the following critical developmental aspects: 1) the developing brain has heightened sensitivity toward the interactive learning that technology offers, and (2) adolescent culture is ingrained in multiple technology applications, spanning web/Internet, smartphone/texting, mobile apps, and social media (Lenhart et al. 2010). Findings from a Pew Internet and American Life Project (Lenhart et al. 2010) indicate that the majority (93%) of teenagers between the ages of 12 and 17 years use the Internet, with most using for social networking connection, entertainment, and news/information. The field has benefited from immense research and practice-based information on how to effectively address adolescent substance use issues (Winters et al. 2011); however, we have a more limited understanding of the current research on the use, utility, and impacts associated with the adoption of technology applications for addressing adolescent substance abuse issues within SUD treatment settings.

Technology to Aid Screening and Prevention

There are many potential applications of technology for screening and prevention in the adolescent population, both prior to SUD onset and along the treatment continuum. While controversial, advanced genetic testing is one potential advancement in the prevention and screening of adolescents prior to onset. Specifically, studies have found functional differences in the μ opioid receptors of individuals with an expressed G allele on the OPRM1 gene, which has been linked with higher sensitivity to alcohol and increased prevalence of alcohol use disorders (Ray and Hutchison 2004). Furthermore, reward deficiency syndrome (RDS) and its group of addictive disorders have been observed in connection with the undersynthesis of dopamine D_2 receptors by the DRD2 gene, which is highly involved in one's reward system and sensations of pleasure (Heber and Carpenter 2011; Noble 2003). Together, technological advancements have led to the development of the Genetic Addiction Risk Score, or GARS, which is a polygenetic test for the RDS phenotype associated with dysfunctional reward behaviors and psychiatric disorders (see Blum et al. 2014).

In a world of evolving technologies, non-invasive DNA sampling for genetic screening purposes is now more economical, efficacious, and unobtrusive than ever before (Rogers et al. 2007). Clinicians and researchers agree that when one is screening for and diagnosing lifetime incidence of SUDs, combinations of biometric and psychometric measures are more accurate than either measure in isolation (Lennox et al. 2006), and the same holds true for preemptive preventive screening. Also, in the realm of screening and prevention, researchers have recently been exploring the possibility of using algorithms to analyze social media trends associated with risks of SUD development and have used Instagram data to identify patterns of deep learning associated with risk for alcohol abuse (Hassanpour et al. 2019). Just as public schools and health care providers have begun implementing Screening, Brief Intervention, and Referral to Treatment (SBIRT) practices for prevention and early intervention (Curtis et al. 2014), genetic and other novel forms of screening may hold future promise to alert parents and caregivers of the potential hereditary or behavioral risks for their youth developing a SUD.

Technological Considerations for Adolescents Along the Treatment-Recovery Continuum

There is growing use of technology-based applications for the delivery of SUD treatment for adolescents. In particular, some studies have explored how the use of technology can help address key barriers related to access, engagement, and compliance that have been commonly cited in adolescent studies as major issues. Research supports that technology-based applications (offered as therapeutic agents) might be of particular interest among adolescents challenged by behavioral health complexities to overcome some of the barriers faced when seeking help, because of the high levels of anonymity, easy access independent of time and location, and the potential of such approaches to be perceived as less stigmatizing (Bauer and Moessner 2013). A recent study exploring interest in the use of technology for delivering relapse prevention found that both adolescents and counselors alike expressed much interest in online relapse prevention, with 84% of the clients rating their satisfaction with the program greater than 5 on a 7-point Likert scale (Trudeau et al. 2012).

A feature that adolescents really liked in this study's prototype was text messaging, while counselors liked the utility online relapse prevention programs have for helping adolescents secure healthy social networks with other peers also engaging in relapse prevention (Trudeau et al. 2012). The interest expressed by adolescents in text messaging raises the importance of paying attention to how programs are communicating to adolescents. Specifically, technology has revolutionized and changed norms of communication exchange. For example, the use of mobile devices invites the relay of information via text, pictorial images using emojis, or other graphics interchange formats (GIFs). Additionally, the Internet offers a powerful medium of communication exchange via email, tweeting, posting, chatting, messaging, hashtagging, tagging, uploading pictures and videos, and liking/disliking. This type of communication exchange does not support the traditional models used in treatment settings, because it conflicts with the standard protocols of 1- to 2-hour assessments and 90-minute group formats that are not brief or instant and require a response. The area of interest expressed by counselors—"securing healthy social networks"—has been an Achilles heel for the adolescent addiction field, as treatment studies have shown that peer use and peer pressure are major impediments to adolescent treatment engagement and successful adherence to treatment regimens (Riggs et al. 2007).

The use of technology in adolescent treatment settings also addresses key organizational issues that have been identified as major performance challenges around access (e.g., not offering transportation or flexible evening, drop-in, or weekend hours) and engagement in services among adolescents and families

(Copeland and Martin 2004). In addition, using technology in therapeutic practice offers a way for counselors to build "therapeutic alliance," a critical component of the adolescent-counselor clinical dyad that has been linked to enhanced engagement and behavioral outcomes among adolescents (Winters et al. 2011), such that technology-based approaches allow for maintaining real-time contact via checking in on treatment progress with goals and objectives. For example, Newman et al. (2011) discuss questions raised about potential challenges technology-driven therapies have with therapeutic efficacy due to the minimal relational contact among individuals with drug and alcohol abuse and smoking addiction; they point out that such technological approaches have been found to be beneficial because they enhance the client-provider relationship by helping individuals feel safe to disclose and to be constantly connected or "plugged in." In addition, studies that have tested the utility of mobile phone–based ecological momentary assessment (EMA) methods with adolescents in clinical settings confirm that ongoing technology-monitoring methods can serve as a "clinician extender" and help with monitoring key information related to high-risk situations and triggers in real time, while keeping adolescents feeling accountable (Marsch and Borodovsky 2016).

All technology-based therapeutic applications are not created equal. The use of technology in the substance use field for adolescents is in the infancy stage, with most of the research focused on utility and feasibility and less on clinical treatment outcome studies. A review of the latter by Marsch and Borodovsky (2016) offers important information about key ingredients (i.e., theoretical and empirically driven components) that technology-based applications are built on for effectively addressing adolescent SUDs. One key element is the inclusion of social influence–driven strategies such as integrating norms-based education and using peer-delivered models (Toumbourou et al. 2007). Studies suggest that incorporating social norming information during SUD interventions can help decrease risk behaviors, given that it does more than merely educate about harms; it encourages critical thinking about existing social norms regarding substance abuse and correcting misconceptions regarding risk behaviors within the context of social norms (Neighbors et al. 2004). Additionally, the use of virtual peers within technology-based applications in the behavioral health field broadly has also been found to be effective compared with standard or traditionally based delivery methods such as in-person or generic texts (Eysenbach et al. 2004; Pfeiffer et al. 2011).

Another critical element is the inclusion of motivational enhancement strategies such as interactive, simulated scenarios that offer youth opportunities to engage in decision-making and readiness-for-change exercises, as well as to make autonomous choices through exploring activities from a menu of options. According to adolescent problem behavior theory, motivation-driven interventions are important for adolescents who engage in substance use risk behaviors because they tend to be in precontemplative (in denial of personal risk behaviors) or contemplative (ambivalent toward accepting personal risk behaviors) states that require motivational interventions (Jessor 1991). As such, motivational enhancement strategies allow adolescents the opportunity to explore and resolve ambivalence about risky behavior and the need for change through the inclusion of technology, which can help with dynamically adapting to fluid levels of motivation to change (Dallery et al. 2015; Jessor 1991).

The inclusion of cognitive-behavioral skills–based learning strategies is key as well. Such strategies include teaching specific skills related to resisting opportunities to engage in substance use behavior using virtual role-plays, problem solving, and rehearsal learning in a manner that opens adolescents up allowing them to respond freely. These strategies are especially useful given the reluctance that adolescents have in opening up to counselors without feeling embarrassment or shame, as can be the case during in-person group sessions. Specifically, this approach allows sensitive issues to be dealt with in a personalized, yet confidential manner and promotes honest reporting on sensitive topics (Braciszewski et al. 2018). Marsch et al. (2007) point out that the delivery of such skill-based learning via technology is enhanced through the use of an array of multimedia methods to deliver personalized feedback, videos, audio instruction of techniques or case examples to model use of therapeutic techniques, and printable therapy worksheets. Newman et al. (2011) found benefits of using technological approaches in treatment settings because such approaches enhance the development of skills by promoting self-monitoring and the facilitation of tracking one's own progress in therapy, which positively affects motivation and adherence.

Trials and Empirical Contributions

The literature indicates that mobile phone–based programs, GPS tracking, and wearable sensors are among the primary methods of mobile health (mHealth) technology–based interventions. However, mobile phone–based programs are by and far the most prominent of the currently used technology-based interventions. Dennis et al. (2015) conducted a feasibility study that utilized a mobile phone–based platform to assess EMAs multiple times daily and demonstrated the ability of such data to predict risk of youth participants' relapse in the subsequent week. There have been few full-length trials, but we discuss here three randomized controlled trial pilots for mobile phone–based interventions that reported positive outcomes: Project ESQYIR, which was specifically with a youth sample, and A-CHESS and LBMI-A, both of which have designs that were demonstrated to be effective with adults and that show promise as models for adolescents.

Project ESQYIR (Educating and Supporting inQuisitive Youth in Recovery) was a clinical trial that randomly assigned youth participants, ages 14–26 years, to receive either an experimental mobile texting aftercare intervention or an aftercare-as-usual control intervention for 3 months following discharge from primary substance use treatment (Gonzales et al. 2014). Project ESQYIR employed a disease self-management model that facilitated monitoring, feedback, reminders, social support, and education through automated text messages and prompts for participant response. The project demonstrated efficacy at reducing primary substance use relapse and increasing rates of recovery-related extracurricular and self-help participation when compared with the control intervention (Gonzales et al. 2016). Additionally, Project ESQYIR saw reductions of overall SUD and co-occurring symptomatology in the intervention group as measured by the Global Appraisal of Individual Needs—Short Screener, which has been shown to predict future substance use relapse and recidivism (Smith et al. 2017). Last, Gonzales-Castaneda et al. (in press) performed mediational analyses and discovered that the participants' increased extracurricular activity resulting from Project ESQYIR was the primary mechanism of action facilitating the reduction in substance use.

The adult Addiction-Comprehensive Health Enhancement Support System (A-CHESS; Gustafson et al. 2014) is a mobile phone–based and GPS-equipped application designed to improve continuity of treatment for alcohol dependence. One feature of this mobile application is the Weekly Check-In, which gathers information shown to predict substance use relapse and may provide an opportunity to give critical support to individuals at times of heightened risk. An additional adult program is the Location-Based Monitoring and Intervention for Alcohol Use Disorders (LBMI-A), or "Buddy" as referred to by the users in its trial (Dulin et al. 2014). LBMI-A demonstrated efficacy at increasing percentage of days abstinent during the trial and showed that overall drinks per week and heavy drinking days decreased the more the participants utilized the application. Together, A-CHESS and LBMI-A provide evidence for the feasibility and efficacy of mobile phone–based programs with adults, which in turn has provided insight into the implementation and targeted services needs of similar programs for adolescents.

While mobile phone–based platforms are the most common form of technological integration in the recovery continuum to expand the scope of treatment, wearable devices and digital phenotyping are beginning to be utilized more frequently (Ferreri et al. 2018). Like mobile phones, which extend the scope of treatment, wearable health devices expand the reach of biometric monitoring and the wealth of data available for diagnosis and progress tracking, thereby improving treatment outcomes, improving quality of life, and decreasing the overall cost of health care (Yilmaz et al. 2010). Wearable sensors, often in the form of a bracelet, are able to track vitals (i.e., heart rate, blood pressure, blood glucose, and cardiac or respiratory activity) as well as cognitive states and physiological arousal through electrochemical sensors with results comparable to those of an electroencephalogram or electrocardiogram (Dubad et al. 2018; Windmiller and Wang 2013). Additionally, transdermal alcohol sensors are able to actively monitor and detect alcohol consumption accurately in a timely manner and have been shown to reduce relapse, especially when paired with other behavioral interventions (Barnett et al. 2011). Last, given their limited ability for emotion regulation due to developmental limitations in the frontal cortex (Volkow and Fowler 2000), emotional volatility is a primary risk factor for adolescent SUD episodes, and, therefore, mobile mood-monitoring applications have immense utility with youth for high risk for SUD (Dubad et al. 2018).

Digital phenotyping is a form of live evaluation used in psychiatric and behavior change interventions that compiles data from smartphones and wearable devices to approximate patterns of risk (Insel 2017). Wearable devices can track symptoms of chronic disease in real time, providing feedback to patients and providers in order to initiate early action and minimize harm during a relapse episode (Steinhubl et al. 2015). Platforms that employ wearable sensors and self-report data through a mobile application have developed an mHealth model that can predict risk of substance use relapse based on a myriad of pre-dictor variables that are tracked continuously. Although pilot programs have had moderate success and have demonstrated feasibility, more research is necessary to explore the efficacy of combined technological approaches (e.g., mobile application combined with GPS and wearable biosensors) in comparison with other treatment modalities and combinations of technological integration. As the number of independent studies on mHealth interventions continues to grow, the need for meta-analysis becomes more apparent, as just over 50% of the existing trials have reported positive outcomes (Nesvåg and McKay 2018).

Technology Applications for Adolescents in Recovery

For most, recovery is a long process with phases overlapping a variety of SUD manifestations and spanning periods of treatment, remission, and relapse; the process starts when the individual first recognizes the detrimental impact of his or her using behaviors, contemplates change, and then begins making steps toward that change (Dennis and Scott 2007). The Substance Abuse and Mental Health Services Administration (SAMHSA) released a working definition of recovery in 2012: *recovery* was defined as a process of change to obtain health and well-ness, while seeking one's full potential and living a self-directed life supported by four major dimensions: health, home, community, and purpose (Substance Abuse and Mental Health Services Administration 2012). Although not all adolescents go through treatment before entering recovery, the majority of mobile phone–based interventions have been implemented during outpatient treatment, the final stage in a step-down treatment model before being discharged from all levels of care and fully reintegrated in society (Kampman and Jarvis 2015). This is primarily for logistical and methodological reasons to structure a controlled trial but also because organizational support is a necessary component for sustained adherence to such programs (Nesvåg and McKay 2018).

Although adolescent service needs have not been studied exclusively, findings from adult samples reveal that housing, relationships with family and others, and especially employment and education are top concerns for individuals in recovery (Laudet and White 2010). These findings are consistent with SAMHSA's four dimensions of recovery, but it is expected that the order of priority varies for adolescents, with social and relational aspects (i.e., community) being paramount (Riggs et al. 2007). The utility of mobile-based interventions at facilitating social support was demonstrated when A-CHESS was accessed most for social networking purposes among its available functions (Gustafson et al. 2014); this indicates that mobile platforms could meet this relational/community service need for adolescents outside the scope of treatment. Additionally, Project ESQYIR provides a unique contribution to the field because it not only studied an adolescent sample but also employed the intervention exclusively during recovery, as opposed to during primary or outpatient treatment as has been the case in most other trials (Gonzales et al. 2014). Further supporting the efficacy of mHealth for adolescents in recovery, Gonzales et al. (2016) found that the adolescents in Project ESQYIR's experimental texting group had sustained improvements in self-help and extracurricular involvement compared with the control group at 6 and 9 months following completion of the texting intervention.

A recent meta-analysis evaluating outpatient treatment for adolescents found that cognitive-behavioral therapy (CBT) and motivational enhancement therapy, as well as family and behavioral therapies, demonstrated the best outcomes (Tanner-Smith et al. 2013), findings that provide insight into the respective approaches to employ via mHealth for adolescents in recovery. These findings are encouraging because Watts et al. (2013) has found efficacy for CBT in mobile platforms for adults with depression that could be similarly employed for youth with SUD. Additionally, Earley (2017) discusses new patents that are pending for mHealth in the private sector, such as David Gastfriend's DynamiCare RecoveryMind Training, which integrates contingency management as a form of behavioral modification, as well as the typical mHealth functions (i.e., monitoring, feedback, GPS, psychoeducation, goal setting, and scheduling). Multiple simultaneous approaches are more effective than any single approach, and, therefore, it is recommended that one use mobile technology to target and facilitate multiple facets of an adolescent's recovery by maintaining contact, monitoring, engaging, locating through GPS, incentivizing, and networking through social media or otherwise (Farabee et al. 2016).

Future Directions

Although the use of technology for behavioral interventions and therapies has become an emerging approach for supporting the delivery of treatment for adolescent populations challenged with SUDs, there are future directions for study that warrant consideration. One area of future research is the use of contingency management strategies in technology-based therapeutic interventions with adolescents. Contingency management has been identified as a critical element of successful programs supported by decades of research showing the efficacy of using incentives and rewards for influencing desired behavioral change (Stitzer and Petry 2006). To date, such studies have only been conducted with adult clinical samples. For instance, Alessi and Petry (2013) have tested the feasibility and utility of a mobile phone–based contingency management intervention with individuals with alcohol use disorder and found high satisfaction among drinkers and counselors alike, as well as longer duration of abstinence compared with control subjects. In addition, Budney et al. (2015) demonstrated the cost-effectiveness of using contingency management protocols when offered with computer-delivered CBT/MET for reducing cannabis use, with a savings of $175 on average per participant.

More research is needed in the area of family systems involvement in adolescent treatment using technology approaches. Processes within the family system (parents and caregivers) have been established as key influences affecting adolescent engagement and treatment outcomes that involve monitoring and communication (Tobler and Komro 2010). A few studies have investigated the utility of an online program for parents of adolescents in treatment called "Parenting Wisely," which targeted improving communication and disciplinary skills of parents and resulted in reduced substance abuse and other behavior problems with their children (Becker et al. 2017). In addition, more work is needed around exploring the utility of peer support–driven online resources for youth. A specific area to explore is the extent to which activity level in online support groups determines outcomes among adolescents who use alcohol and drugs, given that most work has been done among youth who smoke tobacco (Woodruff et al. 2007). The impact of including a professional health care/treatment clinician (e.g., "The Doctor Is In" chatroom) and how this affects motivation to change due to perceived help needs to be explored further (Dallery et al. 2015).

Another area of growing interest that warrants future study is the utility of technology applications for adolescents in rural, remote areas without ready access to services (Jackmon et al. 2016). The U.S. Department of Agriculture Economic Research Service currently estimates that more than 70% of individuals in rural areas use the Internet, with more than 50% maintaining home Internet service (Stenberg et al. 2009). Web-based technology permits communities to utilize preexisting resources (i.e., Internet), thus requiring less capital investment for start-up, reducing cost of program implementation by lessening labor-intensive components and other costly resources, and increasing accessibility to prevention methods. Such a call for using technology-based methods in health care prevention efforts is the cornerstone of recent funding initiatives by the U.S. Department of Health and Human Services.

Finally, more research is needed on the utility and impact of using technology as supplemental aids to regular, in-person treatment among adolescents. There is growing interest in using technology to aid with addressing co-occurring behavioral needs among substance-abusing adolescents, such as polysubstance use or continued use of "other substances" like tobacco and alcohol while in treatment for other illicit drug use, HIV/STD risks, and medication compliance for adolescents with opioid use disorder receiving medication-assisted treatment. Technology can also be used in helping track relapse factors, such as mood, with wearable physiological sensors and engagement in nondrug activities based on tagging locations for such activity via GPS (Dallery et al. 2015). In addition, more research is needed on the integration of technology approaches for delivering non-clinical-based services that are important components of care, such as implementing assessment and case management protocols.

Conclusion

Overall, technology applications such as mHealth, mobile phone–based interventions, wearables, and GPS have demonstrated feasibility and utility among adults and hold great promise for adolescents despite scarce empirical evidence. The limited trials on that segment of the population have demonstrated successful outcomes, warranting further investigation and future application. Technology has the potential to accommodate the barriers for youth in recovery and cater both to the unique culture of our current adolescent generation and to the vast demands of the today's Information Age. Commonalities between most technology applications for adolescents across the SUD continuum involve personalization, monitoring, feedback, support, social facilitation, goal setting, and psychoeducation on relapse prevention, conflict resolution, emotional coping, communication, and disease management, with more recent applications integrating GPS and wearable sensors. Further, cognitive-behavioral, behavioral, and motivational therapies such as contingency management, as well as medication-assisted treatment, are being implemented and evaluated concurrently with mHealth modalities. Some of the more radical approaches to screening and monitoring certainly are not without controversy, but given the growing costs to society related to substance use and given the increasing fatality rates with the introduction of new synthetic substances, more rigorous approaches may be warranted in the future. In conclusion, technology for adolescents in recovery is rapidly evolving, but given the relative paucity of randomized controlled trials, this remains an area requiring future exploration.

Key Points

- New technologies continue to become more readily available and economical.

- Extant, but limited, studies have demonstrated feasibility and efficacy of such programs at improving primary substance use outcomes.

- Mobile phone–based platforms accommodate typical treatment barriers for youth associated with stigma, scheduling, and inaccessibility, and maximize connectivity by capitalizing on the technology-enthralled culture of the current adolescent generation.

- The most common mobile-based platforms include multiple components to promote behavior change and consist of some combination of self-report ecological momentary assessments, GPS, and/or biometric monitoring.

References

Alessi SM, Petry NM: A randomized study of cellphone technology to reinforce alcohol abstinence in the natural environment. Addiction 108(5):900–909, 2013 23279560

Barnett NP, Tidey J, Murphy JG, et al: Contingency management for alcohol use reduction: a pilot study using a transdermal alcohol sensor. Drug Alcohol Depend 118(2–3):391–399, 2011 21665385

Bauer S, Moessner M: Harnessing the power of technology for the treatment and prevention of eating disorders. Int J Eat Disord 46(5):508–515, 2013 23658102

Becker SJ, Hernandez L, Spirito A, et al: Technology-assisted intervention for parents of adolescents in residential substance use treatment: protocol of an open trial and pilot randomized trial. Addict Sci Clin Pract 12(1):1, 2017 28049542

Blum K, Oscar-Berman M, Demetrovics Z, et al: Genetic Addiction Risk Score (GARS): molecular neurogenetic evidence for predisposition to reward deficiency syndrome (RDS). Mol Neurobiol 50(3):765–796, 2014 24878765

Braciszewski JM, Wernette GKT, Moore RS, et al: A pilot randomized controlled trial of a technology-based substance use intervention for youth exiting foster care. Children and Youth Services Review 94:466–476, 2018

Budney AJ, Stanger C, Tilford JM, et al: Computer-assisted behavioral therapy and contingency management for cannabis use disorder. Psychol Addict Behav 29(3):501–511, 2015 25938629

Copeland J, Martin G: Web-based interventions for substance use disorders: a qualitative review. J Subst Abuse Treat 26(2):109–116, 2004 15050088

Curtis BL, McLellan AT, Gabellini BN: Translating SBIRT to public school settings: an initial test of feasibility. J Subst Abuse Treat 46(1):15–21, 2014 24029623

Dallery J, Jarvis B, Marsch L, et al: Mechanisms of change associated with technology-based interventions for substance use. Drug Alcohol Depend 150:14–23, 2015 25813268

Dennis M, Scott CK: Managing addiction as a chronic condition. Addict Sci Clin Pract 4(1):45–55, 2007 18292710

Dennis ML, Scott CK, Funk RR, et al: A pilot study to examine the feasibility and potential effectiveness of using smartphones to provide recovery support for adolescents. Subst Abus 36(4):486–492, 2015 25310057

DeWit DJ, Adlaf EM, Offord DR, et al: Age at first alcohol use: a risk factor for the development of alcohol disorders. Am J Psychiatry 157(5):745–750, 2000 10784467

Dubad M, Winsper C, Meyer C, et al: A systematic review of the psychometric properties, usability and clinical impacts of mobile mood-monitoring applications in young people. Psychol Med 48(2):208–228, 2018 28641609

Dulin PL, Gonzalez VM, Campbell K: Results of a pilot test of a self-administered smartphone-based treatment system for alcohol use disorders: usability and early outcomes. Subst Abus 35(2):168–175, 2014 24821354

Earley PH: RecoveryMind Training: A Neuroscientific Approach to Treating Addiction. Las Vegas, NV, Central Recovery Press, 2017

Eaton DK, Kann L, Kinchen S, et al: Youth risk behavior surveillance—United States, 2005. J Sch Health 76(7):353–372, 2006 16918870

Eysenbach G, Powell J, Englesakis M, et al: Health related virtual communities and electronic support groups: systematic review of the effects of online peer to peer interactions. BMJ 328(7449):1166, 2004 15142921

Farabee D, Schulte M, Gonzales R, et al: Technological aids for improving longitudinal research on substance use disorders. BMC Health Serv Res 16(1):370, 2016 27509830

Ferreri F, Bourla A, Mouchabac S, et al: E-addictology: an overview of new technologies for assessing and intervening in addictive behaviors. Front Psychiatry 9:51, 2018 29545756

Gonzales R, Ang A, Murphy DA, et al: Substance use recovery outcomes among a cohort of youth participating in a mobile-based texting aftercare pilot program. J Subst Abuse Treat 47(1):20–26, 2014 24629885

Gonzales R, Hernandez M, Murphy DA, et al: Youth recovery outcomes at 6 and 9 months following participation in a mobile texting recovery support aftercare pilot study. Am J Addict 25(1):62–68, 2016 26689171

Gonzales-Castaneda R, McKay JR, Steinberg J, et al: Testing mediational processes of substance use relapse among youth who participated in mobile texting aftercare project. Substance Abuse (in press)

Gustafson DH, McTavish FM, Chih M-Y, et al: A smartphone application to support recovery from alcoholism: a randomized clinical trial. JAMA Psychiatry 71(5):566–572, 2014 24671165

Hassanpour S, Tomita N, DeLise T, et al: Identifying substance use risk based on deep neural networks and instagram social media data. Neuropsychopharmacology 44(3):487–494, 2019 30356094

Heber D, Carpenter CL: Addictive genes and the relationship to obesity and inflammation. Mol Neurobiol 44(2):160–165, 2011 21499988

Insel TR: Digital phenotyping: technology for a new science of behavior. JAMA 318(13):1215–1216, 2017 28973224

Jackmon W, Blaalid B, Chester-Adam H: Child and adolescent drug abuse prevention: a rural community-based approach. S D Med No:49–54, 2016 28817850

Jessor R: Risk behavior in adolescence: a psychosocial framework for understanding and action. J Adolesc Health 12(8):597–605, 1991 1799569

Kampman K, Jarvis M: American Society of Addiction Medicine (ASAM) national practice guideline for the use of medications in the treatment of addiction involving opioid use. J Addict Med 9(5):358–367, 2015 26406300

Laudet AB, White W: What are your priorities right now? Identifying service needs across recovery stages to inform service development. J Subst Abuse Treat 38(1):51–59, 2010 19631490

Lenhart A, Purcell K, Smith A, et al: Social Media and Mobile Internet Use Among Teens and Young Adults: Millennials. Washington, DC, Pew Internet & American Life Project, 2010

Lennox R, Dennis ML, Scott CK, et al: Combining psychometric and biometric measures of substance use. Drug Alcohol Depend 83(2):95–103, 2006 16368199

Marsch LA, Borodovsky JT: Technology-based interventions for preventing and treating substance use among youth. Child Adolesc Psychiatr Clin N Am 25(4):755–768, 2016 27613350

Marsch LA, Bickel, W, Grabinski, M: Application of interactive, computer technology to adolescent substance abuse prevention and treatment. Adolescent Medicine: State of the Art Reviews 18(2):342–356, xii, 2007

Neighbors C, Larimer ME, Lewis MA: Targeting misperceptions of descriptive drinking norms: efficacy of a computer-delivered personalized normative feedback intervention. J Consult Clin Psychol 72(3):434–447, 2004 15279527

Nesvåg S, McKay JR: Feasibility and effects of digital interventions to support people in recovery from substance use disorders: systematic review. J Med Internet Res 20(8):e255, 2018 30139724

Newman MG, Szkodny LE, Llera SJ, et al: A review of technology-assisted self-help and minimal contact therapies for anxiety and depression: is human contact necessary for therapeutic efficacy? Clin Psychol Rev 31(1):89–103, 2011 21130939

Noble EP: D2 dopamine receptor gene in psychiatric and neurologic disorders and its phenotypes. Am J Med Genet B Neuropsychiatr Genet 116B(1):103–125, 2003 12497624

Pfeiffer PN, Heisler M, Piette JD, et al: Efficacy of peer support interventions for depression: a meta-analysis. Gen Hosp Psychiatry 33(1):29–36, 2011 21353125

Ray LA, Hutchison KE: A polymorphism of the mu-opioid receptor gene (OPRM1) and sensitivity to the effects of alcohol in humans. Alcohol Clin Exp Res 28(12):1789–1795, 2004 15608594

Riggs PD, Thompson LL, Tapert SF, et al: Advances in neurobiological research related to interventions in adolescents with substance use disorders: research to practice. Drug Alcohol Depend 91(2–3):306–311, 2007 18038460

Rogers NL, Cole SA, Lan HC, et al: New saliva DNA collection method compared to buccal cell collection techniques for epidemiological studies. Am J Hum Biol 19(3):319–326, 2007 17421001

Smith DC, Bennett KM, Dennis ML, et al: Sensitivity and specificity of the GAIN short-screener for predicting substance use disorders in a large national sample of emerging adults. Addict Behav 68:14–17, 2017 28088053

Steinhubl SR, Muse ED, Topol EJ: The emerging field of mobile health. Sci Transl Med 7(283):283rv3, 2015 25877894

Stenberg PL, Morehart MJ, Vogel SJ, et al: Broadband Internet's value for rural America (Economic Research Report ERR-78. Washington, DC, Economic Research Service, U.S. Dept of Agriculture, August 2009. Available at: https://www.ers.usda.gov/publications/pub-details/?pubid=46215. Accessed July 24, 2019.

Stitzer M, Petry N: Contingency management for treatment of substance abuse. Annu Rev Clin Psychol 2:411–434, 2006 17716077

Substance Abuse and Mental Health Services Administration: SAMHSA's Working Definition of Recovery: 10 Guiding Priniciples of Recovery. Rockville, MD, Center for Behavioral Health Statistics and Quality, Substance Abuse and Mental Health Services Administration, 2012

Substance Abuse and Mental Health Services Administration: Key Substance Use and Mental Health Indicators in the United States: Results From the 2016 National Survey on Drug Use and Health (HHS Publ No SMA 17-5044, NSDUH Series H-52). Rockville, MD, Center for Behavioral Health Statistics and Quality, Substance Abuse and Mental Health Services Administration, 2017

Tanner-Smith EE, Wilson SJ, Lipsey MW: The comparative effectiveness of outpatient treatment for adolescent substance abuse: a meta-analysis. J Subst Abuse Treat 44(2):145–158, 2013 22763198

Tobler AL, Komro KA: Trajectories of parental monitoring and communication and effects on drug use among urban young adolescents. J Adolesc Health 46(6):560–568, 2010 20472213

Toumbourou JW, Stockwell T, Neighbors C, et al: Interventions to reduce harm associated with adolescent substance use. Lancet 369(9570):1391–1401, 2007 17448826

Trudeau KJ, Ainscough J, Charity S: Technology in treatment: are adolescents and counselors interested in online relapse prevention? Child Youth Care Forum 41(1):57–71, 2012 23930049

Volkow ND, Fowler JS: Addiction, a disease of compulsion and drive: involvement of the orbitofrontal cortex. Cereb Cortex 10(3):318–325, 2000 10731226

Watts S, Mackenzie A, Thomas C, et al: CBT for depression: a pilot RCT comparing mobile phone vs. computer. BMC Psychiatry 13:49, 2013 23391304

Windmiller JR, Wang J: Wearable electrochemical sensors and biosensors: a review. Electroanalysis 25(1):29–46, 2013

Winters KC, Botzet AM, Fahnhorst T: Advances in adolescent substance abuse treatment. Curr Psychiatry Rep 13(5):416–421, 2011 21701838

Woodruff SI, Conway TL, Edwards CC, et al: Evaluation of an Internet virtual world chat room for adolescent smoking cessation. Addict Behav 32(9):1769–1786, 2007 17250972

Yilmaz T, Foster R, Hao Y: Detecting vital signs with wearable wireless sensors. Sensors (Basel) 10(12):10837–10862, 2010 22163501

Co-occurring Disorders in Youth

The population of adolescents diagnosed with substance use disorders (SUDs) is heterogeneous. One of the largest subgroups comprises those with one or more co-occurring psychiatric disorders. This condition is commonly referred to as *dual diagnosis*, although it might be a condition involving multiple diagnoses, including psychiatric and/or SUDs (e.g., attention-deficit/hyperactivity disorder (ADHD) and depression and/or alcohol and cannabis use disorders simultaneously). Dual diagnosis is the rule rather than the exception, with a prevalence of 70%–80% in clinical samples of youth (Kaminer 2016). Co-occurring psychiatric disorders have an impact on the development, course, and treatment outcomes of SUD. The opposite is also true because there is a bidirectional effect. To prevent repetition in the chapters included in this section, we address here issues pertaining to SUDs and various co-occurring psychiatric disorders as a group: 1) the etiology and nature of the association, 2) diagnostic considerations and assessment challenges, and 3) clinical and service provision implications.

The Etiology and Nature of the Association

The longitudinal relationship between co-occurring psychiatric disorder and SUD during adolescence cannot be simplistically attributed to a single potential model. Five explanatory models have been proposed: 1) a self-medication model of psychiatric symptomatology leading to a secondary substance use; 2) a disease model in which the primary SUD is the cause of a secondary psychopathology; 3) a bidirectional model in which multiple factors are involved in triggering and maintaining co-occurring psychiatric disorder and SUD; 4) a common factor model, proposed to independently increase the neurobiological risk for both co-occurring psychiatric disorder and SUD; and 5) an unrelatedness model that suggests a co-probability of otherwise unrelated disorders co-occurring. Finally, combinations of these models may interact in different ways for diverse subgroups of youth. Regardless of the model, our view of the research is that SUD is not the sole or primary cause of the initiation of psychiatric symptoms.

What is the supporting evidence for these models? Although the idea that self-medication plays a significant role in the co-occurrence of these disorders is highly popular among both clients and professionals, the reported validity of the self-medication model has been low. The bidirectional and disease models, both of which suggest that SUD plays a central role in the onset and course of dual diagnosis, are not supported by epidemiological data. According to the Epidemiologic Catchment Area study conducted with community samples of individuals ages 18–30 years, in three out of four cases the psychiatric disorder preceded the substance use (Christie et al. 1988). But the issue of the order of co-occurring psychiatric disorder and SUD is complex. A recent systematic review and meta-analysis of cannabis and co-occurring psychiatric disorder suggests that the high prevalence of cannabis use in adolescents and perhaps the growing potency of Δ-9-tetrahydrocannabinol might contribute to the development of depression (odds ratio [OR] = 1.37) and suicidality (ideation OR = 1.50; attempt OR = 3.46), but not anxiety disorders, later during young adulthood (Gobbi et al. 2019). These data may support the bidirectional model.

Genome-wide association studies have shown overlapping genetic involvement in some psychiatric disorders. A large database of human genotypes and phenotypes is available (www.ncbi.nlm.nih.gov/gap). The progress in genetic studies provides support for the common factor, or shared liability, model as a pivotal hypothesis for co-occurring disorders (Groenman et al. 2017). The diagnostic presentation consisting of SUD and co-occurring psychiatric disorder(s), including personality disorder, reflects the relative salience of behavioral and emotional components of psychological dysregulation (Tarter and Horner 2016). Furthermore, the Transmissible Liability Index (TLI) is a unidimensional intergenerational trait encompassing both internalizing and externalizing features that reflects the relative salience of behavioral and emotional components of psychological dysregulation. This unidimensional risk trait is the result of neural circuitry in frontal cortex, striatum, and limbic system (Tarter and Horner 2016). More than 75% of TLI variance is heritable.

Youth dual diagnosis might affect the development, trajectories, and natural and treatment outcomes of one or both co-occurring disorders because of the unique dynamic trajectories of trait variables, such as impulsivity, sensation seeking, hopelessness, and anxiety sensitivity (Conrod 2016). The importance of this conceptual paradigm might be associated with the allostatic hypothesis that emphasizes the secondary psychopathology that emerges after prolonged substance use, including the compensatory use of other drugs (Koob and Le Moal 2008). The term *rebound effect* has been used to explain biological and behavioral processes that provoke an effect by which substance use may produce or increase psychiatric symptoms (the association specifically between relapse and co-occurring psychiatric disorders) (Tomlinson et al. 2006). This effect contributed to the development of the spiral bidirectional hypothesis of the allostatic model.

The opiate epidemic of the last decade can be partially explained by the allostatic model. The progression from occasional to chronic use of cannabis and other drugs is a shift from substance use as a positively reinforced reward-seeking behavior to a negatively reinforced compulsive behavior. With respect to comorbid psychopathology, the model suggests that negative mood states related to substance use cycles evolve into chronic conditions (e.g., internalizing disorders). Progression to co-use or substitution of other substances leading to the use of opiates or cocaine is an anticipated expanded effort to achieve relief from reward deficiency and negative mood states.

Diagnostic Considerations

Most studies examine psychiatric comorbidity in terms of categorical classification and as a static patient characteristic that affects drug use severity and outcomes. The stability or change of diagnostic status among adolescents with co-occurring psychiatric disorders has not been systematically examined, impeding our understanding of how co-occurring disorders affect trajectories of relapse and recovery. The amount and direction of change typically vary across disorders, and much of the shift occurs between subthreshold and threshold status (Costello et al. 2003). Complicating matters is that youth with SUDs, including subdiagnostic SUDs, are also at increased risk for other psychiatric symptoms and diagnoses (Shrier et al. 2003). Psychosocial impairments that do not meet full DSM diagnoses of 29 well-defined disorders were identified as common among youth (Angold et al. 1999).

The Great Smoky Mountains Study examined presence of DSM-IV diagnoses in 1,420 adolescents 9–13 years of age in the community annually until age 16 years, when 36.7% had symptoms that met criteria for at least one psychiatric disorder. Social anxiety, panic, depression, and SUDs increased in prevalence, whereas disorders such as ADHD decreased (Costello et al. 2003). There were comorbidities between anxiety, depression, and SUD, as well as between conduct disorder, ADHD, and SUD. Disruptive behavior disorders and depression were associated with a higher rate and earlier onset of substance use and abuse in both sexes. Despite differences in prevalence of psychopathology, both sexes showed more similarities than differences in the course of early substance use and abuse and its associations with psychopathology (Costello et al. 1999). Findings from a study examining the stability of co-occurring disorders among adolescents in treatment for SUD are consistent with an epidemiological study such as the Great Smoky Mountains Study. There was evidence for both continuity and change in diagnostic status (Hawke et al. 2008). Continuity was greatest for youth with externalizing disorders and for youth who were symptomatic at baseline. However, a considerable number of youths with internalizing disorders improved in terms of their current psychiatric symptoms and diagnostic disorder. These changes included both subthreshold and threshold status.

Once the duration of the disorder reaches a certain point, recovery becomes substantially less probable over the ensuing time period. Understanding the temporal sequencing for onset and maintenance of comorbidity might promote treatment planning. For example, little is known about factors associated with the persistence (i.e., length of the index episode) of cannabis use disorder over time. Farmer et al. (2016) reported that any primary internalizing disorder was significantly and negatively associated with the duration of cannabis use disorder. This finding became a trend ($P<0.06$) after the study authors controlled for putative confounders. This finding of a modest protective factor against longer cannabis use disorder duration is consistent with findings previously reported, including that those with depression are less likely to use cannabis for self-medication. The opposite is true with the secondary emergence of both internalizing and externalizing disorders and/or other SUDs. The presence of both internalizing and externalizing disorders are significantly and positively associated with the duration of any SUD (Farmer et al. 2016).

Clinical and Service Implications

Adolescents with co-occurring psychiatric disorders present many intervention challenges. Such youth are associated with greater problem severity, poorer prognosis, increased treatment challenges, and greater unmet need for treatment compared with youth with either a single SUD or a single behavioral disorder (Clark et al. 2008; Kessler et al. 2005; Priester et al. 2016). Furthermore, trajectories of relapse and recovery may be influenced by fluctuations in diagnostic status related to co-occurring psychiatric disorders and may intersect with use of psychotropic medications, severity of substance use, and utilization of mental health and substance use services. Barriers for integrating treatment services for the dually diagnosed include 1) the historical separation of substance abuse and mental health services; 2) the limited number of clinicians and researchers who focus on dually diagnosed youth; and 3) the tendency to exclude youth with SUD from medication clinical trials of psychiatric disorder. Piecemeal unidimensional treatments targeting a single diagnosis of either the co-occurring psychiatric disorder or the SUD (or vice versa) have a higher risk of failure than integrated treatments that target both disorders. There is a growing clinical consensus for a necessity to develop, test, disseminate, and coordinate intervention protocols aiming for both the SUD and the co-occurring psychiatric disorder.

In this part of the manual (Chapters 17–21), the authors provide further specific information pertinent to the nature of and how to treat several specific co-occurring psychiatric disorders in youth with SUDs.

References

Angold A, Costello EJ, Farmer EM, et al: Impaired but undiagnosed. J Am Acad Child Adolesc Psychiatry 38:129–137, 1999

Christie KA, Burke JD, Regier DA, et al: Epidemiologic evidence for early onset of mental disorders and higher risk of drug abuse in young adults. Am J Psychiatry 145:971–975, 1988

Clark DB, Thatcher DL, Tapert SF: Alcohol, psychological dysregulation, and adolescent brain development. Alcohol Clin Exper Res 32:375–385, 2008

Conrod PJ: Personality-targeted interventions for substance use and misuse. Current Addict Rep 3:426–436, 2016

Costello EJ, Erkanli A, Federman E, Angold, A: Development of psychiatric comorbidity with substance abuse in adolescents: effects of timing and sex. J Clin Child Psychol 28:298–311, 1999

Costello EJ, Mustillo S, Erkanli A, et al: Prevalence and development of psychiatric disorders in childhood and adolescence. Arch Gen Psychiatry 60:837–844, 2003

Farmer RA, Kosty DB, Seeley JR, et al: Association of comorbid psychopathology with the duration of cannabis use disorders. Psychol Addict Behav 30:82–92, 2016

Gobbi G, Atkin T, Zytynski T, et al: Association of cannabis use in adolescence and risk of depression, anxiety, and suicidality in young adulthood: a systematic review and meta-analysis. JAMA Psychiatry Feb 13, 2019 (Epub ahead of print)

Groenman AP, Janssen TWP, Oosterlaan J: Childhood psychiatric disorders as risk factor for subsequent substance abuse: a meta-analysis. J Am Acad Child Adolesc Psychiatry 56:556–569, 2017

Hawke JM, Kaminer Y, Burke R, et al: Stability of comorbid psychiatric diagnosis among youths in treatment and aftercare for alcohol use disorders. Subst Abuse 29(2):33–41, 2008

Kaminer Y (ed): Youth Substance Abuse and Co-occurring Disorders. Arlington, VA, American Psychiatric Publishing, 2016

Kessler RC, Berglund P, Demler O, et al: Lifetime prevalence and age-of-onset distributions of DSM-IV disorders in the National Comorbidity Survey Replication. Arch Gen Psychiatry 62:593–602, 2005

Koob FG, Le Moal M: Addiction and the brain antireward system. Ann Rev Psychol 59:29–53, 2008

Priester MA, Browne T, Lachini A, et al: Treatment access barriers and disparities among individuals with co-occurring mental health and substance use disorders: an integrative literature review. J Subst Abuse Treat 61:47–59, 2016

Shrier LA, Harris SK, Kurland M, et al: Substance use problems and associated psychiatric symptoms among adolescents in primary care. Pediatrics 111:e699–705, 2003

Tarter RE, Horner MS: Developmental pathways to substance use disorder and co-occurring psychiatric disorders in adolescents, in Youth Substance Abuse and Co-occurring Disorders. Edited by Kaminer Y. Arlington, VA, American Psychiatric Publishing, 2016, pp 1–20

Tomlinson KL, Tate SR, Anderson KG, et al: An examination of self-medication and rebound effects: psychiatric symptomatology before and after alcohol or drug relapse. Addict Behav 31:461–474, 2006

17

Assessment and Treatment of Co-occurring Internalizing Disorders

Depression, Anxiety Disorders, and PTSD

Yifrah Kaminer, M.D., M.B.A.

Kristyn Zajac, Ph.D.

Ken C. Winters, Ph.D.

T he objectives of this chapter are, first, to enhance practitioners' understanding of the relationship between concomitant substance use disorder (SUD) and comorbid internalizing disorders, including unipolar depression, anxiety disorders, and posttraumatic stress disorder (PTSD), and, second, to increase the knowledge regarding assessment and coordinated treatment of adolescents with these comorbid disorders. In each section we address the characteristics, epidemiology, assessment, and treatment of the specific internalizing disorder among youth with SUD.

Depression

Epidemiology and the Association Between SUD and Co-occurring Depression

The comorbidity of SUD with unipolar depression in adolescents is well established. Developmentally, adolescence is a time when the prevalence of both depression and substance use increases in nonreferred community samples. Co-occurring adolescent depression is a public health concern in its own right. The median age at onset of unipolar depression has been dropping, and a secular trend of a shift to an earlier age at onset for major depression has been reported. In the mid-1990s, only 8.3% of adolescents were diagnosed with major depressive disorder (MDD). According to results from the 2017 National Survey on Drug Use and Health (Center for Behavioral Health Statistics and Quality 2018), 12.8% of adolescents ages 12–17 had a major depressive episode (MDE). Almost a third of those with MDE had been using psychoactive drugs, compared with 13% without MDE. Depression is second only to disruptive behaviors (e.g., attention-deficit/hyperactivity disorder, conduct disorder) as the most frequent co-occurring psychiatric disorder among adolescents with SUD. Among adults 18–30 years of age, the reported cumulative odds ratio (OR) between MDD, dysthymia, and SUD was 1.7–2.0 (Christie et al. 1988). Comorbidity rates of 24%–50% were reported in clinical samples (Curry and Hersh 2016). Comorbid depression is associated with more severe alcohol or drug disorders, more substance-related problems, poorer social competence, and lower quality of life (Becker and Curry 2007). In depressed samples, alcohol and substance abuse are each associated with longer episodes of depression as well as elevated risk for suicidal behaviors, including suicidal ideation, suicide attempts, and completed suicide. Depressed suicide attempters with alcohol use disorder (AUD) are more impulsive and tend to make more lethal attempts than those without AUD (Sher et al. 2007). For further information on suicidal behavior screening, assessment and interventions, see Chapter 18 in this manual.

It is noteworthy that there are publications that support the view that internalizing disorders are a "protective factor" in the trajectory of SUD. Arendt et al. (2007) discussed enhanced risk for cannabis use and argued that a) internalizing disorders are associated with elevated behavioral inhibition; b) behavioral inhibition may counteract reward seeking associated with negative consequences; c) individuals with internalizing disorders are less likely to affiliate with deviant peers, and these persons may experience cannabis to be less reinforcing; and d) cannabis use may lead to intensification of distressing internalizing symptoms, thus making continued use less likely.

Importance of Subthreshold Disorders

Similarly to the general findings by Angold et al. (1999) on the clinical importance of subthreshold diagnosis, Lewinsohn and colleagues (2000) argued that the clinical significance of depressive symptoms does not depend on crossing the major depressive diagnostic threshold. They established that adolescents who have significant depressive symptoms but whose symptoms do not meet strict DSM-IV criteria for MDD, such as subthreshold depression or depressive disorder not otherwise specified, have greater psychosocial impairment, elevated rates of psychiatric comorbidities and SUD, and increased suicidality. Carrellas et al. (2017) reported that a depressive state does not have to reach diagnostic levels to complicate treatment of SUD. It has been estimated that 5%–29% of adolescents have significant depressive symptoms that do not meet diagnostic criteria. Furthermore, individuals with significant depressive symptoms are at increased risk for both subsequent episodes of depression and SUD. Hill et al. (2014) reported that a third of adolescents with a subthreshold diagnosis developed MDD during a follow-up period. Therefore, youth with fewer than five symptoms of depression necessary for a MDD diagnosis according to the most updated diagnostic criteria, DSM-5 (American Psychiatric Association 2013), can benefit from treatment to alleviate clinically significant depressed mood.

Assessment of Depression in Youth With SUD

The psychiatric assessment of adolescents with SUD should routinely include screening questions about depressive symptoms. Symptoms include depressive or sad mood, irritability, anhedonia, and suicidality. Symptoms should be considered clinically significant if they are present for extended periods of time, affect the teenager's daily psychosocial or academic functioning, and are above and beyond what is expectable for the adolescent's chronological and psychological age. Validated rating scales that screen for depression utilizing either parent report or self-report are used to quantify depressive symptoms. If screening suggests significant depressive symptoms, a thorough clinical evaluation should be completed to determine the presence of a depressive disorder and other comorbid psychiatric and medical conditions.

The most frequently used interview in adolescent depression treatment research has been the Schedule for Affective Disorders and Schizophrenia for School-Age Children—Present and Lifetime Version (K-SADS-PL; Kaufman et al. 1997). The Diagnostic Interview Schedule for Children (DISC; Shaffer et al. 2000) is a structured psychiatric interview with parent and child versions. It includes most common child/adolescent mental disorders, using DSM criteria. A Voice DISC version allows self-administration.

Whereas the diagnostic assessment can determine the presence of a depressive disorder and any comorbid disorders, as well as their onset, sequence, and offset, such interviews are limited in determining current severity of symptoms. For assessment of severity and change, especially before, during, and after treatment, a clinical interview involving rating scales is more useful. The prototype of such a scale in the area of adolescent depression is the Children's Depression Rating Scale, Revised (CDRS-R; Poznanski and Mokros 1996). Fourteen interview items pertaining to the past week are administered to the teen and then the parent. The evaluator synthesizes data on each item, makes a best-estimate rating, and completes three observational items. Scores range from 17 to 114. The CDRS-R has high reliability. A minimum raw score of 40 is required for clinical depression. Calculation of a score is done as follows: baseline score minus current score divided by baseline score minus 17 times 100 (e.g., $(45-35)/(45-17) \times 100$. A 50% reduction in score is considered to be indicative of a remission.

Self-report scales are often used as secondary outcome measures in adolescent depression and can be readily used as a comorbidity measure in substance abuse treatment studies. Self-reports do not take long to complete, and they can be used repeatedly to track change. One of the most commonly used self-report scales is the Beck Depression Inventory–II (BDI-II; Beck et al. 1996). The BDI-II consists of 21 items, each rated on a 0–3 scale, that ask about specific symptoms over the past 2 weeks. Like the CDRS-R, then, it is sensitive to change over relatively short periods of time. It has excellent internal consistency.

Treatment of SUD and Co-occurring Depression

Little is known about how depression influences youth SUD treatment outcomes and vice versa. Clinical care systems usually treat these disorders separately (Hawkins 2009). Adolescents with combined depression and SUD have higher rates of perceived service needs and receive more treatment services as compared with adolescents with noncomorbid disorders.

Primary Depression Treatment

Only a few treatment studies in adolescents have examined the relations between depression and SUD when depression was the primary focus, and most excluded alcohol-abusing youth (e.g., Treatment for Adolescents With Depression Study Team 2003). Goldstein et al. (2009) examined data from the multisite Treatment of Resistant Depression in Adolescents (TORDIA). All subjects were diagnosed with MDD. Although youth with SUD were excluded from the study, 25% reported substance use three or more times during the study. Among MDD responders there was a significant improvement in substance-related impairment. MDD response at 12 weeks was best for adolescents with low 12-week substance-related impairment, regardless of whether they had had high or low substance-related impairment at baseline. MDD response was significantly lower among teens with high 12-week substance-related impairment (Goldstein et al. 2009). Continued alcohol or other drug problems have been shown to be associated with poorer depression treatment response, and the onset of a SUD after recovery from major depression increases risk of depression recurrence (Curry et al. 2012).

Primary SUD Treatment

There is some evidence that SUD treatment alone can lead to a change in co-occurring depression. This is attributed to similar mechanisms of behavior change while utilizing cognitive-behavioral therapy (CBT). Cognitive restructuring is both a tool and a proximal outcome to address SUD, as well as depressed coping skills. Hawke et al. (2008) followed adolescents treated with CBT for SUD. At 1-year follow-up, depression diagnoses were significantly reduced, despite this disorder not being addressed in treatment. Given the long follow-up period, the depression may have remitted. The Cannabis Youth Treatment (CYT) study objective was to compare the efficacy of five psychosocial interventions on reduction of use among a large ($N=600$) cohort of adolescents (ages 12–18 years) with cannabis use disorder (Dennis et al. 2004). A recent secondary analysis of CYT data revealed that depression was common among these youth. Considerable rates of depressive symptoms and MDD were found at baseline (18% and 70%, respectively). There was a significant linear decrease in cannabis use, as well as in the depression score, across the five quarterly time points from baseline to 12-months posttreatment follow-up. The higher the baseline depression score, the more frequent was baseline frequency of cannabis use, and the larger the decrease in both cannabis use frequency and depressive symptoms across time. Finally, within subjects, severity level of depressive symptoms was predicted only by previous depressive symptoms, and not cannabis use. Likewise, cannabis use was not predicted by depressive symptoms (Arias et al. 2018).

A comprehensive review of 13 adolescent SUD treatment studies examined how co-occurring depression affects treatment retention and outcomes (Hersh et al. 2014). Three studies examined retention, and each one reported a different finding (i.e., negative effect, positive effect, or nonsignificant effect). Eleven studies investigated the influence of co-occurring depression on SUD treatment outcome. Across these studies, the relationship between depression and substance abuse treatment outcome varied, also exerting a negative, positive, or nonsignificant effect. It is problematic to conclude a general finding from the review. There was considerable variability across the studies in terms of study hypotheses and methodology. The studies differed in settings (e.g., emergency department, residential, outpatient, day treatment), treatment approach (e.g., 12-step, motivational interviewing, family therapy), measurement methods (e.g., structured interviews, self-report scales, chart reviews), type of depression (i.e., MDD, dysthymia, symptomatic), demographics, and duration of treatment. Outcomes ranged across substance use frequency, substance-related problems, time to relapse, and quality of life. Together, the studies highlight that depression does not have a simple relationship with substance-related treatment outcomes (Hersh et al. 2014).

Treatment of Both Co-occurring Disorders

In a randomized trial, adolescents received treatment for both SUD and co-occurring depression in either a sequenced or a coordinated manner (Rohde et al. 2014). Three sequences of delivering two empirically supported interventions for depression and SUD were evaluated: treat depression first, treat SUD first, or treat both concurrently. The intervention employed for depression was a group intervention (Clarke et al. 1999) and for SUD, functional family therapy (Waldron and Brody 2010) adapted for SUD. All treatment sequences exhibited an early strong depression remission effect that was maintained through 1-year follow-up. However, no evidence of a differential depression response across sequences was found. A stronger depression response occurred for adolescents with MDD compared with those with dysthymia and depression not otherwise specified. Using the same data set, the authors examined the number and nature of depression response profiles through 1-year posttreatment as well as what factors might predict profile membership (Rohde et al. 2018). A four-class solution emerged, with groups designated mildly depressed responders (57%), depressed responders (19%), depressed nonresponders (13%), and depressed with recurrence (11%). The strongest predictor of nonresponse was low family cohesion, whereas recurrence was associated with hopelessness, suicide attempts, and starting treatment near the end of the school year. This study suggests that treatments for SUD alone do not adequately address the need of all youth with co-occurring depression.

Integrative Treatment

Three reports addressed a combination of pharmacological (fluoxetine) and behavioral treatment in an integrative model to address youth with comorbid major depression, using double-blind, placebo-controlled trials. In a study by Riggs et al. (2007), all subjects ($N = 126$) received CBT for SUD concurrent with the medication trial. Fluoxetine showed superior efficacy compared with placebo for remission of depression at and after 13 weeks of treatment. Those adolescents whose depression remitted, regardless of medication group assignment, reported significantly reduced drug use, whereas nonremitters showed no change in drug use. This might be attributed to the CBT effects. Cornelius et al. (2009) reported the lack of a significant difference between groups. Subjects in both the fluoxetine and the placebo groups showed significant improvement in both depressive symptoms and a level of alcohol consumption. These findings may be the result of a limited sample size ($N = 50$) or due to the noteworthy efficacy of the CBT/motivational enhancement therapy (MET) provided to all participants. Finally, following a randomized placebo-controlled trial, fluoxetine was not found to be superior to placebo in alleviating either depressive symptoms or decreasing rates of positive drug screens (Findling et al. 2009).

Rapid and Early Depression Response

Ilardi and Craighead (1994) reviewed CBT studies with depressed adults and concluded that the majority of improvement occurs in the first 4 weeks of treatment, before the cognitive interventions specific to CBT are even introduced. Moreover, these rapid early treatment responders tend to maintain their response. A similar finding was reported in a treatment study for depressed alcohol- or drug-abusing adolescents (Riggs et al. 2007). By week 4, 28% of these adolescents were "responders" on depression, even though they were receiving only CBT for substance abuse and pill placebo for depression. Kaminer and Curry (2018) reached a similar conclusion as reported by Rohde et al. (2014) that a significant proportion of depressed youth respond early to treatment. Approximately 40% of adolescents ages 13–21 years with SUD and co-occurring depression showed a rapid clinical response 4 weeks after onset of CBT targeting SUD only (Kaminer and Curry 2018). In this study response was defined as a 50% reduction in the CDRS-R raw score, plus a Clinical Global Impression—Improvement scale (CGI-I; Guy 1976) rating of "very much" or "much" improved; remission was defined the absence of significant depression symptoms; and recovery was indicated by a score of 28 or less on the CDRS-R that lasted at least 2 months.

Whether rapid, early depression response in depressed adolescents with SUDs is attributable to acquiring general CBT skills such as cognitive restructuring, thought challenging, activity scheduling and alike, in addition to nonspecific therapeutic factors, these adolescents may not need a continued depression-specific intervention to retain a favorable response. Further research is necessary to determine what differentiates rapid depression responders from poor responders (i.e., late responders or nonresponders) as well as what adaptive treatment is efficacious for continued care of poor responders. A design in which only nonearly depression responders then receive depression-specific intervention is consistent with recommendations to use adaptive treatments to improve outcome research with alcohol- or drug-abusing adolescents. A promising research approach relevant here is the sequential multiple assignment randomized trial (SMART) design. This intervention model utilizes individual variables (e.g., severity, preferences) to adapt the intervention, and then after short-term outcome is measured, nonresponders are re-randomized to readapt the intervention (Lei et al. 2012). To learn more about adaptive treatment, see Chapter 12 in this manual.

Case Vignette

Jim (a composite case from our experience) is a 15-year-old Caucasian male who, following an arrest for drug dealing, was referred by a juvenile drug court social worker for psychiatric and substance abuse evaluation and treatment. Jim started smoking marijuana at age 13 after his older brother introduced the drug to him. Jim gradually escalated his use of marijuana over the past 3 years and presently smokes 1–2 joints daily. He reports a calming effect from the marijuana and frequently goes to school "high." Beginning this year, Jim has occasionally worked for a drug dealer distributing marijuana to students on the grounds of his high school where he is a sophomore. He started smoking cigarettes at age 11 and is now smoking a half pack per day. He started drinking alcohol at age 13, and in the last year he has been consuming one 6-pack of beer per night on Friday and Saturday to intoxication. All of Jim's friends are drug and/or alcohol users. Jim is an average student whose grades have gradually deteriorated since seventh grade. Despite a Full Scale IQ of 106, he must make a considerable effort to complete his work in school. He currently has a C– average, and attendance has been compromised. He is now repeating ninth grade.

When Jim was 11 years old his mother died in a car accident. She was in treatment for unipolar depression. When he was 14 years old, he was diagnosed with depression after he reported intense symptoms dating to the loss of his mother consisting of daily anhedonia and boredom, irritability, and uncontrollable anger, especially when he perceived himself as being provoked. He was referred to an anger management group but did not attend. He was prescribed sertraline but took it only briefly. He did not disclose his substance use.

Jim lives with his biological father, who works as an electrician; a 13-year-old sister; and his 19-year-old brother who dropped out of high school, is unemployed, and is a heavy cannabis user. Upon evaluation, Jim reports feeling depressed, irritable, and anhedonic. He completes the BDI, and a total score of 26 (moderate depression) is obtained. He believes marijuana "works better" in calming himself. Upon evaluation Jim is not motivated to abstain from drug use yet but is willing to discuss a treatment option in order to avoid legal consequences and have his pending charges dropped. No suicidal ideation is evident, and no symptoms of bipolar illness are present on mental status examination.

Treatment Goals

The goals for Jim's treatment should be realistic and obtainable. Realistic expectancies, including that treatment is a process and not an event, should be conveyed to both Jim and his father. Although the ultimate goal is abstinence, recovery often involves periods of improvement, followed by relapse, and changes in symptom severity.

Treatment Setting

Since Jim is not suicidal or dangerous, treatment can occur in an outpatient setting. After 3 years of continuous cannabis abuse, he is at risk of withdrawal once he stops using cannabis. A duration of 12 weeks is recommended for a first treatment episode of cannabis use disorder.

Treatment for SUD

Psychosocial treatment strategies that have shown promise in reducing SUD among adolescents are reviewed in Chapters 13 through 15 of this manual.

Because Jim demonstrates little motivation for change and the status of his coping skills to resist substance use in high-risk situations is unknown, we recommend an integrated intervention of MET/CBT. In this context, *motivational* means addressing readiness for behavior change toward abstinence.

A therapeutic contract is recommended. Periodic urinalyses to monitor abstinence with consequences for negative or positive urines are also recommended. A contract negotiated early in treatment between Jim, his father, and the clinician included changes in curfew times, allowance, or other incentives in the form of entertainment items (e.g., CDs, DVDs, movie tickets) and clothing. Adjustments may follow during treatment based on progress. An effort to engage Jim's father as an ally in treatment is important in order to encourage Jim to achieve and maintain abstinence as well as to contain the drug-using activities of Jim's older brother at home.

Psychosocial and Pharmacological Treatment for Comorbid Depression

Jim has symptoms that meet criteria for MDD on clinical assessment. CBT is recommended for Jim's depression and focuses on increasing positive activities, improving problem-solving skills, and learning how to restructure unrealistic negative thoughts. Given his lack of suicidal ideation and moderate severity of depressive symptoms, it is not mandatory to begin antidepressant medication immediately. Since evidence suggests that depression in adolescents is influenced by psychosocial variables, and given the high placebo response rates in clinical trials for youth depression, a period of "watchful waiting" with ongoing monitoring of his clinical status is indicated. Suggestions for lifestyle management, including increased engagement with non-drug-involved peers, daily exercise, and the creation of a daily activity schedule to increase pleasurable activities, are to be encouraged.

Two weeks after the onset of treatment for SUD and with the prompting of his father, Jim agrees to an antidepressant trial "to see if it would help." After a risk-benefit discussion with Jim and his father, fluoxetine is initiated at 10 mg/day, and the dosage is increased to 20 mg/day after 1 week. Three weeks after medication was initiated, Jim reports a BDI score of 18 (a 31% improvement over baseline). He requests to continue his combined medication/psychosocial treatment. Jim adheres to his recommended treatment for 2 months with significant improvement in SUD and depression. He then becomes noncompliant with scheduled visits and medication. Six months later his father reports that Jim has relapsed and is smoking marijuana daily, although he is not depressed. Jim refuses to return to treatment. Our clinic is maintaining contact with his father in order to enable access to treatment.

Conclusion

Future treatment studies should consider how change in depressive symptoms over time is related to changes in substance use. Mediators and moderators, including demographic and treatment settings variables, should be studied. A computer-assisted, evidence-based treatment (CBT/MET) strategy has been found efficacious for adults with SUD and co-occurring depression (Glasner et al. 2018). However, reports on a similar intervention for youth have not yet been published. This approach should be available for youth in a developmentally oriented perspective.

Anxiety Disorders

Anxiety disorders influence the development, course, treatment, and outcomes of SUDs in adolescents. Anxiety disorders are among the most common mental disorders in adolescents and are highly prevalent among adolescents with SUDs (Blumenthal et al. 2011). The diverse range of problems represented by anxiety disorders complicates their relationships with substance use and SUDs (Kushner et al. 2000). The link between adolescent SUDs and some anxiety disorders is relatively clear and has contributed to plausible and empirically supported models for understanding their comorbidity. Yet other anxiety disorders have not been found to have a clinically meaningful relationship to adolescent SUDs (Clark et al. 1994b).

Characteristics and Epidemiology

The DSM-5 diagnostic system includes the following anxiety disorders: separation anxiety disorder, selective mutism, specific phobia, social phobia, panic disorder, agoraphobia, and generalized anxiety disorder. The removal of obsessive-compulsive disorder (OCD) and PTSD into separate categories a major change from DSM-IV to DSM-5. (For purposes of this chapter, we will include OCD in our discussion of the anxiety disorders.) Anxiety disorders, which make up the most common class of psychiatric disorder across the life-span, typically begin much earlier than other commonly occurring classes of mental disorders (Kessler et al. 2009). Specific phobia is consistently estimated to be the most common lifetime anxiety disorder, with prevalence estimates usually in the 6%–12% range (Kessler et al. 2009). Several studies have noted that anxiety disorders occur more often in adolescent females than in adolescent males (Back et al. 2014).

Separation anxiety disorder is defined by excessive anxiety about separation from parents or other attachment figures. *Simple phobias* include persistent fear of other well-defined objects or situations (e.g., insects or heights). *Social anxiety disorder* (or *social phobia*) is defined by the persistent fear of embarrassment in situations involving social scrutiny. In the most severe and generalized form, social anxiety may include virtually all social situations and be associated with disabling avoidance. *Panic disorder* is defined by relatively short periods of intense fear that are not the result of exposure to a feared situation. Panic disorder is often accompanied by *agoraphobia,* a fear of being in situations from which it may be difficult to escape in the event of incapacitating symptoms. *Generalized anxiety disorder* involves excessive, unrealistic, and persistent worry about a number of life circumstances. In *obsessive-compulsive disorder,* obsessions are persistent thoughts that are experienced as intrusive, and compulsions are repetitive and intentional behaviors performed in response to obsessions.

The relative rates of specific anxiety disorders in adolescent community samples (Clark et al. 1994b) provide a context for examining their comorbidity with SUD. Social phobia has been found to occur in about 1.5% of adolescents, although this figure excludes those with milder forms of performance anxiety. Separation anxiety disorder occurs in about 4% of preadolescent children, and the rate declines during the course of adolescence. In community samples of adolescents, simple phobias occur in about 5%, and panic disorder, OCD, and generalized anxiety disorder all occur in about 1%. Agoraphobia is also uncommon. Among affected adolescents, multiple anxiety disorders occur in about 25% (Clark et al. 1994b), and the overlap of social phobia, separation anxiety disorder, and generalized anxiety disorder has been noted to be particularly common in clinical samples (Clark et al. 2005). A depressive disorder also commonly accompanies anxiety disorders. The OR between alcohol use disorders and panic disorder, phobic disorders, and OCD is 2.4, 2.1, and 1.4, respectively (Helzer and Pryzbeck 1988).

Anxiety Disorders and SUD

Demonstrated anxiolytic effects of licit and illicit substances would, to some extent, provide supportive evidence for a model proposing that substance involvement is a way for the user to cope with an anxiety disorder. Yet the theory that adolescents with anxiety disorders consume abused substances for their anxiolytic effects and thereby develop SUD is not consistent with data from adolescent samples. Benzodiazepines, for example, have proven anxiolytic effects and produce a dependence syndrome, but benzodiazepine abuse and dependence are uncommon among adolescents (Clark 2012). The evidence for anxiolytic effects of other more commonly abused substances is less clear. The effects of alcohol on anxiety are complex and depend on dose, individual differences, anxiety type, and use circumstances (Kushner et al. 2000). Stimulants, on the other hand, can lead to or exacerbate anxiety disorders.

The influences of anxiety disorders on substance use and related problems likely vary by developmental stage, substance type, stage of substance involvement, and anxiety symptom characteristics. For example, children with anxiety disorders may be risk averse and may therefore show a delay in early adolescent drug and alcohol experimentation. Anxiety disorders have been found to inhibit tobacco use initiation while being associated with higher rates of daily smoking and nicotine dependence (McKenzie et al. 2010). After a substance is tried and adverse consequences do not occur, individuals with anxiety disorders may have an acceleration of the development of substance-related problems. More complex and comprehensive models need to be developed that take into consideration the mechanisms of interactions among different anxiety disorders, specific substances, and developmental stage.

There are also differential influences based on the specific anxiety disorder. Among *adults* with substance dependence, Compton and colleagues (2000) found that phobic disorders predated SUD onset by an average of over 10 years, whereas generalized anxiety disorder showed a similar onset age and more typically had its onset after SUD. Most recently, the specificity of social anxiety disorder as a risk factor for adolescent SUD has been established after depression and other anxiety disorders were controlled for (Buckner et al. 2008). Other anxiety and mood disorders have not been found to be associated with subsequent adolescent SUD. There is, however, little published information on the sequences of disorders for adolescents with SUD and comorbid anxiety disorders.

Anxiety symptoms and disorders have been found to predict substance use and related disorders in adolescents. In a prospective study of community adolescents, baseline social phobia predicted the onset of hazardous alcohol use, and panic disorder predicted persistent alcohol abuse and dependence (Zimmermann et al. 2003). The Oregon Adolescent Depression Project found that social anxiety disorder at baseline (adolescence) was associated with 6.5 greater odds of cannabis dependence (but not abuse) and 4.5 greater odds of alcohol dependence (but not abuse) at follow-up (early adulthood) after controlling for relevant variables (e.g., gender, depression, conduct disorder) and other anxiety disorders (Buckner et al. 2008). A similar finding was found in a large New Zealand birth cohort, although several significant covariates indicate the relationship is complex (Goodwin et al. 2004; Lopez et al. 2005). As we noted earlier, some anxiety disorders are associated with a delay of the onset of substance use and with diminished substance involvement severity (Kushner et al. 2000; Myers et al. 2003).

Assessment of Anxiety Disorders in Youth With SUDs

As recommended by the American Academy of Child and Adolescent Psychiatry (AACAP), assessment of anxiety and anxiety disorders is a necessary component of the psychiatric evaluation of adolescents and is clinically useful in evaluating adolescents with SUDs (Connolly et al. 2007). Assessment instruments that are designed for adolescents and have favorable psychometric properties are available to identify and evaluate anxiety disorders. Tools that briefly screen for anxiety disorders may be particularly useful in the context of the multiple demands placed on the initial assessment for addiction treatment. For example, Screen for Child Anxiety Related Emotional Disorders (SCARED) is a psychometrically sound 41-item instrument that assesses child or parent report of a child's DSM-IV anxiety disorder symptoms (Clark et al. 2005). The multiscale Spence Children's Anxiety Scale (SCAS; Spence 1998) is another psychometrically strong measure; this child self-report measure evaluates symptoms relating to diagnostic categories of anxiety disorders (separation anxiety, social phobia, OCD, panic/agoraphobia, and generalized anxiety). Although often difficult to achieve, a period of abstinence from alcohol and other drugs is very useful in evaluating anxiety disorders in adolescents with SUD, because substantial improvement may occur early in the course of treatment without specific interventions.

Interview methods appropriate for adolescents, such as the K-SADS-PL, include content to assess for anxiety disorders. A computer-assisted structured diagnostic interview has been developed for the National Survey on Drug Use and Health (NSDUH) for determining DSM-IV mental disorder diagnoses, including anxiety disorders and SUD (Jordan et al. 2008). Semistructured interviews, which are preferred by some because of their flexibility, are intended to be administered by clinically experienced and thoroughly trained interviewers.

Self-administered or interview-based instruments providing graded severity ratings are often more sensitive change indicators than are diagnostic assessments. For example, SCARED scores may be utilized as a broad change indicator (see, e.g., Clark et al. 2005). The assessment of global anxiety (such as with the Hamilton Anxiety Rating Scale [Clark and Donovan 1994]) provides a useful guide for severity and change with treatment that applies across anxiety disorders. The clinician-rated Pediatric Anxiety Rating Scale (PARS) includes a 7-item anxiety severity rating scale that has been shown to have good psychometric properties and sensitivity to treatment effects (Clark et al. 2005). The State-Trait Anxiety Inventory for Children may also be used to determine global anxiety (Kirisci et al. 1996). Focusing on specific anxiety dimensions may also be useful; several psychometrically sound scales are appropriate for the assessment of social anxiety in adolescents (Clark et al. 1994a).

The presence of comorbid anxiety disorders and SUD in adolescents has been found to be associated with decrements in multiple psychosocial and health dimensions (Clark and Kirisci 1996). Consultation with the primary care physician may be helpful in determining whether medical conditions or medication side effects may be contributing to symptoms.

Treatment of SUD and Comorbid Anxiety Disorders

Treatment for anxiety disorders ideally includes all treatment modalities that may improve outcomes (Connolly et al. 2007). Candidate intervention modalities for treating anxiety disorders include education of the adolescent and parents, family therapy, individual psychosocial interventions, and pharmacotherapy.

Other considerations in treatment planning are the potential contribution of SUD to exacerbation of anxiety symptoms and the potential for anxiety disorders to alter response to addiction treatment. Simultaneous treatment for SUD and anxiety disorders, while challenging, is clinically necessary.

Psychosocial Treatment

One type of psychosocial treatment for anxiety disorders is family based. Whereas educational activities and effective communication with parents are standard and necessary elements of treatment with adolescents, the extent and focus of family interventions may vary. In the treatment of youth SUD, adequate parental supervision, emotional support, and favorable role modeling contribute to fostering an environment wherein formal treatment might lead to successful outcomes (Clark et al. 2005). Family interventions for anxiety disorders in children and adolescents, on the other hand, often focus on fostering independence (Connolly et al. 2007). The appropriate balance between parental involvement and adolescent autonomy at a given time in the course of treatment depends on the adolescent's self-regulation capabilities, peer characteristics, developmental considerations, and parental strengths and limitations.

Empirically demonstrated approaches for anxiety disorders have generally utilized CBT approaches (Connolly et al. 2007). In a comprehensive review, CBT has been shown to be effective for a range of anxiety and depressive disorders (Banneyer et al. 2018), and outcome studies indicate that CBT confers long-term benefit (Kendall et al. 2004). Individual and group CBT approaches have proved successful (Manassis et al. 2002), and CBT combined with medication and exposure modeling may be superior to CBT alone (Higa-McMillan et al. 2016). The elements of CBT that are thought to be important include exposure to feared stimuli, cognitive restructuring and relaxation training, with specific features emphasized for particular anxiety disorders (Connolly et al. 2007).

In sum, psychosocial interventions for adolescent SUD are preferred over pharmacological interventions for initial treatment. Treatments targeting anxiety disorders have long been advocated as an approach to diminishing the probability of relapse (James et al. 2013).

Pharmacotherapy

Pharmacological approaches to adolescent anxiety disorders include traditional tricyclic antidepressants, selective serotonin reuptake inhibitors (SSRIs), serotonin-norepinephrine reuptake inhibitors (SNRIs), benzodiazepines, and buspirone (Leonte et al. 2019). SSRIs have been demonstrated to be helpful for children and adolescents with common clinical presentations of separate or overlapping anxiety disorders (Kodish et al. 2011). The effects of SSRIs on anxiety disorders in children and adolescents have also been shown to continue over an extended period (Clark et al. 2005; Leonte et al. 2019; Walkup et al. 2008). Sertraline was found to be associated with a greater symptom reduction compared with placebo, and a combination of CBT and sertraline reduced the severity of anxiety disorders in children and adolescents and was superior to each intervention alone (Walkup et al. 2008). For adults, paroxetine has been shown to be helpful for the treatment of comorbid social phobia and SUD, with decreased symptoms of social anxiety and reduced reliance on alcohol to engage in social situations (Thomas et al. 2008). However, these relationships are rather complex. Although paroxetine reduced symptoms of social anxiety, it did not reduce drinking in those who were not seeking treatment for alcohol problems. Paroxetine led to significantly superior results compared with a placebo group for youth with social phobia (Wagner et al. 2004).

Compared with SSRIs, the other medication classes have disadvantages. Tricyclic antidepressants can have adverse cardiac effects in children and adolescents, and close monitoring is clinically prudent. In addition, the evidence for the effectiveness of tricyclic antidepressant medications for anxiety disorders in children and adolescent is not compelling (Connolly et al. 2007). Because of the risk of abuse and dependence, benzodiazepines are contraindicated in adolescents with SUD. In conclusion, SSRIs are the mainstay of pharmacotherapy for adolescent anxiety disorders.

Integrative Interventions

At this time, recommendations for comorbid anxiety disorders and SUD in adolescents are based on little empirical study. For adolescents with comorbid anxiety disorders and SUD, the integration of treatment options relies on clinical judgment. Because many adolescents do not achieve prolonged abstinence (Winters et al. 2018), the treatment of anxiety disorders may need to proceed under less than ideal circumstances. Both psychosocial and pharmacological treatments are available for adolescents with anxiety disorders, and their integration into addiction treatment does not pose undue problems. Comprehensive treatment guidelines for adolescents with comorbid anxiety disorders and

SUD are unfortunately not supported by an empirical literature and therefore need to be guided by clinical judgment.

Conclusion

Anxiety disorders among adolescents vary in terms of their prevalence, features, relevance to adolescent SUD, and treatment implications. Some anxiety disorders overlap in their symptoms, and combination of disorders represent commonly observed syndromes. Similarly, the overlap between some anxiety disorders and depression may indicate a syndrome rather than independent conditions. The heterogeneity among anxiety disorders is important to acknowledge and to take into consideration in clinical and research applications.

Additional research needs to be done to determine the extent to which anxiety disorders are relevant for adolescent SUD etiology and treatment. Clinical and community studies have suggested that some anxiety syndromes lead to SUD, some substances cause anxiety in adolescents, and substance-induced anxiety may induce long-term changes.

Multifaceted models of the comorbidity between SUD and anxiety disorders need to be developed, tested, and refined. For example, the pharmacological effects of some medications might lead to neurobiological changes that exacerbate anxiety disorders, such as downregulation of the γ-aminobutyric acid (GABA)/benzodiazepine complex receptors (Clark 2012).

Treatment needs to proceed under less than ideal conditions with an unsatisfactory knowledge base. The treatment of adolescents with comorbid anxiety disorders and SUD does not benefit from a rich knowledge base, and thus approaches gleaned from other populations, including adolescents with no comorbid disorders and adults with anxiety disorders, should be applied based on clinical judgment.

Adolescent Posttraumatic Stress Disorder

Characteristics and Epidemiology

PTSD requires not only a pattern of symptoms and psychosocial impairment but also a history of exposure to a stressor. To qualify for PTSD based on DSM-5, the following criteria must be present: exposure to a traumatic event, such as (actual or threatened) serious injury, death, or sexual violence (exposure can be direct, witnessed, or indirect); persistent reexperiencing of the traumatic event (e.g., unwanted upsetting memories, nightmares); avoidance of trauma-related stimuli; negative thoughts or feelings that began or worsened after the trauma (e.g., negative affect); trauma-related arousal and reactivity that began or worsened after the trauma (e.g., irritability, hypervigilance, sleep difficulties); and symptoms lasting more than a month that interfere with normal functioning.

Most persons with PTSD do not have all of these symptoms: at least one of each of the first three categories and at least two of the fourth category are all that is required for a PTSD diagnosis. Substance use serves as an avoidance symptom of PTSD, and several PTSD symptoms (e.g., irritability, poor concentration, risky/destructive behavior) are also impairments often involved in SUD. PTSD may be further classified using the dissociation subtype, characterized by feelings of depersonalization or derealization related to PTSD symptomatology. A significant change between DSM-IV and DSM-5 was the reclassifying of PTSD from the anxiety disorders section to a new diagnostic category called "Trauma and Stressor-Related Disorders." This change was made due to the considerable research linking PTSD with a wide range of negative emotions (e.g., anger, shame) in addition to anxiety.

As many as two in three adolescents report having been exposed to traumatic stressors at some point in their lives, including directly experiencing or witnessing violence, abuse, injury, or loss (McLaughlin et al. 2013), war and terrorism (Pat-Horenczyk et al. 2007), and life-threatening disasters (see Masten and Narayan 2012 for a review). Trauma-exposed adolescents are at risk not only for PTSD but also for MDD, substance use and SUD, and related behavioral and psychosocial problems (e.g., depression, suicidality, delinquent behaviors) (Ford et al. 2010; Kilpatrick et al. 2003).

Epidemiological studies have estimated the lifetime prevalence of PTSD using DSM-IV criteria in the general adolescent population to be around 5% (e.g., McLaughlin et al. 2013), which is comparable to estimates from similar studies with adults (Pietrzak et al. 2011). Prevalence estimates among troubled adolescents range are approximately five times as high in psychiatric and SUD clinical samples and among youth in the juvenile justice system (Dierkhising et al. 2013; Havens et al. 2012; Lubman et al. 2007). PTSD involves severe impairment across multiple biopsychosocial domains and often has a chronic course when not effectively treated (Perkonigg et al. 2005).

SUD is a common comorbidity of PTSD among persons of all ages, and specifically for adolescents. In the National Survey of Adolescents (Kilpatrick et al. 2003), 24% of girls and 30% of boys who had PTSD also had a SUD, and 25% of girls and 14% of boys who had SUD had comorbid PTSD. These comorbidity levels suggest that a substantial subgroup of adolescents (approximately 1.5% in the community) have comorbid SUD and PTSD. Youth at greatest risk for comorbid SUD and PTSD were those who had witnessed violence, had been sexually or physically assaulted, had a parent with substance use problems, or were older (Kilpatrick et al. 2003).

In clinical samples receiving treatment for PTSD or SUD, the rate of co-occurring PTSD and SUD is high. For example, among adolescents seeking treatment for substance use, up to 39% reported trauma-related symptoms, and these symptoms were related to more severe substance use problems (Chan et al. 2008). Another study found that adolescents with comorbid PTSD in SUD treatment had approximately four times as many additional comorbid psychiatric disorders (on average, two other diagnoses), more severe depression, twice as many SUD diagnoses (on average, two SUDs), more frequent use of and dependence on multiple types of substances (on average 7.5 types), as well as more relationship problems, unprotected sex, and self-harm, compared with adolescents without PTSD in SUD treatment (Lubman et al. 2007).

PTSD often has onset prior to SUD. Epidemiological research on PTSD and SUD in adolescents is limited, but several studies indicate that PTSD typically precedes and predicts onset of SUDs, but not vice versa. For example, in a community sample of adolescents, anxiety disorders in general predicted later onset (up to 4 years later) of AUD, but PTSD was the only diagnosis that predicted later onset of all SUDs (Wolitzky-Taylor et al. 2012). Further, SUDs did not predict later onset of PTSD. Two community studies found that approximately two-thirds of older adolescents and adults with comorbid PTSD and SUD had onset of PTSD prior to the SUD (Epstein et al. 1998; Kessler et al. 1995). PTSD also increases the risk of marijuana or hard drug use among adolescents (Kilpatrick et al. 2000).

Assessment of PTSD in Youth With SUDs

Screening to identify adolescents with SUDs who are likely to have comorbid PTSD is the first step in assessment. Experts recommend that youth be screened for PTSD in primary care settings and suggest assessment of trauma exposure with a single question (e.g., "Since the last time I saw you, has anything really scary or upsetting happened to you and your family?"; Cohen et al. 2008). Positive responses should be followed up with a brief assessment of PTSD symptoms, such as an abbreviated version of the UCLA PTSD Reaction Index (Pynoos et al. 1998), which is a self-report measure of PTSD symptoms. A second option for screening is the Child Trauma Screening Questionnaire (CTSQ; Kenardy et al. 2006), another brief self-report measure. The CTSQ is only 10 items and has been studied in adolescents up to age 16. See the review by Eklund and colleagues (2018) for additional screening measures.

Following a positive screen for PTSD among youth with a SUD, a more thorough assessment should be conducted that includes both history of (and current) exposure to traumatic stressors as well as symptom severity and diagnosis. Although a number of validated questionnaires and interviews can be used to assess PTSD symptoms efficiently and accurately with adolescents, the gold standard is the UCLA PTSD Reaction Index. For PTSD diagnostic assessment, the most detailed and widely used is the Clinician Administered PTSD Scale for Children and Adolescents (CAPS-CA; Pynoos et al. 2015). Both the UCLA PTSD Reaction Index (UCLA PTSD Reaction Index for DSM-5; Kaplow et al. 2019) and the CAPS-CA (CAPS-CA-5; Pynoos et al. 2015) have been updated to reflect DSM-5 criteria. The UCLA provides a brief but thorough assessment of trauma history as well as 27 items on which the youth (or a parent) can numerically rate how troubling each PTSD symptom has been, plus 4 additional items that assess for the dissociative subtype. The UCLA's brevity allows for regular readministration during treatment to check on treatment progress. For a diagnosis of PTSD to be made, a clinician-administered structured interview like the CAPS-CA is necessary, in order to probe sufficiently to determine the presence and severity of each symptom and degree of impairment.

Assessment of comorbid psychiatric disorders and associated risk factors is also critical, because adolescents with comorbid SUD and PTSD are more likely than those with SUD alone to have these impairments. Hawke and colleagues (2009) determined that sexual abuse history, comorbid psychiatric symptom severity, and suicidal ideation were strongly associated with the presence of PTSD among youth receiving psychosocial treatment for SUD. Assessment of potential protective factors is another important but often overlooked step in developing a complete clinical formulation and treatment plan. Protective factors that may reduce symptom severity and enhance sustained recovery include positive (nonconflictual) social support, developmentally appropriate parental monitoring, self-efficacy, development and adherence to regular healthy routines and activities, and strong emotion regulation skills (e.g., Saxe et al. 2007).

Treatment of SUD and Comorbid PTSD

The scientific evidence for effective treatment of comorbid SUD and PTSD with adolescents is limited, but a few promising treatments have emerged in the last decade. The AACAP practice guidelines for both SUD and PTSD note that the disorders often co-occur, but the guidelines do not provide any treatment recommendations for comorbid SUD and PTSD. Treatment for adolescents with co-occurring SUD and PTSD therefore must be guided by approaches developed for adults as well as emerging results from research with adolescent samples.

Among adults with SUD, PTSD has been found to be a complicating factor in some studies, predicting high rates of relapse and low rates of treatment success, but other studies have failed to find this relationship or have even found the opposite (see Hildebrand et al. 2015 for a review). In treatment studies, improvements in PTSD symptoms have been found to be more strongly associated with improvement in SUD symptoms than vice versa (see, e.g., Hien et al. 2010). Overall, research with adult populations strongly suggests that concurrent and integrated approaches to PTSD and SUD are preferred over sequential approaches or approaches that focus on either PTSD or SUD alone (McCauley et al. 2012). Consistent with these research findings, adult patients with comorbid SUD and PTSD tend to express a preference for treatment that simultaneously or concurrently addresses both disorders in an integrated rather than compartmentalized or sequential way (see, e.g., Back et al. 2014). Of note, despite evidence that PTSD and SUD are best treated simultaneously, few clinicians working with adolescents adhere to this approach in practice, and many clinicians who treat adolescent PTSD are not sufficiently trained in SUD treatment (Adams et al. 2016).

Studies on the influence of PTSD on SUD treatment retention and outcome, or the influence of SUD on PTSD treatment retention and outcome, also have mixed results in adolescent samples. One study found that adolescents with and without high levels of PTSD symptoms responded equally well to substance use treatment, and those with high levels of PTSD who continued to use substances showed greater reductions in substance use than those without PTSD symptoms (Williams et al. 2008). Jaycox and colleagues (2004) reported that adolescents in inpatient SUD treatment were more likely to end treatment early if they had a history of traumatic stress but did not endorse sufficient symptoms to qualify for a PTSD diagnosis (compared with those with no reported trauma history or those with PTSD). A more recent study found that history of maltreatment predicted greater motivation for SUD treatment, higher treatment engagement, and greater self-awareness related to problematic substance use among youth (Rosenkranz et al. 2012), but this study did not explicitly examine PTSD symptoms.

Psychosocial Treatment

Several models for treatment of comorbid SUD and PTSD have been found to be efficacious for adult populations. A recent meta-analysis concluded that cognitive-behavioral treatments that were delivered individually (vs. a group format) and delivered concurrently with a substance use intervention were most likely to have a positive effect on PTSD symptoms (Roberts et al. 2015). Approaches to PTSD included in this category were exposure therapy and trauma-focused CBT. Little evidence was reported for the effectiveness of approaches that do not explicitly focus on trauma. This review also found high rates of dropout across studies of integrated PTSD/SUD treatments as well as few positive effects on substance use outcomes, highlighting the challenges faced in identifying effective treatments for this population.

Research on integrated PTSD/SUD treatments for adolescents has lagged behind research for adults, but a few approaches have shown promise. Seeking Safety, a psychosocial intervention originally designed for women with comorbid SUD and PTSD, has been adapted for adolescent girls. A pilot clinical trial with 33 adolescent girls found effects of Seeking Safety on sexual concerns/ distress and problems with anorexia, somatization, and depression (Najavits et al. 2006). Seeking Safety provides 25 sessions of psychoeducation about PTSD and SUD and their interrelationship; training in skills for changing cognitions, behaviors, and relationships; and case management to help recipients address current stressors and access resources. Attendance was low (on average fewer than half of the sessions were attended), and there were no significant effects on PTSD or SUD specifically. Additional studies of Seeking Safety have yet to be published. A second treatment, Risk Reduction through Family Therapy, was designed for adolescent victims of childhood sexual abuse and builds on components of trauma-focused CBT (TF-CBT) and multisystemic therapy to target trauma-related symptoms and substance use risk (Danielson et al. 2012). An initial randomized pilot study found effects of RRFT on substance use, depression, and PTSD symptoms, and a larger clinical trial is currently under way. Mindfulness-based cognitive therapy (MBCT) has been evaluated with adolescents who have co-occurring PTSD symptoms and substance use (Fortuna et al. 2018). An open trial found that adolescents receiving MBCT demonstrated reductions in PTSD, depression, and marijuana use. However, only 62% of participants completed treatment, and additional studies of MBCT have not yet been published. To summarize, a few emerging treatments for adolescent PTSD/SUD have undergone preliminary evaluations, but additional research is needed to determine their effectiveness.

In the absence of established models for integrated treatment of co-occurring PTSD/SUD, providers should consider provision of simultaneous treatment of the two disorders, using evidence-based treatments for each disorder. The gold standard for PTSD treatment among youth is TF-CBT (see Cary and McMillen 2012 for a review). Although TF-CBT has extensive validation for children with PTSD, fewer studies have included adolescents. Further, TF-CBT has not been explicitly studied with a comorbid PTSD/SUD sample. However, given the dearth of data on effective interventions, provision of TF-CBT in conjunction with evidence-based SUD treatment is a reasonable approach for clinicians working with this population. Similarly, prolonged exposure therapy has been shown to be effective in treating PTSD in adolescent samples (see, e.g., Foa et al. 2013) and has also been found to be safe and effective when integrated with substance use treatment among adults (Mills et al. 2012).

Pharmacotherapy

Pharmacotherapy for children and adolescents with PTSD is in the early stages of development, with no U.S. Food and Drug Administration (FDA)–approved indications. Unlike pharmacotherapy findings for adult PTSD, for which two SSRIs, paroxetine and sertraline, have been FDA approved, randomized controlled trials (e.g., Stoddard et al. 2011) have failed to find significant positive effects of SSRIs on PTSD for youth samples. Thus, the AACAP does not recommend the use of SSRIs in the absence of psychotherapy (Cohen et al. 2010). In addition, no trials of SSRIs have been conducted with youth who have comorbid PTSD/SUD. Several other classes of medications have been found to be effective for PTSD symptoms among some children and adolescents (e.g., α- and β-adrenergic agents, antipsychotics, anticonvulsants/mood stabilizers, non-SSRI antidepressants), but only in open-label trials and not specifically with youth with SUD. Thus, at this point, medication therapy is considered adjunctive to psychosocial treatments in adolescent PTSD.

The endocannabinoid system plays a role in the control of emotions. Cannabis use has been reported to reduce feelings of stress, tension, and anxiety (Korem et al. 2016). Although medical cannabis has been approved as a treatment for PTSD in some medical marijuana states, there are only anecdotal reports supporting its use for this disorder. Several clinical studies are under way, and no studies in adolescents have been reported.

Case Vignette

McKayla is a 16-year-old girl who was court-mandated to receive an evaluation and treatment for PTSD after her fifth confinement in juvenile detention with legal charges, including felony assault, destruction of property, possession of illegal substances and alcohol, and repeated violations of probation. McKayla was placed on house arrest and ordered to resume attendance at the alternative school from which she had been truant or suspended for more than two-thirds of the past 18 months. She was placed in residential treatment for polysubstance abuse three times, each time being sent back to detention prior to completing the program because of aggressive behavior toward peers and staff. McKayla and her family, including her mother and father and four younger siblings, have received three types of in-home family intervention, which she and her parents agreed led to some improvement in McKayla's willingness to abide by family rules but only temporary reductions in drinking and smoking marijuana.

Evaluations ordered by the court noted that McKayla had experienced sexual abuse by an uncle and adult neighbor from ages 5 to 7, which she did not disclose until she was 13. McKayla was subsequently raped at age 14 by a young adult male whom she met while associating exclusively with adults rather than peers her own age. She was in supportive counseling for a few months after disclosure of the sexual abuse and after the rape, stopping when by her own account, "I had nothing more to say, and the counselor thought I was doing fine."

McKayla has a positive screen with the UCLA PTSD Reaction Index, although she says that she has gotten so used to living with the bad memories and "using whatever I can to avoid them," that "it really doesn't bother me." On the trauma events portion of the UCLA, she discloses the sexual molestation and rape, as well as a traumatic loss of a friend who overdosed, and gang-related physical assaults. On the CAPS-CA, McKayla initially says that she does not have bad memories of even the worst of these experiences (which she identifies as the rape) and that she does not have to avoid them anymore because she just never lets them bother her. On further inquiry, she says that the memories of her traumatic events actually are "always just in the back of my mind, I just tell myself they've gone away." She admits that she avoids going to school because that is where the physical assaults occurred "and I have to see those same fools every day, looking at me like they're laughing and about to jump me again if I'm not careful." McKayla describes nightmares of being attacked, anger, jumpiness, and "my mind going blank" when preparing to go to school, always having to keep her guard up (hypervigilance), and not being able to let anyone get close to her or to enjoy activities she used to find rewarding. Although she does not report flashbacks or memory gaps regarding the traumatic events, McKayla is diagnosed with PTSD with severe impairment in school and social functioning.

McKayla notes that her PTSD symptoms have been much worse since not being able to drink or use drugs because of the court-ordered random drug screens and escalating legal sanctions. She says she does not miss the "high" associated with using as much as the relief that drugs and alcohol temporarily offer from the PTSD symptoms. She reports that the coping skills she learned in SUD treatment "just don't cut it when I get to feeling really bad." She believes she cannot stop using unless there is a way to reduce the frequency and intensity of what she now understands are symptoms of PTSD.

Treatment Goals

The PTSD assessment indicates that McKayla will be most likely to commit to a goal of abstinence if treatment enables her to cope successfully with, and diminish the severity of, her PTSD symptoms. She may then be motivated to consider sober choices for dealing with stressors without using drugs/alcohol or reacting with anger and aggression, and for seeking out and engaging in relationships and activities that provide her with safety, social support, and opportunities for achievement and self-efficacy.

Treatment Setting

Although McKayla is in very serious trouble legally and at school, the legal sanctions and supervision have increased her safety, and she has parents who are invested in supporting her recovery. Outpatient treatment is a reasonable least restrictive option, with close coordination with her probation officer and school social worker.

Psychosocial Treatment

McKayla is provided with concurrent trauma-focused therapy and SUD treatment, with intensive parental involvement. McKayla and her parents receive psychoeducation explaining how PTSD, SUD, and aggressive behavior share the common feature of biologically based stress reactivity that begins as a healthy adaptation to trauma but becomes a serious emotional and behavioral problem. McKayla is taught coping skills for managing reactivity to reminders of trauma (e.g., being at school, encountering hostile peers) by regulating her emotions. The SUD recovery skills she learned previously (e.g., drug refusal, cognitive reappraisal, assertiveness) are reinforced as she learns how to maintain sufficient emotional equilibrium to use those skills in an effective manner. In addition, McKayla's parents are taught how to monitor her drug and alcohol use as well as how to provide positive reinforcement for her continued abstinence. As a family, McKayla and her parents identify prosocial behaviors that McKayla can do instead of spending time with peers who use alcohol and drugs. In individual and family therapy, McKayla is helped to gradually create personal narratives ("tell the story") of the rape and the worst physical assault and to share these with her parents in a therapeutic manner that enables them to feel a stronger bond and genuine hope for the future.

With practice and encouragement from her parents, McKayla is able to master her new coping skills and is able to go to school and deal with peer and other stressors without becoming "too angry to think straight." Facing her traumatic memory in therapy provides her with some relief of her reexperiencing and avoidance symptoms, and her sleep gradually improves over time. Although she continues to have periodic spikes in anger and cravings for alcohol or drugs, McKayla feels increasingly confident that she can cope with those reactions ("It's just my stress alarm; no one's gonna die").

Conclusion

Treatment for youth with comorbid SUD and PTSD involves the challenge of addressing two mutually exacerbating conditions. PTSD symptoms are likely to be precipitated or intensified by substance use, particularly by the patterns of problematic use in SUD, despite the youth intending to use alcohol or other substances to reduce the severity of intrusive memories and hyperarousal. In this light, substance use is a form of PTSD avoidance symptom, which can in turn lead to increased dysphoria, emotional numbing, and social detachment, which are further symptoms of PTSD. The severity of SUD is likely to be intensified by PTSD symptoms, in the form of increased cravings, impulsive use or overuse of substances, or association with peers who use substances to cope with distress. SUD may also lead to additional exposure to traumatic stressors in the form of severe accidents or violence.

Assessment, therefore, should include a careful review of the history of substance use and SUD, as well as of exposure to traumatic stressors and the onset of PTSD symptoms. Treatment is best delivered with an integrative approach addressing PTSD and SUD simultaneously. Promising models of integrative PTSD/SUD and SUD/PTSD treatment have been developed for youth (e.g., RRFT) and offer the clinician a starting point for providing an evidence-based approach in real world practice. Research on the neurobiology of PTSD and SUD has identified a number of potential targets for biological interventions that may lead to additional advances in pharmacotherapy. In the meantime, the treatment of comorbid SUD and PTSD depends largely on careful clinical testing of specific hypotheses about the interplay of the specific symptoms of the two disorders with each individual youth, use of treatments that have been found to be efficacious for (noncomorbid) PTSD and SUD, and the application of promising combined approaches to treatment.

Key Points

- The treatment of youth substance use disorder (SUD) and co-morbid depression and/or anxiety disorders should be conducted simultaneously.

- Mild depression accompanying SUD responds to cognitive-behavioral therapy (CBT). Moderate to severe depression requires an integrative approach, including pharmacotherapy.

- Treatment of SUD accompanied by social phobia should be conducted individually and not in a group setting until significant improvement of this anxiety disorder has been reached.

- Identifying cues that trigger posttraumatic stress disorder (PTSD)–related hyperarousal or avoidance reactions can enhance treatment of substance use problems with adolescents.

- Conducting trauma-focused CBT, including exposure therapy, for PTSD concurrently with therapy for SUD can enhance the latter treatment.

References

Adams ZW, McCauley JL, Back SE, et al: Clinician perspectives on treating adolescents with co-occurring post-traumatic stress disorder, substance use, and other problems. J Child Adolesc Subst Abuse 25(6):575–583, 2016 27840568

American Psychiatric Association: Diagnostic and Statistical Manual of Mental Disorders, 5th Edition. Arlington, VA, American Psychiatric Association, 2013

Angold A, Costello EJ, Farmer EM, et al: Impaired but undiagnosed. J Am Acad Child Adolesc Psychiatry 38(2):129–137, 1999 9951211

Arendt M, Rosenberg R, Fjordback L, et al: Testing the self-medication hypothesis of depression and aggression in cannabis-dependent subjects. Psychol Med 37(7):935-945, 2007 17202003

Arias AJ, Burleson JA, Kaminer Y, et al: Examining the relationship between depression and cannabis use in youth being treated for a cannabis use disorder. Presented at the 2nd Annual Research Society on Marijuana Meeting, Fort Collins, CO, July 2018

Back SE, Killeen TK, Teer AP, et al: Substance use disorders and PTSD: an exploratory study of treatment preferences among military veterans. Addict Behav 39(2):369–373, 2014 24199930

Banneyer KN, Bonin L, Price K, et al: Cognitive behavioral therapy for childhood anxiety disorders: a review of recent advances. Curr Psychiatry Rep 20(8):65, 2018 30056623

Beck AT, Steer R, Brown G: The Beck Depression Inventory, 2nd Edition. San Antonio, TX, Psychological Corporation, 1996

Becker SJ, Curry JF: Interactive effect of substance abuse and depression on adolescent social competence. J Clin Child Adolesc Psychol 36(3):469–475, 2007 17658989

Blumenthal H, Leen-Feldner EW, Badour CL, et al: Anxiety psychopathology and alcohol use among adolescents: a critical review of the empirical literature and recommendations for future research. J Exp Psychopathol 2(3):318–353, 2011 23243493

Buckner JD, Schmidt NB, Lang AR, et al: Specificity of social anxiety disorder as a risk factor for alcohol and cannabis dependence. J Psychiatr Res 42(3):230–239, 2008 17320907

Carrellas NW, Biederman J, Uchida M: How prevalent and morbid are subthreshold manifestations of major depression in adolescents? A literature review. J Affect Disord 210:166–173, 2017 28049101

Cary CE, McMillen JC: The data behind the dissemination: a systematic review of trauma-focused cognitive behavioral therapy for use with children and youth. Child Youth Serv Rev 34:748–757, 2012

Center for Behavioral Health Statistics and Quality: 2017 National Survey on Drug Use and Health: Detailed Tables. Rockville, MD, Substance Abuse and Mental Health Services Administration, 2018

Chan YF, Dennis ML, Funk RR: Prevalence and comorbidity of major internalizing and externalizing problems among adolescents and adults presenting to substance abuse treatment. J Subst Abuse Treat 34(1):14–24, 2008 17574804

Christie KA, Burke JD Jr, Regier DA, et al: Epidemiologic evidence for early onset of mental disorders and higher risk of drug abuse in young adults. Am J Psychiatry 145(8):971–975, 1988 3394882

Clark DB: Pharmacotherapy for adolescent alcohol use disorder. CNS Drugs 26(7):559–569, 2012 22676261

Clark DB, Donovan JE: Reliability and validity of the Hamilton Anxiety Rating Scale in an adolescent sample. J Am Acad Child Adolesc Psychiatry 33(3):354–360, 1994 8169180

Clark DB, Kirisci L: Posttraumatic stress disorder, depression, alcohol use disorders and quality of life in adolescents. Anxiety 2(5):226–233, 1996 9160627

Clark DB, Beidel DC, Turner SM, et al: Reliability and validity of the Social Phobia and Anxiety Inventory for adolescents. Psychological Assessment 6:135–140, 1994a

Clark DB, Hirsche BE, Smith MG, et al: Anxiety disorders in adolescents: characteristics, prevalence, and comorbidities. Clin Psychol Rev 14:113–137, 1994b

Clark DB, Birmaher B, Axelson D, et al: Fluoxetine for the treatment of childhood anxiety disorders: open-label, long-term extension to a controlled trial. J Am Acad Child Adolesc Psychiatry 44(12):1263–1270, 2005 16292118

Clarke GN, Rohde P, Lewinsohn PM, et al: Cognitive-behavioral treatment of adolescent depression: efficacy of acute group treatment and booster sessions. J Am Acad Child Adolesc Psychiatry 38(3):272–279, 1999 10087688

Cohen JA, Kelleher KJ, Mannarino AP: Identifying, treating, and referring traumatized children: the role of pediatric providers. Arch Pediatr Adolesc Med 162(5):447–452, 2008 18458191

Cohen JA, Bukstein O, Walter H, et al; AACAP Work Group On Quality Issues: Practice parameter for the assessment and treatment of children and adolescents with posttraumatic stress disorder. J Am Acad Child Adolesc Psychiatry 49(4):414–430, 2010 20410735

Compton WM3rd, Cottler LB, Phelps DL, et al: Psychiatric disorders among drug dependent subjects: are they primary or secondary? Am J Addict 9(2):126–134, 2000 10934574

Connolly SD, Bernstein GA; Work Group on Quality Issues: Practice parameter for the assessment and treatment of children and adolescents with anxiety disorders. J Am Acad Child Adolesc Psychiatry 46(2):267–283, 2007 17242630

Cornelius JR, Bukstein OG, Wood DS, et al: Double-blind placebo-controlled trial of fluoxetine in adolescents with comorbid major depression and an alcohol use disorder. Addict Behav 34(10):905–909, 2009 19321268

Curry J, Silva S, Rohde P, et al: Onset of alcohol or substance use disorders following treatment for adolescent depression. J Consult Clin Psychol 80(2):299–312, 2012

Curry JF, Hersh J: Depressive disorders and substance use disorders, in Youth Substance Abuse and Co-Occurring Disorders. Edited by Kaminer Y. Arlington, VA, American Psychiatric Association Publishing, 2016, pp 131–156

Danielson CK, McCart MR, Walsh K, et al: Reducing substance use risk and mental health problems among sexually assaulted adolescents: a pilot randomized controlled trial. J Fam Psychol 26(4):628–635, 2012 22686269

Dennis M, Godley SH, Diamond G, et al: The Cannabis Youth Treatment (CYT) Study: main findings from two randomized trials. J Subst Abuse Treat 27(3):197–213, 2004 15501373

Dierkhising CB, Ko SJ, Woods-Jaeger B, et al: Trauma histories among justice-involved youth: findings from the National Child Traumatic Stress Network. Eur J Psychotraumatol 4:4, 2013 23869252

Eklund K, Rossen E, Koriakin T, et al: A systematic review of trauma screening measures for children and adolescents. Sch Psychol Q 33(1):30–43, 2018 29629787

Epstein JN, Saunders BE, Kilpatrick DG, et al: PTSD as a mediator between childhood rape and alcohol use in adult women. Child Abuse Negl 22(3):223–234, 1998 9589176

Findling RL, Pagano ME, McNamara NK, et al: The short-term safety and efficacy of fluoxetine in depressed adolescents with alcohol and cannabis use disorders: a pilot randomized placebo-controlled trial. Child Adolesc Psychiatry Ment Health 3(1):3–11, 2009 19298659

Foa EB, McLean CP, Capaldi S, et al: Prolonged exposure vs supportive counseling for sexual abuse-related PTSD in adolescent girls: a randomized clinical trial. JAMA 310(24):2650–2657, 2013 24368465

Ford JD, Elhai JD, Connor DF, et al: Poly victimization and risk of posttraumatic, depressive, and substance use disorders and involvement in delinquency in a national sample of adolescents. J Adolesc Health 46(6):545–552, 2010 20472211

Fortuna LR, Porche MV, Padilla A: A treatment development study of a cognitive and
mindfulness-based therapy for adolescents with co-occurring post-traumatic
stress and substance use disorder. Psychol Psychother 91(1):42–62, 2018
28815876

Glasner S, Kay-Lambkin F, Budney AJ, et al: Preliminary outcomes of a computerized
CBT/MET intervention for depressed cannabis users in psychiatry care. Cannabis 1(2):36–47, 2018

Goldstein BI, Shamseddeen W, Spirito A, et al: Subthreshold substance use and the
treatment of resistant depression in adolescents. J Am Acad Child Adolesc Psychiatry 48(12):1182–1192, 2009 19858762

Goodwin RD, Fergusson DM, Horwood LJ: Association between anxiety disorders
and substance use disorders among young persons: results of a 21-year longitudinal
study. J Psychiatr Res 38(3):295–304, 2004 15003435

Guy Y: ECDEU Assessment Manual for Psychopharmacology, 2nd Edition (DHEW
Publ No 76-388). Rockville, MD, U.S. Department of Health, Education, and
Welfare, 1976

Havens JF, Gudiño OG, Biggs EA, et al: Identification of trauma exposure and PTSD
in adolescent psychiatric inpatients: an exploratory study. J Trauma Stress
25(2):171–178, 2012 22522731

Hawke JM, Kaminer Y, Burke R, et al: Stability of comorbid psychiatric diagnosis
among youths in treatment and aftercare for alcohol use disorders. Subst Abus
29(2):33–41, 2008 19042322

Hawke JM, Ford JD, Kaminer Y, et al: Trauma and PTSD among youths in outpatient
treatment for alcohol and other substance use disorders. J Child Adolesc Trauma
2:1–14, 2009

Hawkins EH: A tale of two systems: co-occurring mental health and substance abuse
disorders treatment for adolescents. Annu Rev Psychol 60:197–227, 2009
19035824

Helzer JE, Pryzbeck TR: The co-occurrence of alcoholism with other psychiatric disorders in the general population and its impact on treatment. J Stud Alcohol
49(3):219–224, 1988 3374135

Hersh J, Curry JF, Kaminer Y: What is the impact of comorbid depression on adolescent substance abuse treatment? Subst Abus 35(4):364–375, 2014 25157785

Hien DA, Jiang H, Campbell ANC, et al: Do treatment improvements in PTSD severity
affect substance use outcomes? A secondary analysis from a randomized clinical trial
in NIDA's Clinical Trials Network. Am J Psychiatry 167(1):95–101, 2010 19917596

Higa-McMillan CK, Francis SE, Rith-Najarian L, et al: Evidence base update: 50 years of research on treatment for child and adolescent anxiety. J Clin Child Adolesc Psychol 45(2):91–113, 2016 26087438

Hildebrand A, Behrendt S, Hoyer J: Treatment outcome in substance use disorder patients with and without comorbid posttraumatic stress disorder: a systematic review. Psychother Res 25(5):565–582, 2015 24967646

Hill RM, Pettit JW, Lewinsohn PM, et al: Escalation to major depressive disorder among adolescents with subthreshold depressive symptoms: evidence of distinct subgroups at risk. J Affect Disord 158:133–138, 2014 24655777

Ilardi SS, Craighead WE: The role of nonspecific factors in cognitive-behavior therapy for depression. Clinical Psychology: Science and Practice 1:138–156, 1994

James AC, James G, Cowdrey FA, et al: Cognitive behavioural therapy for anxiety disorders in children and adolescents. Cochrane Database Syst Rev (6):CD004690, 2013 23733328 [Update in: Cochrane Database Syst Rev (2):CD004690, 2015]

Jaycox LH, Ebener P, Damesek L, et al: Trauma exposure and retention in adolescent substance abuse treatment. J Trauma Stress 17(2):113–121, 2004 15141784

Jordan BK, Karg RS, Batts KR, et al: A clinical validation of the National Survey on Drug Use and Health assessment of substance use disorders. Addict Behav 33(6):782–798, 2008 18262368

Kaminer Y, Curry J: Treatment outcome of adolescent substance use disorders with co-occurring depression. Presentation at the Second Annual Meeting of the Research Society on Marijuana, Fort Collins, Colorado, July 27–29, 2018

Kaplow JB, Rolon-Arroyo B, Layne CM, et al: Validation of the UCLA PTSD Reaction Index for DSM-5: a developmentally-informed assessment tool for youth. J Am Acad Child Adolesc Psychiatry Apr 3, pii:S0890-8567(19)30259-X, 2019 (Epub ahead of print) 30953734

Kaufman J, Birmaher B, Brent D, et al: Schedule for Affective Disorders and Schizophrenia for School-Age Children-Present and Lifetime Version (K-SADS-PL): initial reliability and validity data. J Am Acad Child Adolesc Psychiatry 36(7):980–988, 1997

Kenardy JA, Spence SH, Macleod AC: Screening for posttraumatic stress disorder in children after accidental injury. Pediatrics 118(3):1002–1009, 2006 16950991

Kendall PC, Safford S, Flannery-Schroeder E, et al: Child anxiety treatment: outcomes in adolescence and impact on substance use and depression at 7.4-year follow-up. J Consult Clin Psychol 72(2):276–287, 2004 15065961

Kessler RC, Sonnega A, Bromet E, et al: Posttraumatic stress disorder in the National Comorbidity Survey. Arch Gen Psychiatry 52(12):1048–1060, 1995 7492257

Kessler RC, Ruscio AM, Shear K, et al: Epidemiology of anxiety disorders, in Behavioral Neurobiology of Anxiety and Its Treatment. Edited by Stein MB, Steckler T. New York, Springer, 2009, pp 21–35

Kilpatrick DG, Acierno R, Saunders B, et al: Risk factors for adolescent substance abuse and dependence: data from a national sample. J Consult Clin Psychol 68(1):19–30, 2000 10710837

Kilpatrick DG, Ruggiero KJ, Acierno R, et al: Violence and risk of PTSD, major depression, substance abuse/dependence, and comorbidity: results from the National Survey of Adolescents. J Consult Clin Psychol 71(4):692–700, 2003 12924674

Kirisci L, Clark DB, Moss HB: Reliability and validity of the State-Trait Anxiety Inventory for Children in adolescent substance abusers: confirmatory factor analysis and item response theory. Journal of Child and Adolescent Substance Abuse 5(3):57–69, 1996

Kodish I, Rockhill C, Ryan S, et al: Pharmacotherapy for anxiety disorders in children and adolescents. Pediatr Clin North Am 58(1):55–72, x, 2011 21281848

Korem N, Zer-Aviv TM, Ganon-Elazar E, et al: Targeting the endocannabinoid system to treat anxiety-related disorders. J Basic Clin Physiol Pharmacol 27(3):193–202, 2016 26426887

Kushner MG, Abrams K, Borchardt C: The relationship between anxiety disorders and alcohol use disorders: a review of major perspectives and findings. Clin Psychol Rev 20(2):149–171, 2000 10721495

Lei H, Nahum-Shani I, Lynch K, et al: A "SMART" design for building individualized treatment sequences. Annu Rev Clin Psychol 8:21–48, 2012 22224838

Leonte KG, Puliafico A, Na P, et al: Pharmacotherapy for anxiety disorders in children and adolescents. UpToDate, March 15, 2019. Available at: https://www.uptodate.com/contents/pharmacotherapy-for-anxiety-disorders-in-children-and-adolescents?search=pharmacotherapy-for-anxiety-disorders-in-children-and-adolesce&source=search_result&selectedTitle=1~150&usage_type=default&display_rank=1. Accessed May 14, 2019.

Lewinsohn PM, Solomon A, Seeley JR, et al: Clinical implications of "subthreshold" depressive symptoms. J Abnorm Psychol 109(2):345–351, 2000 10895574

Lopez B, Turner RJ, Saavedra LM: Anxiety and risk for substance dependence among late adolescents/young adults. J Anxiety Disord 19(3):275–294, 2005 15686857

Lubman DI, Allen NB, Rogers N, et al: The impact of co-occurring mood and anxiety disorders among substance-abusing youth. J Affect Disord 103(1–3):105–112, 2007 17291589

Manassis K, Mendlowitz SL, Scapillato D, et al: Group and individual cognitive-behavioral therapy for childhood anxiety disorders: a randomized trial. J Am Acad Child Adolesc Psychiatry 41(12):1423–1430, 2002 12447028

Masten AS, Narayan AJ: Child development in the context of disaster, war, and terrorism: pathways of risk and resilience. Annu Rev Psychol 63:227–257, 2012 21943168

McCauley JL, Killeen T, Gros DF, et al: Posttraumatic stress disorder and co-occurring substance use disorders: advances in assessment and treatment. Clin Psychol (New York) 19(3):283–304, 2012 24179316

McKenzie M, Olsson CA, Jorm AF, et al: Association of adolescent symptoms of depression and anxiety with daily smoking and nicotine dependence in young adulthood: findings from a 10-year longitudinal study. Addiction 105(9):1652–1659, 2010 20707783

McLaughlin KA, Koenen KC, Hill ED, et al: Trauma exposure and posttraumatic stress disorder in a national sample of adolescents. J Am Acad Child Adolesc Psychiatry 52(8):815–830.e14, 2013 23880492

Mills KL, Teesson M, Back SE, et al: Integrated exposure-based therapy for co-occurring posttraumatic stress disorder and substance dependence: a randomized controlled trial. JAMA 308(7):690–699, 2012 22893166

Myers MG, Aarons GA, Tomlinson K, Stein MB: Social anxiety, negative affectivity, and substance use among high school students. Psychol Addict Behav 17(4):277–283, 2003 14640823

Najavits LM, Gallop RJ, Weiss RD: Seeking Safety therapy for adolescent girls with PTSD and substance use disorder: a randomized controlled trial. J Behav Health Serv Res 33(4):453–463, 2006 16858633

Pat-Horenczyk R, Peled O, Miron T, et al: Risk-taking behaviors among Israeli adolescents exposed to recurrent terrorism: provoking danger under continuous threat? Am J Psychiatry 164(1):66–72, 2007 17202546

Perkonigg A, Pfister H, Stein MB, et al: Longitudinal course of posttraumatic stress disorder and posttraumatic stress disorder symptoms in a community sample of adolescents and young adults. Am J Psychiatry 162(7):1320–1327, 2005 15994715

Pietrzak RH, Goldstein RB, Southwick SM, et al: Prevalence and Axis I comorbidity of full and partial posttraumatic stress disorder in the United States: results from Wave 2 of the National Epidemiologic Survey on Alcohol and Related Conditions. J Anxiety Disord 25(3):456–465, 2011 21168991

Poznanski E, Mokros H: Children's Depression Rating Scale—Revised Manual. Los Angeles, CA, Western Psychological Services, 1996

Pynoos R, Rodriguez N, Steinberg A, et al: The UCLA PTSD Index for DSM-IV. Los Angeles, CA, UCLA Trauma Psychiatry Program, 1998

Pynoos RS, Weathers FW, Steinberg AM, et al: Clinician-Administered PTSD Scale for DSM-5—Child/Adolescent Version. National Center for PTSD, 2015. Available at: https://www.ptsd.va.gov/professional/assessment/child/caps-ca.asp. Accessed May 15, 2019.

Riggs PD, Mikulich-Gilbertson SK, Davies RD, et al: A randomized controlled trial of fluoxetine and cognitive behavioral therapy in adolescents with major depression, behavior problems, and substance use disorders. Arch Pediatr Adolesc Med 161(11):1026–1034, 2007 17984403

Roberts NP, Roberts PA, Jones N, et al: Psychological interventions for post-traumatic stress disorder and comorbid substance use disorder: a systematic review and meta-analysis. Clin Psychol Rev 38:25–38, 2015 25792193

Rohde P, Waldron HB, Turner CW, et al: Sequenced versus coordinated treatment for adolescents with comorbid depressive and substance use disorders. J Consult Clin Psychol 82(2):342–348, 2014 24491069

Rohde P, Turner CW, Waldron HB, et al: Depression change profiles in adolescents treated for comorbid depression/substance abuse and profile membership predictors. J Clin Child Adolesc Psychol 47(4):595–607, 2018 26890999

Rosenkranz SE, Henderson JL, Muller RT, et al: Motivation and maltreatment history among youth entering substance abuse treatment. Psychol Addict Behav 26(1):171–177, 2012 21574672

Saxe GN, MacDonald HZ, Ellis BH: Psychosocial approaches for children with PTSD, in Handbook of PTSD: Science and Practice. Edited by Friedman MJ, Keane TM, Resick PA. New York, Guilford Press, 2007, pp 359–375

Shaffer D, Fisher P, Lucas CP, et al: NIMH Diagnostic Interview Schedule for Children Version IV (NIMH DISC-IV): description, differences from previous versions, and reliability of some common diagnoses. J Am Acad Child Adolesc Psychiatry 39(1):28–38, 2000 10638065

Sher L, Sperling D, Stanley BH, et al: Triggers for suicidal behavior in depressed older adolescents and young adults: do alcohol use disorders make a difference? Int J Adolesc Med Health 19(1):91–98, 2007 17458328

Spence SH: A measure of anxiety symptoms among children. Behav Res Ther 36(5):545–566, 1998 9648330

Stoddard FJJr, Luthra R, Sorrentino EA, et al: A randomized controlled trial of sertraline to prevent posttraumatic stress disorder in burned children. J Child Adolesc Psychopharmacol 21(5):469–477, 2011 22040192

Thomas SE, Randall PK, Book SW, et al: A complex relationship between co-occurring social anxiety and alcohol use disorders: what effect does treating social anxiety have on drinking? Alcohol Clin Exp Res 32(1):77–84, 2008 18028529

Treatment for Adolescents With Depression Study Team: Treatment for Adolescents With Depression Study (TADS): rationale, design, and methods. J Am Acad Child Adolesc Psychiatry 42(5):531–542, 2003 12707557

Wagner KD, Berard R, Stein MB, et al: A multicenter, randomized, double-blind, placebo-controlled trial of paroxetine in children and adolescents with social anxiety disorder. Arch Gen Psychiatry 61(11):1153–1162, 2004 15520363

Waldron HB, Brody JL: Functional family therapy for adolescent substance use disorders, in Evidence-Based Psychotherapies for Children and Adolescents. Edited by Weisz JR, Kazdin AE. New York, Guilford, 2010, pp 401–415

Walkup JT, Albano AM, Piacentini J, et al: Cognitive behavioral therapy, sertraline, or a combination in childhood anxiety. N Engl J Med 359(26):2753–2766, 2008 18974308

Williams JK, Smith DC, Gotman N, et al: Traumatized youth and substance abuse treatment outcomes: a longitudinal study. J Trauma Stress 21(1):100–108, 2008 18302171

Winters KC, Botzet AM, Stinchfield R, et al: Adolescent substance abuse treatment: a review of evidence-based research, in Adolescent Substance Abuse: Evidence-Based Approaches to Prevention and Treatment, 2nd Edition. Edited by Leukefeld C, Gullotta T, Staton Tindall M. New York, Springer Science+Business Media, 2018, pp 141–171

Wolitzky-Taylor K, Bobova L, Zinbarg RE, et al: Longitudinal investigation of the impact of anxiety and mood disorders in adolescence on subsequent substance use disorder onset and vice versa. Addict Behav 37(8):982–985, 2012 22503436

Zimmermann P, Wittchen HU, Höfler M, et al: Primary anxiety disorders and the development of subsequent alcohol use disorders: a 4-year community study of adolescents and young adults. Psychol Med 33(7):1211–1222, 2003 14580076

18

Assessment and Treatment of Co-occurring Suicidal Behavior

David B. Goldston, Ph.D.

Angela M. Tunno, Ph.D.

John F. Curry, Ph.D.

Karen C. Wells, Ph.D.

Michelle Roley-Roberts, Ph.D.

Adolescents who use substances and are suicidal are a diverse, high-risk group with multiple comorbidities, life stresses, and developmental trajectories. Care of patients with these clinical presentations is challenging because of multiple treatment needs; comorbid psychiatric problems; legal, academic, and family difficulties; impulsivity; and ambivalence about participating in treatment and changing behavior. Careful assessment, safety monitoring, and integrated treatment are important in their clinical care, but research on treatment in this population is limited.

In this chapter, we review the problem of suicidal behaviors among youth with substance use problems, and the interrelationship between risk for suicidal behaviors and substance use. Then, we discuss issues in the assessment and treatment of suicidal behaviors among youth with substance use problems. Finally, we present a clinical vignette with discussion of a treatment approach.

Definitions of Suicidal Behaviors

Suicide-related terms have been used inconsistently in the literature, impeding progress in research and creating communication difficulties for researchers and practitioners (Posner et al. 2007). In this chapter, we operationally define *suicide* as a fatality that is the result of a self-injurious behavior associated with some intent to die (Crosby et al. 2011). *Suicide attempt* is used to refer to potentially self-injurious behaviors associated with some intent to end one's life (Crosby et al. 2011; Posner et al. 2011). *Suicidal ideation* refers broadly to thoughts about killing oneself, regardless of intention to act on these thoughts. *Nonsuicidal self-injurious behavior* refers to self-harm that is not associated with any intent to die. For example, cutting oneself to relieve tension or taking an accidental overdose of drugs in an effort to get high would not be considered suicidal.

These operational definitions notwithstanding, the classification of suicidal behaviors among individuals who are intoxicated or have substance use problems can be difficult. For example, alcohol or other substance use is related to memory difficulties (Nandrino et al. 2017), and individuals may sometimes find it difficult to remember the intent or motives associated with behaviors while intoxicated. In addition, death via ingestion or injection drug use can be very difficult to classify accurately, particularly in cases when there is no communication of intent (e.g., a "suicide note") and/or when the decedent is known to have a history of depression or suicidal behavior in addition to substance use (Cantor et al. 2001).

Characteristics and Epidemiology of Suicidal Ideation and Behaviors

According to the Youth Risk Behavior Survey (YRBS), in which a self-report questionnaire was administered anonymously to high school students, 17.2%

of adolescents in 2017 reported that they had "seriously considered" killing themselves (i.e., had suicidal ideation) in the last year (Kann et al. 2018). Moreover, 13.6% of high school students reported that they had made a suicide plan in the preceding year. A total of 7.4% of the students said that they had made a suicide attempt in the past year. In addition, 2.4% of students reported suicide attempts that required treatment by a doctor or a nurse (Kann et al. 2018).

The rate of suicide attempts increases as youth enter adolescence, particularly for girls, but then declines again during the transition from adolescence to young adulthood (Lewinsohn et al. 2001). The primary methods of attempted suicide among young people are overdose and cutting (Lewinsohn et al. 1996). Although there is a range of medical consequences associated with adolescent suicidal behavior, the majority of suicide attempts do not result in a high degree of medical lethality (Goldston et al. 2009; Lewinsohn et al. 1996).

Rates of death by suicide are lower than rates of nonlethal suicidal behavior, with an average of 8.80 per 100,0000 12- to 19-year-olds dying by suicide in 2017 in the United States (Centers for Disease Control and Prevention 2019). Nonetheless, suicide is the second leading cause of death in this age group, surpassed only by unintentional injury (i.e., accidents) (Centers for Disease Control and Prevention 2019). Moreover, rates of suicide in the United States for young people ages 15–19 and 20–24 are the highest they have been at any time since the year 2000 (Miron et al. 2019). The main method of death by suicide in the United States for adolescents ages 12–15 is suffocation (including hanging), which accounts for 51.3% of suicides. The main method used in suicide deaths by adolescents ages 16–19 is firearms, accounting for 44.8% of suicides (Centers for Disease Control and Prevention 2019).

There are gender and ethnic differences in rates of suicidal thoughts and behaviors in the United States. Adolescent girls have suicidal ideation and make suicide attempts more often than boys, but adolescent boys have a higher rate of dying by suicide (Centers for Disease Control and Prevention 2019; Kann et al. 2018). Native Americans have the highest rates of suicidal ideation, suicide attempts, and deaths by suicide of all racial and ethnic groups (Centers for Disease Control and Prevention 2019; Goldston et al. 2008). In 2017, a lower percentage of white non-Hispanic female adolescents reported suicide attempts in the last year compared with both black and Hispanic female adolescents (Kann et al. 2018). In addition, rates of suicide deaths are lower for black adolescents than for white adolescents in the same age range (Bridge et al. 2018).

Suicidal Ideation and Behaviors and Substance Use Disorders

Substance/alcohol use and suicidal thoughts and behaviors among youth in clinical settings frequently co-occur (Esposito-Smythers and Goldston 2008). In a longitudinal study of psychiatrically hospitalized adolescents who were then followed through young adulthood, substance use disorders (SUDs) were associated with proximal threefold increased risk for suicide attempts (Goldston et al. 2009). SUDs were also associated with 38% of all repeat attempts, although this risk was mostly associated with comorbid depressive or disruptive behavior disorders (Goldston et al. 2009). SUDs in adolescence and adulthood are also more common among individuals who died by suicide than among case-control subjects (Conner et al. 2019). In particular, mixed drug use, followed by opioid use disorder and intravenous drug use, are associated with the greatest likelihood of suicide (Wilcox et al. 2004). Alcohol use disorder and heavy drinking also are associated with increased risk of suicide.

Relationship Between Alcohol and Substance Use Disorders and Suicidal Behaviors

There are several reasons why adolescent suicidal behaviors and substance use may be related. First, there appear to be shared motives associated with suicidal ideation and substance use. Adolescents may try to kill themselves because they find life circumstances intolerable and experience difficulties coping with associated psychological pain (e.g., depressive symptoms). To this end, they may consider suicide a potential solution or escape from life circumstances and psychological difficulties (Roley-Roberts et al. 2017). Similarly, young people may drink or use other substances to escape from current difficulties and distress (Hufford 2001).

Second, common risk factors may increase the likelihood of suicidal thoughts and behaviors and substance use. For example, aggressive tendencies (Conner et al. 2009; Fite et al. 2007), childhood traumatic events and victimization (Bailey and McCloskey 2005; Roley-Roberts et al. 2017), family environment and stresses (Donaldson et al. 2016; Gould et al. 1996), and psychiatric disorders (Goldston et al. 2009; Hill et al. 2017) are all related to suicidal thoughts or behavior and also to alcohol and substance use.

Third, substance use can indirectly increase risk for suicidal thoughts and behaviors via effects on associated risk factors. For example, alcohol and substance use may contribute to significant depression (Conner et al. 2014), which, in turn, may increase suicide risk. Substance use and related conduct problems may also contribute to arguments and conflicts within families, which, in turn, can be precipitants for depression and suicidal thoughts and behaviors (Conner and Goldston 2007). In addition, substance use can result in more disinhibition, increasing the likelihood of unplanned attempts or acting on self-destructive urges (Bryan et al. 2016).

Fourth, at a biological level, altered serotonergic functioning and serotonin transporter genes have been implicated in individuals who have died by suicide and those who have substance use difficulties (Arango et al. 2001; Pinto et al. 2008). Neuropsychological studies have demonstrated that individuals with chronic substance use and those who have engaged in suicidal behavior often show impaired executive functioning, including decision-making biases in which they focus on short-term rewards rather than long-term rewards (Bridge et al. 2012; Whitlow et al. 2004).

Finally, alcohol and substance use can provide young people with a readily accessible means of attempting suicide (e.g., by overdose; Goldston 2004). For example, a teenager who is using pills recreationally may take multiple pills in an attempted overdose.

Clinical Characteristics of Youth With Both Substance Use Problems and Suicidal Behaviors

Youth who experience co-occurring suicidal behaviors and substance use can present with several clinical challenges (Esposito-Smythers and Goldston 2008). They may be reluctant to enter or to continue in treatment; they may lack motivation to address substance use problems, despite negative consequences in multiple domains; or they may discontinue working on mental and emotional difficulties, once immediate distress has been reduced. Many youth presenting with suicidal thoughts or behaviors and substance use also have academic difficulties, including school suspensions and expulsions, poor attendance, and declining grades. Many youth with substance use problems socialize in peer groups who exhibit delinquent or risk-taking behaviors and often use alcohol or substances. Because of the higher degree of substance use in their peer groups, teens may not recognize the degree to which their own substance use is problematic. Families of youth with these difficulties may have experienced their own adversities and life stresses, may feel frustrated and hopeless regarding attempts to support changes in their child, or may have difficulties monitoring their children as closely as needed.

Assessment of Suicidal Behaviors Among Youth With Substance Use Problems

It is important for clinicians to assess both previous and current suicidal thoughts and behaviors and suicide risk with youth using substances because of their higher risk for suicidal behaviors. Unfortunately, because of fragmented care between mental health and substance use professionals for youth with comorbid psychiatric and SUDs, assessment of suicidal thoughts and behavior may not always occur. Substance use treatment providers sometimes avoid asking about suicidal thoughts and behaviors because they might believe that the mental health professional is assessing for suicide risk while their focus should be limited to substance use. In contrast, mental health professionals sometimes do not assess for suicidal thoughts or behavior when it is not an expected symptom of a presenting problem. Moreover, assessment of suicidal thoughts and behaviors can be anxiety-provoking for even experienced clinicians, who may be uncomfortable working with high-risk clients, or who are unsure of their ability to intervene effectively with this population.

Suicidal behavior among adolescents often goes undetected by parents and caregivers. For example, comparisons of adolescent and parent reports have revealed that parents are often unaware of the suicidal thoughts and behaviors of youth (Foley et al. 2006). Because of the lack of parental knowledge of much adolescent suicidal behavior, it is essential that assessment of suicidal thoughts and behaviors include the adolescent and not rely solely on reports of parents or other adults. Some clinicians may be reluctant to ask youth about suicide because they are concerned that they may give adolescents the idea of suicide by asking about it. However, there have been no iatrogenic effects associated with asking youth about suicide or screening for suicide risk (Gould et al. 2005). Assessment is important for the clinician to ascertain level of risk, implement appropriate safety plans with the adolescents and families, better understand the context of suicidal behaviors for purposes of psychotherapy, and monitor the course of the adolescents' difficulties during treatment.

Self-report measures and interviews can be used as tools to assist in the assessment of suicidal behaviors and risk. However, as suggested by Goldston (2003), these assessments should never be used exclusively in estimating risk and should never supplant clinical judgment. There are generally two types of clinical instruments that may be of most use to clinicians working with substance-using clients in assessing suicidal behaviors and risk. The first set of instruments consists of detection instruments (Goldston 2003), which are used primarily to detect presence or absence and the severity of past and current suicidal thoughts and behaviors. These instruments can be used for both initial and ongoing assessments of suicidal thoughts and behavior during treatment. Detection assessments include semistructured and structured interviews and standardized questionnaires. Perhaps the most widely disseminated detection instrument being used in clinical care, screening, and research is the Columbia–Suicide Severity Rating Scale (C-SSRS; Posner et al. 2011), a measure with well-established psychometric characteristics. There are multiple versions of the C-SSRS for use with different populations or in different contexts; however, across versions, there are questions about thoughts of wanting to die, suicidal thoughts, plans and intentions for suicidal behavior, and histories of suicidal behaviors. Another commonly used brief screener for pediatric clinical populations is the Ask Suicide-Screening Questions (ASQ; Horowitz et al. 2012). This screener, which has high sensitivity and negative predictive value, includes four questions for pediatric patients focused on wishes to be dead, feelings that they or their family would be better off if they were dead, thoughts about suicide, and history of suicide attempts. If patients respond affirmatively to any of those screening questions, they are asked about whether they are currently having thoughts of killing themselves.

Among the most widely used standardized questionnaires are the Suicidal Ideation Questionnaire (SIQ; Reynolds 1988) and the Beck Scale for Suicidal Ideation (BSS; Beck and Steer 1991). Both of these measures have excellent test-retest reliability and are sensitive to change (Goldston 2003). Both the SIQ and the BSS focus primarily on suicidal thoughts, although the BSS has a single item asking about past history of suicide attempts. Hence, it is useful to supplement questionnaires or other assessments focusing primarily on suicidal thoughts with assessments of recent and past suicidal behaviors.

Risk assessment instruments, used primarily to ascertain level of risk of future suicidal behaviors, may also be useful for clinicians. These assessment instruments may focus on adolescent suicidal behavior risk factors, protective factors, or both. Unfortunately, many instruments purported to assess risk of subsequent suicide have not actually been evaluated prospectively (Goldston 2003). Moreover, suicidal behavior arises in many different contexts and is the result of heterogeneous developmental trajectories (Goldston et al. 2016), making it difficult to predict. With that caveat, two instruments that have been evaluated longitudinally and found to have utility in identifying youth at higher risk for suicidal are the Beck Hopelessness Scale (BHS; Beck and Steer 1988) and the Reasons for Living Inventory (RFL-48; Linehan et al. 1983). The BHS assesses hopelessness as a risk factor associated with suicide attempts and has been shown to have predictive validity with youth in clinical populations (Goldston 2003). The RFL-48 focuses on protective factors and has demonstrated validity in predicting adolescent repeat suicide attempts in a clinical sample (Goldston et al. 2001; Linehan et al. 1983). Despite the potential clinical utility of these instruments in prediction, and in identifying possible treatment targets, clinicians should be cautious about relying on information about single risk factors in estimating risk to young clients.

Assessment of Imminent Risk

One primary purpose of clinical assessment is to determine the degree to which an adolescent patient poses imminent risk of harm to himself or herself. For many adolescents, crisis management procedures can be used to de-escalate level of risk so that the adolescent can be effectively treated in the least restrictive setting. For others, a higher level of care may be needed. In determining whether patients are at imminent risk, adolescent report of intent and perceptions of whether the patients can keep themselves safe (and participate in a safety plan) is of primary importance. That said, there are certain situations when adolescents' reports may be influenced by environmental contingencies. For example, an adolescent may deny suicidal intent if he or she is trying to avoid hospitalization.

Clinical judgment of imminent risk should also consider whether the adolescent's family and social environment can provide close monitoring, whether lethal means for attempting suicide are accessible, and whether the adolescent can articulate alternatives to suicidal behavior if crises recur. The adolescent's history of suicidal behavior and risk factors, and whether situational factors contributing to acute risk have been reduced, also need to be considered in assessing imminent risk. For example, if an adolescent reports that he will try to kill himself with a hidden gun the next time his mother yells, but his mother does not believe him and says she fully intends to "give him a piece of her mind" when she gets home, that adolescent would be considered at imminent risk because of intent, availability of method, and the high likelihood that a crisis may occur without intervention.

Functional Assessments

Beyond simply determining presence and severity of or risk for suicidal ideation and behavior, a functional analysis can provide important insight into the context of suicidal thoughts and behavior and possible targets for intervention to reduce risk for future suicidal behaviors (Goldston 2004). In describing the functional analysis, we follow the SORC (stimulus-organism-response-consequence) model described by Goldfried and Sprafkin (1974). In the service of developing integrative and individualized treatment approaches for youth with suicidal thoughts and co-occurring substance use difficulties, the SORC model can be used to identify functional commonalities (e.g., common triggers, risk and protective factors, or consequences) and relationships between substance use and suicidal thoughts and behaviors. In this model, S refers to the antecedent events that precipitate or serve as the "trigger" for substance use and suicidal thoughts or behaviors. O refers to the variables (e.g., feelings, cognitions, history, risk and protective factors) that moderate or mediate relationships between the triggers and the substance use and/or suicidality. For example, an adolescent might not always react to a stressful family interaction (e.g., a trigger) with substance use or suicidal behavior; rather, there may be factors such as depression, anxiety, anger, or low perceived social support that increase the likelihood of the maladaptive behaviors occurring in the presence of environmental triggers. R refers to the behavior or response(s) of interest in the functional analysis (i.e., substance use and suicidality). C refers to the consequences that serve to maintain, reinforce, or decrease the likelihood of the behavior recurring. For example, to the extent that suicidal behavior and substance use are associated with removal or diminution of unpleasant affective states, these behaviors will be negatively reinforced and the likelihood of their recurrence in similar circumstances will increase. As described previously, it is often the case that there are common triggers, risk and protective factors, and even consequences for suicidal and substance-abusing behaviors (Goldston 2004). Identification of these functional commonalities can be of assistance in choosing appropriate treatment targets.

Treatment of Substance Use Disorder and Suicidal Ideation and Suicide Attempts

Psychosocial Interventions

There are few published reports of randomized controlled studies evaluating the efficacy of psychosocial interventions specifically developed for suicidal youth with SUDs. That said, there are several promising psychosocial approaches. Esposito-Smythers and colleagues (2011) developed an integrated cognitive-behavioral therapy (CBT)/motivational interviewing (MI) intervention for suicidal youth with alcohol and/or other substance use problems. With this intervention, parents and youth had their own therapist in a coordinated treatment approach because of the severity and multiplicity of the difficulties of this population. In addition to the integrated intervention, youth and families also received case management assistance and psychiatric referrals for monitoring of medications. The intervention consisted of 6 months of weekly active treatment, 3 months of biweekly maintenance sessions, and three monthly booster sessions. Modules in the CBT/MI intervention for adolescents included safety planning, MI, and cognitive-behavioral skills training. Modules for work with parents included, but were not limited to, monitoring, consequences, beliefs regarding adolescents, and communication with adolescents.

The results with this intervention were very encouraging, with fewer suicide attempts, hospitalizations, emergency room visits, arrests, heavy drinking days, and days using cannabis among youth in the integrated CBT/MI treatment relative to those in enhanced treatment as usual (treatment as usual plus case management and provision of a psychiatrist for medications).

Kaminer and colleagues (2006) compared in-person and telephone relapse prevention aftercare for adolescents with alcohol use disorders following completion of 9 weeks of group CBT. Both aftercare approaches consisted of four sessions of CBT and MI over 3 months focused on alcohol and substance use but not suicidal behaviors or risk. In addition to beneficial effects on substance use outcomes, the in-person CBT/MI aftercare intervention resulted in greater reductions in suicidal ideation relative to the telephone aftercare or no aftercare, although the magnitude of the difference between the groups was small.

Dialectical behavior therapy (DBT) is a variant of combined individual and group CBT developed and shown to be effective for individuals with borderline personality disorder and suicidal or self-harm behaviors (Linehan et al. 2006). DBT includes a focus on skills related to mindfulness, emotion regulation, distress tolerance, and interpersonal effectiveness (Linehan et al. 2006). DBT has been adapted for use with adolescents, including involvement of parents, and focuses on developmentally appropriate issues such as the balance between need for parental monitoring versus the adolescent strivings for autonomy (Rathus and Miller 2002). In a recent randomized trial, DBT was found to be efficacious in reducing suicidal behaviors among adolescents (McCauley et al. 2018). Although DBT has not been evaluated specifically for youth with substance use and suicide risk, DBT as an integrated approach has been shown to reduce drug use among adult women with borderline personality disorder (Linehan et al. 1999).

The Family Intervention for Suicide Prevention (FISP) is a brief, one-session intervention for acutely suicidal youth (Asarnow et al. 2009). The intervention is cognitive-behavioral; involves both youth and parents, together and separately, and emphasizes resilience, connectedness to others, identification of warning signs and triggers of strong emotions as well as coping strategies, development of a safety plan, education about potentially disinhibiting effects of alcohol and drug use, discussion of restriction of potentially lethal means of attempting suicide, linkage to aftercare, and follow-up caring contacts. The

FISP has been demonstrated to improve attendance at initial outpatient appointments (Asarnow et al. 2011), and it is also the first session of the longer Safe Alternatives for Teens and Youth (SAFETY) intervention (a cognitive-behavioral intervention lasting 12 weeks with separate therapists for youth and family), which, in turn, is associated with reduced attempts (Asarnow et al. 2017). The FISP has been adapted for trauma-exposed youth, and a separate addendum for the FISP has been developed that describes an integrated approach for youth who both are suicidal and have substance use problems.

Drawing from these psychosocial studies, and our own work in developing an integrated intervention with MI and CBT approaches for suicidal dually diagnosed youth, we describe several approaches to intervention with the adolescent suicidal behavior and substance use. First, as with all suicidal youth, it is important to begin gathering information about the context of the suicide attempt or crisis, to hear the "story" (Berk et al. 2004). This contextual information can be used to develop a better understanding of substance use and suicide risk, which, in turn, can be used to identify treatment targets. Complementing this emphasis on "understanding the story," MI approaches are useful in helping the adolescent to consider reasons for living and for quitting substance use, as well as highlighting ambivalence and discrepancies between these reasons and current behavioral patterns. MI approaches can also be used with parents, given the importance of parents in monitoring, reinforcing change, and helping adolescents continue in treatment (Logan and King 2001).

It is important to collaboratively develop a safety plan for use when the adolescent is beginning to feel distressed or in danger of hurting himself or herself (Asarnow et al. 2009; Stanley and Brown 2012). With the safety plan, the youth can identify coping thoughts and strategies, as well as safe adults (including the therapist) who may be contacted when the youth is feeling suicidal or unsafe. Safety considerations also should be reviewed with the adolescent's parents, who also are strongly encouraged to remove access to potential means for attempting suicide, including firearms. The therapist should monitor for suicidal ideation and behavior at every treatment session and collaborate in revising the safety plan as needed.

Encouragement of increased participation in pleasant activities other than alcohol and drug use is often emphasized with teens exhibiting suicidal behaviors and substance use. The giving up of previously important social or recreational activities in favor of increased drug use is one symptom of substance dependence in adolescents or adults (American Psychiatric Association 2000). For example, adolescents with comorbid substance use engage in few social activities (Becker and Curry 2007). The therapist can work with the adolescent to help identify and increase pleasant activities, including social activities that are alternatives to substance use, that may serve to reduce depression (through behavioral activation), and underscore reasons for living.

Another approach useful for teens with co-occurring suicidal thoughts and/or behavior and substance use is to focus on enhancing problem-solving skills. Adolescents who are suicidal and depressed show deficiencies in social problem solving (Curry et al. 1992), and problem-solving training is often included in treatment programs for substance use (Latimer et al. 2003). With problem-solving training, the adolescent may learn to relax and try to "step back" before solving problems, to brainstorm about possible alternatives, to identify both positive and negative consequences of different options, to choose a possible solution, and to give oneself credit for methodically thinking through how to handle the situation.

One therapy goal common to CBT approaches is to increase awareness of, and to challenge patterns of, negative thoughts. A patient with suicidal behavior is especially likely to have negative thoughts about the future (hopelessness). Increasing awareness of this negative pattern of thinking and coaching the adolescent to externalize and challenge these thoughts by focusing on reasons for living and future goals serve to counter this pattern. Teenagers may also have distorted thoughts about substance use, for example, focusing only on the positive consequences of use, and minimizing or not considering the problems of substance use. The therapist can help the adolescent cultivate greater awareness of and challenge these distortions in thoughts.

In working with substance-using youth at risk for suicide, it is important to involve the parent(s)/caregivers in a collaborative treatment approach. Parents can be provided information about how to monitor the adolescent for signs of escalating depression, withdrawal, and/or suicidal ideation and behavior; how the disinhibiting effects of alcohol and drug use can increase risk for suicidal behavior; and how the safety plan can be used to address risk. Because lower levels of parent monitoring are related to teen conduct problems, increasing parent monitoring of substance use and peer-group activity, especially early in treatment, may be an important goal. Likewise, monitoring the whereabouts of the teen when he or she is out of the house and aspects of behavior such as curfew adherence can be very important treatment targets.

As parents monitor their teenager more, it may become necessary to develop a plan for administering consequences. Monitoring may reveal that the teen is associating with drug-using peers, is coming home on the weekends intoxicated, or is consistently breaking curfew. Treatment sessions can be devoted to collaboratively developing a plan for the consequences that will be applied when the teenager comes home intoxicated or breaks curfew, or conversely, the consequences when the teen makes positive changes. Likewise, monitoring may reveal that the teen is becoming more depressed and/or experiencing an increase in suicidal ideation. In such cases, in addition to offering support and encouraging use of coping skills or activities that might alleviate distress, the parents may need to implement agreed-on consequences such as increasing monitoring, calling the therapist, or, if the youth cannot be kept safe, arranging for emergency intervention.

Negative communication is another potentially important treatment target in working with parents of substance-using youth who are at risk for suicide. Negative communication between parents and youth may serve as a precipitant of suicidal behavior or substance use, and/or interfere with the goals and content of therapy. If parents and teen engage in hostile, blaming, or verbally aggressive behaviors during therapy sessions, these behaviors might interfere with proactive, collaborative discussions. Alternatively, hostile family communication can result in family members shutting down and withdrawing from one another. Therapeutic work focusing on negative communication patterns may involve directly labeling the negative communication behaviors in session or based on family reports, and teaching and then prompting more effective communication skills, such as active listening and reflecting without necessarily agreeing. As a complement to better communication, parents may be encouraged to acknowledge or praise the adolescent when he or she is attempting to use coping skills or is showing desired behaviors.

One last common area of intervention with parents and teens together involves family problem solving. Problem solving is an important family skill, because unresolved family problems or conflict can trigger recurrence of various mental health problems. Suicidal thoughts and behaviors can result from hopelessness, helplessness, anxiety, and feelings of low self-esteem that arise from overwhelming, unsolved problems. Moreover, the urge to use substances is often prompted by an impulse to reduce or escape from the negative feelings that arise from the inability to solve problems effectively and respectfully as a family. The approach to teaching family problem-solving skills is analogous to the process described above for working individually with the adolescent, with the major difference being that the problem-solving steps are collaborative—the family works together to identify the problem in concrete, nonpejorative terms, brainstorms and evaluates solutions, and agrees together on an ultimate solution.

Pharmacotherapy

No published controlled studies with comparison groups to our knowledge have shown the effectiveness of pharmacotherapy in reducing risk for suicidal behaviors or suicide among adolescents with substance use problems, or to reduce risk for both suicidal behaviors and substance use among adolescents. Pharmacotherapy may clearly be useful in reducing risk factors (e.g., anxiety, depression) for both suicidal behavior and substance use.

Integrative Treatment

There are no published efficacy studies of combined pharmacotherapy and psychosocial treatment approaches for adolescents exhibiting suicidal behavior and substance use. Nonetheless, as described earlier, promising results have been obtained with integrated MI and CBT approaches.

Case Vignette

Cathy is a 15-year-old female who lives with her biological mother and younger brother. She presents for treatment after discharge from the hospital following a suicide attempt by overdose, which was discovered by her mother. Cathy had been drinking when she took the pills in an effort to kill herself because she said she was tired of being depressed, and because she was upset after an argument with her mother about grades. Cathy reported being depressed for approximately 3 years after an incident of sexual abuse. Since then, she has felt poorly about herself and began drinking, using cannabis and experimenting with taking pills. Cathy's mother knew she had been using alcohol and drugs, but she was not fully aware of her daughter's use until the hospitalization. Cathy said that she liked to drink and use pills to feel better because she did not like to feel depressed, but also acknowledged that "partying" was an important part of her social life. Increasingly, Cathy had chosen to give up activities so she could more singularly focus her energies on activities related to alcohol and drug use with the permissive peer group.

In the home, Cathy was often punished by her mother (generally, by being grounded or with restrictions of privileges) because of the lying associated with substance use, breaking of curfew, and sneaking out of the home. Cathy's history revealed that she tended to have intense suicidal ideation when inebriated, particularly when she was feeling anxious about other issues (e.g., school difficulties, problems with peers, conflict with her mother over her friends and substance use). Also, when inebriated, she sometimes had intense memories related to her past sexual trauma. During these times of inebriation, she sometimes was impulsive and had difficulty following her safety plan. Her mother was very frustrated with Cathy and felt increasingly unable to keep her daughter safe. She tried to punish her daughter and lecture her, but Cathy tended to ignore these consequences.

Treatment Goals

The immediate treatment goal is to ensure Cathy's safety. This should include development of a safety plan that identifies strategies or supports when she is feeling suicidal, as well as approaches for reducing access to potential means of suicide. Associated with efforts to reduce suicidal thoughts and risk for suicidal behaviors are the goals of reducing alcohol and substance use, strengthening coping skills, and reducing recurring distress that might be related to suicide and substance use risk. The therapeutic relationship should be collaborative and emphasize empowerment and resilience. Reduction in problems contributing to family conflict, negative thoughts and low self-esteem, lack of involvement in activities other than those focused on substance use, poor problem-solving skills, and lack of effective communication and parental monitoring in the home also likely should be targeted. As a longer-term goal, Cathy and her mother should be encouraged to seek treatment focused on her sexual abuse history, which initially precipitated her pattern of alcohol and drug use.

Treatment Setting

The preferred choice for treatment setting is outpatient, although it is very likely that the patient may need more than the usual 1-hour-per-week psychotherapy session (i.e., either longer or more frequent sessions, as well as emergency sessions when crises occur). If the patient cannot be kept safe, cannot agree to a safety plan, or makes another suicide attempt, psychiatric hospitalization may be an option. If the substance use problems are recalcitrant or worsen, intensive outpatient therapy or residential treatment may be warranted.

Treatment

Initially, and usually separately in psychotherapy, Cathy and her mother will be invited to "tell their story" regarding the events that led up to the suicidal behaviors and current substance use patterns. Building on this information, the therapist should collaboratively develop a safety plan with Cathy and her mother. The therapist will begin working with Cathy and her mother to develop a functional analysis of the context of these problems, common risk factors, and their interrelationship. The therapist will use MI approaches to help establish rapport with Cathy and her mother; to highlight ambivalence; to underscore self-efficacy, positive aspects of her life, and resilience; and to provide a foundation for steps taken toward change.

Over the course of therapy, the therapist will work with Cathy to help her become involved in activities that do not involve drugs and alcohol and, if possible, with new peer groups that are "safer" in terms of the maladaptive behaviors they model and the access to substances that they provide. Particularly given Cathy's low self-esteem and depression, as well as her hopelessness about the future, the therapist will help her to recognize and challenge overly negative thinking; consider her reasons for living, including aspirations for the future; and consider her positive attributes. In tandem with reviewing the events that led up to her current difficulties, the therapist can help Cathy to use better problem-solving skills so she can better consider the alternative behaviors and decisions she can make that might result in better outcomes. Given her trauma history, the therapist may use or recommend trauma-informed approaches (e.g., trauma-focused CBT) to address traumatic stress symptoms related to her earlier abuse, depression, and anxiety. The therapist will work with Cathy's mother to monitor Cathy more closely and to more consistently administer consequences. If possible, the emphasis should be on reward-based consequences for positive steps taken toward change. With the mother and Cathy together, the therapist can help the family improve the negative communication style and approach to resolving conflicts using problem-solving skills. The mother will be encouraged to "catch Cathy" making positive steps and to praise and reward these, and to try to limit angry or blaming communications, even when frustrated because Cathy is not making progress as quickly as hoped or has a setback.

Lastly, as illustrated by Cathy, youth with histories of both suicidal behaviors and substance use often have multiple comorbidities. In addition to the psychotherapeutic approaches, Cathy's treatment may also involve pharmacotherapy aimed at reducing her level of depression and anxiety.

Conclusion

Youth with histories of suicidal thoughts and behaviors as well as substance use problems present challenges for the therapist, with multiple psychiatric comorbidities and family difficulties, as well as risk of recurrent suicidal crises. It is imperative that clinicians closely monitor the adolescent throughout the course of treatment for suicidal thoughts and behaviors and maintain a flexible and individualized approach to intervention. Suicidal thoughts and behavior are often interrelated, with common risk factors and triggers, and substance use may serve to increase the risk for suicidality. Motivational enhancement and cognitive-behavioral skills training approaches, particularly with a relapse prevention focus, have potential utility with this population. Involvement of parents and caregivers is important in monitoring youth, reinforcing change, and collaborating in the intervention process.

Key Points

- Adolescents who use substances are at heightened risk for suicidal thoughts and behavior, and clinicians should routinely monitor for evidence and course of such thoughts and behaviors.

- Substance use and suicidal thoughts and behaviors may have common triggers, risk factors, and motives.

- Youth with suicidal thoughts and behaviors and substance use problems often have multiple psychiatric comorbidities, family difficulties, and life problems, and a flexible approach to treatment is needed with this population.

- Motivational enhancement and cognitive-behavioral skills training approaches with the involvement of parents and caregivers, and an emphasis on relapse prevention, appear to be promising treatment approaches.

References

American Psychiatric Association: Diagnostic and Statistical Manual of Mental Disorders, 4th Edition, Text Revision. Washington, DC, American Psychiatric Association, 2000

Arango V, Underwood MD, Boldrini M, et al: Serotonin 1A receptors, serotonin transporter binding and serotonin transporter mRNA expression in the brainstem of depressed suicide victims. Neuropsychopharmacology 25(6):892–903, 2001 11750182

Asarnow JR, Berk MS, Baraff LJ: Family Intervention for Suicide Prevention: a specialized emergency department intervention for suicidal youths. Professional Psychology: Research and Practice 40(2):118–125, 2009

Asarnow JR, Baraff LJ, Berk M, et al: An emergency department intervention for linking pediatric suicidal patients to follow-up mental health treatment. Psychiatr Serv 62(11):1303–1309, 2011 22211209

Asarnow JR, Hughes JL, Babeva KN, Sugar CA: Cognitive-behavioral family treatment for suicide attempt prevention: a randomized controlled trial. J Am Acad Child Adolesc Psychiatry 56(6):506–514, 2017 28545756

Bailey JA, McCloskey LA: Pathways to adolescent substance use among sexually abused girls. J Abnorm Child Psychol 33(1):39–53, 2005 15759590

Beck A, Steer R: Beck Hopelessness Scale Manual. San Antonio, TX, Psychological Corporation, 1988

Beck A, Steer R: Manual for the Beck Scale for Suicidal Ideation. San Antonio, TX, Psychological Corporation, 1991

Becker SJ, Curry JF: Interactive effect of substance abuse and depression on adolescent social competence. J Clin Child Adolesc Psychol 36(3):469–475, 2007 17658989

Berk MS, Henriques GR, Warman D, et al: A cognitive therapy intervention for suicide attempters: an overview of the treatment and case examples. Cognitive and Behavioral Practice 11(3):265–277, 2004

Bridge JA, McBee-Strayer SM, Cannon EA, et al: Impaired decision making in adolescent suicide attempters. J Am Acad Child Adolesc Psychiatry 51(4):394–403, 2012 22449645

Bridge JA, Horowitz LM, Fontanella CA, et al: Age-related racial disparity in suicide rates among US youths from 2001 through 2015. JAMA Pediatr 172(7):697–699, 2018 29799931

Bryan CJ, Garland EL, Rudd MD: From impulse to action among military personnel hospitalized for suicide risk: alcohol consumption and the reported transition from suicidal thought to behavior. Gen Hosp Psychiatry 41:13–19, 2016 27302719

Cantor C, McTaggart P, De Leo D: Misclassification of suicide—the contribution of opiates. Psychopathology 34(3):140–146, 2001 11316960

Centers for Disease Control and Prevention: Web-Based Injury Statistics Query and Reporting System (WISQARS) Online. National Center for Injury Prevention and Control, March 21, 2019. Available at https://www.cdc.gov/injury/wisqars/index.html. Accessed May 15, 2019.

Conner KR, Goldston DB: Rates of suicide among males increase steadily from age 11 to 21—proposed causes and implications for prevention. Aggression and Violent Behavior 12(2):193–297, 2007

Conner KR, Swogger MT, Houston RJ: A test of the reactive aggression-suicidal behavior hypothesis: is there a case for proactive aggression? J Abnorm Psychol 118(1):235–240, 2009 19222330

Conner KR, Gamble SA, Bagge CL, et al: Substance-induced depression and independent depression in proximal risk for suicidal behavior. J Stud Alcohol Drugs 75(4):567–572, 2014 24988255

Conner KR, Bridge JA, Davidson DJ, et al: Metaanalysis of mood and substance use disorders in proximal risk for suicide deaths. Suicide Life Threat Behav 49(1):278–292, 2019 29193261

Crosby AE, Ortega L, Melanson C: Self-Directed Violence Surveillance: Uniform Definitions and Recommended Data Elements, Version 1.0. Atlanta, GA, Centers for Disease Control and Prevention, National Center for Injury Prevention and Control, 2011

Curry JF, Miller Y, Waugh S, et al: Coping responses in depressed, socially maladjusted, and suicidal adolescents. Psychol Rep 71(1):80–82, 1992 1529081

Donaldson CD, Handren LM, Crano WD: The enduring impact of parents' monitoring, warmth, expectancies, and alcohol use on their children's future binge drinking and arrests: a longitudinal analysis. Prev Sci 17(5):606–614, 2016 27178008

Esposito-Smythers C, Goldston DB: Challenges and opportunities in the treatment of adolescents with substance use disorder and suicidal behavior. Subst Abus 29(2):5–17, 2008 19042320

Esposito-Smythers C, Spirito A, Kahler CW, et al: Treatment of co-occurring substance abuse and suicidality among adolescents: a randomized trial. J Consult Clin Psychol 79(6):728–739, 2011 22004303

Fite PJ, Colder CR, Lochman JE, et al: Pathways from proactive and reactive aggression to substance use. Psychol Addict Behav 21(3):355–364, 2007 17874886

Foley DL, Goldston DB, Costello EJ, et al: Proximal psychiatric risk factors for suicidality in youth: the Great Smoky Mountains Study. Arch Gen Psychiatry 63(9):1017–1024, 2006 16953004

Goldfried MR, Sprafkin JN: Behavioral Personality Assessment. Morristown, NJ, General Learning Press, 1974, pp 295–321

Goldston DB: Measuring Suicidal Behavior and Risk in Children and Adolescents. Washington, DC, American Psychological Association, 2003

Goldston DB: Conceptual issues in understanding the relationship between suicidal behavior and substance use during adolescence. Drug Alcohol Depend 76(suppl):S79–S91, 2004 15555819

Goldston DB, Daniel SS, Reboussin BA, et al: Cognitive risk factors and suicide attempts among formerly hospitalized adolescents: a prospective naturalistic study. J Am Acad Child Adolesc Psychiatry 40(1):91–99, 2001 11195570

Goldston DB, Molock SD, Whitbeck LB, et al: Cultural considerations in adolescent suicide prevention and psychosocial treatment. Am Psychol 63(1):14–31, 2008 18193978

Goldston DB, Daniel SS, Erkanli A, et al: Psychiatric diagnoses as contemporaneous risk factors for suicide attempts among adolescents and young adults: developmental changes. J Consult Clin Psychol 77(2):281–290, 2009 19309187

Goldston DB, Erkanli A, Daniel SS, et al: Developmental trajectories of suicidal thoughts and behaviors from adolescence through adulthood. J Am Acad Child Adolesc Psychiatry 55(5):400.e1–407.e1, 2016 27126854

Gould MS, Fisher P, Parides M, et al: Psychosocial risk factors of child and adolescent completed suicide. Arch Gen Psychiatry 53(12):1155–1162, 1996 8956682

Gould MS, Marrocco FA, Kleinman M, et al: Evaluating iatrogenic risk of youth suicide screening programs: a randomized controlled trial. JAMA 293(13):1635–1643, 2005 15811983

Hill S, Shanahan L, Costello EJ, et al: Predicting persistent, limited, and delayed problematic cannabis use in early adulthood: findings from a longitudinal study. J Am Acad Child Adolesc Psychiatry 56(11):966.e4–974.e4, 2017 29096779

Horowitz LM, Bridge JA, Teach SJ, et al: Ask Suicide-Screening Questions (ASQ): a brief instrument for the pediatric emergency department. Arch Pediatr Adolesc Med 166(12):1170–1176, 2012 23027429

Hufford MR: Alcohol and suicidal behavior. Clin Psychol Rev 21(5):797–811, 2001 11434231

Kaminer Y, Burleson JA, Goldston DB, et al: Suicidal ideation among adolescents with alcohol use disorders during treatment and aftercare. Am J Addict 15 (suppl 1):43–49, 2006 17182419

Kann L, McManus T, Harris WA, et al: Youth Risk Behavior Surveillance—United States, 2017. MMWR Surveill Summ 67(8)(SS-8):1–114, 2018 29902162

Latimer WW, Winters KC, D'Zurilla T, et al: Integrated family and cognitive-behavioral therapy for adolescent substance abusers: a stage I efficacy study. Drug Alcohol Depend 71(3):303–317, 2003 12957348

Lewinsohn PM, Rohde P, Seeley JR: Adolescent suicidal ideation and attempts: prevalance, risk factors and implications. Clinical Psychology: Science and Practice 3(1):25–46, 1996

Lewinsohn PM, Rohde P, Seeley JR, Baldwin CL: Gender differences in suicide attempts from adolescence to young adulthood. J Am Acad Child Adolesc Psychiatry 40(4):427–434, 2001 11314568

Linehan MM, Goodstein JL, Nielsen SL, et al: Reasons for staying alive when you are thinking of killing yourself: the Reasons for Living Inventory. J Consult Clin Psychol 51(2):276–286, 1983 6841772

Linehan MM, Schmidt H 3rd, Dimeff LA, et al: Dialectical behavior therapy for patients with borderline personality disorder and drug-dependence. Am J Addict 8(4):279–292, 1999 10598211

Linehan MM, Comtois KA, Murray AM, et al: Two-year randomized controlled trial and follow-up of dialectical behavior therapy vs therapy by experts for suicidal behaviors and borderline personality disorder. Arch Gen Psychiatry 63(7):757–766, 2006 16818865

Logan DE, King CA: Parental facilitation of adolescent mental health service utilization: a conceptual and empirical review. Clinical Psychology: Science and Practice 8(3):319–333, 2001

McCauley E, Berk MS, Asarnow JR, et al: Efficacy of dialectical behavior therapy for adolescents at high risk for suicide: a randomized clinical trial. JAMA Psychiatry 75(8):777–785, 2018 29926087

Miron O, Yu K, Wilf-Miron R, Kohane IS: Suicide rates among adolescents and young adults in the United States, 2000–2017. JAMA 321(23):2362–2363, 2019 31211337

Nandrino JL, Gandolphe MC, El Haj M: Autobiographical memory compromise in individuals with alcohol use disorders: towards implications for psychotherapy research. Drug Alcohol Depend 179:61–70, 2017 28756101

Pinto E, Reggers J, Gorwood P, et al: The short allele of the serotonin transporter promoter polymorphism influences relapse in alcohol dependence. Alcohol Alcohol 43(4):398–400, 2008 18364363

Posner K, Melvin GA, Stanley B, et al: Factors in the assessment of suicidality in youth. CNS Spectr 12(2):156–162, 2007 17277716

Posner K, Brown GK, Stanley B, et al: The Columbia-Suicide Severity Rating Scale: initial validity and internal consistency findings from three multisite studies with adolescents and adults. Am J Psychiatry 168(12):1266–1277, 2011 22193671

Rathus JH, Miller AL: Dialectical behavior therapy adapted for suicidal adolescents. Suicide Life Threat Behav 32(2):146–157, 2002 12079031

Reynolds WM: Suicidal Ideation Questionnaire: Professional Manual. Odessa, FL, Psychological Assessment Resources, 1988

Roley-Roberts ME, Zielinski MJ, Hurtado G, et al: Functions of nonsuicidal self-injury are differentially associated with suicide ideation and past attempts among child trauma survivors. Suicide Life Threat Behav 47(4):450–460, 2017 27767234

Stanley B, Brown GK: Safety planning intervention: a brief intervention to mitigate suicide risk. Cognitive and Behavioral Practice 19(2):259–264, 2012

Whitlow CT, Liguori A, Livengood LB, et al: Long-term heavy marijuana users make costly decisions on a gambling task. Drug Alcohol Depend 76(1):107–111, 2004 15380295

Wilcox HC, Conner KR, Caine ED: Association of alcohol and drug use disorders and completed suicide: an empirical review of cohort studies. Drug Alcohol Depend 76(suppl):S11–S19, 2004 15555812

Assessment and Treatment of Comorbid Psychotic Disorders

Bipolar Disorder, Schizophrenia, and Drug-Induced Psychotic Disorders

Kara S. Bagot, M.D.

Robert Milin, M.D., F.R.C.P.C.

Desiree Shapiro, M.D.

Daphna Finn, M.D.

Shavon Moore, M.D.

Psychosis and Substance Use Disorders

Cannabis is the most common substance regularly used by adolescents, with nearly 6% of 12th-grade students using daily (Monitoring the Future 2018), and the most prevalent primary substance of misuse that leads to treatment admission (Dennis et al. 2002; Johnston et al. 2018). The onset of schizophrenia is also most common in late adolescence and young adulthood, with first psychotic symptoms often occurring before 20 years of age in 20%–40% of cases (Lehman et al. 2004).

Substance use disorder (SUD) is the most common comorbid disorder in schizophrenia, including first-episode psychosis (FEP). Although SUD prevalence rates among individuals with schizophrenia are two times greater than those in the general population (Tucker 2009; Wade et al. 2006), patients with schizophrenia or FEP may have co-occurring cannabis use disorder (CUD) and stimulant use disorder at rates more than 10 times the rates in the general population (Sara et al. 2013, 2014), and one-third of those diagnosed with FEP also use cannabis (Bahorik et al. 2014). In clinical samples of patients with schizophrenia, current prevalence rates of SUD range from 20% to 40%, with some studies showing lifetime prevalence rates of between 50% and 80% (Tucker 2009; Westermeyer 2006). Similar rates of lifetime, and even higher rates of current, comorbid SUD have been found in adolescent-onset schizophrenia and FEP. In FEP, current rates of SUD have been reported to be as high as 60% (Lambert et al. 2005; Milin 2008). Among transition-age youth (ages 18–25 years), up to 50% of those with FEP and comorbid CUD, and greater than 65% of those with FEP and comorbid stimulant use disorder, had polysubstance use disorder (Ouellet-Plamondon et al. 2017). Younger age and male gender are the most consistent predictors of SUD, especially drug misuse (Wade et al. 2005).

It is also important to note that patients with schizophrenia show remitting rates of comorbid SUD over the course of illness as evidenced by the difference between lifetime and current prevalence rates. Remission rates are influenced by substance (alcohol having higher rates than cannabis and other drugs) and severity (abuse having higher rates than dependence) (Westermeyer 2006). Those who discontinue use have been shown to have a better prognosis than episodic or persistent users, achieving outcomes similar to those of non-users, including improvement in negative symptoms (Weibell et al. 2017), which are difficult to treat.

A gap in the literature exists in regard to prevalence and trajectory of psychotic SUDs in minority adolescents and children. Wu et al. (2011) found that African American youth were more likely to be diagnosed with psychotic disorders and more likely to be hospitalized for any psychiatric diagnosis than

Caucasian youth, but the authors found no differences in SUD diagnoses between the two groups. Other studies have found longer duration of untreated psychosis among Caucasian adolescents as compared with their African American counterparts (Dominguez et al. 2013).

It has been postulated that adolescence may be a unique period of vulnerability for the concurrent development of psychotic disorders and SUD. It is suggested that specific psychosocial challenges and neurodevelopmental brain changes may increase the risk of onset of both psychosis and drug abuse in vulnerable adolescents (Mallet et al. 2017; van Nimwegen et al. 2005). Indeed, earlier age at onset of psychosis, particularly with cannabis use, may be due to cannabis's actions on the developing brain (Galve-Roperh et al. 2009). The endocannabinoid system is implicated in brain maturation, with endocannanoids and cannabinoid receptors reaching peak levels during adolescence (Schneider 2008). Cannbinoid receptors influence γ-aminobutyric acid (GABA) and glutamate neurotransmitter systems, which modulate dopamine neurons. Animal models suggest that repeated Δ-9-tetrahydrocannabinol (THC) exposure may lead to receptor sensitization in striatal and prefrontal regions, resulting in decreased levels of dopamine and psychosis (Kuepper et al. 2010). Additionally, individuals with schizophrenia or FEP and preceding regular cannabis use demonstrate fewer neurological soft signs related to impaired motor coordination, sensory integration, and planning of complex motor movements, and better cognitive functioning as compared with those with schizophrenia without premorbid cannabis use (Mallet et al. 2017; Yücel et al. 2012). However, those with schizophrenia who use cannabis after psychosis onset demonstrate worse neurocognitive performance and worsening of neurological soft signs as compared with those without cannabis use (D'Souza et al. 2005). This suggests a specific phenotype of schizophrenia with a differing neurodevelopmental trajectory in which cannabis exposure plays an important role in gene-environment interaction in neurodevelopment.

Association Between Cannabis Use and Psychotic Disorders

There is a growing body of evidence from international longitudinal and cohort studies supported by a meta-analysis that cannabis use in a dose-dependent relationship increases the risk of clinically relevant psychotic disorders, including schizophreniform disorder, schizophrenia, and FEP. The pooled analysis of more than 66,000 individuals found an odds ratio (OR) of 3.9 for psychosis for those with heavy cannabis use as compared with those who never used, and a median OR of 2.0 for any cannabis users. An examination of these relationships by type of psychosis demonstrated pooled ORs of 3.6 for psychotic symptoms and 5.1 for schizophrenia or another psychotic disorder (Marconi et al. 2016). An earlier meta-analysis found an increased risk of psychosis of 40% for those who ever used cannabis, and a dose-dependent effect with a risk of psychosis between 50% and 200% for those who used cannabis most frequently (Moore et al. 2007).

A similar significant relationship has been found for cannabis and schizophrenia, with accumulating evidence that cannabis use is an independent risk factor for the development of schizophrenia in adulthood, and especially in vulnerable individuals. Findings across studies are consistent with an overall two- to threefold increase in the risk of developing schizophrenia with cannabis use in a dose-dependent manner, and of greater risk with onset of use in adolescence (Arseneault et al. 2002; Bagot et al. 2015). Adolescent cannabis use is associated with an increased risk of psychotic disorders even after prodromal symptoms, parental psychosis, and other substance use are controlled for (Mustonen et al. 2018). This increased risk is comparable to those of better-known associations, including cigarette smoking and hypercholesterolemia in developing lung cancer and heart disease, respectively (D'Souza 2007).

Notwithstanding these findings, evidence to date does not necessarily support a causal link between cannabis use and schizophrenia; nevertheless, it warrants serious consideration (Degenhardt et al. 2003; Radhakrishnan et al. 2014). Moore and colleagues (2007) in their analysis concluded that there was now sufficient evidence to warn young people that cannabis use may increase their risk for developing a psychotic illness later in adulthood. Cannabis use in a dose-dependent relationship is a significant independent risk factor in the complex interaction of genetic liability and environmental factors that leads to the expression of schizophrenia in young adults and adolescents (Arseneault et al. 2002; Henquet et al. 2005b; Marconi et al. 2016). Genes that have been found that influence both dopamine D_2 receptors, implicated in psychosis, and the endocannabinoid system include the AKT1 C/C genotype and the COMT gene (Di Forti et al. 2014; Henquet et al. 2009; van Winkel and Genetic Risk and Outcome of Psychosis (GROUP) Investigators 2011). Further, certain

COMT variants have been shown to interact with environmental factors such as childhood trauma to increase vulnerability to psychosis among cannabis users (Alemany et al. 2014; Vinkers et al. 2013).

Clinical studies demonstrate a temporal relationship, with substance misuse preceding the onset of psychosis/schizophrenia, although it may occur concurrently with the onset or post-onset of schizophrenia. Heavy cannabis use has been associated with an earlier age at onset of schizophrenia (Bagot et al. 2015; D'Souza et al. 2009). The clinical implication of this finding is considerable, given that early age at cannabis use onset is associated with early FEP/psychotic disorder and poorer prognosis. Although alcohol has not been meaningfully linked to an earlier age at onset of schizophrenia, there are increased rates of alcohol use among individuals with psychotic disorders (Abdel-Baki et al. 2017; Koskinen et al. 2009).

Comorbid SUD imparts a significant negative effect on the course and outcome of schizophrenia and has been frequently associated with increased risk of psychotic relapse, criminality, violence, suicidality, depression, homelessness, unemployment, greater utilization of hospital-based services, treatment nonadherence (including to pharmacotherapy), and illness severity (including more positive [e.g., hallucinations and delusions] and negative [e.g., apathy and flat affect] symptoms and poorer treatment response) (Abdel-Baki et al. 2017; Barak et al. 2008; Lambert et al. 2005; Ouellet-Plamondon et al. 2017; Weibell et al. 2017). Similar findings of poorer clinical outcomes have also been found for persisting comorbid SUD in longitudinal studies of FEP, including increased rates of relapse and hospitalization, decreased remission rates, and poorer functional outcomes (Lambert et al. 2005; Wade et al. 2006). Wade and colleagues (2007) also demonstrated a relationship between substance severity and psychosis outcomes, with heavy substance use associated with poorer symptomatic and functional outcomes as compared with those with mild substance use. CUDs were markedly prevalent in the high-severity SUD group and significantly more so than in the low-severity SUD group. Cannabis misuse and severity have also been strongly implicated in poorer clinical outcomes in prospective studies of recent-onset psychosis/schizophrenia in young adulthood (Grech et al. 2005; Hides et al. 2006). Comorbid alcohol use and alcohol use disorders (AUDs) among those with psychosis have been associated with suicidality and depression, poorer quality of life, poorer medication adherence and social functioning, and greater hospital service utilization (Barak et al.

2008; Ouellet-Plamondon et al. 2017). Finally, comorbid stimulant use disorder has been shown to worsen positive and negative symptoms, other comorbid psychiatric symptoms, quality of life, functioning (including employment status), hospitalization rates, and medication adherence (Ouellet-Plamondon et al. 2017).

Although the focus of this chapter is on youth, it is important to address the contribution of cannabis use to variation in the incidence of psychotic disorders among adults. In a multicenter case-control study involving 11 sites across Europe and Brazil, the investigators concluded that differences of frequency of daily use and in use of high-potency (THC≥10%) cannabis contributed to striking variations in increased incidence of psychotic disorders compared with non-user control subjects (Di Forti et al. 2019).

In summary, comorbid SUD, with cannabis misuse playing a principal role, and severity of use convey a more debilitating course of illness/outcome in FEP and are associated with an earlier age at onset of schizophrenia and other related psychotic disorders.

Assessment and Differential Diagnosis

Acute or chronic intoxication with diverse substances may produce similar psychotic symptoms and clinical features. Similar presentations may also be seen with substance withdrawal with heavy and prolonged use of alcohol and sedative/hypnotics and anxiolytics. These substances may produce psychotic symptoms in individuals without serious mental health disorders that are similar to those found in those with schizophrenia. Psychoactive substances may also affect individuals with primary psychotic disorders, whereby psychotic symptoms may be exacerbated, changed, or temporarily decreased. Substance-induced psychotic symptoms are, by far, most commonly transient and resolve within several hours to days. However, there is some evidence to suggest that chronic and heavy use of stimulants, cocaine, hallucinogens, phencyclidine (PCP), and cannabis may result in more prolonged psychotic reactions that may last for weeks or longer (Milin 2008).

It is important to distinguish between substance-induced psychotic disorder (SIPD) and substance intoxication or withdrawal with perceptual disturbance. The former diagnosis should be made when psychotic symptoms are more prominent than one would expect with intoxication or withdrawal and when the severity of symptoms warrants independent clinical attention. The latter diagnosis includes hallucinations or delusions that may occur in the course of intoxication or withdrawal with intact reality testing (the individual is aware that the hallucinations are an effect of the substance).

The differential diagnosis between SIPD and a primary psychotic disorder with concurrent SUD is often challenging, with a history of significant substance misuse being typically common to both conditions. A diagnosis of schizophrenia and related disorders may be reliably made in the presence of symptoms of schizophrenia and the absence of substance misuse within the preceding month, even with a history of prior SUD (Mueser et al. 1992). However, periods of extended abstinence of a month or longer are often difficult to achieve. Clinicians, therefore, may need to consider the onset, course, and other features of presentation. The differential diagnosis is inherently even more difficult to make during adolescence/young adulthood, when both schizophrenia and SUD commonly have their onset. Other factors to consider include the effect of substance use and cessation on psychotic symptoms, the severity of psychotic symptoms in relation to the degree of substance use, and the characteristic symptoms produced by the principal substance of misuse in relation to the full spectrum of positive and negative symptoms of schizophrenia. The clinical presentation may be further confounded by a pattern of multiple substance misuse. Whenever possible, urine drug analyses including quantitative levels may be helpful in gauging the role of substance use.

When the clinician is assessing concurrent psychotic and substance-related disorders, it is important to explore both the cross-sectional and the longitudinal course of the illness. Collateral and family history, where possible, is often helpful in assessing the course of illness and differentiating etiology, especially in adolescents and young adults.

Several significant predictive factors have been found to distinguish between SIPD and primary psychotic disorders with concurrent substance use. SIPD has been associated with drug dependence, parental history of SUD and visual hallucinations, and more diagnostic instability. Approximately 25% of individuals may go on to develop a primary psychotic disorder. Primary psychotic disorders are associated with more total psychopathology, including both positive and negative symptoms, and family history of parental mental illness, and tend to remain diagnostically stable (Caton et al. 2005, 2007).

In a Danish longitudinal cohort study (Arendt et al. 2005), the incidence rate estimated for cannabis-induced psychotic disorder was 2.7 per 100,000 person-years, a relatively uncommon event. However, of the patients who received a diagnosis of cannabis-induced psychotic disorder (CIPD) with no prior history of psychosis, nearly 50% subsequently received a diagnosis of a schizophrenia spectrum disorder on follow-up of at least 3 years. The conversion risk rate for CIPD has been shown to be almost twice that of noncannabis SIPD conversion (Starzer et al. 2018). Younger age was associated with increased risk of conversion to schizophrenia.

Similar rate ratios for family history of general psychiatric and psychotic disorders have been found for both cannabis-induced psychosis and schizophrenia spectrum disorders (Arendt et al. 2008). This suggests that cannabis-induced psychosis is neither a random occurrence nor a benign condition.

In summary, there is no certain way to differentiate a SIPD from a primary psychotic disorder with concurrent SUD except in cases of an acute brief episode of psychosis lasting 48 hours or less (Arendt et al. 2008). Distinguishing these disorders relies, for the most part, on clinical judgment based on current and longitudinal history of psychotic symptoms, substance use, and knowledge of the course of illness of schizophrenia and the pharmacological properties of the principal substance in question. This differentiation is made even more complex in adolescence/young adulthood by the severity of SUD and the early age at onset, and by the often unclear course of premorbid symptoms, with both abrupt and insidious onset of psychosis. Several predictive factors have been identified as being helpful in the differential diagnosis: diagnosis of drug dependence, parental mental illness and/or substance use, visual hallucinations and severity of psychotic/psychiatric symptoms, and drug-induced psychotic disorder requiring treatment. The serious clinical implications warrant longitudinal follow-up of SIPD, and specifically cannabis-induced psychosis, in adolescents and young adults, given the diagnostic instability and the role of SIPD as a cogent marker for schizophrenia. However, it is not uncommon for cannabis users to report transient psychotic symptoms (Green et al. 2003), whereas substance or cannabis-induced psychosis is a relatively uncommon disorder made in individuals requiring clinical attention/treatment.

Treatment

Symptoms and history often overlap for SIPD and FEP, so it is for providers to decide on the most appropriate treatment interventions. At first presentation, substance-induced psychosis may look identical to a primary psychotic illness (Goerke and Kumra 2013). Comorbid substance use is common, and diagnostic certainty at the initial evaluation stages is rare. Patients with SIPD have shown a greater rate of remission than those with primary psychotic disorders at 1-year follow-up (Caton et al. 2006). The American Psychiatric Association (Lehman et al. 2004) practice guidelines for the treatment of patients with SUD note that individuals with certain substance-induced psychotic symptoms may benefit from the short-term use of antipsychotic medication. There are limited data on the optimal treatment of young patients with psychosis and substance use; however, there is increasing support for treating substance-induced psychotic reactions that persist beyond a reasonable period of abstinence without significant improvement of psychotic symptoms as a functional psychotic disorder. In youth being treated for FEP, persistent substance use was found to have a 2.6 times increased risk of disengagement. Providers should prioritize substance use and incorporate social networks into treatment (Schimmelmann et al. 2006). Among patients 16 years and older who were followed over 7 years in an observational database of FEP patients, those with drug-induced psychosis were more likely than those with schizophrenia to lose contact with services (Crebbin et al. 2009), highlighting the need to promote engagement with this high-risk group. In addition to medication nonadherence, there are higher rates of hospitalization in patients with schizophrenia and comorbid substance use (Lang et al. 2010). Continued substance use in the setting of psychosis is linked to poorer engagement in care and poor remission rates; therefore, early and integrated interventions, both psychosocial and pharmacological, are recommended (Lambert et al. 2005).

Pharmacotherapy remains the mainstay of treatment of schizophrenia and other related psychotic disorders with or without comorbid SUD. Clinically, second-generation antipsychotics (SGAs), with their dopamine (D_2) and 5-HT$_{2A}$ receptor blockade leading to antipsychotic effects and reduction of the extrapyramidal symptoms associated with first-generation antipsychotics, remain the first choice of treatment for adolescents and young adults with FEP. Youth may be more sensitive to side effects and may be more reluctant to take psychotropic medications, so care must be taken to involve the youth in addition to the family to ensure proper psychoeducation and exploration of the meaning of the prescription, goals of treatment, and estimated length of time on the medication. To date, six SGAs—risperidone (Risperdal), lurasidone (Latuda), olanzapine (Zyprexa), paliperidone (Invega), quetiapine (Seroquel), and aripiprazole (Abilify)—have received U.S. Food and Drug Administration (FDA) approval for the treatment indication of schizophrenia in adolescents. In FEP, SGAs are typically initiated at a low dosage, and the dosage is gradually titrated to response within a standard therapeutic dosage range. Close monitoring for adverse effects is required, especially in adolescents and those with comorbid SUD, because adverse effects may be potentiated by active substance abuse.

In patients with schizophrenia-related disorders, studies have found associations of comorbid SUD with higher antipsychotic dosage and poorer response to antipsychotic treatment even when there is adherence to medication. Comorbid SUD is also associated with nonadherence with pharmacotherapy, further exacerbating its negative influence on outcome (Hunt et al. 2002). Similarly poorer treatment response and adherence have been found for patients with FEP with a lifetime history of comorbid SUD (Green et al. 2004). Interestingly, in one study, medication adherence was linked to a modest reduction in cannabis relapse in patients with recent-onset psychosis predominantly receiving SGA (Hides et al. 2006). Long-acting injectable (LAI) antipsychotic medication in FEP patients with comorbid SUD should be considered to increase medication adherence. Risperidone, aripiprazole, paliperidone, and olanzapine are SGAs with LAI medication options.

The highest standard of care for FEP involves specialized early intervention (SEI) treatment services. Common elements of SEI services include assertive case management, use of low-dose SGA medication regimens, close monitoring of treatment progress, family intervention, and individual and group psychotherapeutic and cognitive-behavioral interventions. The typical duration of these intensive treatment programs ranges from 18 months to 2 years. The improved relative benefit of SEI to routine care has been identified through high rates of remission, low relapse rates, better control of symptoms, and greater adherence and retention in treatment, as well as, to some extent, by broadly defined improved outcomes of functioning and quality of life over the course of intensive treatment (Albert et al. 2017; Malla et al. 2005). The optimal duration of SEI services and their long-term effectiveness remain to be determined. Five-year follow-up studies of SEI services for patients with FEP found that positive clinical outcomes were not sustainable with transition to routine care following programs of 2 years and 15 months, respectively (Bertelsen et al. 2008; Linszen et al. 2001). Studies of FEP patients receiving SEI have shown a significant and meaningful reduction in SUD over the course of treatment. Reduction in SUD has been associated with improved clinical outcome, and SEI has been shown to be significantly more likely to reduce SUD than routine care (Lambert et al. 2005; Petersen et al. 2005a, 2005b). According to the National Institute for Health and Care Excellence (NICE) guidelines of the United Kingdom, for psychosis in youth, family interventions, cognitive-behavioral therapy (CBT), and medications should be thoughtfully considered. Integrated treatments supported by research have included motivational interventions, CBT, group, contingency management, residential care, and psychopharmacology (Cleary et al. 2009; Drake et al. 2008). Consideration should be taken to address developmental, cognitive, and emotional aspects to providing care. Key aspects of psychological treatment should include reducing distress, improving functioning, using alternative coping strategies, and self-monitoring symptoms and response to symptoms (National Collaborating Centre for Mental Health 2013).

According to the Recovery After an Initial Schizophrenia Episode (RAISE) study (www.nimh.nih.gov/health/topics/schizophrenia/raise/what-is-coordinated-specialty-care-csc.shtml), *coordinated specialty care* (CSC) is a treatment program for individuals with FEP that promotes recovery, shared decision making, individualized treatment, and a team of providers who can assist with educational or employment support, assertive case management, work or education goals, and individual and group treatments (Kane et al. 2016). In a recent study evaluating outcomes for a statewide CSC in participants ages 16–30 with non-affective psychosis, significant improvements were identified in education, employment, and decreased hospitalization rates (Nossel et al. 2018).

Tobacco, alcohol, and cannabis use are common in youth with FEP. Using data from the RAISE Early Treatment Program, Oluwoye et al. (2019) found that compared with nonsmokers, tobacco smokers had worsening illness, greater medication nonadherence, and lower quality of life during treatment. Alcohol and cannabis use during treatment also influenced clinical outcomes negatively, but tobacco smokers had the worst clinical outcomes (Oluwoye et al. 2019).

In a comprehensive meta-analysis of 10 randomized controlled trials (RCTs) comparing early intervention services with treatment as usual in early psychosis, 6–24 months of early intervention services, which included coordinated and integrated treatment, showed superior outcomes in terms of psychiatric hospitalization during the treatment period, global functioning, involvement in school or work, and treatment discontinuation (Correll et al. 2018). Findings supported family involvement in improving symptomatic and functional outcomes and vocational or educational rehabilitation in improving both school and work involvement.

In summary, treatment of adolescents and young adults with FEP and comorbid SUD remains quite challenging, with clinicians being faced with a variety of confounding and competing factors over time, including problematic treatment acceptance and adherence. The advent of SEI and the addition of integrated SUD treatment hold considerable promise in improving outcomes for this complex population. Families, communities, schools, and other natural supports should be called on to encourage treatment and sobriety. Patients with persisting substance abuse/dependence or SUD relapse would be encouraged to further engage in SUD-specific treatment, preferably a combination of individual motivational enhancement therapy/CBT integrated into an overall treatment plan that includes psychoeducation, relapse prevention strategies, groups, and incentive-based interventions. Longer-term follow-up is advisable given the reality that many youth, without adequate tools, supports, and access to care, may resume substance use later in their life.

Case Vignette

A.D., a 16-year-old biracial male with a history of polysubstance use and hypertrophic cardiomyopathy with predominant septal hypertrophy, is admitted to the child and adolescent psychiatric inpatient service because of worsening psychotic symptoms. Upon interview, he has difficulty recollecting the purpose for admission; his primary concern is of increased episodes of "spacing out" in which he "loses consciousness" for a few seconds and has no recollection of his actions during the blackout period. He endorses paranoia worsening over the prior 2 years; he thought unfamiliar people were out to get him, which frequently forced him to isolate himself indoors. He endorses auditory and visual hallucinations but refuses to elaborate beyond describing voices that are "just complaining about things." A.D. also reports having the ability to make shapes transform into unrelated objects when "I relax my eyes" and to read others' minds via nonverbal cues.

A.D. reports current/recent use of mushrooms, "sid" (lysergic acid diethyl-amide [LSD]), and "weed" (marijuana), with weed being the primary substance of use. He was using more than 2 pounds of weed per month (28–40 g/day) for the preceding year. Additionally, he made his own edibles, including butter that he incorporated into foods such as cheeses and pizza, and concentrated cannabis ("dabs"). A.D. reports waking up in the morning and immediately packing a "mole" (marijuana and tobacco combined) to smoke; he describes then being too stoned to be productive the remainder of the day. He also reports that the addition of tobacco provides a calming effect; he feels "dumbed down" instead of "laughing and appearing high like taking Adderall 5 mg." He uses alone primarily and will "only" use up to a "quad" (7 g) with his "associates" because he does not want to appear stoned in public and get into any legal trouble.

Past Substance Use History

A.D. reports a history of use of cannabis (smoked, vaped, and eaten); LSD; methamphetamine; barbiturates; opiates such as Vicodin, heroin, and fentanyl; kratom; cocaine; benzodiazepines (Ativan, Xanax bars); and alcohol (infrequently). He reports initiation of substance use in 6th grade with cigarettes, with escalation in 7th grade to daily marijuana use, and fentanyl use.

Past Psychiatric History

A.D. had two prior psychiatric inpatient admissions in the past year for suicide attempt and paranoia and homicidal ideation toward peers. He was drug seeking (opiates and stimulants) on both prior admissions. A.D. was previously prescribed olanzapine 5 mg, with which he was noncompliant secondary to a side effect of vivid dreams, and the medication was subsequently discontinued because of prolonged QTc. Prior psychotic symptoms resolved with periods of no drug use while patient was admitted, and with psychotropic medications.

Past Medical History

A.D. has a history of hypertrophic cardiomyopathy with predominant septal hypertrophy and a history of poor compliance with cardiology appointments and recommendations regarding activity and medication.

Hospital Course

A.D. is admitted for 9 days. Symptoms during his admission include hallucinations, paranoid delusions, internal preoccupation, and mild negative symptoms of constricted affect and slowed conversational responses. After cardiology consultation and literature review, it is felt that aripiprazole will carry a low risk of QT prolongation and best address his mood, impulsivity, and psychotic symptoms. A.D. is started on aripiprazole 2.5 mg daily, with titration of the dosage up to 5 mg by mouth daily. QTc on day of discharge is somewhat elevated at 472 ms. He demonstrates a good response in terms of his psychotic symptoms and is felt to be at his baseline function on discharge. A.D. also notes marked improvement in his mood symptoms during the course of admission. He is also started on gabapentin 300 mg by mouth bid during admission to address his symptoms of marijuana withdrawal (irritability, aggression, depressed mood, insomnia). A.D. reports a significant decrease in symptoms by day 3.

Commentary

We have described here a case of substance-induced psychosis and treatment challenges secondary to medical comorbidity. Psychopharmacology remains limited in regard to treatment options for children and adolescents with medical comorbidities. When related medical issues prevent prescribing first-line medications, patients are left with suboptimal outcomes. Particularly concerning adverse effects of antipsychotics include increased risk for seizures, QT segment prolongation, tachycardia, and hypotension, and these effects can be amplified if caused by polysubstance use. QT prolongation is observed with both typical and atypical antipsychotics but most significantly with ziprasidone and thioridazine. However, the QTc with ziprasidone is only about 10 ms longer than with risperidone, quetiapine, or olanzapine. The effect seems to be partially dose related but is also seen more in patients with a genetic predisposition, such as congenital long QT syndrome. There is overall a much lower prevalence of antipsychotic-related long QT syndrome in children; it is thought that the decreased prevalence in children may be due to the relative absence of ischemic heart disease in this population compared with adults (Rasimas and Liebelt 2012).

Cannabis use is associated with decreased adherence to antipsychotic treatment during the first 2 years after FEP, even when potential confounders such as other illicit drug use and clinical and demographic characteristics are controlled for. This is especially problematic after FEP during the "critical period" in which relapses are common and shown to correlate with poorer long-term outcomes. Chronic antipsychotic treatment results in substantial cardiometabolic effects that can be seen in the first 6 months in drug-naïve patients, in particular with risperidone and olanzapine (Arango et al. 2014). These effects are in addition to the health risks associated with chronic cannabis use. Studies have had inconsistent findings regarding weight change with cannabis use, with some showing an inverse relationship between cannabis use and weight gain. A recent longitudinal study found cannabis use in adolescence to not be associated with weight change into midlife but to be inversely associated with decreased physical activity level (Jin et al. 2017). In addition, a cross-sectional analysis using National Health and Nutrition Examination Survey data found an increased risk of metabolic syndrome and hypertension with each year increase in cannabis use, even after adjustment for tobacco and alcohol use (Yankey et al. 2016). Activation of the endocannabinoid system has been shown to stimulate appetite and food intake, and regular THC exposure results in morphological changes in the CB1 receptor–rich orbitofrontal cortex involved in termination of food intake (Jin et al. 2017).

Bipolar Disorder and Substance Use Disorders

Strength of the Association Between Bipolar Disorder and SUDs

Epidemiological studies have consistently reported that bipolar disorder (BD) is the most highly associated disorder with SUD, except for antisocial personality disorder (Salloum and Thase 2000). Specifically, both the Epidemiologic Catchment Area study and the National Comorbidity Survey reported 6- to 10-fold elevated rates of SUD in bipolar patients compared with the general population; there is a lifetime history of SUD in approximately 50% of bipolar patients (Kessler et al. 1997; Regier et al. 1990). This specificity of risk for SUD extends to broader diagnoses of BD, including subthreshold hypomania (Angst et al. 2006; Glantz et al. 2009; Merikangas et al. 2008).

In the National Epidemiologic Survey on Alcohol and Related Conditions, a representative sample of more than 42,000 adult respondents in the United States, mania and hypomania were associated with markedly elevated rates of SUD. Episodes classified as substance induced were excluded from the analyses. Participants with a history of mania were 6 times more likely to have alcohol dependence and 14 times more likely to have another SUD during the previous 12 months (Grant et al. 2004). Specifically, the lifetime prevalence of mania in respondents with SUD (other than AUD) ranged from 8.9% to 33.4% (depending on the class of substance), while that of hypomania ranged from

3.7% to 13.4%. These rates are much higher than those reported for the general population in that sample (i.e., 3.31% for mania and 2.33% for hypomania) (Conway et al. 2006).

In a Canadian cross-sectional study of adolescents ages 13–19 with a bipolar I, bipolar II, or not otherwise specified NOS diagnosis, the lifetime prevalence of SUD (primarily AUD and CUD) was 33% (Scavone et al. 2018). SUD was associated with a greater number of stressful life events, more self-reported impulsivity and parent-reported anger and depression, and a higher lifetime prevalence of conduct disorder, oppositional defiant disorder, panic disorder, and assault of others. Comorbid BD and SUDs have also been associated with high rates of legal problems, unwanted pregnancies, HIV infection risk behaviors, and abortion in adolescents (Goldstein et al. 2008b; Meade et al. 2008).

Clinical studies have reported similarly high rates of SUD among patients with BD (Cassidy et al. 2001; Merikangas et al. 2008). Overall, AUD followed by CUD are the most frequent SUDs, and it is estimated that a substantial proportion of BD patients with AUD also abuse at least one other substance. It is estimated that BD patients also have a fourfold increased risk of sedative-hypnotic and opioid use disorders, although these disorders occur less frequently than AUD and CUD (Salloum and Thase 2000).

In one prospective epidemiological study, cannabis use increased the risk of later manic symptoms, even after adjustment was made for the use of other substances and the presence of prior depressive, manic, and psychotic symptoms. The findings were suggestive of a dose-response relationship between frequency of cannabis use and mania outcome; however, considerably more research is needed to establish a causal link between them (Henquet et al. 2006). In addition to SUD increasing the risk for subsequent development of BD, the reverse is also often observed. Among adolescents ages 12–17 in the Course and Outcome of Bipolar Youth (COBY) study who had symptoms that met criteria for bipolar I disorder, bipolar II disorder, or BD not otherwise specified without SUD at intake, first-onset SUD developed among 32% (Goldstein et al. 2013). Subjects were followed up for an average of 4.25 ± 2.11 years; thus, the lifetime rates of SUD are likely significantly higher. The most robust predictive factor for the development of SUD was lifetime alcohol experimentation at intake. Other significant factors were lifetime oppositional defiant disorder and panic disorder, family history of SUD, low family cohesiveness, and absence of antidepressant treatment at intake; BD subtype was not predictive. Higher hypomanic or manic symptom severity in the preceding 12 weeks predicted greater likelihood of SUD onset. Of note, lithium exposure in the preceding 12 weeks predicted lower likelihood.

A registry study of childhood- or adolescent-onset BD demonstrated that in 98.3% and 75% of these populations, respectively, the criteria for SUD were not met at the time of BD onset (Kenneson et al. 2013). Risk factors for the development of SUD in this population were lifetime oppositional defiant disorder (hazard ratio [HR] = 2.0), any lifetime anxiety disorder (HR = 3.1), adolescent-onset BD (HR = 1.7), and suicide attempts (HR = 15.4). SUD was not predicted by BD type (I, II, or subthreshold), family history of bipolar disorder, hospitalization for a mood episode, attention-deficit/hyperactivity disorder (ADHD), or conduct disorder. Males were more likely to develop SUD. Ultimately the prevalence of secondary SUD among those with early-onset BD was 43.1%.

An earlier analysis by Merikangas et al. (2008) of the Zurich Cohort Study showed a strong association between BD and subsequent onset of alcohol abuse (OR = 9.1) and dependence (OR = 21.1). Furthermore, manic symptoms were found to be a risk factor for the future development of AUD, CUD, and benzodiazepine use disorder (Merikangas et al. 2008).

These studies underscore that BD increases the risk for subsequent development of SUD. SUDs are well known to have a negative impact on the course of illness and outcomes in patients with BD. (For a comprehensive review, see Salloum and Thase 2000.) Briefly, comorbid SUD has been associated with an earlier age at onset, shortening of cycle length, delayed time to recovery, shortened time to relapse, higher number of recurrences, and more mixed and rapid-cycling presentations, as well as more chronicity, disability, cognitive impairment, and mortality attributed to increased suicide risk and more medical complications. Furthermore, SUD is strongly associated with treatment nonadherence, a factor correlated with the poor outcomes cited above.

First-Episode and Early-Onset Bipolar Patients and SUD

Early-onset BD, particularly BD of adolescent onset, has a strong association with SUD (Joshi and Wilens 2009). Unfortunately, psychiatric patients with

SUD tend to be diagnosed later than those without substance abuse, potentially delaying treatment (Toftdahl et al. 2016).

In a 24-month prospective study of patients admitted for a first mania/mixed bipolar I episode, Baethge et al. (2005) reported a 33% prevalence of SUD (mostly substance dependence) at baseline, with 40% having polysubstance use and 60% with monosubstance use disorders. Polysubstance users were younger, less educated, more likely to present in a mixed state, and more likely to have a positive family history of psychiatric illness compared with first-episode patients without SUD. On follow-up, cannabis-dependent patients spent more time in mania, whereas alcohol-dependent patients spent more time depressed. Overall, morbidity was much greater among polysubstance users. The University of Cincinnati First-Episode Mania Study reported a lifetime prevalence of 42% and 46% for AUD and CUD, respectively (Strakowski et al. 2007). SUDs in this cohort were associated with treatment noncompliance and a longer time to recovery. In another study reported by DelBello et al. (2007), the rate of either an AUD or a CUD at baseline was only 15%; however, the age of the cohort was much younger (mean = 15 years at enrollment) than the previous study.

In the initial data from the large cohort of adolescents diagnosed with BD selected from the COBY study, prior to the follow-up period described in the previous section, Goldstein et al. (2008b) described a lifetime rate of SUD at 16%. CUD was the most prevalent, with a lifetime rate of 12% and 73% of those with a SUD. AUD had a prevalence of 8% in the adolescent BD cohort, and 50% of all those with a SUD. Finally, 5% of all BD adolescents and 30% of those with SUD met lifetime criteria for both CUD and AUD. In this study, BD anteceded SUD in 60% of subjects; both conditions had their onset concurrently in an additional 10%. Conduct disorder, suicide attempt, and age were significant positive predictors of SUD in these BD adolescents. Further, adolescents with BD and comorbid SUD were more likely to report trouble with police, teenage pregnancy, and abortion.

A case-control study of 10- to 18-year-olds examined the relationship between BD and SUD, including nicotine dependence and other psychiatric comorbidity. Wilens et al. (2008) reported a higher age-adjusted rate of any SUD among BD subjects compared with control subjects (HR = 8.68). In particular, there was a higher rate of alcohol abuse (HR = 7.66), drug abuse (HR = 18.5), drug dependence (HR = 12.1), and cigarette smoking (HR = 12.3). The association between BD and SUD remained significant after the study authors controlled for other comorbidities, including conduct disorder, ADHD, and anxiety disorders. Furthermore, adolescent-onset BD, compared with pediatric-onset BD, was strongly associated with an elevated risk of SUD (Joshi and Wilens 2009). In 67% of subjects, the onset of BD preceded the onset of SUD, and an additional 24% experienced the onset of BD and SUD within the same year.

Daily cigarette smoking occurs at a very high rate in adult BD patients and has been associated with elevated cardiovascular morbidity, as well as psychosis, suicidal behavior, and other SUDs. Goldstein et al. (2008a) investigated cigarette smoking in more than 400 subjects ages 7–17 participating in the COBY study. They reported that 11% of these BD youth smoked at least 1 cigarette daily at study entry (daily group), and an additional 14% of subjects reported a lifetime history of smoking (ever group). The mean age at regular-smoking onset among the daily group was estimated at 12.9 years. BD onset occurred prior to or in the same year as regular cigarette smoking in 69% of the subjects. A regression analysis comparing ever-smoked to never-smoked subgroups of BD youth found that age, lifetime SUD, lifetime suicide attempt, and a positive family history of SUD were most strongly associated with having ever smoked. The authors concluded that compared with epidemiological studies, the lifetime prevalence of ever smoking may be similar to that in nonclinical samples, while youth with a BD diagnosis show an increased rate of daily smoking compared with youth in the general population.

Cigarette smoking has been reported as highly prevalent in inpatient samples of patients with first-episode mania. Heffner et al. (2008) reported that over 45% of first-episode patients diagnosed with BD had smoked cigarettes within 30 days of admission. The mean age at smoking onset was estimated as 14 years. Current smokers were more likely to report recent alcohol and marijuana use and to have symptoms that met criteria for AUD and CUD. Almost 40% of the subjects indicated a lifetime history of both cannabis and cigarette use, with the majority (over 65%) initiating use of both within the same year. For subjects with a lifetime history of regular alcohol and cigarette use (over 35%), most initiated use of cigarettes first.

Temporal Association Between Bipolar Disorder and SUD

Studies report that most psychiatric illnesses typically have their onset earlier than does SUD, although this temporal relationship is less clear for mood disorders. Most studies, particularly those with a longitudinal prospective design, report that the onset of BD precedes or is concurrent with the onset of the SUD, especially if the onset of the mood disorder is defined as the first manifestation of the syndrome (Angst et al. 2006; Merikangas et al. 2008). In a report by Angst and colleagues (2006) investigating the temporal sequence of bipolar II disorder and AUD, the affective episodes preceded SUD in the majority of cases. The onset of BD was typically prior to age 20, whereas the use of alcohol was "a minor problem" during that age range. However, very rapidly over the next decade AUD became a substantial comorbid diagnosis.

In Duffy et al. (2012), a longitudinal prospective study of more than 200 offspring of BD parents, the study authors found an elevated lifetime SUD prevalence of 24%, with CUD being most common. A bidirectional relationship was seen for BD and SUD, with each disorder showing about a threefold predictive risk for the other. Furthermore, SUD predicted a significant increased risk of developing psychotic symptoms. It was concluded that SUD is a common comorbidity arising during the early course of BD even before the first activated/major mood episode.

A systematic review and meta-analysis of cannabis use and mania symptoms, though based on limited studies, found preliminary evidence that cannabis use may worsen the expression of manic symptoms in those with BD and may act as a risk factor in the incidence of manic symptoms (Gibbs et al. 2015).

Of note, a history of SIPD may increase one's chances of later developing BD (or may simply be a precursor to the condition). In a recent landmark study described earlier in this chapter (Arendt et al. 2005) (see section "Assessment and Differential Diagnosis"), researchers tracked nearly 7,000 Danish subjects over the course of 20 years and showed that in 32% of individuals with any substance-induced psychosis, there was conversion to schizophrenia or BD. The majority of these conversions were to schizophrenia (26% vs. 8% for BD); for half of those whose diagnosis converted to BD, the conversion occurred within 4.5 years. For BD, the type of substance used and age at onset of substance-induced psychosis did not affect conversion rates; however, this may have been due to the lower sample size of this population and insufficient statistical power. Interestingly, personality disorders and self-harm following the incident substance-induced psychotic episode were associated with higher rates of conversion to both schizophrenia and BD (Starzer et al. 2018).

Explaining the Association Between Bipolar Disorder and SUD

The association between BD and SUD has not as yet been worked out, although a number of possibilities have been discussed. Although there may be some shared genetic linkage (Johnson et al. 2009), there is generally good agreement that the association cannot be clearly explained by a shared genetic diathesis (Merikangas et al. 2008; Winokur et al. 1995). That is, there is no difference in familial loading for SUDs among the relatives of patients with BD and SUD compared with BD patients without SUD. Put another way, there is no evidence of the independent transmission of SUDs in patients with BD and their family members, and SUDs in these families typically occur as secondary complications to the BD. Therefore, most discussion has focused on causal models and pathways.

There is some evidence to support the view that patients use substances to self-medicate specific symptoms. In a study by Lorberg et al. (2008), youth with BD reported initiating substances to treat mood symptoms, while non-mood-disordered control subjects used substances to get high. This model would require a match between specific symptoms and the properties of the substance used. In a prospective study of 166 first-episode patients, Baethge and colleagues (2008) reported that cannabis use selectively and strongly preceded or coincided with activated episodes, while alcohol use preceded or coincided with depression. As discussed by Salloum and Thase (2000), anergic depressive symptoms may be indicative of hypofunction of dopaminergic circuits, and dopamine has a central role in the highly reinforcing effects of alcohol and other drugs of abuse, including opiates and cocaine. Therefore, there are several examples implicating neurotransmitter systems involved both in the pathophysiology of BD and in the neurobiology of SUDs.

Another possibility is that certain temperamental, personality, and behavioral factors are associated with the risk of SUD as well as BD. Specifically, arousal, novelty seeking, impulsivity, happiness, and nervousness have been reported as highly predictive of alcohol consumption (Merikangas et al. 2008) and characteristic of those at risk for and diagnosed with BD (Cassano et al. 1992). Moreover, anxiety symptoms and disorders occur frequently in BD and also have a well-recognized association with SUD. The possibility that unstable personality characteristics and anxiety might mediate the relationship between BD and subsequent SUD would also explain the comprehensive risk for a number of different substances in BD.

The variable pattern of substance use between individuals with the same diagnosis (BD) and over time (with cannabis increasing in popularity relative to alcohol in younger age groups) suggests that there are likely several mechanisms underlying the association between BD and SUD. In addition to large-scale studies describing general trends, smaller detailed longitudinal studies of individual patients can clarify certain associations. In one such qualitative study of SUD in BD patients, Healey et al. (2009) reported that patients' reasons for substance use derived from their own personal experiences and that personal experience of alcohol and drugs was idiosyncratic; that is, some found that specific substances enhanced activated episodes, while others found a dampening effect. Furthermore, subjects' experiences and beliefs around the effects of substances on their mood symptoms were formulated early in the course of illness and provided evidence of early self-medication and self-titration. In addition, some subjects stopped taking prescribed medication and used substances in order to feel a part of the normal peer group (social conformity). The latter point may be of particular relevance early in the course of illness, when experimentation with substances is a common adolescent experience and at the same time a developmental and clinical course stage at which acceptance of an illness is most challenging. Yet effective, early treatment may have its largest impact preventing the substantial burden of illness associated with comorbid BD and SUD, including suicidality, depression, psychosis and functional impairment (Cardoso et al. 2017).

Treatment

Treatment of BD in youth encompasses psychosocial and psychotherapeutic interventions with family, individual, group, and community involvement. Most patients will also require pharmacological interventions for mood stabilization. Many treatment guidelines exist, including contributions from the Child and Adolescent Bipolar Foundation, NICE, American Academy for Child and Adolescent Psychiatry, and the Canadian Network for Mood and Anxiety Treatments (Cox et al. 2014; Yatham et al. 2018). Among youth, treatment of acute mania has a stronger evidence base than treatment of bipolar depression or comorbid psychiatric illness, or maintenance treatment. SGAs are effective for youth with mania; however, youth are sensitive to metabolic risks with these medications (Goldstein et al. 2012). Outcome may be significantly improved if the mood stabilizer chosen for prophylactic indications is selected based on the patient profile (Grof 2003; Grof and Müller-Oerlinghausen 2009). Selective response reflects the heterogeneity of BD; for example, responders to lithium experience illness characterized by an episodic remitting course, with good quality of remission both clinically and on psychological testing, and have a family history of recurrent mood disorders but not chronic psychotic illnesses (Alda 2004). Evidence suggests that at least a subgroup of BD youth early in the course of illness may respond very well to selected monotherapy based on the nature of the clinical course (episodic vs. nonepisodic) and the family history (recurrent mood disorders vs chronic psychosis) and the response to mood stabilizers in other family members (Duffy 2014; Duffy et al. 2009).

BD in children is commonly misdiagnosed as ADHD because there are high rates of ADHD among children with mania. Clinical presentation in those with mania and ADHD can be confusing and can be complicated by substance use. It is important to assess for symptoms specific to BD, such as hypersexuality, psychosis, periodicity, and seasonality (Cassano et al. 2000). In a study by Stephens et al. (2014) looking at risk and protective factors associated with SUD in adolescents with first-episode mania, those who had been prescribed stimulants had reduced risk (by nearly 25%) of developing SUD.

There is a lack of information about the treatment of BD with comorbid SUD in adults, and even more so in adolescents. According to a review of studies from 1966 to 2010, there is a lack of evidence-based literature to guide treatment for specific SUDs comorbid with mood disorders. There is more support for treatment of alcohol, cannabis, and cocaine and comorbid bipolar illness, compared with other substances. Psychotherapies were considered an essential aspect of care (Beaulieu et al. 2012).

The current standard of care for BD with or without SUD is pharmacotherapy, in particular SGAs and mood stabilizers. In the United States, lithium, risperidone, olanzapine, asenapine, aripiprazole, and quetiapine are FDA approved for the mixed/manic phase of BD in youth. The olanzapine-fluoxetine combination and lurasidone are approved for the depressive phase of illness. The olanzapine-fluoxetine combination for treatment of bipolar depression in youth was shown to be effective in a recent RCT (Detke et al.

2015). Lurasidone monotherapy (20–80 mg/day) was well tolerated and decreased depressive symptoms in youth with BD in a placebo-controlled study (DelBello et al. 2017). Initial monotherapy is recommended in the acute treatment of mania or a mixed state. SGAs have shown higher response rates than anticonvulsants. There is a paucity of data on maintenance treatment of youth with bipolar disorder. Aripiprazole and other SGAs, including asenapine and ziprasidone, have shown promise for maintenance therapy, and lamotrigine may be useful in adolescent populations. Lithium and divalproex are often used, but more research should be conducted for all of these agents (Stepanova and Findling 2017).

Findling (2005), in his review of treatment of pediatric BD, found BD monotherapy to be associated with symptom reduction, although many of these patients do not achieve full remission. Combination pharmacotherapy may hold some advantage in initial treatment but not necessarily in maintenance therapy. Combination treatments are common after initial monotherapy has been tried, but more studies are needed to determine efficacy. In a RCT combining divalproex and quetiapine in 30 adolescents with bipolar I disorder, the combination treatment was more effective (based on the Young Mania Rating Scale) when compared with divalproex and placebo alone (DelBello et al. 2002). Open-label studies have shown support for combination treatments of lithium and divalproex as well as risperidone and lithium or risperidone and divalproex (Findling and Kuich 2008; Stepanova and Findling 2017).

Few RCT studies examining the effectiveness of pharmacotherapies in patients with comorbid BD and SUD exist. Valproate was studied using a 24-week randomized, double-blind, placebo-controlled, parallel-group design in adults with BD and alcoholism receiving treatment as usual with lithium and psychosocial intervention (Salloum et al. 2005). The study authors found that adjunctive valproate improved alcohol use outcomes but not symptoms of depression or mania. Kemp et al. (2009) compared lithium with lithium and divalproate (Depakote) in adults with rapid-cycling BD and comorbid SUD using a 6-month double-blind RCT of maintenance therapy for BD. Attrition rates were high, and no benefit was found for combined pharmacotherapy over monotherapy. Quetiapine has been linked to decreased alcohol use and craving in one open-label study of participants with co-occurring disorders

(Martinotti et al. 2008). In adult patients with bipolar I disorder, recent hospitalization, and SUD, short-term treatment with olanzapine was associated with less substance use and craving (Sani et al. 2013). In a review of 13 pharmacotherapy trials for treatment of BD and SUD, there was support for valproate and naltrexone in reducing substance use; citicoline was associated with a decrease in cocaine use. The review encourages more research to guide clinical practice (Salloum and Brown 2017).

There are no well-accepted guidelines on pharmacotherapeutic interventions with youth suffering from comorbid BD and SUD. Geller and colleagues (1998) investigated, in a RCT, 6 weeks of lithium treatment in a group of 25 adolescents presenting with bipolar spectrum disorders and comorbid substance dependence receiving interpersonal therapy. Lithium resulted in a reduced number of positive drug urine screens and increased scores on the Children's Global Assessment Scale in comparison to placebo. Topiramate, adjunctive to quetiapine, has been studied in adolescents with mania and co-occurring CUD in an RCT lasting 16 weeks. Compared with the placebo group, those adolescents taking topiramate (average dose = 175 mg/day) had significantly less cannabis use in addition to less weight gain and appetite, and greater rate of excitement (DelBello et al. 2011).

A frequently reported issue in treating BD is nonadherence to medication regimens. Treatment nonadherence has been associated with poorer treatment outcome, including relapse (Manwani et al. 2007). Nonadherence is exacerbated if the patient has comorbid SUD and may result in delayed recovery (Cerullo and Strakowski 2007). Preliminary findings have suggested that alcohol abuse may be associated with the duration of bipolar depression and cannabis with the duration of mania (Strakowski et al. 2000).

Psychoeducation, CBT, family-focused therapy, peer support, and interpersonal and social rhythm therapy are all psychological treatments with an evidence base in BD. FFT has demonstrated efficacy in reducing depressive episodes in youth and young adults according to four RCTs (Miklowitz and Chung 2016). FFT may be a promising intervention for youth with bipolar illness and SUD (Miklowitz 2012). Adult studies of the effects of psychosocial therapies on patients with BD and comorbid SUD are few. Weiss and colleagues developed a CBT-based manualized therapy termed "integrated group therapy" specifically designed for patients with both BD and comorbid substance dependence. They conducted an RCT of 20 weeks of integrated group therapy compared with group drug counseling for adults with BD and current substance dependence receiving mood stabilizers. Integrated group therapy reduced substance use and increased symptoms of depression and mania in comparison to group drug counseling (Weiss et al. 2007). In Salloum and Brown's (2017) review of treatment trials for BD and SUD, there were three psychotherapy trials, and integrated psychosocial interventions were most helpful in reducing substance use. In a qualitative review of substance use co-morbidity in BD investigating psychosocial interventions, none of the eight trials gave clear evidence for management. Integrated group therapy was useful for substance use outcomes (Gold et al. 2018).

Prevention of SUD among people with BD could result in reduced morbidity and improved quality of life. In one review of SUDs among youth with BD, adolescents with BD were more likely to have SUD, and these youth were at a higher risk for illness recurrence, suicidality, treatment nonadherence, legal involvement, and early pregnancy. Strategies for lessening the burden of SUD among people with BD include screening for SUD at a young age, education and family involvement, and prevention strategies (Goldstein and Bukstein 2010).

There remains a significant gap in the evidence-based knowledge and treatment of BD in adolescents with and even without SUD. Unfortunately, there is no robust research to guide clinicians caring for youth with co-occurring mood disorders and SUDs. Few conclusions can be drawn from the limited treatment studies of adults with BD and comorbid SUD. It remains important to address stabilization of the underlying primary disorder, in this case BD, to understand the nature of the relationship with SUD and, if necessary, to include specific treatment for the SUD, with the promise of benefit of integrated treatment for both disorders. Early diagnosis of BD with treatment and screening for SUD is paramount.

Case Vignette

E., a 16-year-old male, presents to the emergency room after being brought in by police for concerning and odd behaviors. In the emergency department, E. is found to be talkative, is unable to sit down, and is very focused on getting back to basketball practice and school. Per the police report, E. was found in the night intrusively asking strangers questions in a mall. When ignored, he became upset and agitated and started to yell, and this behavior prompted the authorities to be called. Patient thought that he had done nothing wrong and that the strangers were rude for not answering his questions and refusing to let him try on items of their clothing. Patient was not dressed appropriately and had no identification or money with him. After a history is collected from patient and family, it is discovered that patient has not been sleeping well for almost 1 week after a weekend party with peers. Parents state that E. was talking more and "not making sense." He required multiple prompts to eat dinner and stay in his room. E.'s teachers expressed concerns to the counseling office and patient was given passes to do his work outside of the classroom. The school commented that patient appeared stressed and overworked, which was not unreasonable given that the term was about to end and many assignments and tests were scheduled. The biggest concern came from E.'s basketball coach, who reported that E. was not following along with plays and was getting easily distracted. E.'s coach saw that other players were trying to keep E. "quiet" and "huddled around him in order to keep me from seeing what he was doing or saying." The coach called E.'s parents at their home to let them know E. should take a break from school.

E. is admitted to the adolescent psychiatric unit with concerns about his odd behaviors, his abrupt change from previous healthy functioning, and his inability to coherently contribute to a safe and realistic plan for discharge. While on the inpatient unit, the patient is hyperfocused on exercise and vigorously works out while others do recreational groups and activities. He exhibits intense eye contact, some mild paranoia about being wrongfully accused of a crime, and poor insight into his mental status changes. He admits to using synthetic marijuana at a party, and he later admits that he has been selling marijuana and other drugs for extra money. The patient is noted to have labile mood, poor sleep, increased goal-directed behaviors, and difficulty following along in interviews and groups on the unit. He is, at times, overly friendly with peers on the unit and takes offense if someone makes any comments about his exercises. There is no evidence of thought insertion/withdrawal, ideas of reference, bizarre delusions, or hallucinations. E.'s family shares that the patient has a history of being moody at times in the past and may have had depressive episodes after acute psychosocial stressors in which E. would "stay in his room for weeks." In terms of family history, there is a first-degree relative who struggled with substances and out-of-state extended family members who may have been psychiatrically hospitalized. There is an extended family history of recurrent mood disorder, with some affected individuals developing comorbid SUD. There is no family history of schizophrenia or primary SUD.

Within 24 hours of admission, the patient begins to calm down with low-dose risperidone. He returns to his baseline functioning within 3 days, and he and his family are eager for discharge. A family meeting is held to discuss psychoeducation, possible diagnoses, and recommendation for close mental health follow-up and substance cessation. Family is certain that substances caused the patient's symptoms despite education about possible other diagnoses, including bipolar illness.

E. seeks treatment for a few weeks after discharge and eventually is lost to follow-up. One year later, he is again brought to the ER by police because of bizarre behaviors in a public setting. Collateral information collected is significant for two major depressive episodes and multiple subthreshold manic and depressive episodes in the time frame between hospitalizations. Whenever the patient would become easily irritable or difficult to understand, or had sleep changes, his parents would assume he was using substances, and this would lead to punishment and conflict. School supports decreased, and the patient was labeled as "troubled." He could no longer play on sports teams and friends began to exclude him, leading to fights on campus with eventual expulsion. The patient states that he did use marijuana and alcohol after his first hospitalization to "change" his mood, but over the last 3 months, the patient reportedly stopped using marijuana or other substances of abuse because of his lack of money and depressed mood; he also denies any drug sales. The episode that prompted return to the hospital was notable for lack of sleep, distractibility, grandiosity, increase in goal-directed behaviors, expansive affect, and irritability. The patient is diagnosed with bipolar illness, and risperidone is again used to manage the acute manic symptoms. Extensive education is provided to the patient and his family about his diagnosis and treatments. After discharge, E. is more engaged in care and focused on health care promotion goals.

Commentary

This patient vignette illustrates a number of key points:

1. The presentation on admission was confusing because the patient had not yet disclosed acute substance intoxication.
2. The patient did not remain engaged in mental health or substance use treatment after his first hospitalization, but he continued to have mood episodes.
3. The delay in treatment led to significantly worse outcomes given his school expulsion and family focusing on punishment rather than treatment.

Prior to E.'s first hospitalization, there were concerning mood episodes and irritability as well as a family history of mental illness. The family's focusing mostly on the substance use potentially prevented accurate tracking of the episodic nature of E.'s illness and delayed diagnosis. E. admitted to using drugs to alter his mood, and this can be seen in youth with bipolar illness. The lengthy period of sobriety was helpful in later determining the diagnosis of BD, but the diagnosis could have been made earlier with more vigilant monitoring. The patient should have been followed closely after his first hospitalization and symptoms should have been tracked, along with implementation of psychosocial interventions, including family involvement, substance treatment, and proper psychoeducation. A strong therapeutic alliance with a mental health team, involvement of E. in treatment planning, and regular monitoring of mood, recovery, sleep, functioning, diet, exercise, and stress may have decreased the burden of his illness.

Key Points

- Substance use disorders (SUDs) are the most common comorbid disorders in first-episode psychosis (FEP) and schizophrenia and have a significant negative impact on outcome.

- Cannabis use (in particular early-onset use and high dosage) has been linked to an increased risk for psychosis/schizophrenia-related disorders in young people.

- Cross-sectional, longitudinal, and family history with knowledge of the inherent pharmacological properties of substances of abuse will assist in differentiating substance-induced psychotic disorder from a primary psychotic disorder with comorbid SUD.

- Optimal treatment for FEP patients with comorbid SUD includes specialized early intervention services with integrated SUD-focused treatment. Treatment for FEP should be initiated even though drug-induced psychosis cannot be excluded.

- Clinical course and family history are essential to making an accurate diagnosis of bipolar disorder early in the course of illness and to differentiate a primary from a secondary SUD.

References

Abdel-Baki A, Ouellet-Plamondon C, Salvat É, et al: Symptomatic and functional outcomes of substance use disorder persistence 2 years after admission to a first-episode psychosis program. Psychiatry Res 247:113–119, 2017 27888680

Albert N, Melau M, Jensen H, et al: Five years of specialized early intervention versus two years of specialized early intervention followed by three years of standard treatment for patients with a first episode psychosis: randomised, superiority, parallel group trial in Denmark (OPUS II). BMJ 356:i6681, 2017 28082379

Alda M: The phenotypic spectra of bipolar disorder. Eur Neuropsychopharmacol 14 (suppl 2):S94–S99, 2004 15142614

Alemany S, Arias B, Fatjó-Vilas M, et al: Psychosis-inducing effects of cannabis are related to both childhood abuse and COMT genotypes. Acta Psychiatr Scand 129(1):54–62, 2014 23445265

Angst J, Gamma A, Endrass J, et al: Is the association of alcohol use disorders with major depressive disorder a consequence of undiagnosed bipolar-II disorder? Eur Arch Psychiatry Clin Neurosci 256(7):452–457, 2006 16917682

Arango C, Giráldez M, Merchán-Naranjo J, et al: Second-generation antipsychotic use in children and adolescents: a six-month prospective cohort study in drug-naïve patients. J Am Acad Child Adolesc Psychiatry 53(11):1179–1190, 1190.e1–1190.e4, 2014 25440308

Arendt M, Rosenberg R, Foldager L, et al: Cannabis-induced psychosis and subsequent schizophrenia-spectrum disorders: follow-up study of 535 incident cases. Br J Psychiatry 187:510–515, 2005 16319402

Arendt M, Mortensen PB, Rosenberg R, et al: Familial predisposition for psychiatric disorder: comparison of subjects treated for cannabis-induced psychosis and schizophrenia. Arch Gen Psychiatry 65(11):1269–1274, 2008 18981338

Arseneault L, Cannon M, Poulton R, et al: Cannabis use in adolescence and risk for adult psychosis: longitudinal prospective study. BMJ 325(7374):1212–1213, 2002 12446537

Baethge C, Baldessarini RJ, Khalsa HM, et al: Substance abuse in first-episode bipolar I disorder: indications for early intervention. Am J Psychiatry 162(5):1008–1010, 2005 15863809

Baethge C, Hennen J, Khalsa HM, et al: Sequencing of substance use and affective morbidity in 166 first-episode bipolar I disorder patients. Bipolar Disord 10(6):738–741, 2008 18837869

Bagot KS, Milin R, Kaminer Y: Adolescent initiation of cannabis use and early onset psychosis. Subst Abus 36(4):524–533, 2015 25774457

Bahorik AL, Newhill CE, Queen CC, et al: Under-reporting of drug use among individuals with schizophrenia: prevalence and predictors. Psychol Med 44(1):61–69, 2014 23551851

Barak Y, Baruch Y, Achiron A, Aizenberg D: Suicide attempts of schizophrenia patients: a case-controlled study in tertiary care. J Psychiatr Res 42(10):822–826, 2008 18479709

Beaulieu S, Saury S, Sareen J, et al; Canadian Network for Mood and Anxiety Treatments (CANMAT) Task Force: The Canadian Network for Mood and Anxiety Treatments (CANMAT) task force recommendations for the management of patients with mood disorders and comorbid substance use disorders. Ann Clin Psychiatry 24(1):38–55, 2012 22303521

Bertelsen M, Jeppesen P, Petersen L, et al: Five-year follow-up of a randomized multicenter trial of intensive early intervention vs standard treatment for patients with a first episode of psychotic illness: the OPUS trial. Arch Gen Psychiatry 65(7):762–771, 2008 18606949

Cardoso TA, Jansen K, Zeni CP, et al: Clinical outcomes in children and adolescents with bipolar disorder and substance use disorder comorbidity. J Clin Psychiatry 78(3):e230–e233, 2017 28068464

Cassano GB, Akiskal HS, Savino M, et al: Proposed subtypes of bipolar II and related disorders: with hypomanic episodes (or cyclothymia) and with hyperthymic temperament. J Affect Disord 26(2):127–140, 1992 1447430

Cassano GB, McElroy SL, Brady K, et al: Current issues in the identification and management of bipolar spectrum disorders in "special populations." J Affect Disord 59 (suppl 1):S69–S79, 2000 11121828

Cassidy F, Ahearn EP, Carroll BJ: Substance abuse in bipolar disorder. Bipolar Disord 3(4):181–188, 2001 11552957

Caton CLM, Drake RE, Hasin DS, et al: Differences between early phase primary psychotic disorders with concurrent substance use and substance-induced psychoses. Arch Gen Psychiatry 62(2):137–145, 2005 15699290

Caton CLM, Hasin DS, Shrout PE, et al: Predictors of psychosis remission in psychotic disorders that co-occur with substance use. Schizophr Bull 32(4):618–625, 2006 16873441

Caton CLM, Hasin DS, Shrout PE, et al: Stability of early phase primary psychotic disorders with concurrent substance use and substance-induced psychosis. Br J Psychiatry 190:105–111, 2007 17267925

Cerullo MA, Strakowski SM: The prevalence and significance of substance use disorders in bipolar type I and II disorder. Subst Abuse Treat Prev Policy 2:29, 2007 17908301

Cleary M, Hunt GE, Matheson S, et al: Psychosocial treatments for people with co-occurring severe mental illness and substance misuse: systematic review. J Adv Nurs 65(2):238–258, 2009 19016921

Conway KP, Compton W, Stinson FS, et al: Lifetime comorbidity of DSM-IV mood and anxiety disorders and specific drug use disorders: results from the National Epidemiologic Survey on Alcohol and Related Conditions. J Clin Psychiatry 67(2):247–257, 2006 16566620

Correll CU, Galling B, Pawar A, et al: Comparison of early intervention services vs treatment as usual for early phase psychosis: a systematic review, meta-analysis, and meta-regression. JAMA Psychiatry 75(6):555–565, 2018 29800949

Cox JH, Seri S, Cavanna AE: Clinical guidelines on long-term pharmacotherapy for bipolar disorder in children and adolescents. J Clin Med 3(1):135–143, 2014 26237252

Crebbin K, Mitford E, Paxton R, et al: First-episode drug-induced psychosis: a medium term follow up study reveals a high-risk group. Soc Psychiatry Psychiatr Epidemiol 44(9):710–715, 2009 19183816

Degenhardt L, Hall W, Lynskey M: Testing hypotheses about the relationship between cannabis use and psychosis. Drug Alcohol Depend 71(1):37–48, 2003 12821204

DelBello MP, Schwiers ML, Rosenberg HL, et al: A double-blind, randomized, placebo-controlled study of quetiapine as adjunctive treatment for adolescent mania. J Am Acad Child Adolesc Psychiatry 41(10):1216–1223, 2002 12364843

DelBello MP, Hanseman D, Adler CM, et al: Twelve-month outcome of adolescents with bipolar disorder following first hospitalization for a manic or mixed episode. Am J Psychiatry 164(4):582–590, 2007 17403971

DelBello MP, Welge J, Adler CM, et al: Topiramate for adolescents with co-occurring cannabis use and bipolar disorders. Presented at the Annual Meeting of the American Academy of Child and Adolescent Psychiatry, Toronto, Ontario, Canada, October 18–23, 2011

DelBello MP, Goldman R, Phillips D, et al: Efficacy and safety of lurasidone in children and adolescents with bipolar I depression: a double-blind, placebo-controlled study. J Am Acad Child Adolesc Psychiatry 56(12):1015–1025, 2017 29173735

Dennis M, Babor TF, Roebuck MC, et al: Changing the focus: the case for recognizing and treating cannabis use disorders. Addiction 97 (suppl 1):4–15, 2002 12460125

Detke HC, DelBello MP, Landry J, et al: Olanzapine/Fluoxetine combination in children and adolescents with bipolar I depression: a randomized, double-blind, placebo-controlled trial. J Am Acad Child Adolesc Psychiatry 54(3):217–224, 2015 25721187

Di Forti M, Sallis H, Allegri F, et al: Daily use, especially of high-potency cannabis, drives the earlier onset of psychosis in cannabis users. Schizophr Bull 40(6):1509–1517, 2014 24345517

Di Forti M, Quattrone D, Freeman TP, et al: The contribution of cannabis use to variation in the incidence of psychotic disorder across Europe (EU-GEI): a multicenter case-control study. Lancet Psychiatry 6(5):427–436, 2019 30902669

Dominguez MD, Fisher HL, Major B, et al: Duration of untreated psychosis in adolescents: ethnic differences and clinical profiles. Schizophr Res 150(2–3):526–532, 2013 24025696

Drake RE, O'Neal EL, Wallach MA: A systematic review of psychosocial research on psychosocial interventions for people with co-occurring severe mental and substance use disorders. J Subst Abuse Treat 34(1):123–138, 2008 17574803

D'Souza DC: Cannabinoids and psychosis. Int Rev Neurobiol 78:289–326, 2007 17349865

D'Souza DC, Abi-Saab WM, Madonick S, et al: Delta-9-tetrahydrocannabinol effects in schizophrenia: implications for cognition, psychosis, and addiction. Biol Psychiatry 15;57(6):594–608, 2005 15780846

D'Souza DC, Sewell RA, Ranganathan M: Cannabis and psychosis/schizophrenia: human studies. Eur Arch Psychiatry Clin Neurosci 259(7):413–431, 2009 19609589

Duffy A: Interventions for youth at risk for bipolar disorder. Current Treatment Options in Psychiatry 1(1):37–47, 2014

Duffy A, Milin R, Grof P: Maintenance treatment of adolescent bipolar disorder: open study of the effectiveness and tolerability of quetiapine. BMC Psychiatry 9:4, 2009 19200370

Duffy A, Horrocks J, Milin R, et al: Adolescent substance use disorder during the early stages of bipolar disorder: a prospective high-risk study. J Affect Disord 142(1–3):57–64, 2012 22959686

Findling RL: Update on the treatment of bipolar disorder in children and adolescents. Eur Psychiatry 20(2):87–91, 2005 15797690

Findling RL, Kuich K: Bipolar disorders, in Clinical Manual of Child and Adolescent Psychopharmacology. Edited by Findling RL. New York, Guilford, 2008, pp 229–263

Galve-Roperh I, Palazuelos J, Aguado T, et al: The endocannabinoid system and the regulation of neural development: potential implications in psychiatric disorders. Eur Arch Psychiatry Clin Neurosci 259(7):371–382, 2009 19588184

Geller B, Cooper TB, Sun K, et al: Double-blind and placebo-controlled study of lithium for adolescent bipolar disorders with secondary substance dependency. J Am Acad Child Adolesc Psychiatry 37(2):171–178, 1998 9473913

Gibbs M, Winsper C, Marwaha S, et al: Cannabis use and mania symptoms: a systematic review and meta-analysis. J Affect Disord 171:39–47, 2015 25285897

Glantz MD, Anthony JC, Berglund PA, et al: Mental disorders as risk factors for later substance dependence: estimates of optimal prevention and treatment benefits. Psychol Med 39(8):1365–1377, 2009 19046473

Goerke D, Kumra S: Substance abuse and psychosis. Child Adolesc Psychiatr Clin N Am 22(4):643–654, 2013 24012078

Gold AK, Otto MW, Deckersbach T, et al: Substance use comorbidity in bipolar disorder: a qualitative review of treatment strategies and outcomes. Am J Addict 27(3):188–201, 2018 29596721

Goldstein BI, Bukstein OG: Comorbid substance use disorders among youth with bipolar disorder: opportunities for early identification and prevention. J Clin Psychiatry 71(3):348–358, 2010 19961811

Goldstein BI, Birmaher B, Axelson DA, et al: Significance of cigarette smoking among youths with bipolar disorder. Am J Addict 17(5):364–371, 2008a 18770078

Goldstein BI, Strober MA, Birmaher B, et al: Substance use disorders among adolescents with bipolar spectrum disorders. Bipolar Disord 10(4):469–478, 2008b 18452443

Goldstein BI, Sassi R, Diler RS: Pharmacologic treatment of bipolar disorder in children and adolescents. Child Adolesc Psychiatr Clin N Am 21(4):911–939, 2012 23040907

Goldstein BI, Strober M, Axelson D, et al: Predictors of first-onset substance use disorders during the prospective course of bipolar spectrum disorders in adolescents. J Am Acad Child Adolesc Psychiatry 52(10):1026–1037, 2013 24074469

Grant BF, Dawson DA, Stinson FS, et al: The 12-month prevalence and trends in DSM-IV alcohol abuse and dependence: United States, 1991–1992 and 2001–2002. Drug Alcohol Depend 74(3):223–234, 2004 15194200

Grech A, Van Os J, Jones PB, et al: Cannabis use and outcome of recent onset psychosis. Eur Psychiatry 20(4):349–353, 2005 16018929

Green AI, Tohen MF, Hamer RM, et al; HGDH Research Group: First episode schizophrenia-related psychosis and substance use disorders: acute response to olanzapine and haloperidol. Schizophr Res 66(2–3):125–135, 2004 15061244

Green B, Kavanagh D, Young R: Being stoned: a review of self-reported cannabis effects. Drug Alcohol Rev 22(4):453–460, 2003 14660135

Grof P: Selecting effective long-term treatment for bipolar patients: monotherapy and combinations. J Clin Psychiatry 64 (suppl 5):53–61, 2003 12720485

Grof P, Müller-Oerlinghausen B: A critical appraisal of lithium's efficacy and effectiveness: the last 60 years. Bipolar Disord 11 (suppl 2):10–19, 2009 19538682

Healey C, Peters S, Kinderman P, et al: Reasons for substance use in dual diagnosis bipolar disorder and substance use disorders: a qualitative study. J Affect Disord 113(1–2):118–126, 2009 18571735

Heffner JL, DelBello MP, Fleck DE, et al: Cigarette smoking in the early course of bipolar disorder: association with ages-at-onset of alcohol and marijuana use. Bipolar Disord 10(7):838–845, 2008 19032716

Henquet C, Krabbendam L, Spauwen J, et al: Prospective cohort study of cannabis use, predisposition for psychosis, and psychotic symptoms in young people. BMJ 330(7481):11, 2005a 15574485

Henquet C, Murray R, Linszen D, et al: The environment and schizophrenia: the role of cannabis use. Schizophr Bull 31(3):608–612, 2005b 15976013

Henquet C, Krabbendam L, de Graaf R, et al: Cannabis use and expression of mania in the general population. J Affect Disord 95(1–3):103–110, 2006 16793142

Henquet C, Rosa A, Delespaul P, et al: COMT ValMet moderation of cannabis-induced psychosis: a momentary assessment study of "switching on" hallucinations in the flow of daily life. Acta Psychiatr Scand 119(2):156–160, 2009 18808401

Hides L, Dawe S, Kavanagh DJ, et al: Psychotic symptom and cannabis relapse in recent-onset psychosis. Prospective study. Br J Psychiatry 189:137–143, 2006 16880483

Hunt GE, Bergen J, Bashir M: Medication compliance and comorbid substance abuse in schizophrenia: impact on community survival 4 years after a relapse. Schizophr Res 54(3):253–264, 2002 11950550

Jin LZ, Rangan A, Mehlsen J, et al: Association between use of cannabis in adolescence and weight change into midlife. PLoS One 12(1):e0168897, 2017 28060830

Johnson C, Drgon T, McMahon FJ, et al: Convergent genome wide association results for bipolar disorder and substance dependence. Am J Med Genet B Neuropsychiatr Genet 150B(2):182–190, 2009 19127564

Johnston LD, Miech RA, O'Malley PM, et al: Monitoring the Future: National Survey Results on Drug Use: 1975–2017: Overview, Key Findings on Adolescent Drug Use. Ann Arbor, MI, Institute for Social Research, The University of Michigan, 2018

Joshi G, Wilens T: Comorbidity in pediatric bipolar disorder. Child Adolesc Psychiatr Clin N Am 18(2):291–319, vii–viii, 2009 19264265

Kane JM, Robinson DG, Schooler NR, et al: Comprehensive versus usual community care for first-episode psychosis: 2-year outcomes from the NIMH RAISE Early Treatment Program. Am J Psychiatry 173(4):362–372, 2016 26481174

Kemp DE, Gao K, Ganocy SJ, et al: A 6-month, double-blind, maintenance trial of lithium monotherapy versus the combination of lithium and divalproex for rapid-cycling bipolar disorder and co-occurring substance abuse or dependence. J Clin Psychiatry 70(1):113–121, 2009 19192457

Kenneson A, Funderburk JS, Maisto SA: Risk factors for secondary substance use disorders in people with childhood and adolescent-onset bipolar disorder: opportunities for prevention. Compr Psychiatry 54(5):439–446, 2013 23332720

Kessler RC, Crum RM, Warner LA, et al: Lifetime co-occurrence of DSM-III-R alcohol abuse and dependence with other psychiatric disorders in the National Comorbidity Survey. Arch Gen Psychiatry 54(4):313–321, 1997 9107147

Koskinen J, Löhönen J, Koponen H, et al: Prevalence of alcohol use disorders in schizophrenia—a systematic review and meta-analysis. Acta Psychiatr Scand 120(2):85–96, 2009 19374633

Kuepper R, Morrison PD, van Os J, et al: Does dopamine mediate the psychosis-inducing effects of cannabis? A review and integration of findings across disciplines. Schizophr Res 121(1–3):107–117, 2010 20580531

Lambert M, Conus P, Lubman DI, et al: The impact of substance use disorders on clinical outcome in 643 patients with first-episode psychosis. Acta Psychiatr Scand 112(2):141–148, 2005 15992396

Lang K, Meyers JL, Korn JR, et al: Medication adherence and hospitalization among patients with schizophrenia treated with antipsychotics. Psychiatr Serv 61(12):1239–1247, 2010 21123409

Lehman AF, Lieberman JA, Dixon LB, et al; American Psychiatric Association; Steering Committee on Practice Guidelines: Practice guideline for the treatment of patients with schizophrenia, second edition. Am J Psychiatry 161(2, suppl):1–56, 2004 15000267

Linszen D, Dingemans P, Lenior M: Early intervention and a five year follow up in young adults with a short duration of untreated psychosis: ethical implications. Schizophr Res 51(1):55–61, 2001 11479066

Malla AK, Norman RMG, Joober R: First-episode psychosis, early intervention, and outcome: what have we learned? Can J Psychiatry 50(14):881–891, 2005 16494257

Mallet J, Ramoz N, Le Strat Y, et al: Heavy cannabis use prior psychosis in schizophrenia: clinical, cognitive and neurological evidences for a new endophenotype? Eur Arch Psychiatry Clin Neurosci 267(7):629–638, 2017 28190094

Manwani SG, Szilagyi KA, Zablotsky B, et al: Adherence to pharmacotherapy in bipolar disorder patients with and without co-occurring substance use disorders. J Clin Psychiatry 68(8):1172–1176, 2007 17854240

Marconi A, Di Forti M, Lewis CM, et al: Meta-analysis of the association between the level of cannabis use and risk of psychosis. Schizophr Bull 42(5):1262–1269, 2016 26884547

Martinotti G, Andreoli S, Di Nicola M, et al: Quetiapine decreases alcohol consumption, craving, and psychiatric symptoms in dually diagnosed alcoholics. Hum Psychopharmacol 23(5):417–424, 2008 18425995

Meade CS, Graff FS, Griffin ML, et al: HIV risk behavior among patients with co-occurring bipolar and substance use disorders: associations with mania and drug abuse. Drug Alcohol Depend 92(1–3):296–300, 2008 17850993

Merikangas KR, Herrell R, Swendsen J, et al: Specificity of bipolar spectrum conditions in the comorbidity of mood and substance use disorders: results from the Zurich cohort study. Arch Gen Psychiatry 65(1):47–52, 2008 18180428

Miklowitz DJ: Family treatment for bipolar disorder and substance abuse in late adolescence. J Clin Psychol 68(5):502–513, 2012 22504610

Miklowitz DJ, Chung B: Family-focused therapy for bipolar disorder: reflections on 30 years of research. Fam Process 55(3):483–499, 2016 27471058

Milin R: Comorbidity of schizophrenia and substance use disorders in adolescents and young adults, in Adolescent Substance Abuse: Psychiatric Comorbidity and High-Risk Behaviors. Edited by Kaminer Y, Bukstein O. New York, Routledge, Taylor & Francis Group, 2008, pp 355–378

Moore THM, Zammit S, Lingford-Hughes A, et al: Cannabis use and risk of psychotic or affective mental health outcomes: a systematic review. Lancet 370(9584):319–328, 2007 17662880

Mueser KT, Bellack AS, Blanchard JJ: Comorbidity of schizophrenia and substance abuse: implications for treatment. J Consult Clin Psychol 60(6):845–856, 1992 1460148

Mustonen A, Niemelä S, Nordström T, et al: Adolescent cannabis use, baseline prodromal symptoms and the risk of psychosis. Br J Psychiatry 212(4):227–233, 2018 29557758

National Collaborating Centre for Mental Health: Psychosis and Schizophrenia in Children and Young People: Recognition and Management. Leicester, UK, British Psychological Society, 2013

Nossel I, Wall MM, Scodes J, et al: Results of a coordinated specialty care program for early psychosis and predictors of outcomes. Psychiatr Serv 69(8):863–870, 2018 29759055

Oluwoye O, Monroe-DeVita M, Burduli E, et al: Impact of tobacco, alcohol and cannabis use on treatment outcomes among patients experiencing first episode psychosis: data from the national RAISE-ETP study. Early Interv Psychiatry 13(1):142–146, 2019 29356438

Ouellet-Plamondon C, Abdel-Baki A, Salvat É, et al: Specific impact of stimulant, alcohol and cannabis use disorders on first-episode psychosis: 2-year functional and symptomatic outcomes. Psychol Med 47(14):2461–2471, 2017 28424105

Petersen L, Jeppesen P, Thorup A, et al: A randomised multicentre trial of integrated versus standard treatment for patients with a first episode of psychotic illness. BMJ 331(7517):602, 2005a 16141449

Petersen L, Nordentoft M, Jeppesen P, et al: Improving 1-year outcome in first-episode psychosis: OPUS trial. Br J Psychiatry Suppl 48:s98–s103, 2005b 16055817

Radhakrishnan R, Wilkinson ST, D'Souza DC: Gone to pot—a review of the association between cannabis and psychosis. Front Psychiatry 5:54, 2014 24904437

Rasimas JJ, Liebelt EL: Adverse effects and toxicity of the atypical antipsychotics: what is important for the pediatric emergency medicine practitioner. Clin Pediatr Emerg Med 13(4):300–310, 2012 23471213

Regier DA, Farmer ME, Rae DS, et al: Comorbidity of mental disorders with alcohol and other drug abuse. Results from the Epidemiologic Catchment Area (ECA) Study. JAMA 264(19):2511–2518, 1990 2232018

Salloum IM, Brown ES: Management of comorbid bipolar disorder and substance use disorders. Am J Drug Alcohol Abuse 43(4):366–376, 2017 28301219

Salloum IM, Thase ME: Impact of substance abuse on the course and treatment of bipolar disorder. Bipolar Disord 2(3 Pt 2):269–280, 2000 11249805

Salloum IM, Cornelius JR, Daley DC, et al: Efficacy of valproate maintenance in patients with bipolar disorder and alcoholism: a double-blind placebo-controlled study. Arch Gen Psychiatry 62(1):37–45, 2005 15630071

Sani G, Kotzalidis GD, Vöhringer P, et al: Effectiveness of short-term olanzapine in patients with bipolar I disorder, with or without comorbidity with substance use disorder. J Clin Psychopharmacol 33(2):231–235, 2013 23422396

Sara G, Burgess P, Malhi GS, et al: Differences in associations between cannabis and stimulant disorders in first admission psychosis. Schizophr Res 147(2–3):216–222, 2013 23684162

Sara GE, Burgess PM, Malhi GS, et al: Stimulant and other substance use disorders in schizophrenia: prevalence, correlates and impacts in a population sample. Aust N Z J Psychiatry 48(11):1036–1047, 2014 24819935

Scavone A, Timmins V, Collins J, et al: Dimensional and categorical correlates of substance use disorders among Canadian adolescents with bipolar disorder. J Can Acad Child Adolesc Psychiatry 27(3):159–166, 2018 30038653

Schimmelmann BG, Conus P, Schacht M, et al: Predictors of service disengagement in first-admitted adolescents with psychosis. J Am Acad Child Adolesc Psychiatry 45(8):990–999, 2006 16865042

Schneider M: Puberty as a highly vulnerable developmental period for the consequences of cannabis exposure. Addict Biol 13(2):253–263, 2008 18482434

Starzer MSK, Nordentoft M, Hjorthøj C: Rates and predictors of conversion to schizophrenia or bipolar disorder following substance-induced psychosis. Am J Psychiatry 175(4):343–350, 2018 29179576

Stepanova E, Findling RL: Psychopharmacology of bipolar disorders in children and adolescents. Pediatr Clin North Am 64(6):1209–1222, 2017 29173781

Stephens JR, Heffner JL, Adler CM, et al: Risk and protective factors associated with substance use disorders in adolescents with first-episode mania. J Am Acad Child Adolesc Psychiatry 53(7):771–779, 2014 24954826

Strakowski SM, DelBello MP, Fleck DE, et al: The impact of substance abuse on the course of bipolar disorder. Biol Psychiatry 48(6):477–485, 2000 11018221

Strakowski SM, DelBello MP, Fleck DE, et al: Effects of co-occurring cannabis use disorders on the course of bipolar disorder after a first hospitalization for mania. Arch Gen Psychiatry 64(1):57–64, 2007 17199055

Toftdahl NG, Nordentoft M, Hjorthøj C: Prevalence of substance use disorders in psychiatric patients: a nationwide Danish population-based study. Soc Psychiatry Psychiatr Epidemiol 51(1):129–140, 2016 26260950

Tucker P: Substance misuse and early psychosis. Australas Psychiatry 17(4):291–294, 2009 19301164

van Nimwegen L, de Haan L, van Beveren N, et al: Adolescence, schizophrenia and drug abuse: a window of vulnerability. Acta Psychiatr Scand Suppl 427(427):35–42, 2005 15877720

van Winkel R; Genetic Risk and Outcome of Psychosis (GROUP) Investigators: Family based analysis of genetic variation underlying psychosis-inducing effects of cannabis: sibling analysis and proband follow-up. Arch Gen Psychiatry 68(2):148–157, 2011 21041608

Vinkers CH, Van Gastel WA, Schubart CD, et al; Genetic Risk and OUtcome of Psychosis (GROUP) Investigators: The effect of childhood maltreatment and cannabis use on adult psychotic symptoms is modified by the COMT Val[158]Met polymorphism. Schizophr Res 150(1):303–311, 2013 23954148

Wade D, Harrigan S, Edwards J, et al: Patterns and predictors of substance use disorders and daily tobacco use in first-episode psychosis. Aust N Z J Psychiatry 39(10):892–898, 2005 16168016

Wade D, Harrigan S, Edwards J, et al: Substance misuse in first-episode psychosis: 15-month prospective follow-up study. Br J Psychiatry 189:229–234, 2006 16946357

Wade D, Harrigan S, McGorry PD, et al: Impact of severity of substance use disorder on symptomatic and functional outcome in young individuals with first-episode psychosis. J Clin Psychiatry 68(5):767–774, 2007 17503988

Weibell MA, Hegelstad WTV, Auestad B, et al: The effect of substance use on 10-year outcome in first-episode psychosis. Schizophr Bull 43(4):843–851, 2017 28199703

Weiss RD, Griffin ML, Kolodziej ME, et al: A randomized trial of integrated group therapy versus group drug counseling for patients with bipolar disorder and substance dependence. Am J Psychiatry 164(1):100–107, 2007 17202550

Westermeyer J: Comorbid schizophrenia and substance abuse: a review of epidemiology and course. Am J Addict 15(5):345–355, 2006 16966190

Wilens TE, Biederman J, Adamson JJ, et al: Further evidence of an association between adolescent bipolar disorder with smoking and substance use disorders: a controlled study. Drug Alcohol Depend 95(3):188–198, 2008 18343050

Winokur G, Coryell W, Akiskal HS, et al: Alcoholism in manic-depressive (bipolar) illness: familial illness, course of illness, and the primary-secondary distinction. Am J Psychiatry 152(3):365–372, 1995 7864261

Wu LT, Gersing K, Burchett B, et al: Substance use disorders and comorbid Axis I and II psychiatric disorders among young psychiatric patients: findings from a large electronic health records database. J Psychiatr Res 45(11):1453–1462, 2011 21742345

Yankey BN, Strasser S, Okosun IS: A cross-sectional analysis of the association between marijuana and cigarette smoking with metabolic syndrome among adults in the United States. Diabetes Metab Syndr 10 (2, suppl 1):S89–S95, 2016 27049971

Yatham LN, Kennedy SH, Parikh SV, et al: Canadian Network for Mood and Anxiety Treatments (CANMAT) and International Society for Bipolar Disorders (ISBD) 2018 guidelines for the management of patients with bipolar disorder. Bipolar Disord 20(2):97–170, 2018 29536616

Yücel M, Bora E, Lubman DI, et al: The impact of cannabis use on cognitive functioning in patients with schizophrenia: a meta-analysis of existing findings and new data in a first-episode sample. Schizophr Bull 38(2):316–330, 2012 20660494

Assessment and Treatment of Co-occurring Externalizing Disorders

Attention-Deficit/Hyperactivity Disorder and Disruptive Behavior Disorders

Martha J. Ignaszewski, M.D.

K.A.H. Mirza, M.B., F.R.C.P.C.

Oscar G. Bukstein, M.D., M.P.H.

Attention-deficit/hyperactivity disorder (ADHD) and disruptive behavior disorders (DBDs)—oppositional defiant disorder (ODD) and conduct disorder (CD)—are the most common co-occurring group of psychiatric diagnoses in young people with substance use disorders (SUDs) (Bukstein et al. 2005; Wolraich et al. 2011). Research has shown that there is an association with these externalizing mental health disorders in adolescents with SUDs and increased rates of future substance-related disorders, as well as significant negative impact in personal, societal, and economic costs (Groenman et al. 2017). In this chapter we focus on the comorbidity of ADHD, DBDs, and SUDs in adolescence and the role of DBD symptomatology in the development of SUDs and its influence on the course and prognosis. We also address the treatment and outcome literature.

Epidemiology

Studies show that dual diagnosis of SUD and psychiatric disorders is common, with 64%–88% of adolescents with SUD having at least one comorbidity (Brewer et al. 2017). Numerous studies have established high comorbidity of substance use and externalizing disorders. Recent meta-analyses have shown an overall prevalence rate of 28% of ADHD in substance use (Brewer et al. 2017) and a prevalence of 44% of undiagnosed ADHD in treatment-seeking SUD patients (Zulauf et al. 2014). These rates are in excess of the estimated 5%–12% prevalence of ADHD in developed countries, with lower rates in adults (National Institute for Heath and Care Excellence 2018; Zulauf et al. 2014). ADHD in SUD populations confers a 3.5 times higher risk of additional comorbidities (van Emmerik-van Oortmerssen et al. 2014).

Similarly, ODD and CD also co-occur with substance use. Although rates of CD have decreased in males in the last 25 years (Johnston et al. 2018), it continues to be the most common externalizing disorder in adolescents with SUD, at 69% (Brewer et al. 2017). ODD is present in half of children with ADHD, combined presentation, and a quarter of children with ADHD, predominantly inattentive presentation. CD also co-occurs in about a quarter of children and adolescents with ADHD, combined presentation (American Psychiatric Association 2013).

The comorbidity of DBD with SUD is associated with earlier drug use, heavier use, and higher risk of development of SUD. Even after treatment, psychiatric comorbidities are associated with worse withdrawal, earlier relapse, and receiving additional outpatient or inpatient treatment. There are also higher rates of familial dysfunction and parental rates of SUD, academic compromise, and risk of legal involvement.

Relationship Between ADHD and Substance Use Disorders

In a meta-analysis reviewing 37 studies with more than 762,187 participants, results identified 97 effect sizes from which to assess prospective risk of developing substance-related disorders (Groenman et al. 2017). Findings showed that children with ADHD were twice as likely to develop alcohol use disorder, had 2.5 times higher risk for nicotine-related use, and had 1.5–2.5 times higher risk for developing any SUD.

A comparison of adolescents with ADHD and a sample of adolescents without ADHD revealed an earlier onset of substance use (57.9% with early use compared with 41.9%) (Molina et al. 2018). Younger age at first use of alcohol, cigarettes, marijuana, or other illicit drugs predicted rapid onset of use disorders and higher adult rates of SUD (Molina et al. 2018). Differential risk for ADHD subtypes is noted by research showing that inattentive subtype of ADHD is associated only with increased risk of development of alcohol use disorder, with an 8%–10% increase in likelihood of alcohol or nicotine use for every increase in attentive symptoms (Groenman et al. 2017).

In examining functional outcomes of adults diagnosed with ADHD in childhood, the 16-year follow-up of the Multimodal Treatment of ADHD (MTA) study revealed that persistent ADHD symptoms predicted substance use and negative clinical outcomes. Even those youth who no longer had symptoms that met ADHD diagnostic criteria had negative outcomes, although such outcomes were reduced when compared with those who did not receive treatment (Hechtman et al. 2016). Comorbid SUD and ADHD is associated with a greater severity of SUD with more severe clinical features, with higher risk of chronicity of use, and portends a more complicated course with low rates of treatment (Hasin and Grant 2015), higher levels of depression, more need for hospitalization, and a greater risk of suicidal ideation (van de Glind et al. 2013).

Controversy continues as to whether ADHD alone poses a significant risk for later SUDs or whether this relationship disappears when co-occurring CD is considered (Groenman et al. 2017; Zulauf et al. 2014). In some reports, ADHD and CD in isolation, as well as SUD-ADHD comorbidity, appear to be related to significantly higher rates of substance use, though not use disorders (Rodgers et al. 2015). ADHD specifically was found to be associated with a significantly higher rate of alcohol use, though with more alcohol use in comorbid conditions, but was not associated with rates of illicit drug use (Zulauf et al. 2014); other studies have shown this association only with cigarette smoking and nicotine use disorder (Kollins et al. 2006). Nicotine may be used to alleviate some of the symptoms of ADHD, though cigarette smoking is known to be a risk factor for other substance misuse, with four to five times increased likelihood of progressing to heavy cigarette use and marijuana use (Miranda et al. 2016). Increased rates of SUDs in individuals with ADHD were also reported in a 2016 meta-analysis, which showed that while individuals with ADHD had higher rates of substance use as well as SUD compared with control subjects, these differences did not reach statistical significance except in alcohol dependence (Erskine et al. 2016). In contrast, another meta-analysis did not report any statistically significant effect of comorbid CD on SUD, finding ADHD primarily related to higher risk of all SUDs studied. Similarly, controlling for comorbid ODD and CD did not have a significant effect size on meta-regression for SUD in ADHD, though ADHD did influence the severity of substance-related outcomes later in life for those who had childhood ADHD (Groenman et al. 2017). These findings suggest that concomitant ODD or CD influences only in part the severity of substance-related outcomes later in life for those who had childhood ADHD.

Causal pathways or mechanisms that may explain the relationship between ADHD and SUD include the following:

1. Poor executive function may prompt poor decision making around substance use in adolescence.
2. Impulsivity may directly increase risk of SUD through poor response inhibition when the individual is presented with substance use cues.
3. Poor coping skills noted in those with ADHD may contribute to rates of use.
4. Self-medication of ADHD through the use of various substances may play a role.

These findings highlight the importance of using "remission" as a goal for ADHD treatment, which may be protective against development of further comorbidity (Hechtman et al. 2016).

Relationship Between Oppositional Defiant Disorder/Conduct Disorder and Substance Use Disorders

The robust association of CD and substance use/SUDs is well supported in the literature, most recently in a meta-analysis of eight studies of community-based trials of ODD or CD showing a significantly increased risk for SUD in ODD or CD, with an overall odds ratio (OR) of 3.18 (Groenman et al. 2017).

Individuals with CD were at twice the risk for developing alcohol-related disorder (OR = 1.73), four times the risk for developing nicotine-related disorder (OR = 4.22), four times the risk for developing any drug-related disorder (OR = 4.24), and almost five times the risk for developing any SUD (OR = 4.86).

Research reveals a bidirectional relationship between SUD and DBDs, with SUD-DBD comorbidity predicting serious delinquent acts and ultimately SUDs in the future. Findings from the Pittsburgh Youth Study, a prospective longitudinal study following males from age 7 to 20, revealed that frequency of alcohol and marijuana use resulted in greater risk for delinquency, and illicit drug use was associated with violent behavior (White et al. 2018). Substance use could increase speed of movement through the pathways for the development of antisocial behavior. In the Pittsburgh Youth Study, serious alcohol use predicted increased rates of progression to serious delinquency, with 18.1% progression within 5 years and 36.2% progression within 10 years, representing a 10-fold increased risk of violence compared with non-users by age 20 (White et al. 2018). Similar rates were seen in frequent marijuana users, with 22.7% progression within 5 years and 43.6% progression within 10 years, and a fivefold risk of progression to violence compared with non-users by age 20. Illicit or "hard" drug users showed a 1.7 risk of developing violent behaviors compared with non-users, though only 14.4% of the former population used hard substances. Moderate use of alcohol and cannabis did not statistically separate from non-use, though frequent use reached statistical significance compared with moderate use (White et al. 2018).

Other reports have revealed that heavier drinking during adolescence is associated with concurrent and future disruptive behavior, although this relationship did not persist for increased drinking during emerging adulthood (White et al. 2015). These findings suggest that legal and normative levels of alcohol use diminish any relationship between disruptive behavior and drinking. Illicit drug use is a persistent risk factor for future violent behavior across all developmental ages, and this is consistent with the evidence that a history of CD behaviors generally precedes substance onset, and severity and early age at onset of such behaviors may increase the risk of SUD, with higher rates of SUD in delinquent youth than in the general population.

As with many forms of psychopathology, the etiology of comorbid CD-SUD is likely to be a combination of genetic predisposition and exposure to environmental risk factors (Arcos-Burgos et al. 2012; Rutter et al. 2006). Environmental effects emerge from maladaptive interactions with family, school, peers, and the community, and risk factors may be quite similar for both CD and SUD (Hasin and Grant 2015). Substance use may result in additional problems, with poor judgment and association with delinquent peers that lead to illegal acts and aggression (White et al. 2018). DBDs are associated with more severe substance abuse at baseline, disruptions in family and social relations, and poorer treatment engagement (Brewer et al. 2017; Zulauf et al. 2014). Early-onset SUD predicts severity of SUD, reduced efforts to seek treatment, and prolonged duration of SUD in adulthood (Zulauf et al. 2014). Updated conceptualizations of mental health disorders as clusters of transdiagnostic factors have led to the labeling of ADHD, CD, ODD, and SUD as externalizing disorders (Eaton et al. 2015) that can be considered to be related syndromes, sharing common pathophysiology, psychopathology, and genetic factors (Arcos-Burgos et al. 2012).

Assessment

Clinicians dealing with an externalizing disorder–SUD comorbidity should develop skills in assessing for ODD, CD, and developmentally expected manifestations and impairments associated with adolescent and adult forms of ADHD, including the use of appropriate instruments and rating scales for a diagnosis of ADHD. The diagnosis of ADHD and/or CD in adolescents with SUDs is made within a comprehensive evaluation (Bukstein et al. 2005; Pliszka and AACAP Work Group on Quality Issues 2007). The acute status of the patient's SUD use may obscure the diagnosis of ADHD, in part because the subject may have difficulty distinguishing drug-induced cognitive status from drug-free cognitive status. Similarly, CD behaviors may be the result of drug-seeking behaviors, such as stealing and/or lying to maintain a drug use habit. Hyperactivity, agitation, impulsivity, attentional difficulties, aggression, and other antisocial behaviors may also be the result of intoxication or withdrawal from various substances. Features associated with ADHD and CD include low frustration tolerance; lack of task persistence; conflictual relations with peers, adults, and authorities; contact with the legal system; and increased rates of mood and anxiety disorders.

In the overwhelming majority of cases, ODD, CD and ADHD will pre-cede the development of SUD, therefore a premorbid history will often result in one or more of these diagnoses. Review of past records (psychological/psychiatric evaluations and/or report cards/school records), as well as information from other informants (parents and teachers), is often critical because both adolescents and adults with ADHD may have poor insight into their level of ADHD symptoms and resulting impairments.

Youth should be seen separately for a confidential interview. The attitude of the clinician should be flexible, empathic, and nonjudgmental in order to engage the young person in the assessment process and to obtain a valid estimate of substance abuse. However, caution should be taken with drug-seeking adolescents with SUDs who may feign ADHD symptoms or history and insist on stimulant treatment, further emphasizing the need for responsible adult informants. Accurate self-report may be challenging to obtain, especially when there are strong incentives to underreport deviant behaviors (e.g., in forensic settings) or to respond in a socially desirable manner (e.g., in clinical settings). The presence of an externalizing disorder should prompt special consideration in the inquiry and assessment of substance use behavior because extremely antisocial youth have much higher responses of "faking good" or normal patterns of substance use than clinical samples (Stein and Graham 2005), and may also be at higher risk of "faking bad" on screens for ADHD due to drug-seeking behavior (Hirsch and Christiansen 2018; Niesten et al. 2015).

Given the high prevalence of ADHD and CD in patients in addiction treatment, all adolescents in treatment for SUDs should be screened and, if needed, fully evaluated for a diagnosis of ADHD and CD. There are a number of well-validated rating scales for adolescents with ADHD (Chang et al. 2016; Pliszka and AACAP Work Group on Quality Issues 2007) and with ODD (Steiner et al. 2007). Although rating scales are often used for antisocial behaviors, clinicians commonly use broad-spectrum measures such as the Child Behavior Checklist (including Youth Self-Report and Teacher's Report Form; https://aseba.org), the Strengths and Difficulties Questionnaire, and the Disruptive Behavior Disorders Rating Scale (Lavigne et al. 2016). It is important to receive both parent and teacher reports of ADHD, ODD, and CD symptoms from the DSM-5 criteria (American Psychiatric Association 2013).

Treatment

Recent and past reviews have presented consensus guidelines applicable for the assessment and treatment of adolescents with SUDs and externalizing disorders (Bukstein et al. 2005; National Institute for Heath and Care Excellence 2018; Pliszka and AACAP Work Group on Quality Issues 2007; Steiner et al. 2007). Although integrated, multimodal treatment of both substance misuse and externalizing disorders has been found to be useful in clinical practice and dual diagnosis treatment is recommended, many treament centers do not fully address comorbid psychatric disorders such as ODD, CD, and ADHD. Reports indicate that only one-third of adolescents in SUD treatment reported receiving mental health treatment in the past year, with only 50%–60% of adolescent addiction programs offering concurrent mental health treatment (Brewer et al. 2017). Specific treatment for severe SUDs may often be needed before initiation of treatment for ADHD. Once some level of stabilization of substance use has been reached, further assessment and treatment for ADHD/CD should proceed. Despite the impact of comorbid SUD and ADHD/CD in the course and outcome of SUD, at present there are few empirical data to guide treatment.

Psychosocial Interventions

Treatment for CD or ODD often takes the form of targeting risk factors for the development and maintenance of CD (e.g., social and problem-solving skills; family targets, including parental supervision and monitoring). While adolescents with DBDs and SUDs should receive many of the modalities deemed efficacious for adolescents with SUDs in general, several psychosocial treatment modalities deserve special consideration.

Many family therapy modalities for treatment of externalizing disorders have been further adapted for use in substance-using adolescents; these include multisystemic therapy (MST), functional family therapy (FFT), multidimensional family therapy (MDFT), and brief strategic family therapy (BSFT) (Horigian et al. 2016). Familial involvement and family therapies have been extensively studied and are effective at reducing substance use, with a mean effect size of 0.26 (Brewer et al. 2017). Factors predicting optimal treatment outcome include having a supportive environment, especially one provided by parents and peers who do not use substances (Horigian et al. 2016).

MST addresses the multidimensional nature of behavior problems in youth with delinquency and has been specifically adapted for use in substance-abusing adolescents (MST-SA) (Henggeler and Schaeffer 2016; Horigian et al. 2016). Treatment focuses on those factors in each youth's social network that are contributing to his or her antisocial behavior. The ultimate goal of MST is to empower families to build a healthier environment through the mobilization of existing child, family, and community resources. MST is delivered in the natural environment (in the home, school, or community). The typical duration of home-based MST services is approximately 4 months, with multiple, weekly therapist-family contacts. MST targets risk factors in an individualized, comprehensive, and integrated fashion, allowing families to enhance protective factors. MST uses specific, empirically supported treatment techniques, including behavioral, cognitive-behavioral, and pragmatic family therapies. MST has been shown to clinically reduce antisocial behavior and delinquency, with positive outcomes in CD, and is often less costly than treatment as usual (Tan and Fajardo 2017). MST has been found to be more efficacious for severe behavior, and colleagues suggest that the modest effects of MST in less severe behavior disorders may relate to treatment fidelity as well as reduced motivation when treatment is not court mandated (Tan and Fajardo 2017). A randomized trial of MST and MST-SA in adolescents in drug court showed that MST-SA preferentially reduced drug use when compared with traditional MST (Horigian et al. 2016).

FFT is a flexible, individualized treatment that consists of three phases to improve familial communication and reduce dysfunctional patterns; it was initially developed for externalizing behaviors and has been adapted for substance abuse treatment. FFT has shown reductions in both substance use and externalizing disorders in various clinical trials and is being studied for implementation via video teleconference. Similarly, MDFT targets interpersonal and intrapersonal factors to address problematic conditions and processes through three stages to develop new skills and patterns for interaction. The effectiveness of MDFT on reducing substance use and externalizing disorders has been established through multiple randomized clinical trials in both controlled and community-based settings. BSFT combines structural and strategic family therapy theories to disrupt maladaptive family interactions through four domains with specific treatment goals. BSFT has been shown to have positive long-term impact on externalizing behaviors and substance use through multiple randomized clinical trials. Both MDFT and BSFT have been shown to have better substance-related outcomes with therapist adherence to the models (Horigian et al. 2016).

Motivation to engage in treatment is a general problem for adolescents with SUDs and is exacerbated with comorbid DBDs. A 2011 meta-analysis of 21 studies showed that motivational enhancement therapy (MET) or motivational interviewing (MI) produces small but significant effects on substance use behavior (Jensen et al. 2011), with moderate effectiveness in youth with low or no desire to change (Brewer et al. 2017). A 2015 study of 151 psychiatrically hospitalized adolescents with dual diagnoses revealed that the MI group had a longer period until first use of any substance following discharge (36 days, compared with 11 days in the treatment-as-usual group) and less total use of substances (Brown et al. 2015). MI was also associated with reductions in rule-breaking behaviors at 6-month follow-up; however, there was no impact on aggression. Although stand-alone MI is likely insufficient for dual diagnoses, it may help increase overall motivation for treatment and its effectiveness in conjunction with other evidenced-based therapies such as cognitive-behavioral therapy (CBT) (Brewer et al. 2017).

Development of a prosocial lifestyle is perhaps one of the more difficult goals for SUD treatment in adolescents with DBDs (Bukstein et al. 2005). Multiple studies have demonstrated that combined contingency management and CBT may result in increased prosocial activities and early abstinence as well as a reduction in externalizing symptoms (Brewer et al. 2017). Other combined or multimodal interventions demonstrating benefits include the Adolescent-Community Reinforcement Approach (A-CRA), which emphasizes prosocial activities and positive reinforcement. A-CRA has shown improvement in substance use, externalizing symptoms, and social stability (Brewer et al. 2017).

A controversial element of traditional treatment programs is the widespread use of group treatment. Dishion and Dodge (2005) cautioned that group interventions may be potentially harmful through iatrogenic "peer contagion" and "deviancy training" due to exposure to peer antisocial behavior and associated reinforcement. These findings were not corroborated by a 19-study literature review, with 13 studies directly assessing group CBT for substance-abusing adolescents (Hogue et al. 2014). In general, there is no evidence for any systematic severe or unmanageable problems in conducting group therapy (e.g., need to eject subjects, discontinue a session, physical abuse) in outpatient settings that include a significant percentage of adolescents with CD. A systematic review of peer-led interventions for nicotine, alcohol, and drug use prevention, involving 17 studies, showed that peer-led intervention had lower rates of smoking (OR=0.78), alcohol use (OR=0.8), and cannabis use (OR=0.7) (MacArthur et al. 2016). Diverse referral sources may allow for a mix of adolescents that are manageable in a group setting once specific expectations and rules are clearly communicated and a signed behavioral contract for ground rules is introduced. Experienced therapists can competently address inappropriate behavior and other "troubleshooting," particularly in a manual-driven treatment.

Given the high rates of treatment discontinuation and relapse rates in adolescent SUD, many adolescents, particularly those with severe SUDs and DBDs, may need continuing care services. Continuing care evolved from "aftercare," based on evidence that adolescents often display high rates of recidivism back to regular substance use (up to 50% in the first 90 days and 60% or more in the first year) after step-down to a less intensive level of care (Passetti et al. 2016). A review of 10 outcome studies showed that continuing care treatment (involving ongoing family therapy, adolescent group work, residential treatment, and 12- step programming) is associated with clinical improvement and ongoing reductions in substance use (Passetti et al. 2016).

Pharmacotherapy

The pharmacotherapy of CD is largely the treatment of comorbid conditions such as ADHD (discussed below) and treatment of aggression and other extreme manifestations of mood dysregulation. The Treatment Recommendations for the Use of Antipsychotics for Aggressive Youth (Pappadopulos et al. 2003; Schur et al. 2003) provided 14 recommendations on how to treat acute and chronic aggression, as well as an algorithm to guide medication choices. Subsequently, the Treatment of Maladaptive Aggression in Youth Steering Committee developed guidelines for management and treatment of maladaptive aggression in the areas of family engagement, assessment and diagnosis, and initial management, appropriate for use by primary care clinicians and mental health providers (Knapp et al. 2012; Scotto Rosato et al. 2012).

There continue to be a limited number of studies of antipsychotics and mood stabilizers for the treatment of ODD- and CD-related aggression (Pringsheim et al. 2015b), with low-quality evidence to support their use. Risperidone has the highest effect (moderate to large) based on a systematic review and meta-analysis with moderate-quality support for its use. There are no published studies of these agents for the treatment of adolescents with SUDs and aggression or CD comorbidity. Psychostimulants, α-agonists, and atomoxetine have demonstrated benefit in disruptive behaviors occurring in the context of ADHD symptoms, with highest-quality evidence for moderate-to-large effect sizes for ODD, CD, and aggression in youth with ADHD, with and without ODD or CD (Katzman and Sternat 2014; Pringsheim et al. 2015a).

Controlled clinical trials of pharmacological treatment of comorbid SUD and ADHD suggest limited, if any, effects on either substance use or ADHD variables, although there are some exceptions in the adult literature. A meta-analysis of 13 outpatient medication trials in both adolescents and adults demonstrated improved ADHD symptomatology, although with no overall benefit for drug abstinence or behaviors (Luo and Levin 2017). Notably, studies showing an effect in reducing substance use utilized robust doses of stimulants: two randomized controlled trials (RCTs) demonstrated higher substance use treatment retention and a higher proportion of negative drug urine tests (23% vs. 16%). Individuals with dual diagnoses were prescribed a 40% higher dose of methylphenidate compared with dosages used for ADHD alone. Explanatory hypotheses for necessity of higher stimulant dose in dual diagnoses include cross-tolerance to cerebral stimulants and dose tachyphylaxis; suboptimal dosing may explain the limited improvement of ADHD treatment on SUD (Carpentier and Levin 2017). Adequate symptom treatment may increase motivation to remain in treatment; ADHD treatment in comorbid SUD was found to preserve active treatment in 45% of cases compared with 37% in the ADHD-only group (Luo and Levin 2017).

In studies in which the effect did not reach statistical significance or in which a benefit was not found, there was no evidence supporting that ADHD treatment affects susceptibility to future substance use or causes more adverse events. Overall stimulant treatment for ADHD has been demonstrated to be safe and well tolerated and to offer protection against later substance use, particularly in adolescents (Zulauf et al. 2014).

For adolescents, Riggs and colleagues (2011) conducted a 16-week, multisite RCT of 300 adolescents with mixed SUD and ADHD receiving CBT for SUD, and either osmotic release oral system–methylphenidate (OROS-MPH) or placebo. They reported significant improvements in symptoms for both treatment arms based on the primary outcome measures of self-reported ADHD symptoms and substance use, but no group differences regarding improvement in ADHD or SUD. However, in a secondary outcome, they noted greater improvements in parent-reported ADHD symptoms for the OROS-MPH group. A similar study of atomoxetine versus placebo in adolescents with SUD and ADHD yielded no differences between the groups on either substance or ADHD outcomes (Thurstone et al. 2010). A placebo-controlled RCT combining CBT/MI and atomoxetine demonstrated no difference in SUD or ADHD symptoms by 12 weeks (Brewer et al. 2017), though this negative finding was attributed to the large effect from placebo and/or CBT/MI.

Practical treatment of comorbid SUD and ADHD may include one of the empirically proven first-line stimulant treatments, such as methylphenidate, amphetamines, or atomoxetine, that are approved by the U.S. Food and Drug Administration (Harstad et al. 2014). The use of atomoxetine and α-agonists may be considered for preferential use in patients with ongoing illicit substance use. Atomoxetine, a selective norepinephrine reuptake inhibitor, has been reported to have little abuse potential (Pérez de los Cobos et al. 2014). Early clinical experience is encouraging, with atomoxetine providing positive response rates of up to 44% in adult ADHD (Carpentier and Levin 2017) and ADHD remission rates of 59% at 12 weeks in youth populations (Katzman and Sternat 2014). Meta-analytic studies have shown that the effect size of atomoxetine is somewhat lower than that with stimulants, with small to moderate effect for oppositional behaviors in youth with ADHD with and without ODD or CD (Pringsheim et al. 2015a). Longer-term studies yielded effect sizes from 0.6 to 1.3 in children with ADHD (Clemow et al. 2017). A 2017 meta-analysis identified 14 studies assessing atomoxetine in the ADHD population, with significant improvements in symptoms of ADHD and CD/ODD; in addition, atomoxetine was found to protect against relapse in pediatric ADHD with concurrent ODD (Clemow et al. 2017).

There are few studies assessing the efficacy of α-agonists for the treatment of youth ODD, CD, and aggression, and none examining the efficacy in youth with SUDs and ADHD. Treatment with extended-release guanfacine yields a small to moderate effect that is supported in the literature. Clonidine may not offer clinically significant positive effects (Pringsheim et al. 2015a). The abuse potential of these medications is likely to be low (Harstad et al. 2014).

Stimulants remain the most effective treatments for ADHD in all ages (Pringsheim et al. 2015a), and tertiary agents such as bupropion and venlafaxine should be reserved for those patients not responding adequately to the first-line medications. Avoidance of stimulants should be considered in patients with active SUD, especially those with stimulant or cocaine dependence and those not receiving psychosocial treatment for their SUD. Individuals with a prior history of SUD and/or with a reasonable interval of remission of use or symptoms (6–12 months) may benefit from first-line stimulant treatment. The use of longer-acting or extended-release formulations of stimulants is strongly recommended (Crunelle et al. 2018; National Institute for Heath and Care Excellence 2018; Pliszka and AACAP Work Group on Quality Issues 2007; Wolraich et al. 2011). If an inadequate response to nonstimulants is noted, and especially if uncontrolled ADHD symptoms appear to be contributing to relapse or instability of the SUD, stimulant treatment may proceed with careful and frequent monitoring.

In addition to avoiding possible abuse of medications by the patient with comorbid ADHD and SUD himself or herself, the assessment of possible diversion by the patient, family members, or peers should always be considered. Prescriptions of medications should be carefully monitored, with high suspicion directed toward frequent early requests for refills or "lost" prescriptions. Medication should never be provided in isolation from psychosocial treatment directed at the patient's SUD.

Other Considerations

Childhood and Adolescent Stimulant Medication Use as a Risk or Protective Factor for the Development of SUDs

The abuse potential of stimulant medication and the impact of childhood medication treatment on the long-term risk of SUDs is an area of ongoing controversy. Critics of drug treatment point out that methylphenidate and other stimulants have a strikingly similar pharmacological profile to cocaine and that pharmacotherapy may increase the risk of development of substance abuse through a process of sensitization. Route of administration and dosage of stimulants are the most important variables that determine the abuse potential. Oral administration is less reinforcing than intravenous administration or inhalation, either of which delivers methylphenidate to the brain more rapidly, and methylphenidate clears from the brain more slowly than cocaine (Romach et al. 2014). Different methylphenidate formulations possess varying pharmacokinetic properties with different rates of onset, offset, and dopamine transporter occupancy. Clinical studies have revealed lower rates of abuse potential with modified-release versus short-acting methylphenidate (Romach et al. 2014). The lower risk for abuse of extended-release formulations of methylphenidate or amphetamine may also be related to the fact that active immediate-release components cannot be readily extracted by such methods as crushing from preparations of these stimulants and are difficult to use via nasal inhalation or injection (Bjarnadottir et al. 2017).

Despite suggestive evidence for sensitization from animal models, SUDs do not appear to be the result of prior stimulant use for the treatment of ADHD in childhood or early adolescence, and in fact appropriate treatment may reduce risk of developing SUD (Harstad et al. 2014). The literature generally supports the protective effect of ADHD treatment on the development of substance use (Cook et al. 2017), although the effect may be modest. The available clinical literature and findings of significantly lower rates of alcohol and drug use in 159 adolescents with ADHD who were treated and compared with an untreated group suggest that treatment with therapeutic oral doses of stimulants for ADHD do not increase the risk for addictive disorders (Hammerness et al. 2017).

Diversion and Abuse of Stimulant Medication

Stimulant medications are controlled drugs and have the potential for abuse and diversion, either for subjective euphoric effects or for effects on performance. Methylphenidate can be abused intranasally by crushing the tablets and snorting the powder or intravenously by dissolving the powder in water and injecting it. People who take the drug to induce euphoria prefer intranasal and intravenous routes, and there have been case reports of intravenous abuse of methylphenidate and amphetamines in adolescents and young adults (Bjarnadottir et al. 2016). Extended-release preparations of stimulants are probably less easy to misuse in this way than immediate-release tablets; MPH-OROS was demonstrated to be the least preferred intravenous stimulant in the methylphenidate class despite being the most widely available showing reduced abuse potential (Bjarnadottir et al. 2016). The oral route is most frequently used for all prescription stimulants (94.7% for MPH-OROS and 80.7% for Ritalin), with snorting occurring second most commonly (with Ritalin used 39.6% of the time), and injection or smoking occurring in roughly 6% (Cassidy et al. 2015).

Misuse and diversion of psychostimulants is common (Harstad et al. 2014; Kaminer 2013). The objective of abuse is either for "getting high" or for alleged cognitive enhancement ("good grade pills" or "smart pills," the use of which is a prevalent and growing problem, especially among college students) (Bagot and Kaminer 2014; Martinez-Raga et al. 2017; Sahakian and Labuzetta 2013). Oral stimulants are commonly used to enhance performance in sports or cognitive tasks and examinations in students. A systematic review of 21 studies revealed rates of past-year nonprescribed stimulant use of 5%–9% in grade school and high school students and 5%–35% in college-age individuals (Harstad et al. 2014). A university study showed nonmedical stimulant use in 18% of students who were not prescribed stimulants, use of someone else's prescription in 15.6%, and use of higher-than-prescribed doses in 27.6% of students with ADHD. These data are consistent with findings from the 2017 Monitoring the Future study, which noted a reported 16.7% rate of nonmedical use of prescription stimulants by age 18, with 43% of the adolescents prescribed stimulants using them for nonmedical purposes. In this study, 97% of adolescents with nonmedical use of stimulants had also used at least one other substance in the previous year (Johnston et al. 2018). The frequency of nonmedical use of stimulants was twice as high in college-age students (13%) compared with individuals ages 26–49 (6.9%), and prevalence was higher among students in public colleges (12.4%) than among students in private colleges (8.5%).

Between 16% and 24% of students had been asked to sell, give, or trade their prescription stimulant, and 13% reported diverting the medication (Cassidy et al. 2015; Harstad et al. 2014). Males were more likely to divert their prescription, with family and friends identified as the most common source, and with fewer than 20% of stimulants accessed through a "dealer" (Cassidy et al. 2015). A comorbid CD diagnosis is also associated with an increased likelihood of misuse and diversion of stimulants. Individuals have rated that stimulants are "fairly easy" to obtain (mean score of 4 on a scale of 1–5) (Cassidy et al. 2015). Reason for use is most commonly to enhance academic or work performance, then to increase alertness. Interestingly, nonmedical use of stimulants has been negatively associated with academic performance (Weyandt et al. 2016). Only 6.9% of individuals prescribed stimulants reported their motivation for using was "to get high" (Cassidy et al. 2015).

There have been reports of parents with and without substance abuse histories misusing their children's prescription stimulant, with 16% of parents endorsing diverting the medication to another household, frequently themselves, and another 13% endorsing temptation to take their child's medication (Pham et al. 2017). In one instance the son was coached by his mother on symptoms of ADHD to persuade physicians to prescribe methylphenidate (Fulton and Yates 1988).

Nevertheless, risk of diversion and nonmedical use of prescription stimulants is considered low when compared with the risk with other controlled agents such as benzodiazepines or opioid analgesics (Martinez-Raga et al. 2017). Physicians prescribing stimulants should be vigilant to any phenomenon indicative of medication misuse or diversion. History of familial drug abuse should be a reason for caution when prescribing stimulants. Pill counting and meeting with the youth as well as parent(s) one-on-one to inquire about discrepancies might be necessary.

Conclusion

CD, ODD, and ADHD are significant risk factors for development of substance abuse through a number of causal pathways. In adolescents with SUDs, CD and ADHD are among the most common of comorbid disorders. Because of the potential influence of CD and ADHD on the course of SUDs, these problems should be identified and treated with a combination of psychosocial and pharmacological interventions. Active treatment of ADHD is likely to reduce the development of CD and substance abuse, and many adolescents with SUD can take stimulants safely and appropriately. However, in view of the potential misuse of stimulants and diversion of stimulant medication, clinicians, teachers, and other professionals should be made aware of the scope and context of the problem and closely monitor adolescents being treated with these agents.

The choice of medication is dependent on the personal and family history of substance abuse, in particular the potential risk of abuse and diversion. In adolescents with ADHD and active SUD symptoms and behaviors, nonstimulant agents (atomoxetine) or antidepressants (bupropion) may be preferable to stimulants, given the absence of more substantial evidence of stimulant efficacy in this population. For youth with poor response to these agents, those whose SUD has been stabilized, or those with merely a prior history of SUD (assuming nonamphetamine SUD), the use of extended-release or longer-acting stimulants with lower abuse liability and diversion potential is a reasonable option. The role of optimal treatment of ADHD and CD on the course of SUD has yet to be fully studied.

Key Points

- Persistent conduct disorder (CD) is among the most robust predictors of adolescent substance use disorders (SUDs).

- Children with attention-deficit/hyperactivity disorder (ADHD) and CD are at higher risk to develop substance abuse in adolescence and adulthood.

- Treatment of ADHD with medication does not increase the risk; rather, it may be a protective factor against the development of SUD.

- Diversion of stimulants employed for the treatment of ADHD is common either for subjective euphoric effects or for cognitive enhancement that has not yet been confirmed.

- Treatment of comorbid ADHD and CD and comorbid SUD should be multimodal, incorporating specific psychosocial and pharmacological treatments.

- Extended-release stimulants, nonstimulants, or prodrugs, when carefully selected, are preferred to short-acting stimulants, because the first three types are less likely to be misused or diverted.

References

American Psychiatric Association: Diagnostic and Statistical Manual of Mental Disorders, 5th Edition. Arlington, VA, American Psychiatric Association, 2013

Arcos-Burgos M, Vélez JI, Solomon BD, et al: A common genetic network underlies substance use disorders and disruptive or externalizing disorders. Hum Genet 131(6):917–929, 2012 22492058

Bagot K, Kaminer Y: Efficacy of stimulants for cognitive enhancement in non-attention deficit hyperactivity disorder youth: a systematic review. Addiction 109(4):547–557, 2014 24749160

Bjarnadottir GD, Magnusson A, Rafnar BO, et al: Intravenous use of prescription psychostimulants: a comparison of the pattern and subjective experience between different methylphenidate preparations, amphetamine and cocaine. Eur Addict Res 22(5):259–267, 2016 27287610

Bjarnadottir GD, Johannsson M, Magnusson A, et al: Methylphenidate disintegration from oral formulations for intravenous use by experienced substance users. Drug Alcohol Depend 178:165–169, 2017 28651152

Brewer S, Godley MD, Hulvershorn LA: Treating mental health and substance use disorders in adolescents: what is on the menu? Curr Psychiatry Rep 19(1):5, 2017 28120255

Brown RA, Abrantes AM, Minami H, et al: Motivational interviewing to reduce substance use in adolescents with psychiatric comorbidity. J Subst Abuse Treat 59:20–29, 2015 26362000

Bukstein OG, Bernet W, Arnold V, et al; Work Group on Quality Issues: Practice parameter for the assessment and treatment of children and adolescents with substance use disorders. J Am Acad Child Adolesc Psychiatry 44(6):609–621, 2005 15908844

Carpentier PJ, Levin FR: Pharmacological treatment of ADHD in addicted patients: what does the literature tell us? Harv Rev Psychiatry 25(2):50–64, 2017 28272130

Cassidy TA, Varughese S, Russo L, et al: Nonmedical use and diversion of ADHD stimulants among U.S. Adults ages 18–49: a national internet survey. J Atten Disord 19(7):630–640, 2015 23269194

Chang LY, Wang MY, Tsai PS: Diagnostic accuracy of rating scales for attention-deficit/hyperactivity disorder: a meta-analysis. Pediatrics 137(3):e20152749, 2016 26928969

Clemow DB, Bushe C, Mancini M, et al: A review of the efficacy of atomoxetine in the treatment of attention-deficit hyperactivity disorder in children and adult patients with common comorbidities. Neuropsychiatr Dis Treat 13:357–371, 2017 28223809

Cook J, Lloyd-Jones M, Arunogiri S, et al: Managing attention deficit hyperactivity disorder in adults using illicit psychostimulants: a systematic review. Aust N Z J Psychiatry 51(9):876–885, 2017 28639480

Crunelle CL, van den Brink W, Moggi F, et al; ICASA Consensus Group: International consensus statement on screening, diagnosis and treatment of substance use disorder patients with comorbid attention deficit/hyperactivity disorder. Eur Addict Res 24(1):43–51, 2018 29510390

Dishion TJ, Dodge KA: Peer contagion in interventions for children and adolescents: moving towards an understanding of the ecology and dynamics of change. J Abnorm Child Psychol 33(3):395–400, 2005 15957566

Eaton NR, Rodriguez-Seijas C, Carragher N, et al: Transdiagnostic factors of psychopathology and substance use disorders: a review. Soc Psychiatry Psychiatr Epidemiol 50(2):171–182, 2015 25563838

Erskine HE, Norman RE, Ferrari AJ, et al: Long-term outcomes of attention-deficit/hyperactivity disorder and conduct disorder: a systematic review and meta-analysis. J Am Acad Child Adolesc Psychiatry 55(10):841–850, 2016 27663939

Fulton AI, Yates WR: Family abuse of methylphenidate. Am Fam Physician 38(2):143–145, 1988 3407585

Groenman AP, Janssen TWP, Oosterlaan J: Childhood psychiatric disorders as risk factor for subsequent substance abuse: a meta-analysis. J Am Acad Child Adolesc Psychiatry 56(7):556–569, 2017 28647007

Hammerness P, Petty C, Faraone SV, et al: Do stimulants reduce the risk for alcohol and substance use in youth with ADHD? A secondary analysis of a prospective, 24-month open-label study of osmotic-release methylphenidate. J Atten Disord 21(1):71–77, 2017 23264367

Harstad E, Levy S; Committee on Substance Abuse: Attention-deficit/hyperactivity disorder and substance abuse. Pediatrics 134(1):e293–e301, 2014 24982106

Hasin DS, Grant BF: The National Epidemiologic Survey on Alcohol and Related Conditions (NESARC) Waves 1 and 2: review and summary of findings. Soc Psychiatry Psychiatr Epidemiol 50(11):1609–1640, 2015 26210739

Hechtman L, Swanson JM, Sibley MH, et al; MTA Cooperative Group: Functional adult outcomes 16 years after childhood diagnosis of attention-deficit/hyperactivity disorder: MTA results. J Am Acad Child Adolesc Psychiatry 55(11):945.e2–952.e2, 2016 27806862

Henggeler SW, Schaeffer CM: Multisystemic Therapy: clinical overview, outcomes, and implementation research. Fam Process 55(3):514–528, 2016 27370172

Hirsch O, Christiansen H: Faking ADHD? Symptom validity testing and its relation to self-reported, observer-reported symptoms, and neuropsychological measures of attention in adults with ADHD. J Atten Disord 22(3):269–280, 2018 26246589

Hogue A, Henderson CE, Ozechowski TJ, et al: Evidence base on outpatient behavioral treatments for adolescent substance use: updates and recommendations 2007–2013. J Clin Child Adolesc Psychol 43(5):695–720, 2014 24926870

Horigian VE, Anderson AR, Szapocznik J: Family based treatments for adolescent substance use. Child Adolesc Psychiatr Clin N Am 25(4):603–628, 2016 27613341

Jensen CD, Cushing CC, Aylward BS, et al: Effectiveness of motivational interviewing interventions for adolescent substance use behavior change: a meta-analytic review. J Consult Clin Psychol 79(4):433–440, 2011 21728400

Johnston LD, Miech RA, O'Malley PM, et al: Monitoring the Future: National Survey Results on Drug Use: 1975–2017: Overview, Key Findings on Adolescent Drug Use. Ann Arbor, MI, Institute for Social Research, The University of Michigan, 2018

Kaminer Y: Stimulant misuse: is the pursuit of happiness by youth overrated? J Am Acad Child Adolesc Psychiatry 52(12):1255–1256, 2013 24290457

Katzman MA, Sternat T: A review of OROS methylphenidate (Concerta®) in the treatment of attention-deficit/hyperactivity disorder. CNS Drugs 28(11):1005–1033, 2014 25120227

Knapp P, Chait A, Pappadopulos E, et al; T-MAY Steering Group: Treatment of Maladaptive Aggression in Youth: CERT guidelines I. Engagement, assessment, and management. Pediatrics 129(6):e1562–e1576, 2012 22641762

Kollins SH, McClernon FJ, Fuemmeler BF: Association between smoking and attention-deficit/hyperactivity disorder symptoms in a population-based sample of young adults. Arch Gen Psychiatry 62(10):1142–1147, 2006 16203959

Lavigne JV, Meyers KM, Feldman M: Systematic review: classification accuracy of behavioral screening measures for use in integrated primary care settings. J Pediatr Psychol 41(10):1091–1109, 2016 27289069

Luo SX, Levin FR: Towards precision addiction treatment: new findings in co-morbid substance use and attention-deficit hyperactivity disorders. Curr Psychiatry Rep 19(3):14, 2017 28251590

MacArthur GJ, Harrison S, Caldwell DM, et al: Peer-led interventions to prevent tobacco, alcohol and/or drug use among young people aged 11–21 years: a systematic review and meta-analysis. Addiction 111(3):391–407, 2016 26518976

Martinez-Raga J, Ferreros A, Knecht C, et al: Attention-deficit hyperactivity disorder medication use: factors involved in prescribing, safety aspects and outcomes. Ther Adv Drug Saf 8(3):87–99, 2017 28382197

Miranda A, Colomer C, Berenguer C, et al: Substance use in young adults with ADHD: comorbidity and symptoms of inattention and hyperactivity/impulsivity. Int J Clin Health Psychol 16(2):157–165, 2016 30487859

Molina BSG, Howard AL, Swanson JM, et al: Substance use through adolescence into early adulthood after childhood-diagnosed ADHD: findings from the MTA longitudinal study. J Child Psychol Psychiatry 59(6):692–702, 2018 29315559

National Institute for Heath and Care Excellence: Attention deficit hyperactivity disorder: diagnosis and management. March 2018. Available at: https://www.nice.org.uk/guidance/ng87. Accessed May 16, 2019.

Niesten IJM, Nentjes L, Merckelbach H, et al: Antisocial features and "faking bad": a critical note. Int J Law Psychiatry 41:34–42, 2015 25843907

Pappadopulos E, Macintyre Ii JC, Crismon ML, et al: Treatment recommendations for the use of antipsychotics for aggressive youth (TRAAY). Part II. J Am Acad Child Adolesc Psychiatry 42(2):145–161, 2003 12544174

Passetti LL, Godley MD, Kaminer Y: Continuing care for adolescents in treatment for substance use disorders. Child Adolesc Psychiatr Clin N Am 25(4):669–684, 2016 27613345

Pérez de los Cobos J, Siñol N, Pérez V, et al: Pharmacological and clinical dilemmas of prescribing in co-morbid adult attention-deficit/hyperactivity disorder and addiction. Br J Clin Pharmacol 77(2):337–356, 2014 23216449

Pham T, Milanaik R, Kaplan A, et al: Household diversion of prescription stimulants: medication misuse by parents of children with attention-deficit/hyperactivity disorder. J Child Adolesc Psychopharmacol 27(8):741–746, 2017 28686059

Pliszka S; AACAP Work Group on Quality Issues: Practice parameter for the assessment and treatment of children and adolescents with attention-deficit/hyperactivity disorder. J Am Acad Child Adolesc Psychiatry 46(7):894–921, 2007 17581453

Pringsheim T, Hirsch L, Gardner D, et al: The pharmacological management of oppositional behaviour, conduct problems, and aggression in children and adolescents with attention-deficit hyperactivity disorder, oppositional defiant disorder, and conduct disorder: a systematic review and meta-analysis. Part 1: psychostimulants, alpha-2 agonists, and atomoxetine. Can J Psychiatry 60(2):42–51, 2015a 25886655

Pringsheim T, Hirsch L, Gardner D, et al: The pharmacological management of oppositional behaviour, conduct problems, and aggression in children and adolescents with attention-deficit hyperactivity disorder, oppositional defiant disorder, and conduct disorder: a systematic review and meta-analysis. Part 2: antipsychotics and traditional mood stabilizers. Can J Psychiatry 60(2):52–61, 2015b 25886656

Riggs PD, Winhusen T, Davies RD, et al: Randomized controlled trial of osmotic-release methylphenidate with cognitive-behavioral therapy in adolescents with attention-deficit/hyperactivity disorder and substance use disorders. J Am Acad Child Adolesc Psychiatry 50(9):903–914, 2011 21871372

Rodgers S, Müller M, Rössler W, et al: Externalizing disorders and substance use: empirically derived subtypes in a population-based sample of adults. Soc Psychiatry Psychiatr Epidemiol 50(1):7–17, 2015 24907047

Romach MK, Schoedel KA, Sellers EM: Human abuse liability evaluation of CNS stimulant drugs. Neuropharmacology 87:81–90, 2014 24793872

Rutter M, Moffitt TE, Caspi A: Gene-environment interplay and psychopathology: multiple varieties but real effects. J Child Psychol Psychiatry 47(3–4):226–261, 2006 16492258

Sahakian BJ, Labuzetta JN: Bad Moves: How Decision Making Goes Wrong, and the Ethics of Smart Drugs. New York, Oxford University Press, 2013

Schur SB, Sikich L, Findling RL, et al: Treatment recommendations for the use of antipsychotics for aggressive youth (TRAAY). Part I: a review. J Am Acad Child Adolesc Psychiatry 42(2):132–144, 2003 12544173

Scotto Rosato N, Correll CU, Pappadopulos E, et al; Treatment of Maladaptive Aggressive in Youth Steering Committee: Treatment of maladaptive aggression in youth: CERT guidelines II. Treatments and ongoing management. Pediatrics 129(6):e1577–e1586, 2012 22641763

Stein LAR, Graham JR: Ability of substance abusers to escape detection on the Minnesota Multiphasic Personality Inventory-Adolescent (MMPI-A) in a juvenile correctional facility. Assessment 12(1):28–39, 2005 15695741

Steiner H, Remsing L; Work Group on Quality Issues: Practice parameter for the assessment and treatment of children and adolescents with oppositional defiant disorder. J Am Acad Child Adolesc Psychiatry 46(1):126–141, 2007 17195736

Tan JX, Fajardo MLR: Efficacy of multisystemic therapy in youths aged 10–17 with severe antisocial behaviour and emotional disorders: systematic review. London J Prim Care (Abingdon) 9(6):95–103, 2017 29181092

Thurstone C, Riggs PD, Salomonsen-Sautel S, et al: Randomized, controlled trial of atomoxetine for attention-deficit/hyperactivity disorder in adolescents with substance use disorder. J Am Acad Child Adolesc Psychiatry 49(6):573–582, 2010 20494267

van de Glind G, Van Emmerik-van Oortmerssen K, Carpentier PJ, et al; IASP Research Group: The International ADHD in Substance Use Disorders Prevalence (IASP) study: background, methods and study population. Int J Methods Psychiatr Res 22(3):232–244, 2013 24022983

van Emmerik-van Oortmerssen K, van de Glind G, Koeter MWJ, et al; IASP Research Group: Psychiatric comorbidity in treatment-seeking substance use disorder patients with and without attention deficit hyperactivity disorder: results of the IASP study. Addiction 109(2):262–272, 2014 24118292

Weyandt LL, Oster DR, Marraccini ME, et al: Prescription stimulant medication misuse: where are we and where do we go from here? Exp Clin Psychopharmacol 24(5):400–414, 2016 27690507

White HR, Buckman J, Pardini D, et al: The association of alcohol and drug use with persistence of violent offending in young adulthood. J Dev Life Course Criminol 1(3):289–303, 2015 26557473

White HR, Conway FN, Buckman JF, et al: Does substance use exacerbate escalation along developmental pathways of covert and overt externalizing behaviors among young men? J Dev Life Course Criminol 4(2):137–147, 2018 30034995

Wolraich M, Brown L, Brown RT, et al; Subcommittee on Attention-Deficit/Hyperactivity Disorder; Steering Committee on Quality Improvement and Management: ADHD: clinical practice guideline for the diagnosis, evaluation, and treatment of attention-deficit/hyperactivity disorder in children and adolescents. Pediatrics 128(5):1007–1022, 2011 22003063

Zulauf CA, Sprich SE, Safren SA, et al: The complicated relationship between attention deficit/hyperactivity disorder and substance use disorders. Curr Psychiatry Rep 16(3):436, 2014 24526271

21

Behavioral Addictions

Gambling Disorder and Internet Gaming Disorder

Luis C. Farhat, M.D.

Jeffrey Derevensky, Ph.D.

Marc N. Potenza, M.D., Ph.D.

The introduction of behavioral addictions is a relatively new development in psychiatry. Whereas many disorders subsumed under the term *behavioral addictions* have existed for decades and have been addressed by clinicians, it was not until 2013 that the DSM work group, based on a growing body of neuroscience and behavioral research along with large-scale epidemiological studies, suggested adding the term *behavioral addictions* to their official classification of psychiatric diagnoses in DSM-5 (American Psychiatric Association 2013). There was strong empirical support indicating that multiple potentially risky behaviors, besides psychoactive substance ingestion, produce short-term rewards that may result in persistent behaviors despite the individual's understanding and awareness of the concomitant adverse consequences (Grant et al. 2010). Such behaviors, characterized as *behavioral addictions,* have been recognized, to varying degrees and with similar but not identical clinical criteria, by the American Psychiatric Association (2013), the World Health Organization (2018) (WHO), and the American Society of Addiction Medicine (2011).

Although multiple behavioral addictions were suggested for inclusion in DSM-5 by the work group, they concluded that there was sufficient evidence for inclusion of gambling disorder (GD) and that further research was necessary before including disorders relating to gaming, Internet or smartphone use, hypersexuality, and excessive exercise or shopping. However, Internet gaming disorder (IGD) was included in Section III of DSM-5 (the section in which conditions warranting additional research were included). The WHO has elected to include gaming disorder in ICD-11 (World Health Organization 2018).

Underlying behavioral addictions is a failure by affected individuals to resist impulses, drives, or temptations that when engaged in excessively result in negative personal, social, academic, occupational, physical, and/or mental health consequences. Addictions may be characterized by four central features: a) appetitive urges often occurring immediately prior to engagement in the addictive behavior (craving); b) impaired control, which may translate clinically into engaging in a behavior longer than originally intended; c) continued participation despite adverse consequences; and d) compulsive or habitual engagement (Potenza 2006). Griffiths (2005) reported six core elements of behavioral addictions: salience (the activity becomes highly valued and takes precedence over other activities), mood modification (emotional responses that, for example, may elevate depressed states), tolerance (need for increasing behavioral engagement to achieve desired levels of mood modification), withdrawal (unpleasant feelings when cutting down or stopping the activity), conflict (with other activities or persons because of the behavior), and relapse (frequent returning to the behavior).

The past several decades have witnessed a significant and remarkable invigoration of both theoretical and empirical research on adolescent risk behaviors that if engaged in excessively can, directly or indirectly, compromise the individual's mental health and well-being, their physical health, and the life-course trajectories of young people. Importantly, adolescents are a vulnerable population with respect to developing multiple addictive behaviors. Most adults with addictions report onset of use during adolescence, and both the severity and the morbidity of addiction are often inversely proportional to age at onset (Chambers et al. 2003). Much early work focused on adolescent problematic behaviors (substance and alcohol abuse, cigarette smoking, unprotected sexual activity, drinking and driving, and delinquency), all of which may have potentially serious negative shorter- and longer-term consequences for individuals, their families, and society. These risky behaviors often compromise one's "healthy development" and may result in mental health, social, educational, and legal difficulties for adolescents. Given the pervasiveness of the problems, researchers and clinicians have sought a better understanding regarding reasons why individuals engage in these behaviors and related risk factors, both proximal and distal, as well as the identification and assessment of protective factors.

Adolescents' susceptibility to addiction may be related to impulsivity, a behavioral pattern that may arise from differences between the development of promotional and inhibitory brain areas. While promotional brain circuitries may mature more rapidly and function similarly in adolescents and adults, inhibitory motivational circuitries involving the prefrontal cortex may be relatively immature. This resultant imbalance is a possible neurobiological explanation for adolescent impulsive behaviors and vulnerability to developing addictions (Chambers et al. 2003). Considering youth susceptibility to multiple forms of addiction and risk-taking behaviors, mental health professionals should understand behavioral addictions in youth.

In this chapter, we review findings regarding adolescent gambling, problem gambling, and the use of the Internet for gaming. Specifically, regarding adolescent gambling, we consider reasons why behavioral addictions in youth may be considered a growing public health concern by showing how adolescent gambling is a widespread activity that may lead to altered developmental trajectories and potentially severe problems later in life. We discuss potential risk factors for adolescent gambling and problem/pathological/disordered gambling and strategies to decrease gambling-related problems via treatments for adolescent gambling disorders. Regarding technological addictions, we discuss a current understanding and limitations, including existing knowledge gaps, and describe specific findings related to IGD.

Gambling Disorder

Gambling opportunities have increased recently. Traditionally considered an activity only for adults, gambling has become a popular mainstream activity for adolescents in most parts of the world. Whether adolescents are purchasing lottery scratch cards, playing poker or other card games among friends, or wagering on sports, international studies have reported that a growing number of adolescents gamble (Calado et al. 2017).

Despite legal prohibitions from engaging in government-regulated gambling activities (the age varies based on the type of gambling and jurisdiction) in most countries, adolescents have been reported to participate in diverse gambling, including online (Calado et al. 2017). Data indicate that onset of gambling is often early, with children as young as age 9 or 10 engaging in some form of gambling (Calado et al. 2017). However, few parents, teachers, and even mental health professionals perceive gambling to be a serious issue for youth (Derevensky et al. 2014). While most youth who gamble may best be described as social, recreational, occasional, or infrequent gamblers, a small but identifiable number develops a serious gambling problem.

Adolescent Gambling and Problem Gambling

With almost 80% of adolescents reporting having gambled for money at least once during their lifetime, and an appreciable number experiencing gambling-related problems, problem and disordered gambling among adolescents may be becoming a significant public health issue (Derevensky 2012). The types of gambling performed by youth may depend on accessibility and availability. School-age children are particularly prone to engage in gambling among peers (often skill-related forms), purchasing lottery tickets (e.g., scratch-off/instant-win tickets), and sports gambling. As youth get older and have greater access to money and credit cards, they may gamble on video lottery terminals (VLTs), in casinos and online (Derevensky 2012).

Calado and colleagues (2017), in reviewing the adolescent gambling literature, reported that between 0.2% and 12.3% of youth have presentations that meet criteria for problem gambling, notwithstanding assessment differences, thresholding scores, time frames, and accessibility and availability of different gambling activities. Volberg and colleagues (2010) suggested that 4%–8% of young people who gamble exhibit problem/pathological gambling, with a further 10%–15% at risk for a gambling problem. Volberg and colleagues also suggested that in addition to males being more likely to report gambling and experiencing problems, individuals who belong to an ethnic minority may be at a higher risk for problem or disordered gambling. Multiple clinical researchers have reported that youth who engage in online wagering are more prone to experience gambling and gambling-related problems, likely the result of the easy accessibility, affordability, convenience, and anonymity of such wagering (Calado et al. 2017).

Concerns exist that gambling problems may escalate with increased gambling availability and accessibility. However, both adolescent and adult prevalence estimates of gambling disorders have remained relatively stable over time, leading some to hypothesize that individuals may adapt to new gambling environments (an adaptation hypothesis). Yet, gambling has dramatically changed since about 2010. Not only has it become more socially acceptable, easily accessible, and readily available, but technological innovations have revolutionized the industry and the ways people gamble. Online wagering, wagering through one's smartphone, fantasy sports wagering, "prop," in-play, and micro sports betting are a few examples. In some jurisdictions, VLTs are readily available and sports wagering has become more prevalent after the 2018 U.S. Supreme Court decision permitting states to regulate sports wagering.

Many youth, in spite of prohibitions, have managed to access and engage in many forms of gambling (Derevensky 2012). Derevensky and Gainsbury (2016) raised concerns about social casino gaming (simulated forms of gambling that individuals play for points or chips but which may have higher-than-average payout rates). A large percentage of individuals migrate from gambling on online social casino games to actual online gambling as young adults (Kim et al. 2017). King (2018), in reviewing the available literature, pointed to the convergence between gaming and gambling and suggested that some forms of gaming may be a "gateway" to actual gambling. King (2018) concluded, after a review of the available empirical evidence, that simulated gambling during adolescence increases risk of monetary gambling during adulthood. McBride and Derevensky (2012) also reported that playing social casino games was related to more problematic gambling behaviors among adolescents and young adults, similar to findings from the U.K. Gambling Commission.

Other forms of gambling-related activities, such as fantasy sports wagering, appear popular among adolescent males. Marchica and Derevensky (2016), in a large-scale study of adolescents, reported that individuals engaging in fantasy sports wagering frequently reported multiple gambling-related behaviors. An epidemiological survey of public high school students in Connecticut revealed that approximately one in five adolescents had gambled online in the past year. Adolescents who had gambled online (as compared with those who had gambled but not online) were more likely to exhibit at-risk pathological gambling behaviors (Potenza et al. 2011). Understanding how different features of the Internet (e.g., online social games, loot boxes or loot crates in video games, microtransactions in online games) may lead youth to develop gambling problems in the current digital environment warrants further investigation.

Assessing Gambling Problems Among Adolescents and Young Adults

DSM-5 criteria for GD, the gold standard, require that at least four of the following nine criteria be met: 1) increases in the amount of money gambled to generate the same previous effect (tolerance); 2) feelings of irritability or listlessness when not gambling (withdrawal); 3) unsuccessful attempts to cut back or quit gambling; 4) significant preoccupation with gambling; 5) gambling to alleviate negative states or as a form of escape; 6) gambling to regain money recently lost ("chasing"); 7) lying to people regarding one's involvement with gambling; 8) jeopardizing a job or relationship due to involvement with gambling; and 9) dependence on others to provide financial support ("bailout"). The exclusion criterion is that the problematic gambling is not better accounted for by a manic episode.

As a screening tool for gambling problems among adolescents, multiple instruments have been adapted from DSM criteria and adult screening instruments. The South Oaks Gambling Screen—Revised for Adolescents (Winters et al. 1993), the DSM-IV-J (Fisher 1992) and its revision, the DSM-IV-MR-J (Fisher 2000), and the Massachusetts Gambling Screen (Shaffer et al. 1994) have been used in adolescent prevalence studies. Each instrument was modeled on adult screening instruments. More recently, the Canadian Adolescent

Gambling Inventory was specifically developed to assess gambling severity among adolescents. As with adult instruments, there exist common constructs underlying these instruments. The notions of deception (lying), stealing money to support gambling, preoccupation, and chasing losses are common. Similarly, although the number of items and constructs may differ, each criterion item has equal weighting, and a cut score is provided identifying GD for respective instrument.

Considering that gambling and gambling-related problems may be understood along a continuum, researchers have argued that hierarchical categories may best define levels of subsyndromal gambling (e.g., problem gambling). For example, *low-risk gambling* has been used to describe individuals who gamble but whose gambling does not meet any criteria for GD; *at-risk gambling* has been used to describe those whose gambling meets one or two GD criteria; *problem/pathological gambling* has been used to describe those whose gambling meets three or more criteria (Yip et al. 2011).

Risk Factors Associated With Adolescent Gambling Disorders

Males are more likely to gamble and experience gambling problems (Derevensky 2012). Early age at gambling onset, being from a racial/ethnic minority group, having disrupted familial and peer relationships, and having a parent or close family member with a gambling disorder are also possible risk factors (Derevensky 2012). From a psychological perspective, many adolescents with gambling problems report significant mental health concerns, including anxiety disorders, depression, and impulsivity. Adolescents with GD score lower on measures of conformity and self-discipline and report high rates of suicide ideation and attempts. Academically, these adolescents may experience a wide variety of school-related problems, including impaired academic performance, interpersonal difficulties, and conduct-related problems and delinquency. Other possible risk factors associated with youth gambling problems include having an early "big win," with peer gambling behaviors being predictive of gambling problems.

Adolescents with gambling problems appear prone to exhibiting erroneous beliefs, displaying cognitive thinking that may lack knowledge of the independence of events, and reporting an overestimation of their skill when gambling. They typically have poor or maladaptive general coping skills, report a high risk propensity, and exhibit poor resiliency in the face of adversity. Adolescents with gambling problems report more daily hassles and traumatic life events.

Despite these potential risk factors, most adolescents never develop significant gambling problems, suggesting that protective factors may decrease the likelihood of experiencing youth problem gambling. Dickson and colleagues (2008) found that family cohesion, school connectedness, achievement motivation, low risk propensity, and effective coping skills served as protective factors. Lussier and colleagues (2014) reported that youth scoring high on resiliency measures were less likely to experience gambling-related problems. These factors may serve to counteract risk factors through a cancellation process (Dickson et al. 2008; Lussier et al. 2014).

Adolescent gambling and problem gambling may not be stable over time. Although few longitudinal studies have satisfactorily addressed this issue, findings suggest that neither adolescent gambling nor adolescent gambling-related problems are good predictors of adult gambling (Delfabbro et al. 2014). Nevertheless, the impact of adolescent problem gambling is quite pervasive, with these youth experiencing significant mental health, social, interpersonal, educational, familial, and sometimes legal issues (see Derevensky 2012 for a comprehensive discussion). Furthermore, adult gamblers who experienced early gambling problems during adolescence (earlier-onset adult gambling) report more severe gambling symptomatology and increased need for help with gambling-related problems in comparison to individuals who began gambling as adults (later-onset adult gambling). Earlier-onset adult gambling has been linked to substance use disorders, suicidal ideation, and psychiatric hospitalization, in comparison to later-onset groups.

Internet Gaming Disorder

The past two decades have seen technological advances associated with gaming consoles, smartphones, and dramatic changes in the games themselves. It is estimated that more than 90% of children and adolescents spend considerable time playing either video games on a console or games on a computer, smartphone, or other digital device in the United States (Gentile et al. 2017). Király and colleagues (2014) have argued that online video games represent one of the most widespread recreational activities for children, adolescents, and adults, irrespective of culture and gender. The gaming market continues to expand in spite of some concerns, with estimates that it will become a $180 billion market by 2021 (Newzoo 2017). This growing interest in video games should not be interpreted that gaming itself is harmful. On the contrary, video games may satisfy certain psychological needs of the user, including identity expression, a sense of mastery and achievement, and the desire to escape from reality. Video games have been reported to increase visual, spatial, attention, and problem-solving skills; additionally, if games are being played with peers or family members, they may create opportunities for social interaction. Nevertheless, if video games are played excessively, individuals may experience a number of negative consequences, including financial losses (because online games often require money to continue), psychological detachment, sleep deprivation, a lack of personal and social interaction if played alone, depression, anxiety, and decrease in academic performance.

As noted earlier in this chapter, the DSM-5 work group identified IGD as a potential disorder worthy of further investigation, and WHO decided there was sufficient clinical and empirical evidence to include gaming disorder in ICD-11 (World Health Organization 2018) as a disorder due to addictive behaviors. Within ICD-11, gaming disorder is defined as a pattern of gaming behavior ("digital gaming" or "video gaming") characterized by impaired control over gaming, increased priority being given to gaming over other activities to the extent that gaming takes precedence over other interests and daily activities, and a continuation or escalation of gaming despite the occurrence of negative consequences. As part of the clinical criteria, this behavior is not episodic and must be of sufficient severity (both intensity and frequency) to result in significant impairment in personal, familial, social, educational, occupational, or other important areas of functioning. The WHO diagnostic criteria indicate that in most circumstances this behavior must be present for a period of at least 12 months.

IGD, the putative diagnosis defined by the American Psychiatric Association (American Psychiatric Association 2013), requires five of the following nine criteria: 1) preoccupation with games; 2) irritability when gaming is ceased (withdrawal); 3) an increasing amount of time engaged in gaming (tolerance); 4) unsuccessful attempts to control, cut back, or stop video game playing; 5) loss of interest in other activities; 6) continued involvement with using games despite gaming-related social and functional problems; 7) lying to people about involvement with gaming; 8) gaming as a way of relieving dysphoria (gaming as a form of psychological escape); and 9) jeopardizing a relationship or an educational or professional opportunity due to involvement with gaming. Despite similarities in the ICD-11 and DSM-5 criteria, there remains significant inconsistency among experts about how to conceptualize a gaming disorder or gaming addiction. Several gaming researchers report that by using criteria established for substance use and gambling disorders, clinicians and parents may pathologize normal gaming behavior (Griffiths et al. 2016).

Prevalence

A consensus concerning the prevalence rates of a gaming disorder has been difficult to achieve given the significant variability between studies in terms of definition, assessment criteria, geographical considerations, accessibility (related to income and Internet access), and methodological approaches. Several reviews examining prevalence estimates of gaming disorder (Király et al. 2014; Rehbein et al. 2016) suggest that the prevalence among adolescents ranges between 1.5% and 9.9%, with some estimates as high as 25% among U.S. university students (Fortson et al. 2007). Although a gaming disorder may occur at any age, gaming disorders are more typical among children and adolescents (possibly because of more free time). A recent study revealed that excessive gaming time may be dependent on the individual's preference of game genre. Role-playing and shooter-type games may be related to more time spent gaming (Rehbein et al. 2016). Eichenbaum et al. (2015) reported that massively multiplayer online role-playing games (MMORPGs) were highly related to IGD, whereas action and puzzle games were found to be minimally linked. However, if played excessively, the latter games may similarly lead to IGD. One's motivation for gaming may be related to a gaming disorder. For example, youth who engage in games excessively for social reasons versus psychological escape may have fewer negative consequences. However, as gaming frequency and time spent gaming escalate, the likelihood of a gaming disorder increases. Donati et al. (2015) reported that the more game genres performed, the greater the likelihood of a gaming disorder.

Potential Risk Factors for a Gaming Disorder

Individuals with a severe gaming disorder may have a variety of psychosocial problems and psychiatric conditions (e.g., depressive symptomatology, attention-deficit/hyperactivity disorder, mood disorders, anxiety disorders, personality disorders, obsessive-compulsive and related disorders, substance abuse problems, and antisocial and delinquent behaviors) (Mihara and Higuchi 2017). However, it is important to note that there is very little research examining temporal or causal relationships between psychiatric disorders and gaming disorder (King 2018). Furthermore, disordered gaming significantly predicted poorer academic performance, even after researchers controlled for gender, age, and weekly amounts of game playing (Gentile 2009). Long-term effects of violent video games may also predict more aggressive behavior (Gentile et al. 2014). Kuss et al. (2013) have further suggested that understanding one's cultural context is important because it may embed gamers into a "community" of individuals with shared beliefs and practices, endowing their gaming with a particular meaning.

Whether because of gaming's social features, the ability to manipulate and control aspects of the game itself, reward and punishment features (e.g., earning or losing points), the aesthetic quality of the games, the ability to assume an alternate identity with the game characters, or the ability to interact with others, children and adolescents may be particularly drawn to these games. Online gaming has become a space of "virtual socialization" in which players may experience social interactions as an integral part of the gaming process. For some, the increased frequency of gaming represents a need for completion of increasingly more intricate, time-consuming, or difficult goals to achieve satisfaction and the need to rectify perceived gaming inadequacies (King et al. 2018).

Assessing Internet Gaming Disorder

As previously noted, the American Psychiatric Association (2013) articulated nine criteria for clinical diagnosis of a gaming disorder. Yet, the need for common diagnostic criteria has been repeatedly emphasized in the psychological and psychiatric literature. The existence of several screening instruments developed to establish prevalence rates reflects the divergent opinions in the field. However, this situation has not precluded researchers from developing multiple screening instruments and scales. For example, the Internet Gaming Disorder Test (IGD-20) (and its short form, IGDS9-SF, assessing severity of online and offline gaming behaviors), the Internet Gaming Disorder Test–10 (a 10-item scale based on the DSM-5 criteria for IGD), and the Internet Gaming Disorder Scale (both the 9- and 27-item versions) are designed to assess negative consequences associated with a gaming disorder.

Accessibility and availability of online games have never been greater. Given clinical reports, parental concerns, and the vast number of electronic games being developed and played via the Internet and on smartphones, there remains little doubt that youth gaming disorders have become an important social public health issue.

Treatment of Gambling and Gaming Addictions

While it remains beyond the scope of this chapter to go into depth concerning the treatment of disorders due to addictive behaviors, it is important to note that few children and adolescents voluntarily seek treatment for these disorders (Derevensky 2012). Regarding the treatment of adolescent problem gambling, it has been debated whether abstinence versus controlled use should be the appropriate treatment outcome. While one might propose abstinence for gambling, especially for children and adolescents, it is more difficult to make the argument for gaming. Internet or smartphone use (the most popular mediums for game playing) is widespread. In some Asian countries, inpatient treatment is growing, especially for youth with a gaming disorder. Many schools are now prohibiting smartphones in the classroom, with some schools blocking WiFi access for specific gaming, gambling, pornography, and social media sites. With respect to youth gambling, governments around the world are establishing greater age restrictions on regulated forms of gambling.

Traditional forms of treatment for behavioral addictions include cognitive therapy and cognitive-behavioral therapy (CBT), motivational interviewing, family therapy, and online forums and support groups. There currently is no approved psychopharmacological approved treatment for adolescent gambling or gaming disorders. Yau et al. (2014) suggested that a comprehensive treatment program for behavioral addictions should incorporate an integrated approach, drawing on several different therapeutic approaches that focus on addressing symptoms as well as the underlying dynamics that contribute to the addictive behavior. Although Yau and colleagues were discussing treatment of a food addiction, this model would be beneficial in working with youth experiencing other forms of behavioral addictions.

Multiple self-help interventions, typically designed to reduce the barriers associated with seeking treatment (e.g., cost, stigma, difficulties with transportation), have been developed for behavioral disorders. These include teleconferencing, self-directed computer interventions and online support groups, bibliotherapy, workbooks, and more traditional peer-support meetings (e.g., Gamblers Anonymous). CBT, a widely used treatment approach, targets maladaptive cognitions and related behaviors, with an emphasis on understanding the interrelatedness of cognitions, emotions, and behavior. A fundamental aim of CBT is to help the individual identify and change irrational and erroneous beliefs. Petry's eight-session CBT program includes topics such as identifying and managing triggers, conducting a functional analysis of gambling/gaming episodes, increasing the client's participation in alternative activities, dealing with urges and cravings, building interpersonal conflict skills, recognizing and correcting cognitive biases, and relapse prevention (Rash and Petry 2014). Other therapeutic interventions designed for addictive disorders, such as motivational interviewing (Miller and Rollnick 2012), which has support for use with GD, may have practical significance for other behavioral disorders. Mindfulness-based approaches also warrant consideration.

The role that parents have in both preventing and modifying their children's addictive behaviors is important. Gaming, the Internet, and smartphones are commonly used for socializing, communicating, and entertainment. Many parents may be unaware of the extent to which children engage in gaming, gambling, and other Internet-use behaviors until such behaviors become problematic. With respect to gambling, parents should emphasize that this is an adult activity and should not encourage gambling by giving lottery tickets to children and adolescents as birthday or holiday gifts. Concerning gaming, parents should set limits early on and modify or curb excessive use.

Conclusion

Today's youth face different stressors than prior generations. Not only are they dealing with physiological changes, increasing academic demands, social pressures, and a difficult employment market, they are doing so with an online audience. Youth are expected to be "on" 24 hours a day, 7 days a week. While technology has made certain tasks easier, the social pressures placed on youth have increased significantly.

Behavioral addictions often develop during childhood and adolescence and are prevalent among young people. Excessive "screen time" has led to major confrontations with parents over devices. Awareness of behavioral addictions is essential. Setting limits by parents may result in more conflict. Tracking children's screen time may provide parents with a better understanding of the extent of problems.

With time, it is likely that many youth will outgrow these adolescent disorders as they become adults through a process of natural recovery or in some cases through psychological or psychiatric interventions. Nevertheless, the concomitant mental health, academic, social, familial, and interpersonal issues associated with these early behavioral addictions may have long-standing consequences. Although many treatment approaches have emanated from work on substance abuse, each disorder requires an understanding of the child's motivations underlying their behaviors. Further understanding of the developmental trajectories and the risk and protective factors for each of these associated behavioral disorders will ultimately enable the development of best practices for prevention and treatment.

Key Points

- Behavioral addictions are important yet largely understudied disorders among adolescents.

- Addictive behaviors usually co-occur in adolescents, so assessing across domains is important.

- Gambling is common among adolescents, yet identifying gambling problems may be particularly difficult because of certain features of gambling by youth.

- Gambling disorder and Internet gaming disorder are relatively novel conditions and largely understudied; employing the DSM-5 set of criteria for Internet gaming disorder is advisable.

- Treatment of adolescent gambling and other behavioral addictions (e.g., Internet gaming disorder) should consider the comorbidity profile of each individual.

References

American Psychiatric Association: Diagnostic and Statistical Manual of Mental Disorders, 5th Edition. Arlington, VA, American Psychiatric Association, 2013

American Society of Addiction Medicine: Public Policy Statement: Definition of Addiction. Chevy Chase, MD, American Society of Addiction Medicine, 2011

Calado F, Alexandre J, Griffiths MD: Prevalence of adolescent problem gambling: a systematic review of recent research. J Gambl Stud 33(2):397–424, 2017 27372832

Chambers RA, Taylor JR, Potenza MN: Developmental neurocircuitry of motivation in adolescence: a critical period of addiction vulnerability. Am J Psychiatry 160(6):1041–1052, 2003 12777258

Delfabbro P, King D, Griffiths MD: From adolescent to adult gambling: an analysis of longitudinal gambling patterns in South Australia. J Gambl Stud 30(3):547–563, 2014 23595217

Derevensky JL: Teen Gambling: Understanding a Growing Epidemic. New York, Rowman & Littlefield, 2012

Derevensky JL, Gainsbury SM: Social casino gaming and adolescents: should we be concerned and is regulation in sight? Int J Law Psychiatry 44:1–6, 2016 26421603

Derevensky JL, St-Pierre RA, Temcheff CE, et al: Teacher awareness and attitudes regarding adolescent risky behaviours: is adolescent gambling perceived to be a problem? J Gambl Stud 30(2):435–451, 2014 23423729

Dickson L, Derevensky JL, Gupta R: Youth gambling problems: examining risk and protective factors. Int Gambl Stud 8:25–47, 2008

Donati MA, Chiesi F, Ammannato G, et al: Versatility and addiction in gaming: the number of video-game genres played is associated with pathological gaming in male adolescents. Cyberpsychol Behav Soc Netw 18(2):129–132, 2015 25684613

Eichenbaum A, Kattner F, Bradford D, et al: Role-playing and real-time strategy games associated with greater probability of Internet gaming disorder. Cyberpsychol Behav Soc Netw 18(8):480–485, 2015 26252934

Fisher SE: Measuring pathological gambling in children: the case of fruit machines in the U.K. J Gambl Stud 8:263–285, 1992

Fisher SE: Developing the DSM-IV-MR-J criteria to identify adolescent problem gambling in nonclinical populations. J Gambl Stud 16:253–273, 2000

Fortson BL, Scotti JR, Chen YC, et al: Internet use, abuse, and dependence among students at a southeastern regional university. J Am Coll Health 56(2):137–144, 2007 17967759

Gentile D: Pathological video-game use among youth ages 8 to 18: a national study. Psychol Sci 20(5):594–602, 2009 19476590

Gentile DA, Li D, Khoo A, et al: Mediators and moderators of long-term effects of violent video games on aggressive behavior: practice, thinking, and action. JAMA Pediatr 168(5):450–457, 2014 24663396

Gentile DA, Bailey K, Bavelier D, et al: Internet gaming disorder in children and adolescents. Pediatrics 140 (suppl 2):S81–S85, 2017 29093038

Grant JE, Potenza MN, Weinstein A, et al: Introduction to behavioral addictions. Am J Drug Alcohol Abuse 36(5):233–241, 2010 20560821

Griffiths MD: A "components" model of addiction within a biopsychosocial framework. Journal of Substance Use 10(4):191–197, 2005

Griffiths MD, van Rooij AJ, Kardefelt-Winther D, et al: Working towards an international consensus on criteria for assessing internet gaming disorder: a critical commentary on Petry et al. (2014). Addiction 111(1):167–175, 2016 26669530

Kim HS, Wohl MJA, Gupta R, et al: Why do young adults gamble online? A qualitative study of motivations to transition from social casino games to online gambling. Asian J Gambl Issues Public Health 7(1):6, 2017 28890860

King D: Online Gaming and Gambling in Children and Adolescents—Normalising Gambling in Cyber Places. Melbourne, Australia, Victorian Responsible Gambling Foundation, September 2018. Available at: https://responsiblegambling.vic.gov.au/resources/publications/online-gaming-and-gambling-in-children-and-adolescents-normalising-gambling-in-cyber-places-479/. Accessed May 16, 2019.

King D, Herd M, Delfabbro PH: Motivational components of tolerance in Internet gaming disorder. Computers in Human Behavior 78(C):133–141, 2018

Király O, Nagygyörgy K, Griffiths MD, et al: Problematic online gaming, in Behavioral Addictions: Criteria, Evidence, and Treatment. Edited by Rosenberg KP, Feder L. New York, Academic Press, 2014, pp 61–97

Kuss D, Griffiths MD, Binder J: Internet addiction in students: prevalence and risk factors. Computers in Human Behavior 29(3):959–966, 2013

Lussier ID, Derevensky J, Gupta R, et al: Risk, compensatory, protective, and vulnerability factors related to youth gambling problems. Psychol Addict Behav 28(2):404–413, 2014 24274433

Marchica L, Derevensky JL: Fantasy sports: a growing concern among college student-athletes. International Journal of Mental Health and Addictiction 14(2):635–645, 2016

McBride J, Derevensky J: Internet gambling and risk-taking among students: an exploratory study. J Behav Addict 1(2):50–58, 2012 26165306

Mihara S, Higuchi S: Cross-sectional and longitudinal epidemiological studies of Internet gaming disorder: a systematic review of the literature. Psychiatry Clin Neurosci 71(7):425–444, 2017 28436212

Miller WR, Rollnick S: Motivational Interviewing: Helping People Change. New York, Guilford, 2012

Newzoo: Newzoo's 2017 report: insights into the $108.9 billion global games market. June 20, 2017. Available at: https://newzoo.com/insights/articles/newzoo-2017-report-insights-into-the-108-9-billion-global-games-market/. Accessed May 16, 2019.

Potenza MN: Should addictive disorders include non-substance-related conditions? Addiction 101 (suppl 1):142–151, 2006 16930171

Potenza MN, Wareham JD, Steinberg MA, et al: Correlates of at-risk/problem internet gambling in adolescents. J Am Acad Child Adolesc Psychiatry 50(2):150–159.e3, 2011 21241952

Rash CJ, Petry NM: Psychological treatments for gambling disorder. Psychol Res Behav Manag 7:285–295, 2014 25328420

Rehbein F, Kuhn S, Rumpf HJ, et al: Internet gaming disorder: a new behavioral addiction, in Behavioral Addictions: DSM-5 and Beyond. Edited by Petry NM. New York, Oxford University Press, 2016, pp 43–70

Shaffer HJ, LaBrie R, Scanlan K, Cummings T: Pathological gambling among adolescents: Massachusetts Gambling Screen. J Gambl Stud 10:339–362, 1994

Volberg RA, Gupta R, Griffiths MD, et al: An international perspective on youth gambling prevalence studies. Int J Adolesc Med Health 22(1):3–38, 2010 20491416

Winters KC, Stinchfield RD, Fulkerson J: Toward the development of an adolescent gambling problem severity scale. J Gambl Stud 9:371–386, 1993

World Health Organization: International Classification of Diseases, 11th Revision. Geneva, World Health Organization, 2018

Yau YH, Gottlieb C, Krasna L, et al: Food addiction: evidence, evaluation, and treatment, in Behavioral Addictions: Criteria, Evidence, and Treatment. Edited by Rosenberg KP, Feder L. New York, Academic Press, 2014, pp 143–184

Yip SW, Desai RA, Steinberg MA, et al: Health/functioning characteristics, gambling behaviors, and gambling-related motivations in adolescents stratified by gambling problem severity: findings from a high school survey. Am J Addict 20(6):495–508, 2011 21999494

PART V

Special Populations

22

Management of Youth With Substance Use Disorders in the Juvenile Justice System

Kristyn Zajac, Ph.D.

Tess K. Drazdowski, Ph.D.

Ashli J. Sheidow, Ph.D.

Each year, over 31 million youth are involved in the juvenile justice system, and nearly 1 million new youth formally come into contact with the juvenile justice system (Hockenberry and Puzzanchera 2018). These youth are more likely than their non-involved peers to have comorbid behavioral health problems, the most common being substance use. Among adjudicated youth, an estimated two-thirds report a history of substance use (Belenko and Logan 2003), and over one-third have use that meets criteria for a substance use disorder (SUD) (Aarons et al. 2001; Wasserman et al. 2010). Similarly, one study found that 58% of youth receiving substance use treatment were involved in the justice system (Hser et al. 2001).

In addition to high rates of substance use, justice-involved youth have elevated rates of other challenges that differentiate them from non-justice-involved youth. For example, justice-involved youth show high rates of learning disabilities and school failure. As a group, justice-involved youth tend to have intellectual functioning in the low-average to average range, and many show academic deficits in reading, math, and written and oral language due to either learning disabilities or lack of educational engagement (Foley 2001). In a study of juvenile offenders ages 10–20, close to 20% had a specific learning disability, and youth with elevated mental health symptoms were even more likely to have learning problems (Cruise et al. 2011). Justice-involved youth also have high rates of involvement with the child welfare system. More than 60% of youth considered "serious offenders" in juvenile detention have a history of child welfare involvement due to child maltreatment (Langrehr 2011). Youth with a substantiated history of maltreatment have approximately 50% more contacts with the juvenile justice system compared with youth without such a history, and approximately 16% of youth placed in foster care come into contact with the juvenile justice system (Ryan and Testa 2005).

While much of the information presented in other chapters of this manual is also applicable to juvenile offenders, clinicians and other professionals who focus on helping youth should be aware of the distinctive characteristics and needs of youth involved in the juvenile justice system. In this chapter we discuss common risk factors for youth who have juvenile justice system involvement and substance use problems; outcomes for these high-risk youth; substance use screening, assessment, and interventions for justice-involved youth; unique intervention challenges; and the often-overlooked population of transition-age youth with juvenile justice system involvement.

Overlapping Risk Factors for Substance Use and Juvenile Justice System Involvement

Given the high rates of substance use reported by youth in the juvenile justice system, it is not surprising that there are many overlapping risk factors, which often interact to increase risk for negative outcomes. These risk factors are observed throughout a youth's ecology. At the individual level, certain mental health concerns, like externalizing disorders (e.g., oppositional defiant disorder, conduct disorders, antisocial behaviors), learning disabilities/poor academic achievement, hyperactivity, and concentration problems, are related to both substance use (e.g., Molina and Pelham 2003) and justice system involvement (Barrett et al. 2014; Development Services Group 2017). Another shared risk factor is childhood trauma. One study of detained youth found that the vast majority (93%) reported at least one traumatic experience, most reported more than one (84%), and youth with trauma-related mental health problems were more likely to have an SUD (Abram et al. 2013).

At the family level, parental maltreatment, poor family management practices, and favorable parental attitudes toward substance use and violence are consistently related to higher rates of juvenile justice system involvement and substance use (see, e.g., Barrett et al. 2014). Involvement in the foster care system and receiving child welfare services are also known risk factors for both (Barrett et al. 2014). Additionally, having delinquent and substance-using siblings and/or peers, including gang membership, places a youth at risk for both substance use and contact with the justice system. At the community level, school disengagement, poverty, availability of drugs, and exposure to community violence and racial prejudice are linked to both (Henry et al. 2012).

Outcomes for Youth With Substance Use and Juvenile Justice System Involvement

Youth with SUDs are more likely to engage in delinquency and violence, and consequently come into contact with the justice system more often than their non-substance-using peers (Development Services Group 2017). These youth also display more severe delinquent behavior and recidivate more frequently, both as youth and during adulthood, compared with justice-involved youth without substance use problems (Dembo et al. 2007). Substance use in youth offenders is linked to worse educational, occupational, and health outcomes, including elevated risk for HIV and other sexually transmitted infections (Chassin et al. 2014; Rowe et al. 2008). Many of these youth are diagnosed with multiple behavioral health disorders, not just SUDs (Schubert et al. 2011), further complicating treatment needs.

Screening and Assessment Within the Juvenile Justice System

Assessment of substance use problems has gained traction over the past decade, with most states implementing screening and assessment procedures within juvenile justice programs (Wachter 2015a, 2015b). Because the juvenile justice system prioritizes public safety, assessments typically focus on identifying risk factors that can be addressed in treatment or programming to reduce the youth's likelihood of recidivism. Screening and assessment can take place at any point during the youth's involvement in the justice system, and results are used for a variety of purposes (e.g., determining appropriateness for diversion programming, deciding placement during sentencing, defining frequency of community supervision contacts). It is also important to note that while the terms "screening" and "assessment" are frequently used interchangeably, they refer to two different processes. Screenings are typically briefer and therefore more cost-effective and can be used with all youth entering a system or facility. Assessments are used to collect more extensive information once screening has identified a potential problem or risk profile.

Substance use is typically assessed as part of a broader protocol that also evaluates other behavioral health concerns and risk for violence. Screening and assessment tools for substance use problems are discussed in greater detail in Chapter 3 in this manual, but tools specifically developed for justice-involved youth are highlighted below.

Massachusetts Youth Screening Instrument—Version 2

The Massachusetts Youth Screening Instrument–Version 2 (MAYSI-2; Grisso and Barnum 2006) is a 52-item screening tool designed for use in the juvenile justice system. It aims to identify alcohol and drug use, mental health needs, and emotional disturbances. The MAYSI-2 is intended for youth ages 12–17 years and can be used at any entry or transitional placement point. Youth respond to "yes/no" questions, denoting if the item has been true "in the past few months." The measure is scored on six valid and reliable clinical scales: 1) Alcohol/Drug Use, 2) Angry-Irritable, 3) Depressed-Anxious, 4) Somatic Complaints, 5) Suicide Ideation, and 6) Thought Disturbance (this last scale has been found to be valid for males only). Each clinical scale has two cutoff scores: Caution and Warning. A score above the Caution cutoff indicates "possible clinical significance," while a score above the Warning cutoff indicates an exceptionally high score (upper 10%) compared with national norms among justice-involved youth. An additional scale, Traumatic Experiences, assesses exposure to traumatic events. The MAYSI-2 comes with computer scoring software and the capability to read questions aloud to the youth.

Youth Level of Service/Case Management Inventory

The Youth Level of Service/Case Management Inventory (YLS/CMI; Bechtel et al. 2007) is a 42-item tool that assesses risk level, identifies needs that could be targeted by treatment or programming, and informs decisions about community supervision and case management. Eight domains are measured: 1) prior and current offenses/ adjudications, 2) family circumstances and parenting issues, 3) education and employment, 4) peer relations, 5) substance abuse, 6) leisure and recreation, 7) personality and behavior, and 8) attitudes and orientation. Youth are classified as being at low, moderate, high, or very high risk for reoffending based on a combination of these domains.

Youth Assessment and Screening Instrument

The Youth Assessment and Screening Instrument (YASI; Orbis Partners 2011) includes a 33-item Pre-Screen and 88-item Full Assessment of risk, needs, and strengths among youth in the juvenile justice system. The Pre-Screen classifies risk and protective factors as low, moderate, or high. If a youth is identified as being at moderate or high risk, the Full Assessment is administered. The Full Assessment evaluates 10 domains: 1) legal history, 2) family, 3) school, 4) community and peers, 5) alcohol and drugs, 6) mental health, 7) aggression/ violence, 8) attitudes, 9) skills, and 10) employment/use of free time. The YASI includes a review of the official criminal record, a semistructured interview with the youth, and information gathering from key informants (e.g., parents, police, school officials). The YASI recommends specific treatment options based on each youth's needs and guides case management planning.

Structured Assessment of Violence Risk in Youth

The Structured Assessment of Violence Risk in Youth (SAVRY; Borum et al. 2006) includes 6 Protective Factors and 24 Risk Factors items (including substance use problems) and is used to assess offending risk in youth ages 12–18. Risk Factors are rated as low, moderate, or high. Protective Factors are rated as present or absent. Items are rated as "critical" if deemed by the assessor to be strongly related to the youth's offending and in need of immediate intervention. The SAVRY uses a structured professional judgment approach, in which the assessor provides the final Summary Risk Rating (low, moderate, high risk) based on professional judgment and informed by the assessment items.

Other Screening Tools

Recent analyses of states' screening and assessment processes for youth in juvenile justice found that there are many different tools being used. For example, 20 different risk assessments were reported in different juvenile justice systems, with the YLS/CMI and YASI being most common (Wachter 2015b). The MAYSI-2 is the most widely used screening tool for behavioral health needs used in detention centers when mental health screening is required by the state (Wachter 2015a).

Other behavioral health screening tools used in juvenile justice systems include the Mental Health Juvenile Detention Assessment Tool, as well as tools that were not originally developed for the juvenile justice system but have been used in this setting: Global Appraisal of Individual Needs—Short Screener, Problem Oriented Screening Instrument for Teenagers, Strengths and Difficulties Questionnaire, Personal Experience Screening Questionnaire, and the Brief Mental Status Assessment, many of which are discussed further in Chapter 3. Some states have also developed their own screening tools (e.g., Connecticut: Prospective Risk Evaluation of Delinquency in CT [PrediCT]; Florida: Suicide Risk Screening Instrument; Georgia: Department of Juvenile Justice Mental Health Screening).

Whereas risk assessments of reoffending are often completed in juvenile probation settings (Wachter 2015b), screening and assessment for behavioral health problems are most likely to occur in detention and corrections agencies and are less common in probation settings (Wachter 2015a). Efforts to increase screening and assessments for juvenile probationers have yielded mixed results. For example, one study found that implementing a risk/needs assessment reduced formal supervision rates and recidivism and that substance use treatment reduced recidivism for youth with substance use problems, but that youth received similar levels of mental health services regardless of their assessed risk and receiving mental health services did not reduce recidivism (Vincent and Perrault 2018).

Interventions for Youth With Substance Use and Juvenile Justice System Involvement

The juvenile justice system is the largest referral source for treatment of substance use and related antisocial behavior in youth (Ives et al. 2010). Therefore, clinicians who treat adolescents with substance use problems should be familiar with issues specific to justice-involved youth. In the past several decades, treatment has been incorporated throughout the juvenile justice continuum, including within detention centers, community-based supervision, juvenile drug courts, and community reentry programs (National Institute on Drug Abuse 2014). Many of the substance use treatment approaches discussed in previous chapters apply to justice-involved youth, while some other interventions have been designed specifically for this population. Further, certain interventions should be used with caution when justice-involved youth are the target.

Some interventions developed specifically for delinquent adolescents have been found to be ineffective and even detrimental. Unfortunately, some such programs have been widely implemented. These include Scared Straight, or prison visitation programs; guided group interaction; positive peer culture; military-style boot camps; and wilderness challenges (Dodge et al. 2006). Such programs are more likely to have adverse effects under conditions of low supervision or insufficient staff training. One reason for these observed negative effects is the group format of such interventions, which can lead to deviant peer contagion or deviancy training, such that youth exit these programs and engage in more externalizing behaviors, delinquency, and substance use (Dodge et al. 2006). Simply being processed in the juvenile court system increases the chances of future offending, potentially in part because of being exposed to other youth with access to drugs, weapons, and gang affiliations. Therefore, it is important to consider not only the type of intervention but also the format. Some studies suggest that delinquent adolescents can be effectively treated for substance use in group formats when certain precautions are taken (e.g., Burleson et al. 2006; Dennis et al. 2004) (see Chapter 13 in this manual for more details). On the other hand, certain conditions may increase the chance of adverse effects, including detention with youth who committed the same crime, mandated long prison terms, group counseling by probation officers, and younger youth being brought into contact with older delinquent youth (Dodge et al. 2006).

Since youth with SUDs also have high rates of delinquency and justice system involvement (Hockenberry and Puzzanchera 2018), many substance use interventions discussed in previous chapters have been studied specifically with youth in the juvenile justice system. Comprehensive reviews of substance use treatments for adolescents have yielded mixed results for youth in the juvenile justice system (Hogue et al. 2018). For example, motivational interviewing was found to reduce substance use and delinquency in youth adjudicated for a substance-related first offense but was no more effective than treatment as usual. However, Adolescent Community Reinforcement Approach reduced substance use more than treatment as usual among adolescents under community supervision, although this study excluded youth with violent offenses (Hogue et al. 2018).

Some interventions developed specifically for juvenile justice populations, with the main goal of reducing reoffending, have been found to have positive effects on both externalizing behaviors and substance use. These include multisystemic therapy (MST) and functional family therapy (FFT), both of which are intensive family-based treatments targeting risk factors across multiple levels of the youth's ecology (i.e., individual, family, peer, and school) (McCart and Sheidow 2016). Both interventions have positive findings from studies with a range of youth offenders (e.g., chronic and violent juvenile offenders), outcomes (i.e., substance use and delinquent behaviors), and durability of effects (i.e., both short-term and long-term outcomes). These interventions are described further in other chapters.

Importantly, interventions developed either for justice-involved youth with substance use problems or for non-offending adolescents with substance use problems often overlap. For example, juvenile drug courts were introduced in the mid-1990s, and the aim of these courts is to divert youth from incarceration by offering court supervision, mental health and substance use treatment, and regular monitoring. A review failed to find overall support for the effectiveness of juvenile drug courts for reducing recidivism (Sullivan et al.

2016), potentially because of the lack of evidence-based principles employed in many such drug courts (e.g., lack of family involvement, use of educational treatments that have limited efficacy). However, juvenile drug courts have been found to be effective in reducing adolescent substance use and recidivism when courts employ evidence-based interventions such as MST and contingency management (CM) (Hogue et al. 2018). The Office of Juvenile Justice and Delinquency Prevention (2018) has developed Juvenile Drug Treatment Court Guidelines that emphasize a family- and evidence-based, treatment-oriented approach for youth, and a range of clinical and implementation resources from juvenile drug courts are available from the National Council of Juvenile and Family Court Judges (www.ncjfcj.org/our-work/juvenile-drug-courts).

Recently, within the juvenile drug court system, treatments such as CM, ecological family-based treatments (e.g., multidimensional family therapy, FFT), and group cognitive-behavioral therapy have been evaluated separately or in combination. Overall, these treatments have been found in individual studies to reduce substance use in justice-involved youth, though a combination of ecological family-based treatments and CM, known as Risk Reduction Therapy for Adolescents, was not found to improve substance use beyond the effects of juvenile drug court and usual services (Hogue et al. 2018).

Unique Challenges When Intervening With Substance Use in the Juvenile Justice System

Despite the high rates of substance use problems among justice-involved youth, availability of substance use treatment, particularly evidence-based treatment, is woefully limited. This limited availability is likely due to a variety of factors. The juvenile justice system's top priority is public safety rather than rehabilitation of juvenile offenders. Thus, assessment and treatment of substance use and other behavioral health needs are at best secondary concerns, despite evidence that successfully addressing these problems reduces recidivism and thus positively impacts public safety (Hoeve et al. 2014). In addition, a variety of logistical and systems-level barriers prevent youth from receiving effective treatments.

Access to substance use treatment and barriers to care for youth in the juvenile justice system vary based on the youth's placement. A majority of youth are under community supervision rather than in locked settings. Specifically, among youth processed and adjudicated delinquent by the juvenile justice system in 2014, 26% were placed in residential settings, 63% were placed on probation, and 11% received other sanctions (Hyland 2018). However, even though the majority of youth are not detained, most of the substance use treatment services provided to youth involved with the justice system occur in confined settings (Mulvey et al. 2007). These services are most often low intensity, including drug and alcohol education, and are rarely evidence based (Young et al. 2007). Family involvement in substance use treatment, a factor that is a key predictor of successful treatment (Hogue et al. 2018), is infrequently available to incarcerated youth. Lack of family involvement likely limits both treatment effectiveness and maintenance of gains past the time of detention, as the youth often return home to their families. In addition, many treatments in correctional facilities are delivered in a group format, which as mentioned earlier, may have unintended negative consequences (Dodge et al. 2006). Further, there is often a lack of continuity of care as youth transition to treatment providers in the community.

Justice-involved youth with substance use problems who are not in confined settings are most commonly referred to substance use treatment providers in the community. However, in many areas, referral rates to substance use services are low. One study found that only 65% of youth identified as having an SUD received a referral for substance use treatment (Hoeve et al. 2014), leaving a substantial number of youth with unmet treatment needs. Further, many youth who are referred for treatment never actually receive services. Johnson et al. (2004) found that less than half of youth entering the juvenile justice system with a substance use problem actually receive services. A more recent study estimated that only 25% of youth on probation receive treatment services, inclusive of both mental health and substance use treatment, and among those receiving services, only about 25% receive substance use treatment (White 2017). The likelihood of evidence-based care was even lower, with only 6.6% of youth on probation who received services actually getting an evidence-based treatment for either mental health or substance use (White 2017).

Barriers to services in the community include lack of sufficient health care coverage, inability to navigate the health care system, and, for many youth, lack of service providers in their communities. Very few youth involved with the justice system have access to private health insurance to cover the costs of treatment (White 2017). Thus, the costs of substance use treatment services must be covered by other sources, including federal block grants and public insurance (i.e., Medicaid, Children's Health Insurance Program), which covers a substantial proportion of justice-involved youth. Coverage by these programs is stopped but not terminated when a youth is incarcerated; however, reinstatement of this coverage after release can be challenging to navigate and time consuming, leaving gaps in coverage.

Even when youth do have adequate health care coverage and the resources to navigate the health care system, some communities simply do not have sufficient numbers of substance use treatment providers to meet youth's needs (see, e.g., Anderson and Gittler 2005). This shortage of providers is particularly true in rural areas. Justice-involved youth from rural communities are less likely to access substance use treatment (Pullmann and Heflinger 2009). Such youth are less likely to have health care coverage, fewer treatment providers practice in such areas, and many families lack the resources to travel long distances to seek treatment.

In addition to observable barriers to treatment, there is some evidence of bias in terms of identification and treatment of substance use problems in the juvenile justice system. Specifically, rates of referral to and receipt of substance use services among justice-involved youth can be predicted by specific characteristics of youth other than service need. For example, substantial racial disparities exist, such that minority youth in the justice system are less likely to be referred to substance use treatment (see Spinney et al. 2016 for a review). These disparities likely exacerbate other racial disparities, including the overall higher rates of minority youth who come into contact with the juvenile justice system (Hockenberry and Puzzanchera 2018) and lower rates of mental health and substance use treatment access for minority youth regardless of justice involvement (e.g., Kataoka et al. 2002). Age is also a significant predictor of treatment access, with younger adolescents more likely to be referred for treatment, independent of treatment need (e.g., Teplin et al. 2005). Thus, although need for substance use treatment should be the determining factor in referral to and receipt of services, other factors have been shown to influence access among justice-involved youth.

As noted above, even among youth who successfully access treatment, very few receive an evidence-based treatment. Family involvement is a key component of evidence-based substance use treatment for adolescents, even when they are not involved in the juvenile justice system (Hogue et al. 2018). However, one study found that only about a quarter of the treatments received by justice-involved youth had a family component (Chassin et al. 2009). This is problematic because family factors (e.g., parental substance use or criminal behavior, lack of appropriate monitoring and supervision) are strong predictors of both adolescent substance use and the types of delinquent behaviors that lead to justice involvement in youth (Barrett et al. 2014). Thus, targeting family risk factors may be particularly important in the treatment of SUDs among justice-involved youth, and intensive family treatment (e.g., MST, FFT) may be necessary in many cases.

In sum, substance use problems among justice-involved youth often go untreated, and even when treatments are available, they are unlikely to be evidence based. This is not surprising given that this group of youth have multiple competing treatment needs (i.e., delinquent behaviors, substance use, and often co-occurring mental health disorders). Nevertheless, provision of effective and comprehensive substance use treatment for this population is necessary to prevent recidivism and promote positive outcomes for these high-risk youth.

Falling Through the Cracks: Transition-Age Youth

The term *transition-age youth* refers to individuals ages 16–25 years. Compared with youth from all other age groups, transition-age youth report the highest initiation rates and overall use of illicit substances (Substance Abuse and Mental Health Services Administration 2017). Additionally, although transition-age youth make up less than 10% of the U.S. population, they account for 28% of arrests, 26% of probationers, and 28% of the jail population (Justice Policy Institute 2016). The rise in criminal activity is compounded by the transition to adulthood, because the justice system no longer views such behavior with a juvenile lens, and the young person may face criminal rather than juvenile delinquency charges.

Transition-age youth with substance use problems are at risk for poor outcomes. They have a fourfold greater probability of incarceration between ages 18 and 24 compared with those without substance use problems, and transition-age youth offenders with substance use problems are more likely to recidivate and continue offending into adulthood (Hoeve et al. 2014). Despite the great need for substance use services for these individuals, only 2% of transition-age youth with recognized substance use treatment needs report receiving any type of substance services (Substance Abuse and Mental Health Services Administration 2017). Service utilization declines sharply during the transition age because of the multiple barriers to services that occur during this period, including loss of health care coverage and the transition from child to adult service systems. Transition-age youth with justice system involvement face additional barriers, given the known difficulties of receiving substance use services in justice system settings. Further, they have the highest rates of dropout from substance use treatment and evidence the worst treatment outcomes, though these may vary based on type of substance use treatment received (Satre et al. 2004; Sinha et al. 2003; Smith et al. 2011).

For youth who struggle during the transition to adulthood, having multiple problems is the rule rather than the exception. This is compounded by the multiple transitions in life roles that occur during this important developmental period. During this period some of the following social role transitions are expected to occur: leaving home, gaining financial independence, gaining independence in decision making, making a partnership commitment, renegotiating relationships with parents, starting a career, becoming a parent, and engaging with the community and the wider social world. Success in these domains is determined by a complex interplay between youth, their families and neighborhoods, and available opportunities. This transitional period presents challenges for even the most well-adjusted youth as they navigate new roles.

As a result of all these changes, this developmental period is marked by experimentation and instability (Arnett 2005). Therefore, it is not surprising that the highest rates of illicit drug use are reported by transition-age youth (Substance Abuse and Mental Health Services Administration 2017). Arnett (2005) suggested that transition-age youth experiment with drugs and alcohol because they are curious about the experiences of using various substances and want to have a wide range of experiences before they settle into adult life. Additionally, since constructing a stable identity may be confusing and difficult, transition-age youth may use substances to relieve negative feelings stemming from identity confusion. Transition-age youth may also be more likely to use substances because of the stress and negative affect that are associated with disruptions in life (e.g., new residences, romantic partners, educational and vocational settings). This developmental period is also when individuals are most at risk for developing mental health disorders such as depression, generalized anxiety, schizophrenia, and bipolar disorder (Substance Abuse and Mental Health Services Administration 2017), compounding the difficulties that transition-age youth may experience. In addition, transition-age youth with substance use problems are often involved with the justice system, which is poorly equipped to meet their treatment needs.

Transition-age youth in the justice system have multiple barriers to the successful transition to adulthood compared with their non-justice-involved peers, many revolving around the risk factors previously discussed. For example, successful transitions to adulthood increasingly depend on financial and other material support from families well beyond adolescence, an advantage that many justice-involved youth do not have. Justice-involved youth have high rates of learning disabilities and school failure (Cruise et al. 2011), making successful vocational and/or higher education transitions difficult. High rates of involvement with the child welfare system, substantial histories of maltreatment, and increased likelihood of being placed in group home settings (Vidal et al. 2017) leave justice-involved transition-age youth with greatly compromised development and a lack of natural supports for transitioning to adulthood. Further, transferring youth from the juvenile to adult justice system can lead to poor outcomes for youth, including increased likelihood of arrest for future crimes (see Zane et al. 2016 for a review).

Currently, the juvenile justice system is struggling to find a balance between punishing delinquent acts and providing rehabilitative services in the best interest of the youth. Clinicians working with transition-age youth need to be informed of the aforementioned challenges and how they impact treatment provision and be prepared to assist these youth in navigating the various systems and developmental milestones that interact during this important life stage. Unfortunately, even though there is great need, there are no evidence-based practices targeting justice-related behaviors for this age group (McCart and Sheidow 2016). Further, there are no established treatments for substance use problems in general for transition-age youth (Hogue et al. 2018). Therefore, much more support and research are needed to close the gap on the unmet needs for this incredibly vulnerable, and often overlooked, population. The authors of this chapter, along with other investigators, have completed pilot work on adapting evidence-based practices that have been found to be effective in substance-using adolescents who are involved in the juvenile justice system, and are currently conducting a large-scale project to test the effectiveness of Multisystemic Therapy for Emerging Adults for transition-age youth who are involved in the juvenile justice system and have an SUD.

Case Vignette

Jamie, a 17-year-old female, grew up in a low-income neighborhood where community violence was common. Jamie was placed in foster care as a teenager, after allegations that her mother was neglectful as a result of her substance use problems and likely exposed Jamie to physical and sexual abuse from others who came in and out of their house. Once in foster care, Jamie began stealing her foster parents' pain pills and eventually started experimenting with heroin and other street drugs. Jamie's foster parents reported her to the police after discovering that she had stolen large sums of money from them. As a result, Jamie experienced her first contact with the juvenile justice system. While in detention, Jamie was identified as having a substance use problem and was required to attend an educational substance use group, but it only met once a week. After her release from detention, Jamie's caseworker was unable to find her a new foster family, and she was sent to live in a group home. She was referred to substance use treatment but never followed through because there were no drug treatment centers that treated adolescents nearby. Jamie had a hard time adjusting to her new living situation and learned tricks and tips from the other girls about how to access drugs and alcohol in the community and how to fake negative drug screens. She told her probation officer that she was having difficulty sleeping because of disturbing dreams related to childhood trauma. Jamie's probation officer recognized that, along with substance use problems, Jamie was having symptoms related to trauma and was able to schedule her an appointment with a mental health clinic. Unfortunately, after the intake assessment, the therapist discovered that Jamie could not be seen at the clinic because it did not accept Medicaid. While her probation officer was able to get her another appointment at a different clinic, her records were not transferred in time, and Jamie was frustrated that she had to complete another intake appointment and repeat her history to another clinician. Additionally, because of the clinician's high caseload, she was only able to see Jamie every other week and had limited training in substance use treatment. The clinician also primarily worked with adults, and Jamie felt like her therapist did not understand her problems. Then, Jamie had a slip-up and took too many pills when she was hanging out with her friends. While Jamie swore that it was accidental and that she lost track of how many pills she had taken, she was transferred to a residential substance use treatment facility that was 2 hours away from her hometown. Since this drug use was a violation of her probation, her involvement with the justice system was extended.

Commentary

Jamie's experience is all too common among youth with substance use problems in the juvenile justice system. The current system for rehabilitation often fails to address, or even presents barriers to meeting, the multiple needs of such youth. Many of the difficulties faced by Jamie are structural in nature (e.g., lack of substance use providers in her area, the need to rely on Medicaid for health care coverage), likely requiring state or federal policy and funding changes in order to be addressed adequately. Others may be addressed by more intensive services (e.g., MST, FFT) that are unlikely to be found at standard outpatient mental health clinics. Communities could consider investing funds in these evidence-based programs, because they offer cost savings in the long run by preventing the need for out-of-home placements. More attention needs to be paid to coordination of care for multiple needs (i.e., mental health, behavioral, substance use, vocational), since treatment of a single problem is unlikely to result in a positive outcome. Finally, individual clinics and clinicians can take action by seeking training in evidence-based treatments for adolescent substance use, particularly family-based models that are likely to have the greatest impact on justice-involved youth with substance use problems.

Key Points

- Substance use and delinquent behaviors have overlapping risk factors, and substance use predicts worse outcomes for youth involved in the juvenile justice system, including higher rates of recidivism.

- Interventions that include family members and target family-level risk factors for substance use are likely to be particularly important for youth in the justice system

- Group treatments for justice-involved youth should only be provided by experienced therapists to reduce the "deviancy training" effect between the adolescents.

- Youth in the juvenile justice system present unique intervention challenges, including receiving services across multiple providers who oftentimes have different priorities, problems with accessing providers who are trained to work with the specific population, and issues with family engagement.

- Transition-age youth involved in the justice system face even greater difficulties in trying to navigate both the youth and adult systems, and special attention is needed for their unique developmental needs and challenges.

References

Aarons GA, Brown SA, Hough RL, et al: Prevalence of adolescent substance use disorders across five sectors of care. J Am Acad Child Adolesc Psychiatry 40(4):419–426, 2001 11314567

Abram KM, Teplin LA, King DC, et al: PTSD, trauma, and comorbid psychiatric disorders in detained youth. Juvenile Justice Bulletin. Washington, DC, U.S. Department of Justice, Office of Justice Programs, Office of Juvenile Justice and Delinquency Prevention, 2013

Anderson RL, Gittler J: Unmet need for community-based mental health and substance use treatment among rural adolescents. Community Ment Health J 41(1):35–49, 2005 15932051

Arnett JJ: The developmental context of substance use in emerging adulthood. Journal of Drug Issues 35(2):235–254, 2005

Barrett DE, Katsiyannis A, Zhang D, et al: Delinquency and recidivism: a multicohort, matched-control study of the role of early adverse experiences, mental health problems, and disabilities. J Emot Behav Disord 22:3–15, 2014

Bechtel K, Lowenkamp CT, Latessa E: Assessing the risk of re-offending for juvenile offenders using the Youth Level of Service/Case Management Inventory. J Offender Rehabil 45:85–108, 2007

Belenko S, Logan TK: Delivering more effective treatment to adolescents: improving the juvenile drug court model. J Subst Abuse Treat 25(3):189–211, 2003 14670524

Borum R, Bartel P, Forth A: Manual for the Structured Assessment of Violence Risk in Youth (SAVRY). Odessa, FL, Psychological Assessment Resources, 2006

Burleson JA, Kaminer Y, Dennis ML: Absence of iatrogenic or contagion effects in adolescent group therapy: findings from the Cannabis Youth Treatment (CYT) study. Am J Addict 15 (suppl 1):4–15, 2006 17182415

Chassin L, Knight G, Vargas-Chanes D, et al: Substance use treatment outcomes in a sample of male serious juvenile offenders. J Subst Abuse Treat 36(2):183–194, 2009 18657942

Chassin L, Mansion A, Nichter B, et al: To Decrease Juvenile Offending, Make Effective Drug Treatment a Priority. Chicago, IL, MacArthur Foundation, 2014

Cruise KR, Evans LJ, Pickens IB: Integrating mental health and special education needs into comprehensive service planning for juvenile offenders in long-term custody settings. Learning and Individual Differences 21:30–40, 2011

Dembo R, Wareham J, Schmeidler J: Drug use and delinquent behavior: a growth model of parallel processes among high-risk youths. Criminal Justice and Behavior 34(5):680–696, 2007

Dennis M, Godley SH, Diamond G, et al: The Cannabis Youth Treatment (CYT) study: main findings from two randomized trials. J Subst Abuse Treat 27(3):197–213, 2004 15501373

Development Services Group: Intersection Between Mental Health and the Juvenile Justice System. Washington, DC, Office of Juvenile Justice and Delinquency Prevention, 2017

Dodge KA, Dishion TJ, Lansford JE (eds): Deviant Peer Influences in Programs for Youth: Problems and Solutions. New York, Guilford, 2006

Foley RM: Academic characteristics of incarcerated youth and correctional educational programs: A literature review. J Emot Behav Disord 9(4):248–259, 2001

Grisso T, Barnum R: Massachusetts Youth Screening Instrument–Version 2: User's Manual and Technical Report. Sarasota, FL, Professional Resource Press, 2006

Henry KL, Knight KE, Thornberry TP: School disengagement as a predictor of dropout, delinquency, and problem substance use during adolescence and early adulthood. J Youth Adolesc 41(2):156–166, 2012 21523389

Hockenberry S, Puzzanchera C: Juvenile Court Statistics 2016. Pittsburgh, PA, National Center for Juvenile Justice, 2018

Hoeve M, McReynolds LS, Wasserman GA: Service referral for juvenile justice youths: associations with psychiatric disorder and recidivism. Adm Policy Ment Health 41(3):379–389, 2014 23397231

Hogue A, Henderson CE, Becker SJ, Knight DK: Evidence base on outpatient behavioral treatments for adolescent substance use, 2014–2017: outcomes, treatment delivery, and promising horizons. J Clin Child Adolesc Psychol 47(4):499–526, 2018 29893607

Hser YI, Grella CE, Hubbard RL, et al: An evaluation of drug treatments for adolescents in 4 US cities. Arch Gen Psychiatry 58(7):689–695, 2001 11448377

Hyland N: Delinquency Cases in Juvenile Court, 2014. Washington, DC, U.S. Department of Justice, Office of Justice Programs, Office of Juvenile Justice and Delinquency Prevention, 2018

Ives ML, Chan YF, Modisette KC, et al: Characteristics, needs, services, and outcomes of youths in juvenile treatment drug courts as compared to adolescent outpatient treatment. Drug Court Review 7(1):10–56, 2010

Johnson TP, Cho YI, Fendrich M, et al: Treatment need and utilization among youth entering the juvenile corrections system. J Subst Abuse Treat 26(2):117–128, 2004 15050089

Justice Policy Institute: Improving approaches to serving young adults in the justice system. December 2016. Available at: http://www.justicepolicy.org/uploads/justicepolicy/documents/jpi_young_adults_final.pdf. Accessed May 16, 2019.

Kataoka SH, Zhang L, Wells KB: Unmet need for mental health care among U.S. children: variation by ethnicity and insurance status. Am J Psychiatry 159(9):1548–1555, 2002 12202276

Langrehr KJ: Racial distinctions in the psychosocial histories of incarcerated youth. Psychol Serv 8(1):23–35, 2011

McCart MR, Sheidow AJ: Evidence-based psychosocial treatments for adolescents with disruptive behavior. J Clin Child Adolesc Psychol 45(5):529–563, 2016 27152911

Molina BSG, Pelham WE Jr: Childhood predictors of adolescent substance use in a longitudinal study of children with ADHD. J Abnorm Psychol 112(3):497–507, 2003 12943028

Mulvey EP, Schubert CA, Chung HL: Service use after court involvement in a sample of serious adolescent offenders. Child Youth Serv Rev 29(4):518–544, 2007 19907667

National Institute on Drug Abuse: Principles of Drug Abuse Treatment for Criminal Justice Populations: A Research-Based Guide. Washington, DC, National Institutes of Health, U.S. Department of Health and Human Services, 2014

Office of Juvenile Justice and Delinquency Prevention: Juvenile drug treatment court guidelines. 2018. Available at: https://www.ojjdp.gov/Juvenile-Drug-Treatment-Court-Guidelines.html. Accessed May 16, 2019.

Orbis Partners: Validation of the Youth Assessment and Screening Instrument for Use by the Vermont Department for Children and Families. Ottawa, Ontario, Canada, 2011

Pullmann MD, Heflinger CA: Community determinants of substance abuse treatment referrals from juvenile courts: do rural youth have equal access? J Child Adolesc Subst Abuse 18(4):359–378, 2009 20890388

Rowe CL, Wang W, Greenbaum P, et al: Predicting HIV/STD risk level and substance use disorders among incarcerated adolescents. J Psychoactive Drugs 40(4):503–512, 2008 19283954

Ryan JP, Testa MF: Child maltreatment and juvenile delinquency: investigating the role of placement and placement instability. Child Youth Serv Rev 27(3):227–249, 2005

Satre DD, Mertens JR, Areán PA, et al: Five-year alcohol and drug treatment outcomes of older adults versus middle-aged and younger adults in a managed care program. Addiction 99(10):1286–1297, 2004 15369567

Schubert CA, Mulvey EP, Glasheen C: Influence of mental health and substance use problems and criminogenic risk on outcomes in serious juvenile offenders. J Am Acad Child Adolesc Psychiatry 50(9):925–937, 2011 21871374

Sinha R, Easton C, Kemp K: Substance abuse treatment characteristics of probation-referred young adults in a community-based outpatient program. Am J Drug Alcohol Abuse 29(3):585–597, 2003 14510042

Smith DC, Godley SH, Godley MD, et al: Adolescent Community Reinforcement Approach outcomes differ among emerging adults and adolescents. J Subst Abuse Treat 41(4):422–430, 2011 21831564

Spinney E, Yeide M, Feyerherm W, et al: Racial disparities in referrals to mental health and substance abuse services from the juvenile justice system: a review of the literature. Journal of Crime and Justice 39(1):153–173, 2016

Substance Abuse and Mental Health Services Administration: Key Substance Use and Mental Health Indicators in the United States: Results From the 2016 National Survey on Drug Use and Health (HHS Publ No SMA 17-5044, NSDUH Series H-52). 2017. Available at https://www.samhsa.gov/data/sites/default/files/NSDUH-FFR1–2016/NSDUH-FFR1–2016.htm. Accessed May 16, 2019.

Sullivan CJ, Blair L, Latessa E, et al: Juvenile drug courts and recidivism: results from a multisite outcome study. Justice Quarterly 33(2):291–318, 2016

Teplin LA, Abram KM, McClelland GM, et al: Detecting mental disorder in juvenile detainees: who receives services. Am J Public Health 95(10):1773–1780, 2005 16186454

Vidal S, Prince D, Connell CM, et al: Maltreatment, family environment, and social risk factors: determinants of the child welfare to juvenile justice transition among maltreated children and adolescents. Child Abuse Negl 63:7–18, 2017 27886518

Vincent GM, Perrault R: Risk Assessment and Behavioral Health Screening (RABS) Project Final Technical Report. Unpublished. Document No 251912, July 2018. Available at https://www.ncjrs.gov/pdffiles1/ojjdp/grants/251912.pdf. Accessed May 16, 2019.

Wachter A: Mental Health Screening in Juvenile Justice: JJGPS StateScan. Pittsburgh, PA, National Center for Juvenile Justice, 2015a

Wachter A: Statewide Risk Assessment in Juvenile Probation: JJGPS StateScan. Pittsburgh, PA, National Center for Juvenile Justice, 2015b

Wasserman GA, McReynolds LS, Schwalbe CS, et al: Psychiatric disorder, comorbidity, and suicidal behavior in juvenile justice youth. Criminal and Justice Behavior 37(12):1361–1376, 2010

White C: Treatment services in the juvenile justice system: examining the use and funding of services by youth on probation. Youth Violence and Juvenile Justice 17(1):62–87, 2017

Young DW, Dembo R, Henderson CE: A national survey of substance abuse treatment for juvenile offenders. J Subst Abuse Treat 32(3):255–266, 2007 17383550

Zane SN, Welsh BC, Mears DP: Juvenile transfer and the specific deterrence hypothesis: systematic review and meta-analysis. Criminology and Public Policy 15(3):901–925, 2016

23

Maternal Substance Use in Pregnancy

Amy M. Johnson, M.D., F.A.C.O.G.

Courtney Townsel, M.D., M.Sc., F.A.C.O.G.

Substance use in pregnancy is a significant concern at any age, affecting women of all racial, ethnic, and socioeconomic backgrounds. In many cases, abuse disorders may not be identified until the postpartum period. Alcohol and illicit and licit drugs can easily cross the placenta and have an impact on the developing fetus, and this can have long-term health consequences. Over the past 20 years, neonatal abstinence syndrome (NAS) has increased substantially in the United States. While individual substances can be associated with distinct sequelae, in general substance use in pregnancy places the fetus in jeopardy for numerous neonatal conditions, including intrauterine growth restriction, cardiac defects, and respiratory, neurological, infectious, hematological, and feeding problems, as well as prolonged hospital stays and a higher mortality rate (Hwang et al. 2017).

543

Substance use among adolescents significantly increases the incidence of high-risk sexual activity and sexually transmitted diseases (STDs). Although teenage pregnancy rates have decreased in the United States, substance use in adolescents remains a substantial concern. Adolescents who abuse substances report high rates of unplanned pregnancies as well as repeat unintended pregnancies. In a 2011 survey of pregnant teens ages 15–17, 18.3% reported illicit drug use in the prior month (Substance Abuse and Mental Health Services Administration 2013). In adolescents presenting for treatment for opioid use disorder (OUD), 91.9% reported sexual activity, 65% without contraception (Handy et al. 2018). Of those studied, 35% of adolescent patients reported a prior pregnancy and 16% an STD (Handy et al. 2018). Pregnant teens were more likely to report substance abuse in the prior 12 months than nonpregnant teens (with the exception of inhalants). More than half of pregnant teens reported using at least one illicit substance in the prior year—nearly double the rate in nonpregnant teens (Salas-Wright et al. 2015). Pregnant adolescents were also more likely to report the use of alcohol (15.8%), marijuana (14.5%), and controlled substances such as opioids (5.3%) (Salas-Wright et al. 2015). The highest risk of continued use during pregnancy appears to occur in early adolescents, ages 12–14 years old, and in those with a lack of parental involvement. However, the use of both licit and illicit substances does appear to decrease as the pregnancy progresses.

Screening

Universal screening in pregnancy for both prior and current substance use is recommended by several professional organizations, including the American College of Obstetricians and Gynecologists (ACOG), American Academy of Pediatrics (AAP), the U.S. Preventive Services Task Force, and the Centers for Disease Control and Prevention (CDC) (Wright et al. 2016). Substance use screening based solely on factors such as lack of prenatal care, race, ethnicity, or prior adverse pregnancy outcome can lead to significantly lower rates of diagnosis and adds to the culture of complicit or implicit bias providers should avoid (American College of Obstetricians and Gynecologists 2017b). Screening for substance use disorders (SUDs) in pregnancy may consist of maternal interviews and drug toxicology testing. Obtaining a history using open-ended questions in a nonjudgmental fashion is more likely to result in patient disclosure of substance use. Several validated screening questionnaires are available for routine screening for substance abuse in pregnancy (Table 23–1). Substance use screening should occur at the initial prenatal appointment for all patients and then in the subsequent trimesters for women with risk factors such as a positive initial screen for current or past substance use (Wright et al. 2016).

Urine drug testing may be used as an adjunct to screening questionnaires and interviews. Some obstetric practices perform routine urine drug screening on all patients at the initial intake. However, urine drug testing should not be performed without first obtaining patient consent. Pregnant women may decline drug toxicology testing because of fears of reporting of positive test results to authorities, loss of child custody, and denial of welfare benefits after delivery (Pulatie 2008). Obstetric providers should prioritize the patient-practitioner relationship by using positive screening and toxicology test results as an opportunity for intervention, and not to shame or criminalize patients. Women who continue to use substances in pregnancy have better maternal and infant outcomes if they attend routine prenatal appointments. Nondisclosure or refusal to complete urine toxicology screening may have a negative impact on maternal and neonatal outcomes. Universal screening increases proper identification of exposures in pregnancy, allowing for the development of appropriate treatment plans, and provides practitioners the opportunity to observe for evidence of NAS in drug-exposed pregnancies after delivery.

Review of Substances and Pregnancy Risks

Determining the potential effects of each individual substance on the mother or fetus can be difficult. Research is limited by underreporting of prenatal exposure, and polysubstance abuse is frequent. Furthermore, the risk of prenatal drug use depends on not only the type of substance but also the timing of exposure and dose effects. Medication and substance use during the first trimester may increase the risk of congenital abnormalities or spontaneous abortion. Exposure during the second and third trimester, particularly if it is chronic, may increase the risk of poor fetal growth, neurodevelopmental delay, placental abruption (i.e., a shearing of the placenta from the uterine wall), pregnancy loss, and NAS. Additional concerns include maternal malnutrition with poor weight gain, lack of adequate health care, increased risk of infectious diseases,

Table 23–1. Substance use screening in pregnancy

Screening test	Substance	Description
T-ACE[a] (Sokol et al. 1989) Positive screen ≥ 2 points	Alcohol	**Tolerance** (2 points) *How many drinks does it take to feel first effect?*
		Annoyance (1 point) *Have people annoyed you by criticizing your drinking?*
		Cut-down (1 point) *Have you felt you should cut down on your drinking?*
		Eye-opener (1 point) *Have you ever had a drink first thing in the morning to steady your nerves or get rid of a hangover?*
TWEAK[a] (Chan et al. 1993) Positive screen ≥ 3 points	Alcohol	**Tolerance** (2 points) *Requires 3 or more drinks to feel effect*
		Worry (2 points) *Has family or friends worried or complained about your drinking in the past year?*
		Eye-opener (1 point) *Do you sometimes take a drink in the morning when you first get up?*
		Amnesia (1 point) *Has a friend or family member told you about something you said or did while you were drinking that you could not remember?* (blackout)
		Cut down (1 point) *Do you sometimes feel a need to cut down on your drinking?*

Table 23–1. Substance use screening in pregnancy (continued)

Screening test	Substance	Description
AUDIT-C[a] (Bush et al. 1998) Maximum score is 12 Positive screen ≥ 2	Alcohol	*How often do you have a drink containing alcohol?* Never (0), monthly (1), 2–4×/month (2), 2–3×/week (3), ≥4×/week (4)
		How many drinks containing alcohol do you have on a typical day when you drink? 1–2 (0), 3–4 (1), 5–6 (2), 7–9 (3), ≥10 (4)
		How often do you have 6 or more drinks on one occasion? Never (0), <monthly (1), monthly (2), 2–3×/month (3), ≥4×/month (4)
ASSIST[b] (WHO ASSIST Working Group 2002)	Any substance	Categorizes individuals: **High risk** (score ≥27) *Advise, Assess, Assist Arrange referral*
		Moderate risk (score 4–26) *Advise, Assess, Assist*
		Low risk (score 0–3)
4P's Plus[a] (Chasnoff et al. 2007) Associated with a licensing fee Positive screen if admission to use month prior to pregnancy	Any substance	*Problem with alcohol or drugs* **Parents?** **Partner?** In the **Past** have you ever used alcohol? In the month before you knew you were **Pregnant**, how many cigarettes did you smoke? How much alcohol did you drink?

Table 23–1. Substance use screening in pregnancy *(continued)*

Screening test	Substance	Description
SURP-P[a] (Yonkers et al. 2010)	Any substance	*In the month before you knew you were Pregnant how much alcohol (beer, wine, liquor) did you drink?* Never (0), Any (1) *Have you ever felt you need to cut down on your drug or alcohol use?* # of affirmative items = score 0–low risk, 1 = moderate risk, 2–3 = high risk
CRAFFT[a,b] (Knight et al. 2002)	Any substance	Ever ridden in a **Car** driven by you or someone else who was "high" or had been using drugs or alcohol? Do you ever use drugs or alcohol to **Relax**? Do you ever use drugs or alcohol **Alone**? Do you **Forget** things you did while using drugs or alcohol? Have **Friends/Family** ever told you to cut down on alcohol or drug use? Ever gotten in **Trouble** while using alcohol or drugs? (Each positive answer = 1 point)

Note. ASSIST = Alcohol, Smoking and Substance Involvement Screening Test; AUDIT-C = Alcohol Use Disorders Identification Test—Consumption; SURP-P = Substance Use Risk Profile—Pregnancy.
[a]Validated in pregnant women.
[b]Validated in adolescents.

and presence of psychiatric illnesses, all of which can have a negative impact on the fetus.

Opioids

Opioids are a class of drugs that include illegal formulations such as heroin (diamorphine); synthetic forms such as fentanyl; prescription forms such as hydromorphone; and over-the-counter forms such as loperamide, which is used for diarrhea. Opioids act by binding the opioid receptors (μ, δ, and κ), which are responsible for mediating psychoactive and somatic effects. The central nervous system action of opioid drugs has led to their potential for misuse and abuse. Mirroring the U.S. opioid epidemic, the rate of opioid use or dependence in pregnancy rose almost fivefold, from 1.9 to 5.77 per 1,000 pregnancies between 2000 and 2009 (Patrick et al. 2012). It is noteworthy that fatal and nonfatal overdose incidents have been reported among pregnant and postpartum women using opiates (Schiff et al. 2018). Overdoses were lowest in the third trimester and highest 7–12 months after delivery. Women with OUD who received pharmacotherapy had reduced overdose rates in the vulnerable early postpartum period. Incorporating pregnancy recovery centers for pregnant and postpartum women with OUD may improve OUD outcomes (Krans et al. 2018).

Drug withdrawal in newborns caused by exposure in utero is called *neonatal abstinence syndrome* or *neonatal opioid withdrawal* when the maternal drug exposure is to opioids. Opioid use in pregnancy has been associated with numerous poor outcomes for the fetus and infant. These conditions include but are not limited to preterm delivery, birth defects (e.g., neural tube, cardiac, gastroschisis), low birth weight, sudden infant death syndrome (SIDS), and difficulty controlling maternal pain following cesarean birth (American College of Obstetricians and Gynecologists 2017b; Broussard et al. 2011; Yazdy et al. 2013). NAS or neonatal opioid withdrawal entails a spectrum of symptoms in the neonate that typically occur within the first 3 days of delivery or as late as 2 weeks. Caused by the sudden withdrawal from the substance used by the mother, NAS can be a life-threatening condition but typically results in mild to moderate symptoms with a prolonged hospital stay. Infants may exhibit excessive high-pitched crying, poor feeding, mottling of skin, fever, and even seizures (Logan et al. 2013). Initial treatment includes symptomatic and nonpharmacological support but often necessitates treatment with tapering doses of morphine. Symptoms can last up to 6 months after delivery. Because of the growing opioid epidemic in pregnancy, the incidence of NAS has dramatically increased, from 7 to 27 neonatal intensive care unit (NICU) admissions per 1,000 deliveries between 2004 and 2013, and has accounted for an estimated $1.5 billion in additional health care costs (Patrick et al. 2012; Tolia et al. 2015).

Marijuana (Cannabis)

Marijuana is the substance most commonly used during pregnancy in the United States. The psychoactive compound Δ-9-tetrahydrocannabinol (THC) in marijuana binds the cannabinoid receptor CB1 to exhibit the drug's effects. Children exposed in utero to cannabis present with permanent neurobehavioral and cognitive impairments. On a molecular level, repeated THC exposure disrupts endocannabinoid signaling with CB1 receptors. THC alters axon morphology, and this affects the computational power of neural circuitries (Tortoriello et al. 2014).

Self-reported rates of marijuana use average 2%–5%, with rates as high as 15%–28% in young, urban, socioeconomically disadvantaged individuals (Substance Abuse and Mental Health Services Administration 2013). Adolescent girls who use marijuana are more likely to participate in high-risk behaviors such as alcohol use and condomless sex and to surround themselves with negative peer influences, compared with adolescents who abstain from marijuana (Tzilos Wernette et al. 2018). A recent survey in Colorado found that 69% of cannabis dispensaries contacted recommended marijuana by phone to pregnant women who were wondering if it would help with first-trimester morning sickness (Dickson et al. 2018). A longitudinal study of 648 mothers showed that at age 5 children who had been exposed to marijuana (at least 1 joint per day) in the first trimester had a mean IQ that was 6 points lower than that in youth who had not had such exposure (Goldschmidt et al. 2008). At age 10, children in the same cohort who had been exposed to marijuana in the first trimester were about twice as likely to have depression compared with youth who had not been exposed (Gray et al. 2005). Then, at age 14 these youth were about 12 times more likely to have used marijuana compared with youth not exposed in utero and scored significantly lower on tests of school achievement (Day et al. 2006; Goldschmidt et al. 2012). This finding remained significant even after researchers controlled for current parental use of marijuana. Consequently, there is no known safe amount of marijuana use during pregnancy.

It is difficult to draw causal links between in utero or childhood marijuana exposure and subsequent impairments because it is unethical to randomly assign humans in research to a potentially toxic substance versus placebo. However, results from animal studies in which adolescent-phase animals were exposed to either THC (or similar pharmacological agent) or placebo were consistent with those from human studies. Most notable findings included adult deficits in attention, memory, motivation, and social interaction (Rubino and Parolaro 2016).

The ACOG recommends that pregnant women or those considering pregnancy discontinue the use of marijuana because of the potential neonatal risks (American College of Obstetricians and Gynecologists 2017a). Consequences of use include potential negative effects on fetal brain development, low birth weight, increased risk of stillbirth, and increased risk of preterm delivery. In addition, prenatal marijuana use has been associated with the potential for behavioral problems and attention-deficit/hyperactivity disorder (ADHD) in exposed school-age children. Since the legalization of marijuana in the state of Colorado, the rates of cardiac defects (ventricular septal defects and hypoplastic heart) have increased. However, further studies are needed to determine the true effect.

Synthetic marijuana formulations known as "K2" or "Spice" have become popular and are created by spraying various chemicals on plants before drying. These formulations are not marijuana per se, but they bind the same cannabinoid receptors in the central nervous system and other organs. The effects are more profound than those of marijuana and more unpredictable and include paranoia, seizures, hallucinations, aggression, cardiac symptoms (e.g., palpitations, chest pain), and even death (Tournebize et al. 2017). The rate of K2 or Spice use among adolescents ranges from 2% to 3.7% when 8th, 10th, and 12th graders are examined (National Institute on Drug Abuse for Teens 2017). Adolescent females are less likely than adolescent males to use these formulations, but providers should be aware of their growing popularity and harmful effects. Although there is a paucity of data on K2 or Spice exposure in pregnancy, the above maternal effects are certainly detrimental to the fetus. For more information on cannabis, see Chapter 9 in this manual.

Alcohol

No amount of alcohol is considered to be safe at any time in pregnancy. All women should be screened for and educated on the potential negative effects of alcohol use during pregnancy. In utero exposure has been shown to increase the risk of fetal alcohol syndrome (FAS). In 2010 the CDC estimated that in the United States 0.3 of every 1,000 children ages 7–9 years are living with FAS (Denny et al. 2019). However, the National Institutes of Health report that rates could be as high as 1%–5% of school-age children (May et al. 2018). Research and diagnosis can be clouded by the lack of confirmation of maternal alcohol use. Historically, controversy has surrounded the accuracy of the diagnostic criteria in the absence of confirmation of fetal alcohol exposure, and diagnosis is often based on phenotypic findings. The signs of FAS include both physical and developmental conditions, such as low birth weight, abnormal facial features, small head size, poor motor control, speech delay, hyperactive disorders, learning disabilities, and low IQ. Classic facial features include a flat upper lip, philtrum, and midface; smaller eye openings, and skin folds at the corner of the eyes (Warren and Foudin 2001). Infants and children may also exhibit visual and hearing impairment, feeding difficulties, and poor eye-hand coordination skills. A variety of symptoms can occur secondary to alcohol exposure and can be classified within the fetal alcohol spectrum disorders. These include not only FAS but also alcohol-related neurodevelopmental disorder and alcohol-related birth defects. Birth defects can include cardiac anomalies, renal agenesis, bone problems, and neural tube defects. Spontaneous abortions and stillbirths are increased in women who report moderate to heavy alcohol use in pregnancy.

Management options for women with alcohol abuse in pregnancy should be individualized. Behaviorial therapy is a mainstay of treatment. Regarding medication-assisted treatment (MAT), disulfiram, acamprosate, and naltrexone are classified as category C medications in pregnancy (DeVido et al. 2015). In addition, patients should be treated for potential nutritional deficiencies. The diagnosis of alcohol withdrawal syndrome in pregnancy can be delayed in those who do not offer a history of alcohol use because hypertension, tachycardia, headache, delirium, and seizures can be mistaken for preeclampsia or eclampsia. Just as in the nonpregnant state, alcohol withdrawal can be life threatening and should be treated. Pregnant women in withdrawal are at additional risk for placental abruption and hemorrhage. The data surrounding the potential risks of short-term benzodiazepines in pregnancy for the treatment of acute withdrawal are limited. Concern exists for the potential for teratogenic effects when benzodiazepines are used in the first trimester as well as hypotonia and respiratory depression if they are used near the time of delivery. However, given the potentially fatal consequences of withdrawal, pregnant women should receive appropriate care in order to ensure their safety.

Cocaine

Cocaine is an addictive stimulant, derived from coca plant leaves, that leads to dopamine release within the brain, causing the characteristic "high" described by users. There are two chemical forms of cocaine: the water-soluble hydrochloride salt (white powder) and the water-insoluble form known as "crack" or "freebase." In general, the cocaine powder is snorted through the nose or rubbed on a mucous membrane (e.g., gums). This form may also be dissolved and injected into the bloodstream. "Speedball" is a term used when both cocaine and heroin are injected concurrently. Crack cocaine is smoked and can be combined with marijuana or tobacco to be inhaled much as with a cigarette. Understanding the type of drug and how it is administered is important in determining the risk level for the patient. Intravenous drugs and risky sexual behavior that can be seen in cocaine abusers further increase the threat of contracting communicable diseases such as HIV disease and hepatitis C (Cain et al. 2013).

Cocaine abuse in pregnancy is associated with significant negative maternal and neonatal outcomes. In addition to overdose, mothers are at risk of myocardial infarction, cardiac arrhythmias, stroke, and hypertensive crisis. The increased risk of placental abruption places the fetus at considerable jeopardy of stillbirth, preterm delivery, and prematurity. Other risks include precipitous delivery, premature rupture of membranes, and low birth weight (Cain et al. 2013; Cressman et al. 2014). Prenatal cocaine exposure can lead to poorer adolescent functioning, poorer perceptual reasoning, impairment in procedural learning, higher rates of oppositional defiant disorder and ADHD, diminished short-term memory, and impaired language development (Cressman et al. 2014).

Amphetamines

Classified as a stimulant, amphetamines are used to treat various conditions such as ADHD and narcolepsy. Often patients do not realize that prescription amphetamines, such as methylphenidate, have a high potential for tolerance and abuse. Amphetamines and their by-products readily cross the placenta and are concentrated in breast milk. Methylphenidate has been shown to cause adverse events in animal models, but research on prescription use in pregnancy is limited. Prenatal amphetamine exposure has been shown to increase the risk of intrauterine growth restriction, preterm delivery, and low birth weight (Wright et al. 2015). Therefore, prescription use in pregnancy should be individualized to patients in whom the risks of discontinuing the medication to the mother outweigh the potential risks to the fetus.

The use of 3,4-methylenedioxymethamphetamine (MDMA), also known as "Ecstasy" or "Molly," is prevalent in younger women. Lower milestone and motor quality scores at 4 months of life were noted in infants born to women who used MDMA during pregnancy (Singer et al. 2012). Although in one study D-amphetamine use was associated with an increased risk of fetal anomalies, other studies have failed to demonstrate such risk (Heinonen 1977; Milkovich and van der Berg 1977; Nelson and Forfar 1971). Severe hyperthermia can occur with MDMA intoxication. Exposure to high temperatures during the first trimester has been associated with neural tube defects. Other common side effects of acute MDMA intoxication include transient hypertension and tachycardia. Such symptoms could be particularly dangerous in a pregnant patient with preexisting hypertension, gestational hypertension, or underlying cardiac conditions.

Methamphetamines are a more potent version of amphetamines, and use has been on the rise since the 1980s in the general population. Consumption in pregnant women has also increased significantly. Admission rates for treatment of methamphetamine abuse among pregnant women rose from 8% in 1994 to 28% in 2006 (American College of Obstetricians and Gynecologists 2011). In addition to its addictive potential, methamphetamine is associated with maternal seizures, arrhythmias, hyperthermia, and hypertension. These conditions can be especially concerning in a pregnant patient, and use has been associated with placental abruption and preterm delivery as well as fetal and neonatal loss (Gorman et al. 2014). Intrauterine growth restriction has been shown to be 3.5 times more likely in women using methamphetamines during pregnancy, even after confounding factors such as alcohol, maternal weight, and tobacco use are taken into account (Smith et al. 2006). Exposed infants are more likely to require admission to the NICU, have a small head circumference, and suffer from poor latching with breastfeeding (Shah et al. 2012). Case reports indicate a potential for an increased risk of congenital anomalies, including cleft palate, limb defects, and cardiac and central nervous system anomalies as well as gastroschisis (Elliott et al. 2009; Forrester and Merz 2007; Golub et al. 2005). However teratogenic effects have not been confirmed with larger cohort studies. Women using methamphetamines are more likely to seek prenatal care later in the pregnancy or not at all. In addition, poor maternal weight gain is associated with active use.

Phencyclidine/Hallucinogens

Phencyclidine (PCP or "angel dust") was initially developed as an anesthetic for use in the 1950s but was subsequently taken off the market secondary to the side effects of confusion, hallucinations, delirium, and agitation. PCP can induce paranoia, violent behavior, and feelings of impending death and mimics the symptoms of schizophrenia (Fico and Vanderwende 1989). The medication was subsequently used only as a veterinary anesthetic. However, in the 1970s and early 1980s it again emerged as a popular drug of abuse secondary to low cost, readily available ingredients, and ease of manufacturing. More recently, PCP use has been on the rise again. PCP readily crosses the placenta and into breast milk. Although studies are limited by small sample size, in utero exposure to PCP has been associated with numerous adverse neonatal outcomes. Negative effects range from low birth weight and sleep disturbances to temperament problems and, potentially, NAS (Chasnoff et al. 1983; Wachsman et al. 1989). Several potential fetal neurobehavioral effects of PCP use during pregnancy have been reported and include jitteriness, blank staring, and hyperactivity (Golden et al. 1984).

Inhalants

Inhalant use is common among adolescents, with as many as 20% of teenagers reporting at least one prior attempt. Since numerous chemicals can be inhaled, the effects vary significantly. The most concerning side effects of inhalants are arrhythmias, sudden cardiac arrest, seizures, and asphyxiation. Chronic inhalation of volatile substances such as toluene can damage the maternal nervous system, producing effects similar to those of multiple sclerosis. Prenatal exposure of toluene has been associated with decreased birth weight, skeletal abnormalities, and delayed neurobehavioral development (Jones and Balster 1998). There are numerous case reports linking prenatal exposure to inhalant use to fetal craniofacial abnormalities, spontaneous abortion, and decreased fertility. However, more vigorous research is lacking.

Management During Pregnancy

In general, abstinence from substance use in pregnancy and lactation is advocated because of the known associated poor pregnancy outcomes and developmental implications for the exposed fetus. As mentioned previously, all women entering pregnancy should be screened for substance use and abuse. When a pregnant woman screens positive, the offending agent(s) should be identified and the risk(s) of specific use in pregnancy and on neonatal outcomes should be reviewed with the patient. Providers are obligated to observe the principles of medical ethics; beneficence, nonmaleficence, justice, and respect for autonomy (Table 23–2). When a provider identifies an SUD, offering brief interventions or alternatives such as quitting, cutting back, or seeking help is as effective as conventional treatment and can promote reduced use, improve health, and decrease health care costs (American College of Obstetricians and Gynecologists 2015). The concept of confidentiality is especially important in building the physician-patient relationship when caring for adolescents. Trust can increase the willingness of the patient to disclose health-related behaviors like substance use. Physicians must consider the principles of informed consent, adolescent assent, and parental permission when screening for and identifying SUDs among pregnant adolescents (American College of Obstetricians and Gynecologists 2015). State laws vary significantly in regard to the care of both minor and adult pregnant women.

Antepartum Care, Labor, and Delivery

For care of pregnant women with SUDs, a multidisciplinary approach can be beneficial. Providers should consider consultation with addiction medicine services, maternal fetal medicine specialists, behavioral health providers, nutritionists, and social workers. Substance use has been associated with higher rates of STDs and condomless sex. Providers should offer expanded screening for STDs at the initial prenatal visit and again in the third trimester. Patients should be screened for hepatitis C as well as immunity to hepatitis B and offered vaccination if appropriate. In addition, a plan for reliable postpartum contraception should be developed during the antepartum period. Urine toxicology should be performed with patient consent during each trimester or more frequently if requested by addiction or social services. Many women with

Table 23–2. Ethical approach to caring for the pregnant adolescent with substance use disorder

Beneficence	Treat with respect and dignity. Establish a therapeutic alliance.
Nonmaleficence	Avoid stigmatization and humiliation. Show empathy and support.
Justice	Provide equitable, fair nondiscriminatory care. Provide preventive education. Refer for treatment.
Autonomy	Notify patients of toxicology screening prior to performing. Offer hope and resources.

Source. Adapted from American College of Obstetricians and Gynecologists 2015.

SUDs have concurrent depression and anxiety and should be screened and treated for these disorders in pregnancy.

Providers should plan to monitor fetal growth with serial prenatal ultrasounds in women with ongoing substance use because of the high incidence of intrauterine growth restriction in this population. Higher rates of stillbirth have not consistently been observed across substance-exposed pregnancies when compared with pregnancies without drug exposure. Routine antenatal surveillance beginning between 32 and 34 weeks for ongoing SUDs is controversial and should be individualized. Antenatal surveillance may include fetal non-stress tests with amniotic fluid assessment or biophysical profile (Table 23–3). Women with known SUDs do not require preterm (<37 weeks) or early term (37 0/7 weeks–38 6/7 weeks) delivery unless obstetric indications arise (e.g., preeclampsia, preterm premature rupture of membranes, placental abruption, significant intrauterine growth restriction). The mode of delivery should be determined by usual obstetric practice (based on, e.g., fetal position, maternal and fetal status, prior obstetric mode of delivery, and current obstetric complications).

Special Considerations for Opioid Use in Pregnancy

Opioid agonist pharmacotherapy or MAT in combination with counseling and behavioral therapy is the recommended treatment for OUD in pregnancy (American College of Obstetricians and Gynecologists 2017b). Both metha-

Table 23–3.   Antepartum management for pregnancies with substance use disorder

Ancillary consultations (e.g., MFM, social work, nutrition, addiction medicine)

Expanded STD screening

Expanded depression screening

Serial prenatal ultrasounds to assess fetal growth

Antenatal surveillance[a] (e.g., IUGR, preeclampsia, antepartum bleeding)

Note.   MFM = maternal fetal medicine; STD = sexually transmitted disease; IUGR = intrauterine growth restriction.
[a]Routine antenatal surveillance beginning between 32 and 34 weeks for ongoing substance use disorders is controversial and should be reserved for standard obstetric indications.

done (opioid receptor agonist) and buprenorphine (mixed opioid receptor agonist) are used as replacement therapy for patients with opioid dependence. These agents are preferred to medically assisted withdrawal because withdrawal has been associated with higher rates of relapse (American College of Obstetricians and Gynecologists 2017b).

Methadone is dispensed daily through a registered comprehensive opioid treatment program. Maternal methadone dosages usually require up-titration in pregnancy, because of the physiological increased volume of distribution, to avoid withdrawal symptoms (e.g., nausea, abdominal cramps, irritability, anxiety) (American College of Obstetricians and Gynecologists 2017b). Providers should counsel pregnant women receiving MAT that maternal dose and duration of MAT do not predict severity of NAS. Therefore, pregnant women receiving MAT should be maintained on the dose of medication that controls their withdrawal symptoms. Although methadone is currently the most common pharmacotherapy agent in pregnancy, buprenorphine has been shown to result in lower rates of NAS. Women who enter pregnancy while taking methadone should not be switched to buprenorphine because of the potential for withdrawal due to buprenorphine's partial agonist properties. Buprenorphine is available as a monoproduct (Subutex) and in combination with naloxone (Suboxone), an opioid antagonist, to reduce diversion. Studies have found no adverse effects and similar outcomes when comparing buprenorphine alone to the combination of buprenorphine and naloxone. Patients who desire buprenorphine must have access to providers with prescribing privileges. Access remains a considerable barrier to buprenorphine use in many areas throughout the country.

Pregnant women receiving MAT who are in labor should have their medication dose continued and should be offered additional pain relief options (e.g., epidural, spinal). However, mixed agonists/antagonists, such as nalbuphine, should be avoided because use with methadone can lead to acute withdrawal. Consultation with anesthesiology may also be considered at the onset of labor because of increased analgesic requirements and higher drug tolerance in women who are receiving MAT. The pregnancy dose of MAT should be continued during the postpartum period and supplemented as appropriate with anti-inflammatory agents and short-acting opioids for pain control. Pediatric staff must be notified of maternal opioid use to optimally assess the infant for NAS.

Postpartum Period

Active substance use of any kind is discouraged during the postpartum period. Significant safety and legal concerns exist when a parent is caring for a child while using both illicit and licit drugs. Substance use during pregnancy and the postpartum period is associated with substantial neonatal and childhood complications. Children born to women who are substance abusers are more likely to have neurodevelopmental delay, ADHD, and poor performance in school and are at a higher risk of substance abuse themselves. Postpartum use decreases the success for maternal and infant bonding and increases the potential for neglect and child abuse.

Although substance use typically decreases during pregnancy, it often subsequently resumes or increases during the first 1–2 years of the postpartum period. The most likely time period of resumption is the first 6 months (Carroll Chapman and Wu 2013). Because this is a particularly vulnerable time period, providers should consider earlier and more frequent follow-up for at-risk individuals. Routine urine toxicology may be useful because only half of those with a positive toxicology self-reported use. Adolescents with a history of depression are three to six times more likely to resume using substances in the postpartum period.

Reliable contraception is an important part of postpartum care. Both adolescents and substance abusers are at increased risk for unintended and short-interval pregnancy. Long-acting reversible contraception (LARC) is the preferred method. Options include intrauterine devices (IUD; multiple types) and the subdermal progesterone implant. Both progesterone and copper IUDs have been shown to be over 99% effective in preventing pregnancy and can be used continuously for 5–10 years depending on the type. Likewise, the subdermal progesterone implant is equally effective and can be used up to 3–4 years. With LARC, unlike birth control pills (which have poor compliance and higher rates of failure), once the contraception is placed, the patient does not need to worry about contraception for several years. In many instances, LARC can be initiated at the time of delivery. High rates of noncompliance with postpartum care have been noted in this population, and therefore ensuring that the patient leaves the hospital with an effective form of contraception is imperative.

In general, breastfeeding has been shown to have numerous short-term and long-term advantages over formula feeding. Benefits to the infant include a decreased risk of obesity, infection (including respiratory and gastrointestinal), diabetes, and SIDS. However, breastfeeding is typically discouraged in women actively using illicit substances. The risk versus benefit of breastfeeding should be carefully weighed in each individual patient. Determination of activity, the substances in question, and potential coexisting medical conditions (such as HIV infection or hepatitis C) of both the infant and mother should be considered.

The ACOG recommends that women be encouraged to breastfeed if they are stable on their opioid agonists and are no longer using illicit drugs. In the event of a relapse, women should stop breastfeeding (American College of Obstetricians and Gynecologists 2017a). Breastfeeding in women who are receiving methadone or buprenorphine is associated with a decreased risk of NAS, shorter infant hospital stays, and a decreased need for maternal pharmacotherapy (Bagley et al. 2014). In addition, breastfeeding promotes maternal infant bonding and provides passive immunity to the infant. Patients who are enrolled in a substance abuse program and have negative urine toxicology screening may be candidates for breastfeeding.

Both the ACOG and AAP advise against the use of marijuana in breastfeeding women (Ryan et al. 2018). Marijuana crosses the placenta and is concentrated in breast milk. The AAP notes that available data indicate the potential for neurodevelopmental delay and behavioral consequences subsequent to concomitant marijuana use and breastfeeding (Bagley et al. 2014).

The CDC warns that mothers should not breastfeed or feed expressed breast milk to infants if the mother is using illicit drugs such as PCP or cocaine (Centers for Disease Control and Prevention 2018). Cocaine is expressed in high concentrations in breast milk. Newborns are particularly sensitive, because they lack the ability to metabolize the drug, and serious adverse events have been reported including infant intoxication, respiratory distress, and seizures. In addition, cocaine may frequently be contaminated with various other substances. The Academy of Breastfeeding Medicine recommends that women with a history of cocaine use should not breastfeed unless they have negative urine toxicology results at the time of delivery, are in a treatment program, and have abstained from use for at least 90 days.

Methamphetamines have been shown to decrease breast milk supply by reducing prolactin levels. In addition, methamphetamine levels in breast milk are 2.8–7.5 times higher than that found in the maternal plasma (National Library of Medicine 2019). PCP concentrates within breast milk at high levels and can lead to infant intoxication. Therefore, breastfeeding is contraindicated in women actively using methamphetamines or PCP.

Women should continue their opioid agonist pharmacotherapy during the postpartum period because this is a time of particularly high risk for relapse. All women should be screened for postpartum depression, the incidence of which increases in women with SUDs. Thus, it is a particularly important time to reassess patients and ensure that they have access to necessary support systems and health care. Patients may benefit from early and frequent follow-up as well as social services support. In addition, patients and family members should receive overdose training and a naloxone prescription.

Key Points

- Substance abuse in adolescents is a risk factor for unintended pregnancy.

- Substance type, cumulative dose, and timing of use correlate with the potential pregnancy risk(s).

- Although substance use typically decreases during pregnancy, adolescents are at risk for increased use during the first 6 months postpartum.

- Breastfeeding is contraindicated in patients actively using substances.

References

American College of Obstetricians and Gynecologists: Methamphetamine abuse in women of reproductive age. Committee Opinion No 479, March 2011. Available at: https://www.acog.org/Clinical-Guidance-and-Publications/Committee-Opinions/Committee-on-Health-Care-for-Underserved-Women/Methamphetamine-Abuse-in-Women-of-Reproductive-Age?IsMobileSet=false. Accessed May 17, 2019.

American College of Obstetricians and Gynecologists: Alcohol abuse and other substance use disorders: ethical issues in obstetric and gynecologic practice. Committee Opinion No 633, June 2015. Available at: https://www.acog.org/-/media/Committee-Opinions/Committee-on-Ethics/co633.pdf?dmc=1. Accessed May 17, 2019.

American College of Obstetricians and Gynecologists: Marijuana use during pregnancy and lactation. Committee Opinion No 722, October 2017a. Available at: https://www.acog.org/Clinical-Guidance-and-Publications/Committee-Opinions/Committee-on-Obstetric-Practice/Marijuana-Use-During-Pregnancy-and-Lactation?IsMobileSet=false. Accessed May 17, 2019.

American College of Obstetricians and Gynecologists: Opioid use and opioid use disorder in pregnancy. Committee Opinion No 711, August 2017b. Available at: https://www.acog.org/Clinical-Guidance-and-Publications/Committee-Opinions/Committee-on-Obstetric-Practice/Opioid-Use-and-Opioid-Use-Disorder-in-Pregnancy?IsMobileSet=false. Accessed May 17, 2019.

Bagley SM, Wachman EM, Holland E, et al: Review of the assessment and management of neonatal abstinence syndrome. Addict Sci Clin Pract 9(1):19, 2014 25199822

Broussard CS, Rasmussen SA, Reefhuis J, et al; National Birth Defects Prevention Study: Maternal treatment with opioid analgesics and risk for birth defects. Am J Obstet Gynecol 204(4):314.e1–314.e11, 2011 21345403

Bush K, Kivlahan DR, McDonell MB, et al: The AUDIT alcohol consumption questions (AUDIT-C): an effective brief screening test for problem drinking. Ambulatory Care Quality Improvement Project (ACQUIP). Alcohol Use Disorders Identification Test. Arch Intern Med 158(16):1789–1795, 1998 9738608

Cain MA, Bornick P, Whiteman V: The maternal, fetal, and neonatal effects of cocaine exposure in pregnancy. Clin Obstet Gynecol 56(1):124–132, 2013 23314714

Carroll Chapman SL, Wu L: Substance use among adolescent mothers: a review. Child Youth Serv Rev 35(5):806–815, 2013 23641120

Centers for Disease Control and Prevention: Contraindications to breastfeeding or feeding expressed breast milk to infants. January 24, 2018. Available at: https://www.cdc.gov/breastfeeding/breastfeeding-special-circumstances/contraindications-to-breastfeeding.html. Accessed May 17, 2019.

Chan AW, Pristach EA, Welte JW, et al: Use of the TWEAK test in screening for alcoholism/heavy drinking in three populations. Alcohol Clin Exp Res 17(6):1188–1192, 1993 8116829

Chasnoff IJ, Burns WJ, Hatcher RP, et al: Phencyclidine: effects on the fetus and neonate. Dev Pharmacol Ther 6(6):404–408, 1983 6641470

Chasnoff IJ, Wells AM, McGourty RF, et al: Validation of the 4P's Plus screen for substance use in pregnancy validation of the 4P's Plus. J Perinatol 27(12):744–748, 2007 17805340

Cressman AM, Natekar A, Kim E, et al: Cocaine abuse during pregnancy. J Obstet Gynaecol Can 36(7):628–631, 2014 25184982

Day NL, Goldschmidt L, Thomas CA: Prenatal marijuana exposure contributes to the prediction of marijuana use at age 14. Addiction 101(9):1313–1322, 2006 16911731

Denny CH, Acero CS, Naimi TS, Kim SY: Consumption of alcohol beverages and binge drinking among pregnant women aged 18–44 years—United States, 2015-2017. MMWR Morb Mortal Wkly Rep Apr 26; 68(16):365–368, 2019 31022164

DeVido J, Bogunovic O, Weiss RD: Alcohol use disorders in pregnancy. Harv Rev Psychiatry 23(2):112–121, 2015 25747924

Dickson B, Mansfield C, Guiahi M, et al: Recommendations from cannabis dispensaries about first-trimester cannabis use. Obstet Gynecol 131(6):1031–1038, 2018 29742676

Elliott L, Loomis D, Lottritz L, et al: Case-control study of a gastroschisis cluster in Nevada. Arch Pediatr Adolesc Med 163(11):1000–1006, 2009 19884590

Fico T, Vanderwende C: Phencyclidine during pregnancy: behavioral and neurochemical effects in the offspring. Ann N Y Acad Sci 562:319–326, 1989 2545154

Forrester MB, Merz RD: Risk of selected birth defects with prenatal illicit drug use, Hawaii, 1986–2002. J Toxicol Environ Health A 70(1):7–18, 2007 17162495

Golden NL, Kuhnert BR, Sokol RJ, et al: Phencyclidine use during pregnancy. Am J Obstet Gynecol 148(3):254–259, 1984 6695970

Goldschmidt L, Richardson GA, Willford J, et al: Prenatal marijuana exposure and intelligence test performance at age 6. J Am Acad Child Adolesc Psychiatry 47(3):254–263, 2008 18216735

Goldschmidt L, Richardson GA, Willford JA, et al: School achievement in 14-year-old youths prenatally exposed to marijuana. Neurotoxicol Teratol 34(1):161–167, 2012 21884785

Golub M, Costa L, Crofton K, et al: NTP-CERHR Expert Panel Report on the reproductive and developmental toxicity of amphetamine and methamphetamine. Birth Defects Res B Dev Reprod Toxicol 74(6):471–584, 2005 16167346

Gorman MC, Orme KS, Nguyen NT, et al: Outcomes in pregnancies complicated by methamphetamine use. Am J Obstet Gynecol 211(4):429.e1–429.e7, 2014 24905417

Gray KA, Day NL, Leech S, et al: Prenatal marijuana exposure: effect on child depressive symptoms at ten years of age. Neurotoxicol Teratol 27(3):439–448, 2005 15869861

Handy CJ, Lange HLH, Manos BE, et al: A retrospective chart review of contraceptive use among adolescents with opioid use disorder. J Pediatr Adolesc Gynecol 31(2):122–127, 2018 29162530

Heinonen OP: Birth Defects and Drugs in Pregnancy. Littleton, MA, Publishing Sciences Group, 1977

Hwang SS, Diop H, Liu CL, et al: Maternal substance use disorders and infant outcomes in the first year of life among Massachusetts singletons, 2003–2010. J Pediatr 191:69–75, 2017 29050752

Jones HE, Balster RL: Inhalant abuse in pregnancy. Obstet Gynecol Clin North Am 25(1):153–167, 1998 9547765

Knight JR, Sherritt L, Shrier LA, et al: Validity of the CRAFFT substance abuse screening test among adolescent clinic patients. Arch Pediatr Adolesc Med 156(6):607–614, 2002 12038895

Krans EE, Bobby S, England M, et al: The Pregnancy Recovery Center: a women-centered treatment program for pregnant and postpartum women with opioid use disorder. Addict Behav 86:124–129, 2018 29884421

Logan BA, Brown MS, Hayes MJ: Neonatal abstinence syndrome: treatment and pediatric outcomes. Clin Obstet Gynecol 56(1):186–192, 2013 23314720

May PA, Chambers CD, Kalberg WO, et al: Prevalence of fetal alcohol spectrum disorders in 4 US communities. JAMA 319(5):474–482, 2018 29411031

Milkovich L, van der Berg BJ: Effects of antenatal exposure to anorectic drugs. Am J Obstet Gynecol 129(6):637–642, 1977 920764

National Institute on Drug Abuse for Teens: Spice. May 2017. Available at: https://teens.drugabuse.gov/drug-facts/spice. Accessed May 17, 2019.

National Library of Medicine: Drugs and lactation database (LactMed). 2019. Available at: https://www.ncbi.nlm.nih.gov/books/NBK501922/. Accessed May 17, 2019.

Nelson MM, Forfar JO: Associations between drugs administered during pregnancy and congenital abnormalities of the fetus. BMJ 1(5748):523–527, 1971 4396080

Patrick SW, Schumacher RE, Benneyworth BD, et al: Neonatal abstinence syndrome and associated health care expenditures: United States, 2000–2009. JAMA 307(18):1934–1940, 2012 22546608

Pulatie K: The legality of drug-testing procedures for pregnant women. Virtual Mentor 10(1):41–44, 2008 23206742

Rubino T, Parolaro D: The impact of exposure to cannabinoids in adolescence: insights from animal models. Biol Psychiatry 79(7):578–585, 2016 26344755

Ryan SA, Ammerman SD, O'Connor ME; Committee on Substance Use and Prevention; Section on Breastfeeding: Marijuana use during pregnancy and breastfeeding: implications for neonatal and childhood outcomes. Pediatrics 142(3):1–15, 2018 30150209

Salas-Wright CP, Vaughn MG, Ugalde J, et al: Substance use and teen pregnancy in the United States: evidence from the NSDUH 2002–2012. Addict Behav 45:218–225, 2015 25706068

Schiff DM, Nielsen T, Terplan M, et al: Fatal and nonfatal overdose among pregnant and postpartum women in Massachusetts. Obstet Gynecol 132(2):466–474, 2018 29995730

Shah R, Diaz SD, Arria A, et al: Prenatal methamphetamine exposure and short-term maternal and infant medical outcomes. Am J Perinatol 29(5):391–400, 2012 22399214

Singer LT, Moore DG, Fulton S, et al: Neurobehavioral outcomes of infants exposed to MDMA (Ecstasy) and other recreational drugs during pregnancy. Neurotoxicol Teratol 34(3):303–310, 2012 22387807

Smith LM, LaGasse LL, Derauf C, et al: The infant development, environment, and lifestyle study: effects of prenatal methamphetamine exposure, polydrug exposure, and poverty on intrauterine growth. Pediatrics 118(3):1149–1156, 2006 16951010

Sokol RJ, Martier SS, Ager JW: The T-ACE questions: practical prenatal detection of risk-drinking. Am J Obstet Gynecol 160(4):863–868, discussion 868–870, 1989 2712118

Substance Abuse and Mental Health Services Administration: Results from the 2012 National Survey on Drug Use and Health: Summary of National Findings. NSDUH Series H-46, HHS Publ No (SMA) 13-4795. Rockville, MD, Substance Abuse and Mental Health Services Administration, 2013

Tolia VN, Patrick SW, Bennett MM, et al: Increasing incidence of the neonatal abstinence syndrome in U.S. neonatal ICUs. N Engl J Med 372(22):2118–2126, 2015 25913111

Tortoriello G, Morris CV, Alpar A, et al: Miswiring the brain: Δ9-tetrahydrocannabinol disrupts cortical development by inducing an SCG10/stathmin-2 degradation pathway. EMBO J 33(7):668–685, 2014 24469251

Tournebize J, Gibaja V, Kahn JP: Acute effects of synthetic cannabinoids: update 2015. Subst Abus 38(3):344–366, 2017 27715709

Tzilos Wernette G, Bonar EE, Blow FC, et al: Psychosocial correlates of marijuana use among pregnant and nonpregnant adolescent girls. J Pediatr Adolesc Gynecol 31(5):490–493, 2018 29751095

Wachsman L, Schuetz S, Chan LS, et al: What happens to babies exposed to phencyclidine (PCP) in utero? Am J Drug Alcohol Abuse 15(1):31–39, 1989 2923109

Warren KR, Foudin LL: Alcohol-related birth defects—the past, present, and future. 2001. Available at: https://pubs.niaaa.nih.gov/publications/arh25-3/153-158.htm. accessed May 17, 2019.

WHO ASSIST Working Group: The Alcohol, Smoking and Substance Involvement Screening Test (ASSIST): development, reliability and feasibility. Addiction 97(9):1183–1194, 2002 12199834

Wright TE, Schuetter R, Tellei J, et al: Methamphetamines and pregnancy outcomes. J Addict Med 9(2):111–117, 2015 25599434

Wright TE, Terplan M, Ondersma SJ, et al: The role of screening, brief intervention, and referral to treatment in the perinatal period. Am J Obstet Gynecol 215(5):539–547, 2016 27373599

Yazdy MM, Mitchell AA, Tinker SC, et al: Periconceptional use of opioids and the risk of neural tube defects. Obstet Gynecol 122(4):838–844, 2013 24084542

Yonkers KA, Gotman N, Kershaw T, et al: Screening for prenatal substance use: development of the Substance Use Risk Profile-Pregnancy scale. Obstet Gynecol 116(4):827–833, 2010 20859145

Appendix A

Resource Materials on Screening and Assessment Instruments

Print Resources

Buros OK: Mental Measurements Yearbook (Ongoing Book Series). Lincoln, NE, Buros Centers for Testing, 2019. Available at: https://buros.org/mental-measurements-yearbook. Accessed May 17, 2019.

Center for Substance Abuse Prevention: Guide to Risk Factor and Outcome Instruments for Youth Substance Abuse Prevention Program Evaluations (DHHS Publ No SMA 99-3279). Rockville, MD, Substance Abuse and Mental Health Services Administration, 1999

Center for Substance Abuse Treatment: Screening and Assessing Adolescents for Substance Use Disorders, Treatment Improvement Protocol (TIP) Series, No 31 (Publ No SMA 99-3282). Rockville, MD, Substance Abuse and Mental Health Services Administration, 1999

Rush AJ, First MB, Blacker D: Handbook of Psychiatric Measures, 2nd Edition. Washington, DC, American Psychiatric Publishing, 2008

Computerized, Personalized Assessment With Feedback for Substance Abuse

Doumas DM: Web-based personalized feedback: is this an appropriate approach for reducing drinking among high school students? J Subst Abuse Treat 50:76–80, 2015 25448614

Harris SK, Csémy L, Sherritt L, et al: Computer-facilitated substance use screening and brief advice for teens in primary care: an international trial. Pediatrics 129(6):1072–1082, 2012 22566420

Harris SK, Knight Jr Jr, Van Hook S, et al: Adolescent substance use screening in primary care: validity of computer self-administered versus clinician-administered screening. Subst Abuse 37(1):197–203, 2016 25774878

Jasik CB, Berna M, Martin M, et al: Teen preferences for clinic-based behavior screens: who, where, when, and how? J Adolesc Health 59(6):722–724, 2016 27884300

Neighbors C, Lee CM, Lewis MA, et al: Internet-based personalized feedback to reduce 21st-birthday drinking: a randomized controlled trial of an event-specific prevention intervention. J Consult Clinic Psychol 77(1):51–63, 2009 19170453

Olson AL, Gaffney CA, Hedberg VA, et al: Use of inexpensive technology to enhance adolescent health screening and counseling. Arch Pediatr Adolesc Med 163(2):172–177, 2009 19188650

Saitz R, Palfai TP, Freedner N, et al: Screening and brief intervention online for college students: the ihealth study. Alcohol Alcohol 42(1):28–36, 2006 17130139

Appendix B

Parent Resources on Adolescent Substance Use

Website	Description
Partnership for Drug-Free Kids https://drugfree.org/	Parent-focused drug prevention website; provides a comprehensive menu of parent resources to address adolescent substance use.
National Institute on Drug Abuse for Teens https://teens.drugabuse.gov/parents	Wide range of research-informed resources for parents about adolescent drug abuse.
Substance Abuse and Mental Health Services Administration www.samhsa.gov/underage-drinking	Multiple research-based resources to help parents begin and keep up the conversation about the dangers of drinking alcohol and using other drugs at a young age.
Parenting is Prevention www.parentingisprevention.org	Focuses on resources and links for parents to keep their kids drug free. Includes profiles of selected parenting programs and a list of Internet resources on parenting.
Being Adept www.beingadept.org	Parent resources to prevent alcohol and drug abuse among adolescents (especially middle schoolers) through a science-based curriculum that empowers youth and their parents to make informed, healthy choices.

Appendix C

Websites for Self-Help and Mutual-Help Organizations

General Information

HelpGuide: Overcoming Alcohol Addiction: www.helpguide.org/articles/
addictions/overcoming-alcohol-addiction.htm
Treatment 4 Addiction (American Addiction Centers):
www.treatment4addiction.com

Locating Local Mutual-Help Organization Meetings

Alcoholics Anonymous

www.aa.org/pages/en_US/find-aa-resources

Narcotics Anonymous

www.na.org/meetingsearch

Index

Page numbers printed in **boldface** type refer to tables or figures.

Abstinence, as goal of substance abuse interventions, 257, 266–269, **270**

Abuse, as criteria for diagnosis of substance use disorders, 10–11

Academic functioning, and substance use, 183–184, 492–493. *See also* Learning; Schools

Academy of Breastfeeding Medicine, 561

Acamprosate, 148, 552

Accidents, alcohol-associated motor vehicle crashes, 79, 84

"Accurate empathy," as predictor of therapeutic success, 258, 278

Activity goals, and 12-step meetings, 342

Adaptation hypothesis, and gambling disorder, 505

Adaptive treatment, studies of, 264–266

Addiction-Comprehensive Health Enhancement Support System (A-CHESS), 355–356, 358

Addictive disorders, and cannabis use, 185–187. *See also* Behavioral addictions

Adherence, to medication in bipolar disorder comorbid with substance use disorder, 461

Adolescent(s), and adolescence. *See also* Age; College-age students; Substance use; Substance use disorders; Transition-age youth; *specific topics*

as critical developmental period for initiation of substance use, 3–5, 439

definition of, xxv

development of multiple addictive behaviors in, 503

early onset of bipolar disorder and development of substance use disorders in, 453–455

heterogeneity of response to substance use disorder treatment, 259–261

negative consequences of cannabis on, 180, 182–183

negative sequelae of opioid misuse in, 206

pharmacotherapy for alcohol use disorder in, 150–152

prevalence of substance use in, 5–8

problems with inferring safety and efficacy of medication use from adult data, 145

substance-using parents and, 8–9

trajectories of substance use during, 9–10

Adolescent Alcohol and Drug Involvement Scale (AADIS), **59**, 62
Adolescent Community Reinforcement Approach (A-CRA), 266, 290, 309–314, 486, 528
Adolescent Diagnostic Interview (ADI), 63, **64**
Adolescent Drinking Inventory (ADI), 58, **59**
Adolescent Self-Assessment Profile (ASAP), 65, 67, **68**
Adolescent Substance Abuse Goal Commitment questionnaire, 268
Adolescent substance use (ASU). *See* Substance use disorder
Adults. *See also* Age; Transition-age youth
    benefits of Alcoholics Anonymous for, **338–339**
    comorbidity of anxiety disorders with substance use disorders in, 387
    comorbidity of posttraumatic stress disorder with substance use disorders in, 396
    differences from adolescents in preparation for treatment, 257–258
    differences from adolescents in symptoms of substance use disorders, 14
    pharmacotherapy for alcohol abuse in, 145–150
    social roles and transition to, 533
    use of term "emerging," xxv
Advice, and success of therapeutic interventions, 258
African Americans. *See* Race/ethnicity

Aftercare approaches, for suicidal behaviors, 423. *See also* Continuity of care
Age. *See also* Adolescents; Adults; Age at onset; Children; College-age students; Infants; Transition-age youth
    continued use of substances during pregnancy and, 544
    legal drinking age and, 37
    prevalence of substance use disorders in adolescents by, 12
    risk factors for opioid use and, 207
    12-step meetings and, 326
Age at onset
    of attention-deficit/hyperactivity disorder and early onset of substance use, 479
    of cannabis use, 441
    of gambling disorder, 504
    of opioid use, 207, 209, 210
    patterns of substance use and, 5
    of schizophrenia, 438
Aggression, and disruptive behavior disorders, 487–488
Agoraphobia, 386
Alcohol, Smoking and Substance Involvement Screening Test (ASSIST), **547**, 548
Alcoholics Anonymous (AA), 326, 327, 328, **329**, 330, 332, 336, **338–339**, 571
Alcohol use. *See also* Alcohol use disorder
    acute alcohol poisoning and, 128
    attention-deficit/hyperactivity disorder and rates of, 479
    anxiety and, 387
    brief interventions in primary care setting, 87

drug testing and, 103, **104,**
107–109
marijuana use and, 178
motor vehicle crashes, association
with, 79, 84
patterns of in adolescents, 5–6, 7
pharmacological treatment of,
142–152
pregnancy and, 551–553
prevalence of, 141–142
screening instruments for, 58, 62
suicidal behaviors and, 416–417
Alcohol Screening Protocol for Youth, 58
Alcohol use disorder (AUD). *See also*
Alcohol use
baseline assessment reactivity and, 259
bipolar disorder and, 452, 454
continuing care for, 264
DSM-5 criteria for, **85–86**
heterogeneity in development,
course of in adolescents, 15
medications for in adults, 142
pharmacotherapy for in adolescents, 150–152
prevalence of, 141
Alcohol Use Disorders Identification
Test (AUDIT), 63, **82,** 84, 547,
548
All Stars Prevention Program, 39
Alpha-agonists, 489
Alternative medicines, for opioid use
disorder, 219
Alternative peer group (APG) model,
324–325
Ambivalence, during motivational
interviewing process, 279
American Academy of Child and Adolescent Psychiatry (AACAP), 388,
396, 399, 458

American Academy of Pediatrics
(AAP), 77, 87, 99, 168, 211, 544,
560–561
American College of Obstetricians and
Gynecologists (ACOG), 544, 551,
560
American Life Project, 350
American Lung Association, 165
American Psychiatric Association, 445,
502, 509
American Society of Addiction Medicine (ASAM), 212, 502
Amphetamines, **106,** 113–114,
553–555. *See also* Stimulants
Anabolic-androgenic steroids, 115
Anger management, and Adolescent
Community Reinforcement
Approach, 310
Antenatal surveillance, 557, **558**
Antipsychotics
for bipolar disorder comorbid with
substance use disorders,
458–460
for disruptive behavior disorders
comorbid with substance use
disorders, 487–488
for psychotic disorders comorbid
with substance use disorders,
445–446, 450–451
Antisocial behavior
assessment of attention-deficit/
hyperactivity or disruptive
behavior disorders comorbid
with substance use disorders,
482, 483
relationship between substance use
disorders and disruptive behavior disorders, 481
as risk factor for substance abuse, 32

Antisocial personality disorder, 451
Anxiety
    comorbidity of bipolar disorder
        with substance use disorders
        and, 457
    as risk factor for substance abuse,
        29–30
Anxiety disorders
    benzodiazepine abuse and, 246
    comorbidity of with substance use
        disorders, 385–392
Aripiprazole, 459, 460
*ASAM Criteria: Treatment Criteria for
    Addictive, Substance-Related, and
    Co-Occurring Conditions,* 3rd Edi-
    tion (Mee-Lee et al. 2013),
    123–124, **125–126,** 127–135,
    136
Asenapine, 459
Ask Suicide-Screening Questions
    (ASQ), 419
Assertive continuing care (ACC),
    261–263
Assertive outreach, and treatment
    engagement, 131
*Assessing Alcohol Problems: A Guide for
    Clinicians and Researchers* (Allen
    and Wilson 2003), 58
Assessment. *See also* Diagnosis; Screen-
    ing
    of attention-deficit/hyperactivity
        disorder comorbid with
        substance use disorders,
        482–483
    of anxiety disorders in adolescents
        with comorbid substance use
        disorders, 388–389
    ASAM criteria and dimensional,
        125, 127–135

biologically based drug testing and,
    54
clinical interview and, 69
core content of comprehensive,
    55–57
of depression, 377–378
developmental informed approach
    to, 13–14
directive approach and, **281–282**
direct observation and, 54
of disruptive behaviors comorbid
    with substance use disorders,
    482–483
of gambling disorder, 506–507
motivational interviewing and,
    281–282, 284
of nicotine dependence, 162–163
parent reports and, 54
principles of, 52–53
of psychotic disorders in adolescents
    with substance use disorder,
    442–444
of posttraumatic stress disorder in
    adolescents with substance use
    disorder, 394–396
self-report method of, 53
standardized instruments for,
    57–67, **68,** 567–568
of substance use in juvenile justice
    system, 524–527
of suicidal behaviors, 418–422
of treatment outcome, 67
Assessment reactivity (AR), and treat-
    ment outcome, 258–259
Atomoxetine, 192, 489
Attendance, and 12-step organizations,
    326–327, 341, 342–343
Attention, and dimensional assess-
    ment, 129

Attention-deficit/hyperactivity disorder (ADHD)
assessment of in adolescents with substance use disorders, 482–483
methamphetamine and, 237
misdiagnosis of bipolar disorder as in children, 459
prevalence of comorbidity with substance use disorder, 476
relationship between substance use disorders and, 478–480
treatment of comorbid with substance use disorders, 484–490
Avoidance, and comorbidity of posttraumatic stress disorder with substance use disorder, 393
Axonal myelination, and brain development, 182

Baclofen, 149–150
Barbiturates, 178
Barriers
to change and brief motivational interventions, 287
to implementation of contingency management, 294
to interventions for substance use in juvenile justice system, 529–531
to participation in 12-step organizations, 327
to treatment for marijuana use, 192
to treatment planning, 124–127
Baseline assessment reactivity (BAR), 259
Beck Depression Inventory–II (BDI-II), 378
Beck Hopelessness Scale (BHS), 420

Beck Scale for Suicidal Ideation (BSS), 420
Behavior. *See also* Aggression; Antisocial behavior; Behavior therapy; Disruptive behavior disorders; Impulsivity; Mechanisms of behavioral change; Nonsuicidal self-injurious behavior; Reward-related behaviors; Target behaviors; Violent behavior
ASAM criteria and dimensional assessment, **125,** 129–130
comorbidity of bipolar disorder with substance use disorder, 457
family therapy and change in, 306–307
inhibition of and developmentally normative delay in maturation of during adolescence, 4
Behavioral addictions. *See also* Gambling disorder; Internet gaming disorder
core elements of, 502
inclusion of in DSM-5, 501–502
Behavior therapy, and alcohol abuse during pregnancy, 552. *See also* Family behavior therapy; Protective behavioral strategies
Being Adept (website), 569
Benzodiazepines
abuse of, 244–246, 387
agitation from ketamine use and, 239
alcohol use during pregnancy and, 552–553
as contraindicated for adolescents with substance use disorders, 391

Benzodiazepines
    drug testing for, **105**, 110
    marijuana and interactions with,
        178
Benzphetamine, 114
Bidirectional model, of comorbidity
    between psychiatric disorders and
    substance use disorders, 368
Binge drinking, and naltrexone, 147
Biomarkers
    alcohol use and, 103, 107–108
    definition of, 98
    drug testing and available types of,
        100–101
Biomedical conditions, and ASAM cri-
    teria, **125**, 128–129. *See also*
    Medical conditions
Biopsychosocial factors, and compre-
    hensive assessment, 56
Bipolar disorder, comorbidity of with
    substance use disorders, 451–465
Birth defects, and alcohol use during
    pregnancy, 552
Blood alcohol level (BAC), 286
Blood samples, and drug testing, 103,
    109
Blunting, of alcohol craving, 143–144
Borderline personality disorder,
    423–424
Brain
    assessment and development of,
        57
    marijuana use and structural
        changes in adolescent,
        182–183
Breastfeeding, and substance use,
    560–561
Brief family therapy, 36. *See also* Brief
    strategic family therapy

Brief interventions. *See also* Brief moti-
    vation interventions
    in primary care or pediatric setting,
        86–88
    for tobacco use, 163
Brief Mental Status Assessment, 526
Brief motivational interventions (BMI)
    emergency departments and,
        282–288
    evidence base for, 280, 282
    theoretical basis for, 278–280
Brief strategic family therapy (BSFT),
    302, 304, 484, 485–486
Buprenorphine
    breastfeeding and, 560
    drug testing for, **105**, 111
    opioid use disorder and, 213–214,
        215, 216–217, 217–218, 244
    pregnancy and, 558–559
Bupropion, 167, 490
Butane hash oil (BHO), 178, 189

Campbell Collaboration, 34
Canadian Adolescent Gambling Inven-
    tory, 506–507
Canadian Network for Mood and Anx-
    iety Treatments, 458
Cannabidiol (CBD), 177, 178–179
Cannabis. *See* Marijuana
Cannabis-induced psychotic disorder
    (CIPD), 444
Cannabis sativa, and *Cannabis indica*, 176
Cannabis use disorder (CUD). *See also*
    Marijuana
    bipolar disorder and, 452, 454
    clinical course of in adolescents, 15
    comorbidity and duration of, 371
    continuing care for, 263–264,
        265–266

diagnostic criteria for, 185–186
prevalence of, 175
Cannabis Youth Treatment (CYT)
   study, 191, 192, 289, 309,
   379–380
Carbon monoxide, **104**, 110
Cardiovascular system, and marijuana
   use, 187
Case examples
   of bipolar disorder comorbid with
      substance use disorders,
      462–465
   of depression comorbid with sub-
      stance use disorders, 382–385
   of identifying risk levels for sub-
      stance abuse in primary care
      setting, 88–91
   of posttraumatic stress disorder
      comorbid with substance use
      disorders, 399–401
   of schizophrenia comorbid with
      substance use disorders,
      448–450
   of substance use in juvenile justice
      system, 535–536
   of suicidal behaviors comorbid with
      substance use disorders,
      427–429
Catechol-O-methyltransferase
   (COMT) gene, and cannabis use,
   184
CBT-MET5, 36
Cell phones. See also Mobile health
   (mHealth) technology–based
   interventions; Text messaging
   gambling disorder and gaming
      addictions, 512
   tobacco prevention programs and,
      169

Centers for Disease Control and Prevention (CDC), 544, 552, 561
Central nervous system (CNS), and
   cannabis, 176
Certification, in Adolescent Community Reinforcement Approach,
   311
Cessation interventions, for tobacco
   use, 164–168
Change. See also Mechanisms of behavioral change
   ASAM criteria and dimensional
      assessment of, **125**, 130–132
   brief motivational interventions
      and, 284–285, 286–287
   family therapy and behavioral,
      306–307
   harm reduction programs and
      increasing motivation for,
      267–268
   responsibility for and success of
      therapeutic interventions, 258
Chemotherapy, and medical marijuana,
   178
Child and Adolescent Bipolar Foundation, 458
Children. See also Infants
   ingestion of marijuana by as medical
      emergency, 187
   maternal substance abuse and, 559
   misdiagnosis of bipolar disorder as
      ADHD in, 459
Children's Depression Rating Scale—
   Revised (CDRS-R), 378
Children's Global Assessment Scale,
   461
Children's Hospital Colorado, 187
Children of substance-using parents
   (CSUP), 8–9

Child Trauma Screening Questionnaire (CTSQ), 395
Child welfare system, 522
Cigarette smoking. *See* Nicotine; Tobacco use
Cincinnati First-Episode Mania Study, 454
Citicoline, 461
Clinical Global Impression—Improvement scale (CGI-I), 382
Clinical vignettes. *See* Case examples
Clinician Administered PTSD Scale for Children and Adolescents (CAPS-CA), 395
Clonidine, 217, 489
Club drugs, potential health effects of, 229. *See also* GHB (γ-hydroxybutyrate); Ketamine; LSD; MDMA; Methamphetamine
Coaching, and classroom-based prevention interventions, 39
Cocaine
    avoidance of stimulants in cases of dependence, 490
    breastfeeding and, 561
    drug testing for, **105**, 112–113
    pregnancy and, 553
Cognition, and cognitive skills. *See also* Memory
    ASAM criteria and dimensional assessment, **125**, 129–130
    cannabis use and, 183–184
    comprehensive assessment and, 56–57
    protective factors and, 32–33
    smoking cessation and, 165
Cognitive-behavioral therapy (CBT)
    for anxiety disorders comorbid with substance use disorders, 390

cost of, 336–337, 340
    for depression comorbid with substance use disorders, 379, 381–382
    disruptive behavior disorders comorbid with substance use disorders and, 486
    evidence for effectiveness of, 289–290
    for gambling disorder, 512, 513
    group versus individual, 290
    marijuana use and, 190–191
    overview of, 288–289
    suicidal ideation and, 422–423, 424
    technology and, 354, 358
    for tobacco use cessation, 165
    12-step facilitation combined with, 332–333, **334**
Collaborative treatment approach, for suicidal ideation, 425
Collateral informants, and recovery environment, 133
College-age students, and stimulant abuse, 492
Colorado, and liberalization of cannabis policies, 193–194, **195**
Colorado Department of Education, 184
Columbia-Suicide Severity Rating Scale (C-SSRS), 419
Coma, GHB-induced, 234, 235
Combined treatment, as multidomain treatment, 308
Commercialization, of marijuana, 193
Common factor model, of comorbidity between psychiatric disorders and substance use disorders, 368
Communication, suicidal behavior and negative, 426

Communities That Care (CTC), 36–37

Community. *See also* Rural communities

prevention programs based in, 36–37

risk factors for opioid use and, **209**

risk factors for substance use and abuse, 28, **29**

Community Reinforcement Approach (CRA), 309, 310

Comorbidity, of substance use disorders with psychiatric disorders. *See also* Suicide

attention-deficit/hyperactivity disorder and, 478–490

anxiety disorders and, 385–392

bipolar disorder and, 451–465

clinical course of substance use disorders and, 18–19

clinical and service implications of, 371–372

conduct disorder and, 480–490

depression and, 376–385

diagnostic issues, 370–371

nature of association between psychiatric disorders and substance use disorders, 368–370

oppositional defiant disorder and, 480–490

posttraumatic stress disorder and, 392–402

psychotic disorders and, 437–451

treatment of opioid use disorder and, 213

Comprehensive Adolescent Severity Inventory (CASI), 65, **66**

Computer(s). *See* Internet; Technology

Computer-assisted interview (CAI), 53

Conduct disorder (CD), comorbidity of with substance use disorders, 478, 480–490

Confidentiality

management of substance use during pregnancy and, 556

referrals to treatment from primary care settings and, 91–92

screening for substance use in primary care settings and, 79, 88

Conflict, in family as risk factor for substance abuse, 31

Contingency management (CM)

assertive continuing care and, 262

disruptive behavior disorders comorbid with substance use disorders and, 486

implementation of, 292–293

limitations of, 294

marijuana use and, 191

research on effectiveness of, 290–292

smoking cessation and, 166

technology-based interventions and, 359

Continuity of care

adaptive treatment and, 264–266

aftercare for adolescents with substance use disorders and, 261–264

dimensional assessment and, 133

disruptive behavior disorders comorbid with substance use disorders and, 487

future directions for research on, 269

harm reduction programs and, 266–269, **270**

Contraception, and postpartum care, 559–560

Contract(s)
contingency management and, 292,
293
for home drug testing, 99
Contract for Life, 88
Coordinated specialty care (CSC), 447
Coping skills
attention-deficit/hyperactivity disorder comorbid with substance
use disorders and, 480
brief motivational interventions
and, 287–288
cognitive-behavioral therapy and,
288–289
smoking cessation and, 165
Core-elements approach, to family
therapy, 303–304
Cost, and cost effectiveness
annual of abuse and dependence to
U.S. society, 26
contingency management protocols
and, 359
drug testing and, 101
mutual-help organizations and,
332–333, 336–337, 340
substance use during pregnancy
and, 550
Cotinine, 104
Cough and cold medications, abuse of
over-the-counter, 246–247.
See also Dextromethorphan
Course and Outcome of Bipolar Youth
(COBY) study, 452, 454, 455
CRAFFT 2.0, 59, 62, 63, 79, 80, 84, 548
Craving
as criteria for diagnosis of substance
use disorders, 11
pharmacotherapy for alcohol abuse
and, 143–144, 147

Criminal justice system, and substance
use disorders in transition-age
youth, 532–535. See also Juvenile
justice system
Culture, and adaptation of prevention
programs, 41
Customary Drinking and Drug Use
Record (CDDR), 63, 64
Cyanamide, 151
Cytochrome P450 (CYP) enzymes, and
marijuana, 178–179

Dangerousness, assessment for, 129.
See also Safety
DARE initiative, 41
Death
alcohol-related motor vehicle
crashes as leading cause of for
adolescents, 79, 84
opioid use and, 203, 206
rates of by suicide, 415
Decriminalization, of marijuana, 193
Delinquency, as risk factor for substance abuse, 29–30
Dental diseases, and smokeless tobacco,
161
Department of Health and Human Services, 360
Dependence. See also Tolerance
as criteria for diagnosis of substance
use disorders, 10–11
GHB and, 234
ketamine and, 239
MDMA and, 232
methamphetamine and, 236
opioids and, 243
risk for substance use disorders
and subthreshold symptoms
of, 12

Depression
comorbidity of with substance use
disorders, 376–385
marijuana use and, 185
as risk factor for substance abuse,
29–30
Detoxification, and opioid use, 217, 244
Development
adolescence as critical period for initiation of substance use, 3–5
assessment of substance use disorders and, 13–14
effect of parental substance use on
child's, 9
importance of in approach to substance use disorders in adolescents, xxv–xxvi
self-report method of assessment
and, 53
Dextromethorphan, 111–112, 241,
246–247
Diagnosis. *See also* Assessment; Differential
diagnosis; DSM-5; Dual diagnosis
of cannabis use disorder, 185–186
of comorbidity between psychiatric
disorders and substance use
disorders, 370–371
concept of "diagnostic orphans," 12
DSM-IV and DSM-5 criteria for
substance use disorders, 10–11
misdiagnosis of bipolar disorder as
attention-deficit/hyperactivity
disorder in children, 459
of opioid use disorder, 211–212
of tobacco use, 162–163
Diagnostic interview(s), and standardized instruments, 63, **64**, 65
Diagnostic Interview for Children and
Adolescents (DICA-R), 63, **64**

Diagnostic Interview Schedule for Children—Revised (DISC-R), 63, **64**
Dialectical behavioral therapy (DBT),
for suicidal behaviors, 423
Differential diagnosis
of psychotic disorders comorbid
with substance use disorders,
442–444
severity of substance use disorders
and, 55
Digital phenotyping, 356
Directive approach, compared to motivation enhancement therapy,
281–282
Disease model, of comorbidity between
psychiatric disorders and substance use disorders, 368
Disruptive behavior disorders (DBDs).
See Conduct disorder; Opposi-
tional defiant disorder
Disruptive Behavior Disorders Rating
Scale, 483
Dissociation, and comorbidity of posttraumatic stress disorder with sub-
stance use disorders, 393
Disulfiram, 146, 150, 151, 552
Divalproex, 460
DNA sampling, for genetic screening,
351
Dose-response relationship, between
cannabis use and development of
opioid use disorder, 221
Dronabinol, 178, 191
Drug Abuse Screening Test—Adolescents
(DAST-A), 59, 62
Drug-drug interactions, and mari-
juana, 178–179
Drug Enforcement Administration,
233

Drug testing. *See also* Urine drug tests
    alcohol and, 103, **104**, 107–109
    for amphetamine and methamphet-
        amine, **106**, 113–114
    anabolic-androgenic steroids and,
        115
    assessment and, 54
    available biomarkers for, 100–101
    benzodiazepines and, **105**, 110
    cocaine and, **105**, 112–113
    concordance among reports, 100
    dextromethophan and, 111–112
    hallucinogens and, 114
    inhalants and, 115
    in home, 99–100
    marijuana and, **104**, 109–110
    nicotine and, **104**, 110
    opioids and, **105**, 110–111
    overview of by sample source,
        101–103
    phencyclidine and, 115
    properties of common screens,
        104–107
    schools and, 98–99
    social context of, 98
    websites on, 117
Drug Use Screening Inventory—
    Revised (DUSI-R), **60**, 62–63
DSM-IV (*Diagnostic and Statistical
    Manual of Mental Disorders,*
    Fourth Edition)
    criteria for diagnosis of substance
        use disorders, 10–11
    prevalence of substance use disor-
        ders and, 11–13
DSM-5 (*Diagnostic and Statistical
    Manual of Mental Disorders,* Fifth
    Edition)
    anxiety disorders in, 385–386

behavioral addictions in, 501–502
    criteria for alcohol use disorder,
        85–86
    criteria for diagnosis of substance
        use disorders, 10–11, 55–56
    internet gaming disorder as poten-
        tial disorder in, 509
    reclassification of PTSD in, 393
Dual diagnosis, 18, 367. *See also*
    Comorbidity
DynamiCare RecoveryMind Training,
    358

Eating disorders, 483
E-cigarettes, 158–160, 162, 177.
    See also Vaping
Ecological family therapy, 304
Ecological momentary assessment
    (EMA), 353, 355
Education. *See* Academic functioning;
    Learning; Schools; Teaching;
    Training
eHealth programs, 43
Emergency department (ED). *See also*
    Hospitalization
    brief motivational interventions
        and, 282–288
    marijuana use and, 187
    opioid use disorder and, 219
Emerging adults, use of term, xxv
Emotions, ASAM criteria and dimen-
    sional assessment, **125**, 129–130
Empathy, and success of therapeutic
    interventions, 258
Endocannabinoid system (eCB), 176,
    399, 439
Environmental factors
    ASAM criteria and dimensional
        assessment of, **125**, 133–135

prevention programs and, 37–38
risk factors for opioid use and, **209**,
    210
Enzyme-linked immunosorbent assay
    (ELISA), 114
Ephedrine, and methamphetamine,
    235
Epidemiologic Catchment Area study,
    368, 451
Epidemiology. *See also* Prevalence
    of anxiety disorders comorbid with
        substance use disorders,
        385–387
    of benzodiazepine abuse, 245
    of bipolar disorder comorbid with
        substance use disorders,
        451–453
    of cannabis use, 179–180, **181**
    of depression comorbid with sub-
        stance use disorders, 376–377
    of externalizing disorders comorbid
        with substance use disorders,
        478
    of ketamine use, 238
    of LSD use, 240
    of MDMA use, 232
    of methamphetamine abuse, 236
    of opioid use, 205–206, 243
    of over-the-counter medication
        abuse, 247
    of posttraumatic stress disorder
        comorbid with substance use
        disorders, 392–394
    of suicidal ideation and behaviors,
        414–416
Epidiolex, 178
Epigenetic effects, of marijuana use,
    180, 182
Epilepsy, and medical marijuana, 178

Ethics, and care for pregnant adoles-
    cents with substance use disorders,
    557
Ethnicity. *See* Culture; Race/ethnicity
Evidence-based interventions, for opi-
    oid use disorder, 211–213
Executive functioning
    attention-deficit/hyperactivity dis-
        order comorbid with substance
        use disorders and, 480
    cannabis use and, 183–184
Exposure therapy, for posttraumatic
    stress disorder, 397
Externalizing disorders. *See* Attention-
    deficit/hyperactivity disorder;
    Conduct disorder; Oppositional
    defiant disorder

Facebook, 37–38
False positives, and drug testing, 108
Family. *See also* Family history; Family
    therapy; Parents
    Adolescent Community Reinforce-
        ment Approach and, 310
    involvement of in interventions for
        substance use in juvenile jus-
        tice system, 530, 531–532
    problem-solving skills and,
        426–427
    recovery environment and,
        133–135
    risk factors for opioid use and, **209**
    risk factors for substance use and,
        28, **29**, 29–30, 31
    substance-using parents and preven-
        tion efforts or interventions
        for, 9
Family behavior therapy (FBT), 302
Family Check-Up (FCU), 283

Family-focused therapy, 461
Family history
　of cannabis-induced psychosis, 444
　of opioid misuse, **208**
Family Intervention for Suicide Prevention (FISP), 423–424
Family therapy. *See also* Family behavior therapy; Family-focused therapy; Functional family therapy; Multidimensional family therapy
　for anxiety disorders, 390
　behavior change and, 306–307
　core elements of, 303–304
　definition of, 301
　engagement and, 304–305
　for externalizing disorders comorbid with substance use disorders, 484–486
　intervention strategies to improve recovery environment, 134–135
　overview of, 302–303
　relational reframing and, 305–306
　restructuring of family and, 307
　technology-based interventions and, 359
Feedback
　brief motivational interventions and, 285–286
　as predictor of success of therapeutic interventions, 258
Fentanyl, 110–111, 549
Fetal alcohol syndrome (FAS), 552
Fidelity, and implementation of prevention programs, 39–40
Firearms, and suicidal behaviors, 421
First-episode psychosis (FEP), and comorbidity with substance use disorders, 438, 445, 446–447

"Fishbowl-drawing procedure," and contingency management, 293
5As approach, to tobacco cessation, 164
Flavors, in e-cigarettes, 159
Flexibility, and adaptation of prevention programs, 40–41
Flunitrazepam, 244
Fluoxetine, 151, 381, 459
Follow up, and treatment planning, 136. *See also* Aftercare approaches; Continuity of care
Food and Drug Administration (FDA), 142, 145–148, 164, 213, 218
Four-process method, and motivational interviewing, 279
4Ps Plus, **547**
FRAMES (acronym), 258
Functional analysis
　Adolescent Community Reinforcement Approach and, 310
　harm reduction programs and, 268
　of suicidal ideation, 421–422
Functional family therapy (FFT), 302, 304, 380–381, 484, 485, 528

Gabapentin, 148–149, 191
GAIN–Short Screener (GSS), **60**, 62
Gambling disorder, 502, 504–508, 512–513
"Gateway effect," of adolescent marijuana use, 186
Gender
　differences in substance use prevalence by, 7–8, 12
　risk factors for opioid use and, **208**
　suicidal behavior and, 415–416
Generalized anxiety disorder, 386
Genetic Addiction Risk Score (GARS), 351

Genetics
  association between bipolar disorder
    and substance use disorders,
    457
  causal link between cannabis use
    and schizophrenia, 440
  comorbidity between psychiatric
    disorders and substance use
    disorders, 369
  risk factors for opioid misuse, **208**
  technology and advanced testing,
    350–351
GHB (γ-hydroxybutyrate), 233–235
Global Appraisal of Individual Needs
  (GAIN), 62, **64**, 65, 355, 526
Goal setting
  brief motivational interventions
    and, 287
  harm reduction programs and,
    268
  tobacco cessation and, 165
Good Samaritan laws, and opioid overdoses, 218
Graphics interchange formats (GIFs),
  352
Great Smoky Mountains Study, 370
Group therapy
  for bipolar disorder comorbid with
    substance use disorders,
    461–462
  cognitive-behavioral therapy and,
    290
  for disruptive behavior disorders
    comorbid with substance use
    disorders, 486–487
  for youth with substance use and
    juvenile justice system involve-
    ment, 527–528
Guanfacine, 489

Guidelines, for initial clinical interviews
  with adolescents, 69
Guiding Good Choices, 36

Hair drug testing, 102, 109, 110, 111,
  112–113
Hallucinogens, 114, 555. *See also* LSD
Haloperidol, 239
Hamilton Anxiety Rating Scale, 389
Harm reduction (HR) strategies, 191,
  266–269, **270**
Hashish (Ganja), 185
Health care. *See also* Emergency depart-
  ment; Hospitalization; Medical
  conditions; Medical marijuana
  brief interventions in primary care
    setting, 86–88
  case examples of risk levels for sub-
    stance abuse, 88–91
  referrals for substance abuse treat-
    ment, 91–92
  tobacco prevention programs and,
    168–169
Health insurance, and treatment for
  substance use in juvenile justice
  system, 531
HelpGuide (website), 571
Heroin, 186, 205–206, 221, 549, 553
Hilson Adolescent Profile (HAP), 67,
  68
Hippuric acid, 115
Hispanic Americans. *See* Race/ethnicity
HIV, opioid use and risk of, 213
Home-based incentives, and contin-
  gency management, 292–293
Home drug testing, 99–100
Hookah (water pipe), 161
Hooked on Nicotine Checklist
  (HONC), 163

Hospitalization, for schizophrenia and comorbid substance use, 445. *See also* Emergency department; Partial hospitalization program

Hydrocodone, 205, 242

Hypomania, 452

Identity, and transition to adulthood, 533

Imminent risk, and assessment of suicidal behavior, 420–421

Implementation
  of multicomponent treatment, 311–314
  of prevention programs, 38–40
  of 12-step facilitation, **330–331**

Impulsivity
  adolescents' susceptibility to addiction and, 503
  attention-deficit/hyperactivity disorder comorbid with substance use disorders and, 480

Inattentive subtype, of attention-deficit/hyperactivity disorder, 479

Infants, and substance use during pregnancy, 549–550

Information, about 12-step meetings, 340–341

Infrequent use, as posttreatment trajectory, 16

Inhalants
  drug testing for, 115
  pregnancy and, 555

"In-service" training, and prevention programs, 38

Insight, and impact of brain development on assessment, 57

Insomnia, and methamphetamine, 236

Instagram, 351

Integrated treatment
  for anxiety disorders comorbid with substance use disorders, 391–392
  for bipolar disorder comorbid with substance use disorders, 461–462
  for depression comorbid with substance use disorders, 381
  as example of multidomain treatment, 308–309
  for posttraumatic stress disorder comorbid with substance use disorders, 397–398
  for suicidal ideation, 422–423, 424, 427

Integrated TSF (iTSF), 332–333, **334**

Interactive teaching strategies, and prevention programs, 39

Internalizing disorders. *See* Anxiety disorders; Depression; Posttraumatic stress disorder

Internet. *See also* Social media; Technology
  drug testing and, 101–102, 117
  information resources for parents, 569
  online courses in Adolescent Community Reinforcement Approach, 311
  online gambling and, 505–506, 508–512
  prevention programs and, 43, 169
  self-help and mutual help organizations, 571
  treatment delivery and, 352

Internet gaming disorder (IGD), 502, 508–512

Internet Gaming Disorder Scale, 512

Interpersonal skills, as protective factor, 33–34

"Intervention agent," and prevention, 41

Interviews. *See also* Diagnostic interviews
anxiety disorders and, 389
clinical for assessment, 69

Intrauterine devices (IUD), 560

JUUL, 159, 177

Juvenile Automated Substance Abuse Evaluation (JASAF), 67, **68**

Juvenile drug courts, 528–529

Juvenile justice system
characteristics of youth involved with, 521–522
interventions for youth with substance use in, 527–532
referrals to community-based substance use treatment from, 314
risk factors for substance use and, 522–523
screening and assessment for substance abuse in, 524–527
treatment engagement and, 131

Keepin' it REAL program, 41

Ketamine, 115, 237–239

Kiddie Schedule for Affective Disorders and Schizophrenia—Lifetime and Present Episodes (K-SADS-PL), 378, 389

Kratom (*Mitragyna speciosa*), 219

K2 ("Spice"), 178, 189, 551

Learning. *See also* Social learning model
strategies of for prevention programs, 42–43
technology and skill-based, 354

Legal system, and laws. *See also* Criminal justice system; Juvenile justice system
legalization of marijuana and, 76, 109, 130, 177, 179, 188, 189, 192–194
management of substance use during pregnancy and, 556
opioid overdoses and "Good Samaritan" laws, 218

Life contexts, and youth-specific 12-step groups, 321, 324–325

LifeRing, 320, 343

Lithium, 453, 459, 460, 461

Location-Based Monitoring and Intervention for Alcohol Use Disorders (LBMI-A), 355–356

Long-acting reversible contraception (LARC), 560

LSD (lysergic acid diethylamide), 114, 239–241

Lurasidone, 445, 459, 460

Macro-level tobacco control approaches, 161–162

Maintenance treatment, for opioid use disorder, 214–217

Major depressive disorder, and marijuana use, 185

Management, clinical
of opioid use disorder, 211–213
of substance use during pregnancy, 552, 556–561

Mania, in patients with substance use disorders, 452, 453, 455

Manualized family therapy, 303

Marijuana. *See also* Cannabis use disorder; Medical marijuana
addictive disorders and, 185–187

Marijuana *(continued)*
associations between drug testing and self-reports, 100
breastfeeding and, 560–561
cardiovascular system and, 187
cognition and, 183–184
definitions and descriptions of products, 176–178
depression and suicidal ideation, 185
driving under influence of, 188
drug testing and, **104**, 109–110
e-cigarettes and vaporization of, 159–160
emergencies and, 187
endocannabinoid system and, 176
interactions with medications, 178–179
legalization of, 76, 109, 130, 177, 179, 188, 189, 192–194
negative effects of on adolescents, 180, 182–183
opioid use and, 220–222
patterns of substance use by adolescents and, 6, 7
pregnancy and, 550–551
prevalence and epidemiology of use, 179–180, **181**
prevention and treatment of, 189–192
psychosis and psychotic disorders, 184–185, 439–442
risk of manic symptoms and, 452
weight change and, 451
Massachusetts Gambling Screen, 506
Massachusetts Youth Screening Instrument—Version 2, 524–525, 526
Massively multiplayer online role-playing games (MMORPGs), 510

MDMA (ecstasy), **106**, 230–232, 554
Mechanisms of behavioral change (MOBCs), 257–266, 279–280
Media, and tobacco prevention campaigns, 164
Medical conditions, and risk factors for opioid use, 207, **208**. *See also* Biomedical conditions; Health care
Medical marijuana, 178, 193, 220, 221, 399
Medication(s). *See* Pharmacotherapy
Medication-assisted treatment (MAT), for opioid use disorder, 213–214, 557–559
Memory
ASAM criteria and dimensional assessment of, 129
cannabis use and, 183
suicidal behaviors and, 414
Mental Health Juvenile Detention Assessment Tool, 526
Menu, of alternative change options, 258
Mescaline, 114
Methadone
detoxification from opioids and, 244
opioid use disorder in youth and, 213–214, **215**, 216
pregnancy and, 558, 559, 560
Methadone maintenance treatment (MMT), 216
Methamphetamine. *See also* Stimulants
breastfeeding and, 561
as club drug, 235–237
drug testing for abuse of, 113–114
Methylenedioxyamphetamine (MDA), and methylenedioxymethylamphetamine (MDMA), 113

Methylphenidate, 488–489, 491–493, 553–555
Micro-level tobacco control approach, 162
Mindfulness-based approaches, to gambling disorders, 513
Mindfulness-based cognitive therapy (MBCT), 398
Mobile health (mHealth) technology–based interventions, 354–357
Modified Fagerström Tolerance Questionnaire (mFTQ), 163
Monitoring, and suicidal behaviors, 425–426
Monitoring the Future (MTF) study, 5, 6, 7, 8, 179–180, 193, 232, 234, 236, 238, 240, 243, 245, 247, 284
Mood stabilizers, 459, 487–488. *See also* Lithium
Morphine, **105**, 110, 550
Motivation
    for change, 267–268
    disruptive behavior disorders comorbid with substance use disorders and, 486
    mutual-help organizations and, 337, 340
    for quitting tobacco use, 163
Motivational interviewing (MI) and motivational enhancement therapy (MET). *See also* Brief motivational interventions
    cognitive-behavioral therapy combined with, 289
    directive approach compared with, **281–282**
    disruptive behavior disorders comorbid with substance use disorders and, 486

gambling disorder and, 513
harm reduction programs and, 268
initial meeting with adolescent and, 69
marijuana use and, 190–191
readiness to change and, 130
risk assessment in primary care setting and, 89
smoking cessation and, 165–166
substance use in youth involved with juvenile justice system, 528
suicidal ideation and, 422–423, 424
technology and, 354
12-step facilitation combined with, 332–333, **334**
Motor vehicles
    crashes associated with alcohol, 79, 84
    marijuana use and risk while driving, 188, 190
Multicomponent treatment, 308–314
Multidimensional family therapy (MDFT), 290, 302, 304, 484, 485–486
Multimodal Treatment Study of Children with ADHD (MTA), 479
Multiphase optimization strategy (MOST), 266
Multiscale questionnaires, 65, 67, **68**
Multisystemic therapy (MST), 484, 485, 528
Multisystemic Therapy for Emerging Adults, 535
Mutual-help organizations (MHOs). *See also* Self-help organizations; 12-step groups
    cost effectiveness of, 336–337, 340

Mutual-help organizations (MHOs) *(continued)*
   evidence for effectiveness of, 327–332
   social networks and, 320
   studies on participation in, 325–327
   websites for, 571
Myocardial infarction, and marijuana use, 187

Nabilone, 178
Nabiximols, 178
N-acetylcysteine (NAC), 191–192
Nalmefene, 149
Naloxone
   combined with buprenorphine for opioid use disorder, **215,** 216–217
   opioid overdoses and, 218–219
   pregnancy and, 557, 559
Nalbuphine, 559
Naltrexone
   alcohol use during pregnancy and, 552
   bipolar disorder comorbid with substance use disorders and, 461
   opioid use disorder and, 213–214, **215,** 217
   treatment of alcohol use disorder in adolescents and, 146–148, 150, 151–152
Narcotics Anonymous (NA), 326, 327, 328, 331–332, 571
National Cancer Institute, 169
National Comorbidity Study, 451
National Council of Juvenile and Family Court Judges, 529

National Epidemiologic Survey on Alcohol and Related Conditions (NESARC), 221, 451–452
National Health and Nutrition Examination Study, 451
National Highway Traffic Safety Administration, 188
National Institute on Alcohol Abuse and Alcoholism (NIAAA), 77, 87, 144, 145
National Institute on Drug Abuse (NIDA), 216, 312–313, 320
National Institute on Drug Abuse for Teens, 569
National Institute for Health and Care Excellence (NICE), 447, 458
National Institutes of Health, 552
National Survey on Drug Use and Health (NSDUH), 5, 6, 7, 12, 180, 192, 194, 205, 376, 389
Neonatal abstinence syndrome (NAS), 549–550
Neurobiology, and opioids, 204–205
Neurocognitive deficits, and substance use during adolescence, 4–5
Neuropsychological studies, of suicidal behaviors, 417
Neurotoxicity, of MDMA, 232
NIAAA screen (alcohol), **81,** 84
Nicotine. *See also* Tobacco use
   assessment of dependence, 162–163
   drug testing and, **104,** 110
   patterns of substance use by adolescents and, 6, 7
   vaping and changing trends in use of, 76
Nicotine replacement therapy (NRT), 167

No-intervention control condition (NIC), and continuing care, 263
Nonsuicidal self-injurious behavior, 414
Not On Tobacco (NOT) intervention, 165
Nurse Family Partnership program, 36

OARS (acronym), 279
Observation, and assessment, 54
Obsessive-compulsive disorder, 386
Office of Juvenile Justice and Delinquency Prevention, 529
Olanzapine, 446, 451, 459–460, 461
Ondansetron, 151
Open-ended questions, and motivational interviewing, 284
Operant learning, and cognitive-behavioral therapy, 288
Opioid(s), and opioid use. *See also* Opioid epidemic; Opioid use disorder
    definition of misuse, 204
    drug testing for, **105**, 110–111
    epidemiology of, 205–206, 243
    marijuana use and, 186–187
    negative sequelae of misuse by adolescents, 206
    overdose prevention and, 218–219
    pain management and, 220
    pharmacology and neurobiology of, 204–205
    postpartum period and, 561
    pregnancy and, 549–550, 557–559
    prevention of, 210–211
    risk factors for development of misuse, 206–210
    withdrawal from, 127, 242–243

Opioid epidemic, as public health issue, 77, 203–204, 206, 242, 369, 549
Opioid use disorder (OUD). *See also* Opioid(s)
    alternative medicines for, 219
    cannabis use and, 220–222
    clinical management and evidence-based interventions for, 211–213
    definition of, 204
    pharmacotherapy for, 204–205, 213–217, 243–244
    risk factors for in adolescents, 206–210
Oppositional defiant disorder (ODD), comorbidity of with substance use disorders, 478, 480–490
Oregon Adolescent Depression Project, 388
Outcome, of treatment for substance abuse
    abstinence as goal of, 257
    Adolescent Community Reinforcement Approach and, 313
    mechanisms of behavioral change and, 257–266
    12-step process and, **322–323**
Over-the-counter medications. *See also* Dextromethorphan
    drug testing and, 113–114
    "pharming" and, 229–330
Overdoses
    of dextromethorphan, 247
    of MDMA, 232
    of opioids, 218–219, 549
Oxycodone, **105**, 111, 242

Pain reduction, and opioid use, 209–210, 220

Paliperidone, 446
Panic disorder, 386, 388
Parent(s). *See also* Family
    assessment and reports from, 54
    drug testing in home and, 99–100
    gambling disorder and gaming
        addictions, 513
    information resources for, 569
    patterns of substance use in children
        of substance using, 8–9
    prevention programs and, 36
    risk factors for opioid use and, **209**
    stimulant abuse by, 493
    suicidal behavior in adolescents and,
        418–419, 425–427
    support for 12-step meetings,
        342–343
Parenting is Prevention, 569
"Parenting Wisely" (online program),
    359
Paroxetine, 391
Partial hospitalization program (PHP),
    136
Partnership for Drug-Free Kids, 569
Patient-Reported Outcomes Measure-
    ment Information System Nico-
    tine Dependence Item Bank for
    e-cigarettes (PROMIS-E), 163
Pediatric Anxiety Rating Scale (PARS),
    389
Peer(s). *See also* Social networks
    peer-led interventions for disruptive
        behavior disorders comorbid
        with substance use disorders,
        487
    risk factors for opioid use and,
        209
    risk factors for substance abuse and,
        32

technology-based applications and,
    353
Perceptual disorders, and LSD, 240,
    241
Persistent high substance involvement,
    as posttreatment trajectory, 16
Personality traits
    comorbidity of bipolar disorder and
        substance use disorders,
        457–458
    risk factors for opioid use and, **208**
Personal Experience Inventory (PEI),
    67, **68**
Personal Experience Screening Ques-
    tionnaire (PESQ), **60**, 62, 63, 526
Pew Internet Survey, 350
Pharmacotherapy. *See also* Adherence;
    Alternative medicines; Antipsy-
    chotics; Benzodiazepines; Drug-
    drug interactions; Mood stabiliz-
    ers; Opioid(s); Over-the-counter
    medications; Overdoses; Prescrip-
    tion medications; Selective sero-
    tonin reuptake inhibitors; Side
    effects; Tricyclic antidepressants
    Adolescent Community Reinforce-
        ment Approach and, 310
    alcohol abuse and, 142–152
    for anxiety disorders comorbid with
        substance use disorders,
        390–391
    for bipolar disorder comorbid with
        substance use disorders,
        459–461
    for disruptive behavior disorders
        comorbid with substance use
        disorders, 487–490
    management of relapse potential
        and, 133

marijuana use and, 191–192
opioid use and, 204–205,
   213–217, 243–244
opioid withdrawal and, 214,
   217–218
for psychotic disorders comorbid
   with substance use disorders,
   445–446, 450–451
for posttraumatic stress disorder
   comorbid with substance use
   disorders, 398–399
smoking cessation and, 167–168
suicidal behaviors and, 427
PharmChek Laboratories, 103
"Pharming," 229–230
Phencyclidine, 115, 555, 561
PhenX Toolkit, 58
Phone intervention, and continuing
   care, 263. *See also* Cell phones
Physostigmine, 235
Pittsburgh Youth Study, 481
Pod devices, and e-cigarettes, 159
Point-of-care drug screening kits, 101
Poison control centers, and opioid
   overdoses, 219
Polysubstance use
   bipolar disorder and, 454
   first-episode psychosis and, 438
   GHB and, 234
   pattern of among adolescents, 12
Polytobacco use, 158
Poppy seeds, and drug testing, 110,
   111
Positive reinforcement
   Adolescent Community Reinforce-
      ment Approach and, 309
   contingency management and, 292,
      293, 294
Postpartum depression, 561

Postpartum period, and substance use,
   559–561
Posttraumatic stress disorder (PTSD),
   comorbidity of with substance use
   disorders, 392–402
Posttreatment course, of substance use
   involvement, 15–17
Predictors, of clinical course of substance use disorders, 17
Pregnancy
   management of substance use
      during, 556–561
   marijuana use and, 182
   negative impact of substance use
      during, 543, 545, 549–555
   risk factors for substance abuse and,
      29–30
   screening for substance use during,
      544–545
Prescription medications. *See also*
   Benzodiazepines; Opioids
   changing trends in substance abuse
      and, 76
   patterns of substance use by adoles-
      cents and, 6
   overview of misuse, 241
Prevalence. *See also* Epidemiology
   of cannabis use disorder, 175
   of dual diagnosis, 367
   of internet gaming disorder, 510
   of marijuana use, 179–180, **181**
   of posttraumatic stress disorder,
      393
   of schizophrenia comorbid
      with substance use disorders,
      438
   of substance use in adolescents, 5–8,
      11–13
   of tobacco use, 158, 159, 160

Prevention
  adaptation of programs for, 40–41
  of alcohol use, 141–142
  background of efforts on, 26–27
  evidence-based programs for, 34–38
  future of efforts, 41–43
  implementation of programs for,
    38–40
  of marijuana use, 189–190
  of opioid use, 210–211, 218–219
  protective factors and, 32–34
  risk factors and, 27–32
  of substance use disorders in
    patients with bipolar disorder,
    462
  technology and, 350–351
  of tobacco use, 161–162, 163–164
Prilocaine, 112
Principles of Adolescent Substance Use
  Disorder Treatment (National
  Institute on Drug Abuse), 312–
  313
Problem-focused interviews, and comprehensive assessment, 65
Problem Oriented Screening Instrument for Teenagers (POSIT), 61,
  62, 63, 526
Problem-solving skills, and suicidal ideation, 425, 426–427
Project ESQYIR (Educating and Sup-
  porting inQuisitive Youth in
  Recovery), 355, 358
Prolonged exposure (PE) therapy, 398
Protective behavioral strategies (PBS),
  and marijuana use, 191
Protective factors
  for children of substance using par-
    ents, 9
  gambling disorder and, 508

posttraumatic stress disorder comor-
    bid with substance use disor-
    ders and, 395–396
  prevention and, 32–34
Psilocybin, 114
Psychiatric disorders, and risk factors
  for opioid use, 207, 208. See also
  Anxiety disorders; Attention-defi-
  cit/hyperactivity disorder; Comorbidity; Conduct disorder;
  Depression; Oppositional defiant
  disorder; Psychotic disorders
Psychosis. See also Psychotic disorders
  ketamine and, 239
  LSD and, 240
  marijuana use and, 184–185,
    439–442
Psychosocial functioning, and posttreatment course of substance use
  involvement, 15–17
Psychosocial interventions. See also
  Cognitive-behavioral therapy;
  Contingency management; Family
  therapy; Group therapy; Motivational interviewing
  for anxiety disorders comorbid with
    substance use disorders, 390
  for bipolar disorder comorbid with
    substance use disorders,
    461–462
  for disruptive behavior disorders
    comorbid with substance use
    disorders, 484–487
  marijuana use and, 190–191
  for posttraumatic stress disorder
    comorbid with substance use
    disorders, 397–398
  for suicidal ideation, 422–427
  for tobacco cessation, 165

for youth with substance use and
juvenile justice system involvement, 527–529
Psychotic disorders, comorbidity of
with substance use disorders,
437–451. *See also* Psychosis;
Schizophrenia
Public health. *See also* Opioid epidemic
adolescent depression and, 376
approaches to prevention, 26–27
effective intervention for adolescents
with substance use disorders
and, 319
gambling disorder and, 504
opioid overdose deaths and, 204
policies on marijuana and, 194
substance use among adolescents as
concern, 75–76

QT prolongation, and antipsychotics, 450
Quetiapine, 446, 459, 460–461

Race/ethnicity
access to treatment for marijuana
use, 192
comorbidity of psychotic disorders
with substance use disorders,
438–439
differences in substance use prevalence by, 8, 12–13
risk factors for opioid use and, **208**
substance use problems in juvenile
justice system and, 531
suicidal behavior and, 415–416
Random student drug testing (RSDT),
98–99
Real Cost campaign, 164
Reasons for Living Inventory (RFL-48),
420

Rebound effect, and comorbidity
between psychiatric disorders and
substance use disorders, 369
Recovery After an Initial Schizophrenia
Episode (RAISE) study, 447
Referrals, for substance abuse treatment
primary care settings and, 91–92
to substance use treatment from
juvenile justice system, 314,
530
Relapse
ASAM criteria and dimensional
assessment of, **125**, 132–133
risk for after treatment, 16
technology and programs for prevention of, 352
Relational reframing, and family therapy, 305–306
Remission rates, of schizophrenia
comorbid with substance use disorders, 438
Research Domain Criteria (RDoC), 11
Residential treatment, and recovery
environment, 135, 136
Resilience, and protective factors, 33
Retention rates, for Adolescent
Community Reinforcement
Approach, 313
Reward deficiency syndrome (RDS),
351
Reward-related behaviors
development during adolescence
and, 4
opioid misuse and, 209–210
Risk factors, for substance abuse.
See also Protective factors
bipolar disorder and, 453
cannabis use and development of
schizophrenia, 440

Risk factors, for substance abuse
(continued)
gambling disorder and, 507–508
identifying levels of in primary care
setting, 88–91
internet gaming disorder and,
510–511
for opioid misuse, 206–210
prevention and, 27–32
for substance use in juvenile justice
system, 522–523
for suicidal behaviors, 416–417,
420
Risk Reduction through Family Therapy, 398
Risk Reduction Therapy for Adolescents, 529
Risperidone
aggression related to disruptive behavior disorders and, 487–488
bipolar disorder and, 459, 460
cardiometabolic effects of, 451
schizophrenia in adolescents and,
445, 446
Rocky Mountain High Intensity Drug
Trafficking Area, 194
Role-playing, and prevention programs,
42
Rural communities, and access to substance use treatment for justice-
involved youth, 531
Rutgers Alcohol Problem Index
(RAPI), 58, 61

Safety
assessment of substance use in primary care setting and, 92
as priority in juvenile justice system,
529

suicidal behaviors and plans for, 424
SAFETY intervention, for suicidal
behaviors, 424
Saliva drug tests, 102
Scaffolding, and learning strategies for
prevention programs, 43
Schizophrenia
age at onset and, 438
antipsychotics for treatment of substance use disorders comorbid
with, 446
bipolar disorder and, 456
cannabis use and neurological soft
signs in, 439, 440
comorbid substance use disorders
and course or outcome of, 441
marijuana use and risk of, 184, 185,
440
prevalence rates for comorbidity of
with substance use disorders,
438
Schools. See also Academic functioning;
Learning; Teaching
cannabis use and, 184
drug testing and, 98–99
prevention programs in, 35–36, 40
risk factors for opioid use and, 209
risk factors for substance abuse and,
29–30, 31–32
tobacco prevention programs in,
168
treatment engagement and programs based in, 131
Screen for Child Anxiety Related Emotional Disorders (SCARED), 388,
389
Screening. See also Assessment
health maintenance visits and,
78–79

principles of, 52
standardized tools for, 58, **59–61,**
  62–63, 79, **80–83,** 84, 86
for substance use in juvenile justice
  system, 524–527
for substance use in pregnancy,
  544–545, **546–548**
technology and, 350–351
*Screening and Assessing Youth for
  Drug Involvement* (Center for Substance Abuse Treatment 1999), 58
Screening to Brief Intervention (S2BI),
  62, **83,** 84
Screening, Brief Intervention, and
  Referral to Treatment (SBIRT),
  77, 211
Seeking Safety, 397–398
Selective serotonin reuptake inhibitors
  (SSRIs), 391, 399
Self-administered questionnaire (SAQ),
  53
Self-efficacy
  brief motivational interventions
    and, 287–288
  as predictor of therapeutic success,
    258
Self-help interventions, for gambling
  disorder, 513
Self-help organizations, and websites,
  571. *See also* Mutual help organizations; 12-step groups
Self-medication, and comorbidity between
  psychiatric disorders and substance
  use disorders, 368, 457, 480
Self-regulation, acquisition of as goal of
  treatment, 130
Self-reports
  agreement between drug testing
    and, 100

depression and, 378
as method of assessment, 53
problems with underreporting and,
  97–98
suicidal behaviors and, 419
Separation anxiety disorder, 386
Sequential multiple assignment randomized trial (SMART), 266, 382
Sertraline, 391
Settings, for treatment of tobacco use,
  168–169. *See also* Health care;
  Schools
Severity, of substance use disorders
  comprehensive assessment and,
    55–56
  DSM-5 scales for, 11
Sexual behaviors
  opioid use disorder and, 213
  substance use among adolescents
    and, 544
Sexually transmitted diseases (STDs)
  assessment and treatment of, 128
  opioid use in adolescents and, 213
  substance use during pregnancy
    and, 556
  substance use and risk of, 544
Side effects, of medications
  antipsychotics and, 445, 446, 450
  baclofen and, 150
  disulfiram and, 146
  gabapentin and, 149
  GHB and, 234
  methamphetamine and, 236
  nalmefene and, 149
  naltrexone and, 147–148
  topiramate and, 149
Simple phobias, 386
Simple Screening Instrument for Alcohol and Other Drug Abuse, 54

Skill-based learning, and technology, 354

Slow improvers, and posttreatment trajectories, 16

Smart Approaches to Marijuana (SAM), 194

Smartphones. *See* Cell phones

SMART Recovery, 320, 343

SmokefreeTXT, 169

Smokeless tobacco, 161

"Snowball" pattern, of risk, 28

Social learning model, and cognitive-behavioral therapy, 288

Social media
  influence of on early-stage drug use, 37–38
  risks of substance use disorder development and, 351

Social networks. *See also* Peer(s); Social roles; Social skills
  influence of on substance use, 320, 324
  recovery environment and, 16, 135
  12-step organizations and, 333–336, 337, 340

Social phobia, 386, 388

Social roles, and transition to adulthood, 533

Social skills, as protective factor, 32–33

SORC (stimulus-organism-response-consequence), 421–422

South Oaks Gambling Screen— Revised for Adolescents (DSM-IV-J), 506

Specialized early intervention (SEI), 446–447, 448

Specific phobia, 386

"Speedball," 553

Spence Children's Anxiety Scale (SCAS), 388

Spiritual/religious language, and 12-step groups, 321

Stable abstinence, as posttreatment trajectory, 16

Standardized instruments, for assessment, 57–67, **68**, 567–568

State-Trait Anxiety Inventory for Children, 389

Stepped-care models, and treatment planning, 129, 265

Stimulants, diversion and abuse of, 490–493. *See also* Amphetamines; Methamphetamine

Strengths and Difficulties Questionnaire, 483, 526

Structured Assessment of Violence Risk in Youth (SAVRY), 525–526

Subdermal progesterone implants, 560

Subjective responses, to alcohol consumption, 144

Substance Abuse and Mental Health Services Administration (SAMHSA), 113, 211, 218, 357, 569

Substance Abuse Subtle Screening Inventory—Adolescents (SASSI-A), **61,** 62

Substance-induced psychotic disorder (SIPD), 442–444, 456

Substance monitoring contract (SMC), 293

Substance use. *See also* Adolescent(s); Alcohol use; Club drugs; Marijuana; Opioids; Polysubstance use; Prevention; Substance use disorders; Tobacco use; Withdrawal; *specific topics*
  adolescence as critical developmental period for initiation of, 3–5

changing trends in, 76–77
gabapentin and, 149
posttreatment course of involvement with, 15–17
in pregnancy as significant concern, 543
prevalence of in adolescents, 5–8
as public health problem, 75–76
risk factors for, 27–40
trajectories of during adolescence, 9–10
Substance use disorders (SUDs). *See also* Adolescent(s); Alcohol use disorder; Assessment; Cannabis use disorder; Comorbidity; Diagnosis; Opioid use disorder; Prevention; Substance use; Treatment; *specific topics*
DSM-IV and DSM-5 criteria for diagnosis of, 10–11
importance of developmentally informed approach to, xxv–xxvi
prevalence of in adolescents, 11–13
studies of clinical course of adolescent-onset, 14–19
substance use by children of parents with, 8–9
suicidal behaviors and, 416–417
Substance Use Risk Profile—Pregnancy (SURP-P), **548**
Subthreshold disorders, and depressive symptoms, 377
Suicidal Ideation Questionnaire (SIQ), 420
Suicide, and suicidal ideation
clinical characteristics of youth with substance use and, 417–418

definitions of suicidal behaviors, 414
depression comorbid with substance use disorders and, 376
epidemiology of, 414–416
gambling disorder and, 507
marijuana use and, 185
treatment for, 422–429
Sweat drug testing, 102–103
Synaptic pruning, and development of brain, 182
Syndros, 178
Synthetic cannabinoids, 189

T-ACE (alcohol screen), **546**
Target behaviors, and contingency management, 292
"Teachable moment" perspective, and brief motivational interventions, 282
Teaching, and strategies for prevention programs, 39, 42–43
Technology. *See also* Cell phones; Internet; Text messaging
delivery of treatment and, 351–354
future directions in, 358–360
prevention programs and, 43, 350–351
recovery programs and, 357–358
screening and, 350–351
trials of mobile health technology-based interventions, 354–357
Teen Addiction Severity Index (T-ASI), 65, **66**
Teen Intervene, 36
Teen Treatment Services Review, 65
Temperament, and protective factors, 33. *See also* Personality traits

Temporal association, between bipolar disorder and substance use disorders, 455–456

Testosterone, 115

Tetra-hydrocannabinol (THC), 175–176, 176–177, 439, 550

Text messaging. *See also* Cell phones adolescent treatment engagement and, 352
aftercare programs and, 264
smoking cessation programs and, 167, 169

Therapeutic alliance motivational interviewing and, 268
technology-based approaches and, 353

Therapeutic relationship, and treatment engagement, 131–132

Thioridazine, 450

Thoughts, and negative thinking smoking cessation and, 165
suicidal ideation and, 425

Timeline follow-back (TLFB), 53

Tobacco use. *See also* Nicotine anxiety disorders and, 387
attention-deficit/hyperactivity disorder and, 479–480
bipolar disorder and, 455
cessation interventions for, 164–168
diagnosis of, 162–163
negative health effects of, 157–158
noncigarette products and, 158–162
prevalence of, 158
prevention programs and, 163–164
treatment modality and settings, 168–169

Tolerance. *See also* Dependence benzodiazepines and, 245
GHB and, 234

Toluene, 115, 555

Topiramate, 148–149, 461

Training
Adolescent Community Reinforcement Approach and, 311–312
contingency management and, 293

Transdermal alcohol sensors, 356

Transition-age youth, and substance use in criminal justice system, 532–535

Transmissible Liability Index (TLI), 369

Transtheoretical model of change (TTM), 166–167, 278

Trauma-focused cognitive-behavioral therapy (TF-CBT), 397, 398

Treatment. *See also* Barriers; Continuity of care; Integrated treatment; Management; Motivational interviewing; Outcomes; Pharmacotherapy; Prevention; Psychosocial interventions; Referrals; Relapse; Settings; Treatment planning acceptability of method to individuals with substance use disorders, 291
of attention-deficit/hyperactivity disorder comorbid with substance use disorders, 484–490
of anxiety disorders comorbid with substance use disorders, 389–392
of bipolar disorder comorbid with substance use disorders, 458–462

of depression comorbid with substance use disorders, 378–385
of disruptive behavior disorders comorbid with substance use disorders, 489–490
duration of as predictor of clinical course of substance use disorders, 17
of gambling disorder and internet gaming addictions, 512–513
harm reduction versus abstinence as goal of, 266–269, **270**
incorporating elements of 12-step meetings into, 342
mechanisms of behavioral change and outcomes of, 257–266
multicomponent models of, 308–314
progress in research on, 256
of psychotic disorders comorbid with substance use disorders, 444–451
of posttraumatic stress disorder comorbid with substance use disorders, 396–401
self-regulation skills as goal of, 130
strategies to improve patient engagement, 131–132
of suicidal ideation comorbid with substance use disorders, 422–429
technology and delivery of, 351–354
utilization of by adolescents meeting criteria for DSM-IV substance use disorders, 13
Treatment Episode Data Set, 192
Treatment 4 Addiction, 571
Treatment of Maladaptive Aggression in Youth Steering Committee, 487

Treatment planning
ASAM criteria and, 127–135
general principles of, 124–127
matching of services with individual adolescent, 135–136
Treatment Recommendations for the Use of Antipsychotics for Aggressive Youth, 487
Treatment of Resistant Depression in Adolescents (TORDIA), 379
Tricyclic antidepressants, 391
Triggers, for substance use and suicidal thoughts or behaviors, 421
TWEAK (alcohol screen), **546**
Twelve-step facilitation (TSF), 328, 331–332, 340–343
12-step groups. *See also* Alcoholics Anonymous; Mutual-help organizations; Narcotics Anonymous
clinical strategies to increase participation in, 340–343
evidence for effectiveness of, 327–332
life contexts and youth-specific groups, 321, 324–325
moderators and mediators of participation benefits, 332–336
outcome of, **322–323**

UCLA PTSD Reaction Index, 395
Ultrasound, serial prenatal, 557, **558**
U.K. Gambling Commission, 506
U.S. Department of Agriculture (USDA), Economic Research Service, 359–360
U.S. Preventive Task Force, 544
Unrelatedness model, of comorbidity between psychiatric disorders and substance use disorders, 368

Urine drug tests. *See also* Drug testing
    falsification of, 101–102
    GHB and, 234–235
    marijuana and, 109
    MDMA and, 232
    methamphetamine and, 237
    opioids and, 111
    postpartum period and, 559
    pregnancy and, 545, 556
Usual continuing care (UCC), 262

Valproate, 460, 461
Vaping, and marijuana, 177. *See also*
    E-cigarettes; Nicotine
Varenicline, 167
Venlafaxine, 490
Veterans Health Administration
    (VHA), 336
Video games, 508–509
Violent behavior
    relationship between SUDs and dis-
        ruptive behavior disorders, 481
    as risk factor for substance abuse,
        29–30
Virtual peers, and technology-based
    applications, 353

Wearable health devices, 356
Weight change, and cannabis use, 451

Withdrawal, from substance depen-
    dence
    alcohol use and pharmacotherapy
        for, 144–145
    alcohol use during pregnancy and,
        552–553
    ASAM criteria and potential for,
        125, 127–128
    benzodiazepines and, 245
    cannabis use disorder and,
        186
    GHB and, 234
    in infants as result of substance
        use during pregnancy,
        549–550
    opioid use and, 214, 217–218,
        242–243
World Health Organization (WHO),
    141, 218, 502, 509

Youth Assessment and Screening
    Instrument (YASI), 525
Youth Level of Service/Case Manage-
    ment Inventory, 525, 526
Youth Risk Behavior Survey (2017),
    76, 284, 414–415

Ziprasidone, 450
Zurich Cohort Study, 453